HANDBOOK OF POLYMER APPLICATIONS IN MEDICINE AND MEDICAL DEVICES

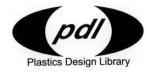

PLASTICS DESIGN LIBRARY (PDL)
PDL HANDBOOK SERIES
Series Editor: Sina Ebnesajjad, PhD
President, FluoroConsultants Group, LLC
Chadds Ford, PA, USA
www.FluoroConsultants.com

The **PDL Handbook Series** is aimed at a wide range of engineers and other professionals working in the plastics industry, and related sectors using plastics and adhesives.

PDL is a series of data books, reference works and practical guides covering plastics engineering, applications, processing, and manufacturing, and applied aspects of polymer science, elastomers and adhesives.

Recent titles in the series

Ebnesajjad, Handbook of Adhesives and Surface Preparation (ISBN: 9781437744613)

Goodman & Dodiuk, Handbook of Thermoset Plastics, 3e (ISBN: 9781455731077)

Kutz, Applied Plastics Engineering Handbook (ISBN: 9781437735147)

Kutz, PEEK Biomaterials Handbook (ISBN: 9781437744637)

McKeen, The Effect of Long Term Thermal Exposure on Plastics and Elastomers (ISBN: 9780323221085)

McKeen, Film Properties of Plastics and Elastomers, Third Edition (ISBN: 9781455725519)

McKeen, Permeability Properties of Plastics and Elastomers, Third Edition (ISBN: 9781437734690)

McKeen, The Effect of Creep and Other Time Related Factors on Plastics and Elastomers, Second Edition (ISBN: 9780815515852)

Sastri, Plastics with Medical Devices, 2e (ISBN: 9781455732012)

Modjarrad and Ebnesajjad, Handbook of Polymer Applications in Medicine and Medical Devices (ISBN: 9780323228053)

Wagner, Multilayer Flexible Packaging (ISBN: 9780815520214)

Woishnis & Ebnesajjad, Chemical Resistance, Volumes 1 & 2—Chemical Resistance of Thermoplastics (ISBN: 9781455778966)

Woishnis & Ebnesajjad, Chemical Resistance, Volume 3—Chemical Resistance of Specialty Thermoplastics (ISBN: 9781455731107)

Ebnesajjad, Handbook of Biopolymers and Biodegradable Plastics (ISBN: 9781455774425)

McKeen, The Effect of Sterilization on Plastics and Elastomers, Third Edition (ISBN: 9781455725984)

Biron Thermoplastics and Thermoplastic Composites, Second Edition (ISBN: 9781455778980)

Sin, Rahmat and Rahman, Polylactic Acid (ISBN: 9781437744590)

Drobny, Ionizing Radiation and Polymers (ISBN: 9781455778812)

Ebnesajjad, Polyvinyl Fluoride (ISBN: 9781455778850)

Fischer, Handbook of Molded Part Shrinkage and Warpage, Second Edition (ISBN: 9781455725977)

Ebnesajjad, Plastic Films in Food Packaging (ISBN: 9781455731121)

Fink, Reactive Polymers, Second Edition (ISBN: 9781455731497)

Niaounakis, Biopolymers Reuse, Recycling, and Disposal (ISBN: 9781455731459)

McKeen, The Effect of UV Light and Weather on Plastics and Elastomers (ISBN: 9781455728510)

Giles Jr., Wagner, Jr., Mount III, Extrusion, Second Edition (ISBN: 9781437734812)

To submit a new book proposal for the series, please contact Sina Ebnesajjad, Series Editor
sina@FluoroConsultants.com

or

Matthew Deans, Senior Publisher
m.deans@elsevier.com

HANDBOOK OF POLYMER APPLICATIONS IN MEDICINE AND MEDICAL DEVICES

Edited by

Kayvon Modjarrad, MD, PhD
Chief, Respiratory Disease Vaccine Development,
United States National Institutes of Health

Sina Ebnesajjad, PhD
President, FluoroConsultants Group, LLC

AMSTERDAM • BOSTON • HEIDELBERG • LONDON • NEW YORK • OXFORD
PARIS • SAN DIEGO • SAN FRANCISCO • SINGAPORE • SYDNEY • TOKYO
William Andrew is an imprint of Elsevier

William Andrew is an imprint of Elsevier
The Boulevard, Langford Lane, Kidlington, Oxford, OX5 1GB
525 B Street, Suite 1800, San Diego, CA 92101-4495, USA

First published 2014

Copyright © 2014 Elsevier Inc. All rights reserved.

No part of this publication may be reproduced or transmitted in any form or by any means, electronic or mechanical, including photocopying, recording, or any information storage and retrieval system, without permission in writing from the Publisher. Details on how to seek permission, further information about the Publisher's permissions policies and our arrangement with organizations such as the Copyright Clearance Center and the Copyright Licensing Agency, can be found at our website: www.elsevier.com/permissions

This book and the individual contributions contained in it are protected under copyright by the Publisher (other than as may be noted herein).

Notices
Knowledge and best practice in this field are constantly changing. As new research and experience broaden our understanding, changes in research methods, professional practices, or medical treatment may become necessary.

Practitioners and researchers must always rely on their own experience and knowledge in evaluating and using any information, methods, compounds, or experiments described herein. In using such information or methods they should be mindful of their own safety and the safety of others, including parties for whom they have a professional responsibility.

To the fullest extent of the law, neither the Publisher nor the authors, contributors, or editors, assume any liability for any injury and/or damage to persons or property as a matter of products liability, negligence or otherwise, or from any use or operation of any methods, products, instructions, or ideas contained in the material herein.

British Library Cataloguing-in-Publication Data
A catalogue record for this book is available from the British Library

Library of Congress Cataloging-in-Publication Data
A catalog record for this book is available from the Library of Congress

ISBN: 978-0-323-22805-3

For information on all William Andrew publications
visit our website at store.elsevier.com

Printed and bound by CPI Group (UK) Ltd, Croydon, CR0 4YY

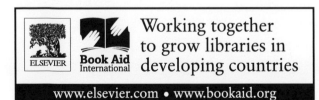

Contents

Preface vii
Author Biographies..ix

1 Introduction 1
Kayvon Modjarrad

2 Application of Plastics in Medical Devices and Equipment 9
Len Czuba

3 Plastics Used in Medical Devices 21
Laurence W. McKeen, PhD

4 Polymeric Biomaterials 55
Wei He and Roberto Benson

5 Biofilms, Biomaterials, and Device-Related Infections....................................77
Paul Stoodley, Luanne Hall-Stoodley, Bill Costerton, Patrick DeMeo, Mark Shirtliff,
Ellen Gawalt and Sandeep Kathju

6 Adhesives for Medical and Dental Applications 103
Sina Ebnesajjad

7 Silicones...131
André Colas and Jim Curtis

8 Review of Research in Cardiovascular Devices 145
Zbigniew Nawrat

9 Endotracheal Tube and Respiratory Care..191
Thomas C. Mort and Jeffrey P. Keck Jr.

**10 Applications of Polyaryletheretherketone in Spinal Implants: Fusion and Motion
Preservation**..231
Steven M. Kurtz, PhD

11 Microbubble Applications in Biomedicine 253
    Sana S. Dastgheyb, PhD Candidate and John R. Eisenbrey, PhD

12 Hydrogels in Regenerative Medicine 279
    Justin M. Saul and David F. Williams

13 Biodegradable Polymers 303
    Zheng Zhang, Ophir Ortiz, Ritu Goyal and Joachim Kohn

**14 Regulations for Medical Devices and Application to Plastics Suppliers: History
    and Overview** 337
    Vinny R. Sastri

Index 347

Preface

The applications of polymer chemistry and plastics engineering to the design and manufacture of medical equipment are evolving at a rapid pace not seen before in the medical device industry. These modern advances, however, reflect decades of incremental progress in biomaterial science. Initially guided by the principles of physiology and chemistry, medical plastics are now influenced by an array of emerging scientific disciplines that include nanochemistry, toxicology, and informatics. The current volume reflects this new interdisciplinary paradigm as it reviews modern innovations in the use of traditional polymers, introduces leading-edge technologies in medical diagnostics and therapeutics, and covers the logistical and regulatory challenges that confront the complex market of medical devices. It is intended as a primer for a broad audience of both medical and engineering professionals who share an interest in this quickly changing, but ever-expanding field.

The book begins (Chapters 2–4) with an overview of the varied applications of synthetic polymers in medical devices. The primary considerations in the design of new biomaterials are reviewed, including biocompatibility, durability, and sterility. The book then shifts (Chapters 5–10) to a specific focus on the medical applications of plastics in the fields of orthopedics, infectious diseases, dentistry, cardiology, pulmonology, critical care, anesthesiology, and neurosurgery. The next section (Chapters 11–13) examines novel applications for medical polymers on a nanoscale and in the contexts of diagnostic ultrasound and tissue engineering. The book concludes (Chapter 14) with a summary of the regulatory policies that influence medical device design and development.

Author Biographies

Dr. Kayvon Modjarrad is an infectious diseases physician, epidemiologist, and immunologist who holds the positions of Staff Clinician at the National Institute of Allergy and Infectious Diseases (NIAID) and the Chief of the Viral Pathogenesis Translational Science Core at the National Institutes of Health (NIH) Vaccine Research Center. After graduating from Duke University, he obtained his MD, MSPH, and PhD through the NIH-funded Medical Scientist Training Program at the University of Alabama at Birmingham School of Medicine and School of Public Health. He completed his medical internship at Yale-New Haven Hospital and his internal medicine residency and clinical infectious diseases fellowship at the Vanderbilt University School of Medicine. He completed his infectious diseases research fellowship at the NIAID. He has authored more than 20 peer-reviewed scientific publications, has served as an associate editor for several scientific journals, and is a member of the Faculty of 1000 advisory board.

Kayvon Modjarrad, MD, PhD

Sina Ebnesajjad is the founder of FluoroConsultants Group, LLC and has been the President of the company since 2006. Sina is the Series Editor of *Plastics Design Library*, published by Elsevier and publications in the areas of plastics, elastomers and adhesives. He retired as a Senior Technology Associate in 2005 from the DuPont Fluoroproducts after nearly 24 years of service. Sina was editor-in-chief of William Andrew Publishing from 2005 to 2007. He earned his master's and PhD degrees in Chemical Engineering from the University of Michigan, Ann Arbor. Sina is author, editor and co-author of fifteen technical books including five handbooks about fluoropolymers technology and applications and three books on adhesives and surface treatment of materials for adhesion.

Sina Ebnesajjad, PhD

1 Introduction

Kayvon Modjarrad
National Institute of Allergy and Infectious Diseases

OUTLINE

1.1 History	2	1.4 Summary	6
1.2 A Historical Example	4	References	6
1.3 Anthology Architecture	6		

Science and technology do not develop seamlessly but rather by major and painful changes in accepted wisdom. Such changes are preceded by a period of profound uncertainty as the accepted solutions become plainly unsatisfactory at solving the problem.
—Thomas S. Kuhn, *The Structure of Scientific Revolutions* [1]

The history of plastics and medical devices traces a complex course of slowly evolving ideas punctuated by moments of intellectual revolution. When viewed from the vantage of retrospect, it becomes apparent that milestones in the progress of biomaterial science represent culminations of gradual shifts in theory and iterative experimentation. This has been as true for methodological developments in polymer chemistry as it has for technological breakthroughs in medical equipment design. The two disciplines, now inextricable from one another, initially advanced along largely separate and occasionally redundant paths. Until the latter decades of the twentieth century, physicians and surgeons modified existing materials to create and refine devices according to their clinical needs while chemists and engineers synthesized materials *de novo* without specific attention to their potential medical applications. In the modern era, however, the lines between the chemical and biological sciences have blurred, paving the way for an interdisciplinary approach toward the design and application of medical plastics.

The current anthology reflects this new paradigm, examining issues surrounding the use of medical plastics through the mutifaceted lens of chemical and biomedical engineering, microbiology, toxicology, nanochemistry, physics, and informatics. Historically, plastics as biomaterials have been reviewed almost entirely in the context of surgical implants. The collection of chapters that follows surveys a broader, newer array of applications for medical plastics that includes diagnostic equipment, product packaging, drug delivery devices, and tissue regeneration. These novel uses for plastics have translated into a surge in the volume of medical devices and equipment being employed around the world. Newer technologies, such as medical molding and packaging, have been responsible for much of the growth in the past several years. However, traditional applications of medical plastics continue to drive the industry forward as well. For example, 300,000 people around the world undergo cardiac valve replacement every year [2]. And in 2011, more than 150 million people wore silicone or hydrogel-based contact lenses, a 25% rise from a decade earlier [3]. The increasing demand for these products has led to an economic resurgence for the field as a whole. Although medical products still only account for 1% of the plastics market share, the consumption of medical devices has tripled in the past decade to become a $300 billion global industry [4]. Over the next several years, the business of biological implants is expected to grow by 7% annually [5]. These trends are in large part a consequence of an aging population, a rising prevalence of chronic diseases, and a shift from invasive surgeries toward minimally invasive implantation procedures.

1.1 History

The emergence of synthetic polymers as a dominant force in medicine, though a recent phenomenon, is rooted in a long history of biomaterials that extends back several millennia. Historical evidence demonstrates that humans have been repurposing natural substances for medical use since the beginnings of civilization. Several thousand years ago, ancient Babylonians and Egyptians were fashioning surgical sutures from flax, hemp, and catgut. The archeological record is relatively quiet on surgical implants, though, until the seventh century AD when Mayans began grafting seashells to their mandibles. Another thousand years would pass before any additional progress was made in biomaterials. In the sixteenth and seventeenth centuries, Renaissance men Leonardo Da Vinci and Rene Descartes proposed their own designs for contact lenses [6]. But theory did not become practice for another two hundred years when the first glass lenses were manufactured for human use. Around this time, in the mid-1800s, the Industrial Age was in full force giving birth to a rapidly rising number of inventions. Even more importantly, scientists and engineers were making their discoveries through repeated experimentation. A new adherence to the scientific method was quickening the pace of biomaterials research, as the seeds of scientific thought grew into practical therapies within the course of several years instead of centuries.

The story of plastics begins here in the mid-nineteenth century (Figure 1.1) when, in 1862, a metallurgist named Alexander Parkes unveiled his eponymous invention, Parkesine, at the London International Exhibition (Figure 1.2). It was a chemically treated celluloid he had patented several years earlier to waterproof clothing fabrics. By adding solvents to a natural product, Parkes was able to create the first artificially modified thermoplastic. Parkes' invention is often heralded as the birth of plastics. However, he owed much to the vulcanization process developed by Charles Goodyear and Thomas Hancock several decades earlier. Parkes, in fact, began his career by improving upon Hancock's methods. And John Wesley Hyatt, a few years after Parkes, invented celluloid by applying the chemical principles of the same predecessors [6]. The work of these pioneers demonstrated proofs of concept that naturally occurring polymers

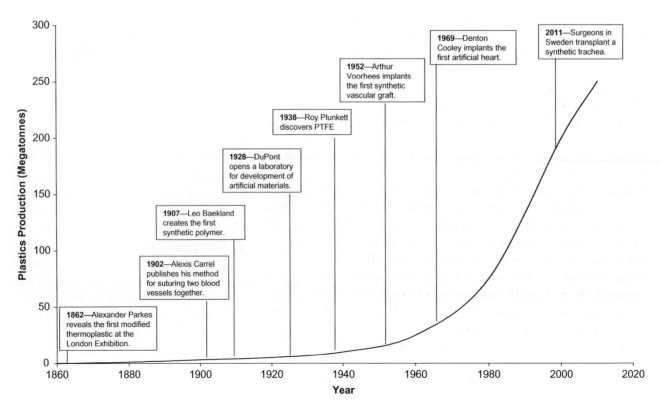

Figure 1.1 A timeline of medical plastic development and production.

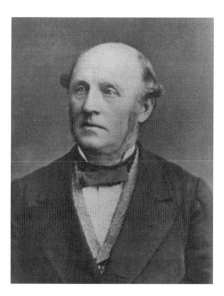

Figure 1.2 Alexander Parkes, inventor of the first modified thermoplastic. (*Science Museum/Science & Society Picture Library*)

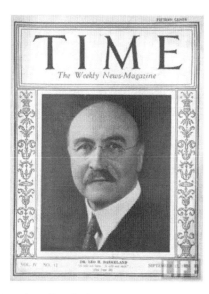

Figure 1.3 Leo Baekeland, inventor of the first entirely synthetic polymer.

could be molded for human use. And though these inventions were innovative in their own right, they still relied on the availability of compounds in the environment.

It wasn't until the turn of the twentieth century that a polymer was synthesized *de novo*. In 1909, Leo Hendrik Baekeland combined formaldehyde and phenol to create a thermostable material that he, like Parkes, named after himself. Bakelite significantly accelerated the growth of the plastics industry by eliminating the need to procure natural products for alteration (Figure 1.3) [7]. By the 1930s, dozens of synthetic polymers were being produced for mass consumption. Textiles, toothbrushes, and furniture were in much larger supply and at a cheaper cost than they had ever been. Within the span of several decades, plastics had moved from a scientific oddity to a household staple. The demand for plastics, however, was far from reaching its peak. Consider the 1941 text, *Plastics*, that opens with a forecast of how humans will live in a world made entirely of plastic.

> *This plastic man will come into a world of colour and bright shining surfaces where childish hands find nothing to break...The walls of his nursery, his bath...all his toys, his cot, the moulded light perambulator in which he takes the air, the teething ring he bites, the unbreakable bottle he feeds from...all will be plastic.... As he grows, he cleans his teeth and brushes his hair with plastic brushes, clothes himself with in plastic clothes, writes his first lesson with a plastic pen and does his lessons in a book bound with plastic...[In the end] His own teeth are gone and wears a denture with silent plastic teeth and spectacles with plastic lenses...until at last he sinks into his grave in a hygienically enclosed plastic coffin.*
> —**Yarsley and Couzens, *Plastics* [8]**

Written at the dawn of World War II, their prediction may have seemed hyperbolic at the time. However, during the war years that followed, plastics production quadrupled from 1 to 4 kilotonnes (now plastics use exceeds 250 megatonnes annually) [9,10]. World War II also drove the expansion of plastics from the home to the battlefield. Parachutes and aircraft parts, gun barrels, and helmets were all taking advantage of the malleable and durable properties of synthetic polymers. Even the Manhattan Project relied on polytetrafluoroethylene (PTFE), or Teflon®, to contain the corrosive byproduct of uranium hexafluoride used to make the atomic bomb [11].

But it wasn't until the post-war period that the plastics industry targeted medicine as its new

Table 1.1 Medical Plastics in Common Use

Polymer	Discovered	Medical Applications
Polytetrafluoroethylene (PTFE, Teflon, Gore-Tex®)	1938	Vascular grafts, catheters, introducers
Poly(ethylene terephthalate) (polyester, Ethibond, Dacron®)	1941	Vascular graft, drug delivery, non-resorbable sutures
Poly(methyl methacrylate) (PMMA)	1877	Bone cement, intraocular lens
Polyurethane	1937	Catheters, tubing, wound dressing, heart valves, artificial hearts
Silicone rubber (polydimethylsiloxane, PDMS)	1943	Catheters, feeding tubes, drainage tubes, introducer tips, flexible sheaths, gas exchange membranes
Polycarbonate	1953	Renal dialysis cartridge, heart–lung machine, trocars, tubing interconnectors
Hydrogels (poly(ethylene oxide), poly(ethylene glycol), poly(vinyl alcohol)		Drug delivery, wound healing, hemostasis, adhesion prevention, contact lenses, extracellular matricies, reconstruction
Polyamides (nylon)	1935	Non-resorbable sutures
Polypropylene (i.e., prolene)	1954	Non-resorbable sutures, hernia mesh

frontier. Other materials, such as metals, had been regularly used as bone and dental implants for decades. However, the union of polymers and medicine could not have occurred any earlier than it did, as neither had yet achieved a level of maturity that would enable fruitful application. Fortunately, mid-twentieth century advances in plastics engineering were matched by concurrent progress in the areas of immunology, microbiology, toxicology, and radiology. Advances in each of these disciplines overcame problems with implanting foreign materials into the human host. With a better understanding of immunology came improvements in the design of biocompatible materials. A deeper appreciation of chemical toxicity translated into definitions for what and how much substance could leach from its site of implantation. And the primary importance of sterility in all clinical products helped to both prescribe safety parameters for plastics and propel the field forward. Since the first use of nylon sutures in the early 1940s through to the present day, medical plastics have evolved considerably to become the broadest class of biomaterials. A catalog of plastics in current clinical use would exceed the scope of this chapter; however, a selected list of the most important examples is provided in Table 1.1. Thus, instead of broadly surveying each development in the history of medical plastics over the last half-century, I will focus on one historically significant case that illustrates the benefits and challenges that follow from the application of plastic solutions to clinical problems.

1.2 A Historical Example

In 1902, a young French surgeon by the name of Alexis Carrel published a manuscript in the *Lyons Medical* journal on his ability to successfully anastamose small caliber blood vessels [12]. Several years earlier, the French President, Sadi Carnot, had been stabbed by an assassin and died by exsanguination. Carrel, a medical student at the time, was convinced that the President would have survived had he been able to restore the integrity of his vasculature. Carrel responded to the tragedy by taking embroidery lessons to develop a technique that would enable two vessels to be sewn together. Sutures had been used for thousands of years to sew wounds, but until the turn of the century, arterial and venous injuries had little remedy. Six years before Carel published his seminal paper, his mentors Jaboulay and Briau demonstrated perfect union of two ends of the carotid artery. Carel improved upon their methods and was awarded the Nobel Prize for this work in 1912 [13]. Other pioneering surgeons quickly moved forward to apply Carel's techniques to arterial bypasses and aneurysms. As the field moved from biologic to synthetic sutures, approximation of blood vessels became more facile. Situations would arise, however, when vessels could not be attached end-to-end. In these instances, patients needed grafts that could replace parts of their vasculature.

Fifty years after Carel began developing and refining his methods in vascular repair, another young surgeon, Arthur Voorhees, made a seminal observation while an intern at Columbia University in New York. From a postmortem examination of an experimental animal, Voorhees noticed that a silk suture left in the animal's heart had become overgrown with endocardial tissue. The observation prompted Voorhees to hypothesize that a cylinder of silk cloth might elicit the same reaction and serve as an arterial prosthesis. He initially experimented on dogs with a silk handkerchief (donated by his wife) but soon moved to Vinyon, the synthetic polyvinyl chloride (PVC) used to make parachutes in World War II. After several years of animal experimentation, Voorhees had the chance, in 1952, to test his device on a human who had suffered an aortic aneurysm rupture [14]. With his tube made of PVC, Voorhees was able to save the patient from an almost certain fatal outcome.

Grafts from human and animal donors had been used previously, but they were in limited supply and ran the risk of host rejection. PVC, on the other hand, was relatively abundant and immunologically inert. But within five years of Voorhees' groundbreaking surgery, PVC was already outdated and replaced by polyethylene terephthalate (PETE) or Dacron®. By the 1960s, this new synthetic polymer had made prosthetic vascular grafts the standard of care for the repair and reconstruction of large diameter (>10 mm) vessels (Figure 1.4) [15]. Compared to its predecessors, PETE was more pliable, durable, and impermeable. Synthetic grafts, in general, were found to be well suited for large vessels (*i.e.* aortic and carotid arteries) with high flow rates and low resistance. When synthetic grafts were used for smaller vessels, however, they had inferior long-term patency as compared to autologous vessels. This limitation is largely due to thrombi that form at the site of anastomosis as a result of endothelial

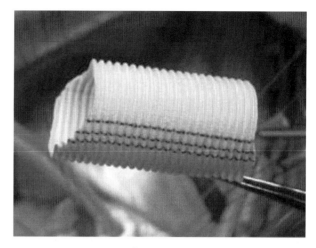

Figure 1.4 A Dacron® vascular graft. *(www.clevelandclinic.org, Lars Svensson, MD, PhD)*

hyperplasia [16]. Expanded PTFE (ePTFE) emerged on the market as an alternative to PETE in 1976 to lower the thrombogenicity and permeability of vascular grafts. They demonstrated little-to-no difference from PETE grafts in patency [17]. Consequently, PETE still constitutes the majority of synthetic vascular grafts (80%). ePTFE has carved a niche, however, in the area of hemodialysis access because of its lower rate of forming aneurysms and greater facility for thrombolysis. Both synthetic graft types have a finite life span depending on the purpose and anatomical location of the graft. Five-year patency is generally 50% for dialysis access and femoro-popliteal grafts but rises to 90% for both PETE and PTFE aortiobifemoral grafts [18]. Arguably, an even greater challenge to the longevity of artificial grafts is their risk of infection; synthetic grafts carry a 2% annual incidence of infection. Although relatively low, this rate is four times that of autologous grafts and has remained unchanged for decades despite advances in sterilization procedures and surgical techniques [19]. Research in antibiotic impregnation of grafts has failed to yield clinically viable products. Despite these limitations, vascular grafts continue to be used with increasing frequency and success [20]. One million vascular grafts are implanted around the world every year, making it a $200 million market in 2012 alone. The storyline of synthetic vasculature, from simple observations in a laboratory to a global industry, recapitulates that of many other medical plastics.

1.3 Anthology Architecture

This book is a hybrid of previously published and newly written chapters, unified by a theme of plastics applications in medical devices and equipment. The content has been chosen to accommodate the background and interests of both medical and engineering professionals. The book's organization loosely reflects the two eras in medical plastics development. The first period, lasting until the 1990s, was characterized by the appropriation of available synthetic polymers for medical purposes. More recently, medical plastics have become more sophisticated as polymers are synthesized for specific use in the clinical arena [21]. Thus, traditional as well as leading-edge clinical applications of synthetic polymers are reviewed. The first half of the book covers medical plastics that have been in use for several decades, while the latter chapters introduce novel applications for synthetic polymers.

This book begins (Chapters 2–4) with an overview of the varied applications of synthetic polymers in medical devices. The primary considerations in the design of new biomaterials are reviewed, including biocompatibility, durability, and sterility. These properties are evaluated for the most widely used polymers in medicine. The book then shifts to a more narrowed focus (Chapters 5–10), discussing specific medical applications in the fields of orthopedics, infectious diseases, dentistry, cardiology, pulmonology, critical care, anesthesiology, and neurosurgery. The next section (Chapters 11–13) examines novel applications for medical polymers on a nanoscale and in the context of diagnostic ultrasound as well as in the burgeoning field of tissue engineering. This book concludes (Chapter 14) with a summary of the economics and regulatory policies that influence medical device design and development.

1.4 Summary

Materials and biologic sciences have been co-evolving over millennia. Plastic, a relatively new class of synthetic substance, has been in use for only 150 years. However, in the last century, the volume and distribution of synthetic polymers in the medical industry has outpaced those of any other biomaterial. Given the complexities of human physiology and immunology, future medical devices—both external and implantable—will rely on synthetic materials that are both versatile and enduring in function. The collection of chapters included in this anthology provides a unique perspective on how far the field of medical plastics has advanced and the directions where it is headed. The journey toward modern biomaterial science is marked by modest observations followed by bold intellectual leaps. The way forward in the field of medical plastics is likely to recapitulate that voyage with increasing speed and reward.

References

[1] Kuhn TS. Historical structure of scientific discovery. Science 1962;136(3518):760.

[2] Etzioni DA, Starnes VA. The epidemiology and economics of cardiothoracic surgery in the elderly. In: Katlic MR, editor. Cardiothoracic surgery in the elderly: evidence based practice. Springer Link; 2011. p. 5–24.

[3] Nichols JJ. Annual report. contact lens spectrum, 2012. 27(January): p. 20–25.

[4] Sastri VR. In: Ebnesajjad S, editor. Plastics in medical devices. Elsevier Science; 2010.

[5] Research TM. Medical plastics market—global industry analysis, size, share, growth, trends, and forecast, 2012–2018, 2013.

[6] Ratner BD, Hoffman AS, Schoen FJ, Lemons JE. Biomaterials science. 2nd ed. Elsevier Science; 2004.

[7] Thomas AW, et al. Leo Hendrik Baekeland. Science 1944;100(2585):22–4.

[8] Yarsley VE, Couzens EG. Plastics. Penguin Books Limited; 1945.

[9] Thompson RC, et al. Our plastic age. Philos Trans Royal Soc B-Biol Sci 2009;364(1526): 1973–6.

[10] Wigotsky V. Medical plastics. Plast Eng 2001;57(1):24.

[11] Foundation CH, Plunkett RJ, 2013 [cited 2013 April 25]. Available from: <http://www.chemheritage.org/discover/online-resources/chemistry-in-history/themes/petrochemistry-and-synthetic-polymers/synthetic-polymers/plunkett.aspx>.

[12] Carrel A. Lai technique operatoire des nastomosis vasculaires et la transplantation des visceres. Lyon Med 1902;98:859–64.

[13] PBS. Innovators & pioneers. red, gold: the epic story of blood, 2013 [cited 2013 April 28]; Available from: <http://www.pbs.org/wnet/redgold/innovators/bio_carrel.html>.

[14] Voorhees Jr. AB, Jaretzki 3rd A, Blakemore AH. The use of tubes constructed from Vinyon "N" cloth in bridging arterial defects. Ann Surg 1952;135(3):332–6.

[15] Ku David N, Allen RC. Vascular grafts. In: Bronzino JD, editor. The biomedical engineering handbook. Boca Raton: CRC Press; 1999.

[16] Cleary MA, et al. Vascular tissue engineering: the next generation. Trends Mol Med 2012;18(7):394–404.

[17] Nishibe T, et al. Optimal prosthetic graft design for small diameter vascular grafts. Vascular 2007;15(6):356–60.

[18] Takagi H, et al. A contemporary meta-analysis of Dacron versus polytetrafluoroethylene grafts for femoropopliteal bypass grafting. J Vasc Surg 2010;52(1):232–6.

[19] Seeger JM. Management of patients with prosthetic vascular graft infection. Am Surg 2000;66(2):166–77.

[20] Metcalfe AD, Ferguson MW. Tissue engineering of replacement skin: the crossroads of biomaterials, wound healing, embryonic development, stem cells and regeneration. J R Soc Interface 2007;4(14):413–37.

[21] Binyamin G, Shafi BM, Mery CM. Biomaterials: a primer for surgeons. Semin Pediatr Surg 2006;15(4):276–83.

2 Application of Plastics in Medical Devices and Equipment

Len Czuba
Czuba Enterprises, Inc.

OUTLINE

2.1 Device Industry Overview	9	2.4.3.4 Technology Innovations	16
2.2 Health-care Trends	10	2.4.4 Ecological and Environmental Concerns and Influence of the Consumer	16
2.2.1 Minimally Invasive Surgeries	10		
2.2.2 Alternate Site Treatment	11	2.5 Market Factors Affecting the Industry	17
2.2.3 Prevention vs. Treatment	12	2.5.1 Concerns Over DEHP and Sometimes Even PVC	17
2.3 From Legacy Materials to Advanced Specialty Polymers for Devices	12	2.5.2 Bisphenol A	17
		2.5.3 The Need for "Green"	18
2.4 Driving Trends Leading to New Material Requirements	13	2.5.4 Globalization of Markets	18
		2.5.5 Globalization of Manufacturing	18
2.4.1 Functionality	13	2.5.5.1 Energy Costs	18
2.4.2 Compatibility	14	2.5.6 Global Influences	18
2.4.3 Cost	15	2.5.6.1 Infectious Diseases (MRSA, SARS, H1N1)	18
2.4.3.1 Material Costs or Process Improvements	15		
2.4.3.2 Light Weighting	15	2.5.6.2 Economic Pressures	19
2.4.3.3 Commoditizing Materials of Construction	15	2.6 Conclusion	19

This chapter will present a look at the medical device market with a particular focus on the materials of construction of devices and what we can expect in new products looking ahead. A deeper look at some other trends that have an effect on the direction of the medical device industry will be done. Finally, consideration will be given to a number of global factors that can have dramatic effect on our industry.

2.1 Device Industry Overview

The medical device industry has roots in the foundation materials of glass intravenous (IV) bottles, rubber tubing, and metal operating room instruments. The development of plastics in the 1930s, 1940s, and 1950s enabled the development of medical devices that overtook and eventually replaced the foundation materials with newer and better materials such as polyvinyl chloride (PVC) for IV bags and tubing, silicone tubing for catheters and balloons, polyolefins for trays and bottles, and fluoropolymers for IV catheters. New polymeric material developments continued to allow a virtual explosion of devices and implements which were able to rely on the excellent properties that were offered by engineering polymers, newer commodity plastics, and improved processing technologies.

As the availability of new products continued to grow, the health-care industry grew as well and by offering life-giving procedures, led to improved health of the population in general. New drugs such as sulfa drugs, penicillin, the Salk polio-vaccine, and insulin all led to the health-care industry being able to provide treatments to a great segment of the overall population, not just the elite, privileged classes or the wealthy. The wide availability of good quality, clean, sterile products at prices that were not absurdly high allowed the widespread growth of smaller hospitals and clinics where the sick and injured could receive medical treatment.

The device industry has grown together with the population expansion following World War II and with the globally expanding baby boomer generation. New technology in materials science, processing, and assembly, and in the health-care community combined to make the global medical device market a $200 billion market in 2008. With a growth rate of 8%, by 2012, the size grew to over $250 billion. The United States is reported to consume between 45% and 47% of the world market for medical devices, while US exports account for an estimated $37 billion, with these products going primarily to Europe (46%) and Japan (12%). The 42% which goes to the rest of the world accounts for approximately 57% of US exports and this segment is growing more rapidly than both the European Union (EU) and Japan as so-called third world or emerging economies begin to consume the basic health-care products for their demanding needs of their populations.

Analysis has shown that the "BRIC" countries of Brazil, Russia, India, and China will be those markets that have the most rapidly growing demand for medical devices. Growth of health care in other parts of the world such as Eastern Europe, the Middle East, and Africa will follow. However, as in any economy, before the general population can be served with a comprehensive health-care system in a country, there needs to be a stable political environment and where basic needs of food, clean water, sanitation, and shelter are available.

Another requirement is the establishment of a health-care delivery infrastructure. It does no good to ship sophisticated or even basic medical devices to parts of the world that have a need for these products if there is no one available to monitor, distribute, and administer the products and to provide for their proper use. Surgical suites cannot effectively operate for more than just the short term in temporary shelters or make-shift buildings. It will take a commitment on the part of the local governments to begin to provide facilities and utilities to the health-care professionals that would then begin dispensing care to the local population.

Evidence of this process is the rebuilding of the war ravaged country of Viet Nam in the late 1970s and 1980s. By no means has this part of Southeast Asia emerged into a sophisticated health-care provider but once stability had been restored, the infrastructure was slowly developed in the population centers, and hospitals and clinics were then able to provide care to their citizens.

2.2 Health-care Trends

Any review of the medical device industry will quickly reveal that several trends are emerging that are shaping the device industry. Three that I will note are:

1. The trend toward minimally invasive surgeries (MIS)
2. The growing popularity of alternate site treatment
3. A strong movement toward prevention vs. treatment of disease.

2.2.1 Minimally Invasive Surgeries

Not many years ago, when a heart patient presented with blocked or restricted arteries, the only course of treatment was to do open heart surgery or coronary artery bypass graft (CABG) surgery. This complicated, expensive, and traumatic surgery required the blood to be circulated by way of blood pumps and tubing through oxygenator devices, while the heart was taken "off-line" allowing the surgeon to replace the occluded blood vessels with harvested vessels usually from the patient's leg. These new vessels were grafted to the heart muscle and bloodstream to "bypass" the occluded vessels effectively restoring normal flow of blood to the heart muscle. The "bypass" surgery required cutting and spreading open the chest of the patient allowing the surgeon access to the heart. Often the recovery from all the steps taken to gain access to the heart muscle took longer than the recovery of the heart surgery itself! Recovery times were counted in weeks in the intensive care unit and hospital rooms and months more at home before normal activity could be resumed.

The development of the heart catheter that was able to deliver a vascular stent or scaffold changed the landscape for treatment of blocked arteries. Cardiovascular surgeons were suddenly able to access the occluded artery using these balloon catheters which were inserted through the femoral artery in the area of the groin. Newly developed imaging technologies gave the cardiovascular surgeon a way to accurately position and deploy a stent in the occluded artery immediately restoring the normal flow of blood through the once occluded artery.

Other products such as multiple instrument access ports allowed for minimally invasive surgeries to be performed within the peritoneal cavity through a single incision in the abdomen. The port would be positioned through the incision and by inflating the cavity using a process called "insufflations," and the surgeon could view inside the body using an endoscope or viewing instrument. The surgeon could then perform procedures such as biopsies, appendectomies, gallbladder procedures, hernia repair, and hysterectomies without the need to open the abdomen beyond the one small incision. Recovery times are greatly reduced, there is far less blood loss, the risk of infections and other complications from the open procedures have been drastically reduced, and the added benefit is that the cost of health care has also dropped.

These new minimally invasive surgical techniques, however, have also led to the development of many new products designed to improve how the procedures are performed. It seems that every medical device company has introduced its own version of the access port and the procedures carry unique names such as Natural Orifice Transluminal Endoscopic Surgery (NOTES). The benefits of MIS are obvious and the amount of new development being done to extend the procedures that are possible with MIS continues to grow.

Orthopedic procedures are possible using MIS with arthroscopy for joint exam and repair being the most commonly used joint repair procedure. Total joint replacement of the hip is now possible with products that rely on endoscopy. And linking this technology with computer-driven robotics has enabled the development of the DaVinci remote surgical system. This takes the possibility of alternate site health care to a new level with the surgeon being able to be remotely located from the patient on whom the procedure is being performed.

2.2.2 Alternate Site Treatment

The norm had for many years been that anyone sick or requiring medical assistance would go to the doctor and likely end up in the hospital for care and treatment. With the emergence of chronic illnesses such as renal or kidney dialysis, it became clear that quality care could be offered to special segments of the population in specially designed outpatient facilities. Doctors' offices became locations where X-rays could be taken, broken bones treated, and minor surgical procedures would be performed. Emergency clinics became satellite locations for the general hospital in the area, and these clinics were staffed with doctors and nurses that in many cases enabled patient care that eliminated the need to even go to the hospital.

Hospitals continue to be the place for major surgeries, intensive care units (ICU), trauma care, and specialty care such as in burns units. Patients that were mobile and otherwise active, however, could get their chronic care by way of the outpatient clinics in conveniently located sites near their homes and communities. Oncology patients could receive the twice or thrice weekly IV infusions at the alternate site, and rehab services, which only had been available at the hospital, were now offered at locations other than the hospital.

The trend to seek health care at locations other than the hospital brings other opportunities for the medical device industry. Products used at the alternate site must be the same good quality as offered by the hospital, but in some cases since the healthcare providers may not have the same level of experience as the hospital staff, the medical devices and equipment need to be made so that new or inexperienced users can reliably and effectively use the product as intended. Products for use in the non-hospital settings should have ease-of-use built into them and the instructions for use must be easy to read and understand.

One final alternate site trend is the tendency to take health care to the home. The cost of health care and the increased restrictions by insurance providers is leading to shorter hospital stays, earlier discharges, and a greater reluctance to admit patients, instead often opting for outpatient treatments. This trend places a greater burden on the family of the patient or requires a mobile healthcare provider to visit and look in on the condition of the patient and sometimes administer medications, therapy, or treat recovering wounds.

When the burden of responsibility falls on the family, medical products and devices must be designed and made so that the non-professional care giver can understand clearly how to use them easily. Often an elderly spouse is the only person available to care for a loved one and if medication containers are difficult to open, if devices are hard to hold and operate, or if the instructions are not clear, it becomes a challenge for the provider to comply as they should.

So to summarize, medical device companies need to consider how their products will be used and by whom. As alternate site delivered medical care becomes more commonplace, products must be made so that even complicated care procedures can be done without a chance of compromising the health of the patient or the care provider.

2.2.3 Prevention vs. Treatment

One final trend that is worth considering in this review is the trend toward prevention of disease or health problems by early diagnosis of a problem and early treatment. Current improvements in diagnosis of a patients' condition can enable the physician to detect the early onset of a problem condition whether that condition is high blood sugar levels pointing toward diabetes, chronic high blood pressure pointing toward heart disease, or the early onset of prostate cancer as indicated by increased prostate specific antigen (PSA) levels.

Effective diagnosis can be done using small samples of blood or urine or other body fluids. These tests are becoming less expensive and therefore are more likely to be done and reimbursed by insurance programs thereby leading to better monitoring of patients' health over the course of their life.

Other more sophisticated diagnostic procedures involve more intensive testing and analysis such as genetic screening. In the case of inherited genetic mutations, genetic testing can detect a patients' likelihood of developing breast cancer. Genetic testing can also determine if a patient has the inherited precursor to breast cancer leading to early and continuous monitoring of their health or leading to those patients seeking preventive surgical intervention such as mastectomies.

Earlier detection of health problems allows earlier treatment of the condition and in many cases the treatment will prevent the full onset of the diseased condition. The patient can avoid the effects of a fully engaged condition and with early treatment the disease may be completely avoided.

This trend toward disease prevention rather than treatment points to the ever-increasing demand for diagnostic products. From instruments that perform the analysis to the containers and reagents that are consumed during the testing to the devices that are used to collect the blood, fluid, and tissue samples, all these require carefully designed and manufactured medical devices. This is a very rapidly growing segment of the industry.

2.3 From Legacy Materials to Advanced Specialty Polymers for Devices

The need for high-quality medical devices has been explained in this chapter, but the construction of these devices has not been addressed. The emergence of PVC, polyolefin polymers, and other traditional commodity plastics was briefly touched upon in Section 2.1. But with the assessment of the trends described in Section 2.2, the full range of medical devices from single use disposables (SUDs) to reusable devices to hardware (e.g., pumps, ultrasonic instruments, heart monitors, and even MRI equipment) all require materials of construction designed to meet the needs of the product and survive the rigors of use, either single use or long-term use. The majority of products made for the device industry are made from commodity polymers or readily available, inexpensive polymeric materials. As the requirements for components or new medical device requirements push the limits of the most generally used materials, new materials are selected that meet the more rigorous requirements.

Examples are higher temperature polymers designed to survive continuous use at elevated temperatures or a polymer that can withstand exposure to aggressive cleaners or solvents now being used to reduce the frequency of hospital acquired infections (HAIs) or materials that can be precisely molded into micro-sized parts with very high tolerance requirements while also surviving the rigors of use.

The primary materials in use continue to be the four mainstay polymers: of polyvinyl chloride (PVC), polypropylene (PP), polyethylene (PE), and polystyrene (PS)—with styrene copolymers of ABS and SAN. But more devices are being made from additional materials which provide improved performance. Some of these materials are PC (polycarbonate), polyethylene terephthalate (PET), or any of the many available polyesters, TPU (thermoplastic urethane), TPE (thermoplastic elastomers), and polyamides (PA, both traditional nylons and amorphous nylons).

With newer devices constantly being developed, the need for new components and new specialty materials continues to increase. At the same time, new polymers and polymer formulations available for use continue to grow. Suppliers are continuing to develop new options that better meet the need for improved performance, allow the use of new technology, and extend the reach of the latest therapies.

An example of a relatively recent new material entering the device industry was the family of materials called liquid silicone rubber (LSR). LSRs allowed component products made from this silicone elastomer formulation to replace the more expensive and more difficult to process gum rubber silicones or different two-part silicone compounds that also were not as easy to process as the LSRs. These new formulations have the superior properties that make silicone so desirable for the medical device industry while also having the ability to be easily injection molded into quality parts. These materials rival the best TPEs as well as the traditional silicone rubber formulations.

There have been new polyolefins developed that can be used as tubing materials for applications which make PVC or silicone unacceptable. These softened olefins have even been considered as PVC replacement materials for such applications as steam sterilized fluid containers. Instruments that must be repeatedly cleaned and sterilized, sometimes multiple times in a day such as dental instruments, can now be made from high-performance polymers such as polyether imide (PEI) or polyether ether ketone (PEEK) polymers. Even some of the commodity polymers are being improved, for example, linear low density polyethylene (LLDPE) is new offered with better clarity, improved heat seal temperature range, and superior seal strength. All these improvements result in better medical devices often at lower manufacturing cost.

2.4 Driving Trends Leading to New Material Requirements

The earlier assessment of trends in health care led to a review of why certain areas of the industry are growing and showed why specific types of medical devices are being developed to meet the needs of the most recent industry trends. This section focuses on the factors that directly affect the devices that are being designed and made to serve the needs of industry. There are four trends listed below that cover how the industry from the suppliers to the convertors to the final device manufacturer are all responding to the needs of the ever-evolving industry.

2.4.1 Functionality

Components of devices must be made in a way that the resultant device or instrument can be used without an operational problem. Newer polymers allow the design of multiple features into one molded component that, for example, may be able to replace metal components or multiple smaller parts. Product redesign and design for manufacturing with the latest materials can bring improved performance to the medical device while reducing the cost of the device.

An example of this is the ability to preprint labeling or bar code information on a film that is then fabricated into a laminate for final manufacture into a fluid container. The critical information contained on the film is printed on an inner layer of the laminate and then sandwiched between outer layers of the laminate. The printing is protected from abrasion or exposure that might damage the printing as it would a label that is printed or affixed to the outside of the container after fabrication. Only with the ability to make dimensionally controlled films, and with the availability of polyurethane adhesives suitable for medical devices, is this technology possible.

Other new adhesives developed to improve the bonding of plastic components can offer better joints while also eliminating the use of volatile solvents. Ultraviolet light-cured adhesives can be used to bond a tubing to a connector while giving superior bonds and a controlled method of application and cure as compared to other methods of bonding. This type of adhesive also enables the use of automation for certain products and with the cost of manufacturing such a critical part of making any medical device, the possibility of eliminating labor by using automation is a meaningful benefit.

Medical devices continue to get smaller and the complications related to making these ever smaller devices and their components present a challenge for both the material and the processes used to make small or micro-components. Multifunctional devices such as the Pill Cam rely on extremely tiny components but together they offer a product that gives remarkable results improving the diagnosis of the condition of a patient's colon.

The Pill Cam is designed to be swallowed by a patient needing a colon exam. Once swallowed, the Pill Cam will track through the body, eventually passing through the entire length of the large intestine, and is then eliminated from the body. During the transit, which is reported to average about 17 hours, it takes two pictures or images of the walls of the large intestine every second. These images are transmitted wirelessly to a receiver outside the body for later analysis. Any irregularity or polyp or lesion can be detected and diagnosed by the surgeon who previously relied on the examination of the colon using a colonoscope. The older procedures called colonoscopies are done on mildly sedated patients in a hospital examination room. This invasive procedure often requires two or three health care professionals and may take up to an hour to complete. The Pill Cam provides this problem by viewing of the entire length of the colon. The resultant set of information available to the surgeon is so large that it often requires retraining to enable the health-care professional to read and understand the dataset obtained from the Pill Cam. This new technology improves the diagnosis accuracy, helps eliminate false positives, or the need for investigatory biopsies, but also is more cost effective and from a patient perspective, a far more comfortable option to the colonoscopy.

One final example of a polymer allowing the improvement of patient care by the use of improved materials and manufacturing technology is the move toward individual specific product labeling that the US FDA (Food and Drug Administration) is implementing. Only with the availability of materials, techniques and equipment can there be a system of UID (unique identification) for devices in the market. Low cost but reliable options will make possible improved device tracking for patients having long-term implantable products or devices.

2.4.2 Compatibility

The term compatibility can be defined in a couple of different ways. The first way is the compatibility of one material with another material which would allow, for example, reliable overmolding of one material onto another material and expecting good adhesion between the two. One example is a housing that needs to be watertight. It incorporates an overmolded sealing gasket directly onto the housing where it would be joined and sealed to the other half of the housing. Unless the materials can be selected each having compatibility with the other, the seal might not perform as expected.

In another example, overmolding was used by an orthopedic instrument company not only to reduce the weight of the tools such as bone hammers and chisels, but also to enhance the performance by giving the user a better gripping surface. These tools are most often used by the surgeon who is gloved and the gloves are not always dry. By using a material that provides improved wet grip characteristics, the reduced weight of the tool, the ergonomic design for finger gripping, and better wet grip made these tools award-winning products. And it was the use of properly selected TPEs that allowed these products to be made effectively. The instruments are repeatedly cleaned and sterilized. The proper selection of the material for compatibility with the process is one of the biggest challenges with this product.

The other use of the term compatibility which is being covered in this review is perhaps more properly termed biocompatibility. But specifically what is meant in this context is the compatibility of the plastic medical device with the health-care need. There are medical devices now available that can be used as joint replacement materials. These materials have been found to provide better long-term outcomes for patients instead of the stainless steel (SS) materials of construction. The implant is made from PEEK polymer that is selected to better match the normal flexibility of the bone into which the implant is secured. When an SS implant is used, the adhesion between the implant and the bone over an extended period of time tends to loosen because the bone has a small amount of flexibility, whereas the SS implant does not flex. This lack of flexibility is called "stress shielding". But using the PEEK polymer as the implant stem, the polymer has close to the same flexibility as the bone and there is a reduced tendency for the implant to loosen over time. This compatibility between bone and polymer makes a more effective medical device and one that will allow better long-term outcomes especially as the average length of implant gets longer with an increase in life span of the general population.

One other similar trend that is dictating the selection of a new medical device material is the concept of resorbability. Resorbable polymers are the newest family of polymers getting serious attention as new products made from them enter the scene. Resorbable polymers have long been used for internal sutures to eliminate the need for a second surgery to retrieve the sutures positioned somewhere under skin. There is an ever-increasing list of new uses for these polymers which include polylactic acid (PLA), poly glycolic acid (PGA), polycaprolactone (PCL) polymers, and all the various copolymers in between. Devices made from these resorbables, when the material is properly selected, provide the mechanical integrity and strength to allow recovery of the patient. But after the bone or tissue heals, the natural process of the body will begin to digest and dissolve the implant. Examples of this family of polymers being used are for bone screws, plates and pins, tissue anchors, sutures, and one of the most recent developments for cardiovascular stents. In theory, any foreign material positioned in the body for an extended length of time has the potential to cause some unexpected complication. But if the long-term implant is made from a material that will gently be digested and metabolized and excreted, there is no foreign body left behind to cause a problem. For this reason, there is a great deal of attention being given to this new class of polymeric materials and the list of new products which are based on these bioresorbables will continue to grow.

2.4.3 Cost

2.4.3.1 Material Costs or Process Improvements

There are few products in the medical device industry that have the luxury of freedom from the cost of material and final product cost in order to be a viable product. The large majority of products are very price sensitive and any way that costs for the final product can be reduced is continually being considered. If for example by using a material with higher temperature properties the time it takes to sterilize the product can be reduced by using a higher sterilization temperature and not affect any other aspect of the product, this would be a very favorable option. The length of time to sterilize and ultimately manufacture the product would be reduced leading to significant cost savings. Large volume products such as IV bags would benefit from such a material improvement.

Any material that can be offered to a device manufacturer that has the potential to reduce the cost of manufacturing can bring an advantage to that product. It could be as simple as easier injection moldability or faster cycle times or something that would help reduce the reject rate or reduce scrap; all these would be considered worthwhile investments to qualify a new material for use in a long-term, high-volume product.

2.4.3.2 Light Weighting

Some products could be made for lower costs and result in savings based on light weighting of the product from both a materials consumed standpoint and reduced transportation costs. The example of the orthopedic instruments mentioned above shows that light weighting or reducing the overall weight of the product gives a functional advantage to those products allowing greater ease of use and resulting in less fatigue in the hands and arms of the surgeons who use these tools often on several patients in a row during their day of surgery.

Light weighting can bring down the ultimate cost of disposal of the used medical devices, not an insignificant cost of doing business in this industry. Smaller product footprint reduced size of packaging and improved shipping and handling costs all result from light weighting or downsizing the medical device as long as there is no commensurate loss in quality or functional performance.

2.4.3.3 Commoditizing Materials of Construction

This last subcategory of trends that helps drive material costs down is a trend to expand the products that a company manufactures but making the components and devices using a common polymer or raw material. As the consumption of a particular polymer grows, the purchase pricing is improved. Additional advantages are that instead of using multiple types of plastics, if one plastic can effectively satisfy the requirements across multiple product lines, then the qualification of new materials is eliminated, there is no need to stock multiple grades or different types of plastics, and the need for incoming testing all those various materials goes away.

All this points to the need for material suppliers to offer materials that have the properties needed for products. If one material can survive exposure to all three of the most common sterilization methods, steam, ethylene oxide gas, and irradiation, then this material would have an advantage over a polymer that is suited to only one or the other or two of the three methods, all else being equal.

One additional consideration for this recommendation is to try if possible to build products on the one material that works. This is that a company becomes familiar with how a material is processed, how it needs to be assembled, and how the product works with that material. This collective knowledge will result in better product, more efficient manufacturing operation, and a reduced product cost.

2.4.3.4 Technology Innovations

New device design and processing technologies can improve products and result in better market share and reduced product costs. Companies that stay current with the latest technology will have the advantage over others that don't. Take for example the move from gated molds with sprue and runner systems to hot runner systems. The cold runner systems generated scrap with every shot that needed to be either discarded or reground and used. Hot runner systems eliminated that loss of material.

Vision systems can be installed on manufacturing cells that provide 100% checking of product to eliminate the concern that one of the products may get into the marketplace that is out of tolerance or otherwise unacceptable. Robotics are now available to move product from one place to another thereby eliminating the need for human handling or other random conveyance systems. This helps keep the component or assembly or device cleaner, free from contamination, and allows for the exact location of that product. Knowing the location of a part allows subsequent steps to be taken in the manufacturing of that product from placing it into a tray, putting a critical label on the product assembling it into a product or packaging it.

By using the latest technology available for manufacturing the medical device, the best possible product will be offered to the customer. Micro-molding, two shot molding, and metal injection molding are all new process technologies that can affect a product and drive that product to the front of the line. Each new development in technology will put new requirements on materials but in the end, these innovations will enable the development and introduction of game-changing new devices.

2.4.4 Ecological and Environmental Concerns and Influence of the Consumer

The final trend that drives new material requirements to be addressed here is the influence of the consumer especially in the current climate of eco-consciousness and environmental awareness. Gone are the days of medical devices being bought based on the personal relationship of the doctor and the company sales representative. No longer are products used because of their appealing color or because of the reputation of the supplier. Buying decisions are being influenced by patients, families of patients, hospital committees that evaluate the products, stockholders or investors of the buying groups, and these days, even politicians are involved. Most medical device manufacturing companies are aware of the need to be environmentally responsible in design of their products, how the products are being manufactured, how these products are used and even how they are discarded after use.

Technologists responsible for the design and manufacturing of medical devices must continue to use the latest materials and process technologies to offer the best products possible. The recent evolution of antimicrobial materials shows a materials technology that at least on first glance seems to have potential to benefit the medical device industry; especially if it actually does reduce the spread of infectious pathogens. The idea of antimicrobial sounds good and is quickly adopted by the general public as an improvement (be it real or just perceived) and it will be up to the device manufacturers to decide on the best way to incorporate such new technology into their products.

To summarize this subcategory of the influence of the consumer on medical device materials, it is important to recognize that there are other players in the scheme of health-care business. Those that will have a significant influence on products that will be a success in the marketplace and those that will not. The consumer of today has information at their fingertips that allows them to be a better informed health-care consumer and empowers them to request and at times even demand the type of product they feel is best. It will benefit the device industry if this influence on products is carefully considered.

2.5 Market Factors Affecting the Industry

Behind the scenes of the medical device industry and health care are the continuing investigations to ensure safety of the general population. Sometimes the investigations are done at universities, sometimes they are done by companies or their competitors and sometimes independent researchers conduct the investigations. Often there are governmental-funded investigations or studies done by activist groups. But no matter who does the investigation and sometimes it does not even matter if the study is done well or not, the results usually will affect the industry, and products in the health-care market will be affected.

2.5.1 Concerns Over DEHP and Sometimes Even PVC

If it were not for the improved ability for blood storage in diethyl hexyl phthalate (DEHP) plasticized PVC coupled with the low-cost superior performance of PVC medical devices, it is not likely that this industry would continue to rely so heavily on this controversial polymer. But flexible PVC is quite a remarkable material meeting so many important needs of the industry from providing safe high-quality inexpensive IV fluid products for patient care, to tubing for conveying the IV fluids, drug therapies and blood, and finally blood collection and storage. There continues to be a drum beat throughout industry alleging that phthalate plasticizers and specifically DEHP poses a danger to those exposed to it from these PVC medical devices. Thousands of studies conducted over more than 40 years of its use have not found reason to stop using f-PVC (flexible polyvinyl chloride). To be precise in this explanation, the studies have not found a problem; but as in any investigation, it is virtually impossible to prove that PVC is safe under all conditions and at every exposure level for every possible population segment. Proving a negative is virtually impossible. At best, industry experts can point to the lack of data showing harmful effects, can further indicate that for billions of uses and in millions of patient infusions, there has not been shown to be any harmful effects in patients exposed to DEHP plasticized PVC, even those listed under the special concerns listing by the FDA. Chemotherapy patients, chronic hemodialysis patients, patients receiving lipid emulsions, and premature infants were all categories of patients that may be more susceptible to adverse effects of high-dose exposure to DEHP. Nevertheless, if alternative materials are available, and if the practitioner were to have concern related to DEHP exposure, it would be a simple matter to use the other materials. But if the choice is between using DEHP plasticized PVC and not giving the patient infusion therapy because alternative materials are unavailable, it would be irresponsible to withhold treatment.

There are strong feelings about this issue and the influence by those holding these opinions has been successful in causing major companies and buying groups to choose to avoid using products that are based on f-PVC. As yet the feedback has not been available regarding the compromise of properties and the effect on patients when using newer materials or the effect of the additional costs of the newer products. It was originally reported that there would be significant savings to the users by switching to the newer materials. This assertion has not yet been verified.

2.5.2 Bisphenol A

Another external factor affecting the medical device community are concerns raised by researchers and voiced in the last five years related to bisphenol A (BPA) coming from plastics. This chemical, a building block for making polycarbonate (PC) plastic, is extracted in minute amounts from containers under certain conditions and potentially finds its way into humans from either certain beverage containers or medical devices which use PC in their construction. The level of BPA found in the bloodstream of mothers and newborn infants was reported to be detectable and higher than expected and the inference was that the chemical came from medical devices. The reason for the concern is that BPA is reported to have hormone-mimicking properties and is therefore said to be a chemical to which humans should not be exposed. The reality of the hazard is not confirmed but in a move toward caution, baby bottle and sport drink container manufacturers have changed the material from PC to alternative materials.

A review of the use of PC in medical devices shows that it is used primarily in connectors and fluid directing components such as manifolds and catheter hubs. The potential exposure of the IV fluids or blood to the PC surfaces is very short duration and the surface area of contact is extremely small leading most device engineers and toxicologists studying the situation to have little concern. The mood of the general public however has caused enough of an uproar that some companies are seeking PC alternative materials. As yet, this situation has not been fully played out.

2.5.3 The Need for "Green"

The consumer is much more aware of the effects of products, including medical devices on the planet, and would like to see products made with renewable resources that reduce the dependence on non-renewable materials. With this in mind, many companies are looking for ways to include renewable materials in their product-line and slowly reduce the amount of non-renewable plastics on which they rely.

It would serve the medical device community well to understand the materials available from companies such as NatureWorks, Metabolix, and Braskem as new products are developed. And every effort to follow the 3Rs—Reduce, Reuse and Recycle—would be to the advantage of every product manufacturing company.

2.5.4 Globalization of Markets

Populations across the face of the earth are becoming more aware of and seeking basic levels of medical care that have become the norm in developed nations. The availability of relatively inexpensive transportation costs makes it possible to expand health-care services to places unreachable only 20 years earlier. With a willing and invested government, basic health care needs can be met with commodity medical devices. As the need becomes apparent, local efforts by local companies in these emerging areas are working to establish manufacturing for medical devices primarily for in-country use.

2.5.5 Globalization of Manufacturing

Multinational companies have been very successful in manufacturing product in parts of the world where low cost labor is available. That product is then shipped to where the market demand exists. Several factors are changing this situation including the rising cost of labor, even in the most remote parts of the world, increasing energy costs affecting transportation of product, and the growing demand for product in every corner of the world. As local manufacturing is established, distant transport is reduced or eliminated. However, the level of quality is expected to be the same as products made in the primary manufacturing plants and if it is, market growth will match the increase in evolving economies.

2.5.5.1 Energy Costs

A major factor affecting globalization of manufacturing is the cost of energy. Transportation costs have already been mentioned as having an influence on where medical devices are made, but another factor is the cost of both raw materials and energy to produce the final product. Further considerations are the requirements for support of the remote operation from corporate headquarters.

2.5.6 Global Influences

2.5.6.1 Infectious Diseases (MRSA, SARS, H1N1)

Several other factors to consider in the global assessment of health care and the medical device industry are the effects of contagious diseases such as avian bird flu, SARS (severe acute respiratory syndrome) and MRSA (methicillin-resistant *Staphylococcus aureus*). These contagious diseases and others can rapidly spread around the world affecting countless numbers of the global population. Products are needed that can help stop the spread of any outbreak and treat patients that contract the disease. Part of the problem is that rarely is any attention given to this problem until there is actually an outbreak. Preventive measures are difficult to justify but unless done, the after-the-fact response is usually too little, too late.

2.5.6.2 Economic Pressures

A final market factor that is worth mentioning is the global economic situation. No longer can one country's economy be considered independent of other countries since there has developed in most parts of the world a global interdependence. When the EU falters, it affects the economy in the Middle East and Asia as well as in the United States. Governmental elections often cause market swings across the world and when conflict or war breaks out, the ripple effect can be seen throughout the world. It is with this in mind that medical device companies now are encouraged to keep a global perspective even if their primary markets are not spread across multiple continents. Companies are advised to be aware of what is happening around the world in order to stay current and relevant in meeting current and future demands of the healthcare needs of people everywhere.

2.6 Conclusion

It is essential that any review of the medical device market includes not only the materials of construction of existing medical devices but also takes into account new materials, new processing technologies, and the ever-changing needs of the marketplace. We exist in a global economy that is constantly changing and only by staying aware of and up to date on influences that affect our industry can a company keep their product mix at the forefront of health-care delivery.

3 Plastics Used in Medical Devices

Laurence W. McKeen, PhD

OUTLINE

3.1 Plastic Compositions 22	*3.2.5 Sterilization Capability* 31
3.1.1 Polymer Properties 22	*3.2.6 Long-Term Durability* 31
3.1.1.1 Linear, Branched, and Cross-linked Polymers 22	*3.2.7 Leachables and Extractables* 32
3.1.1.2 Isomers 22	*3.2.8 Supplemental Tests* 33
3.1.1.3 Molecular Weight 24	*3.2.9 Shelf Life and Aging* 33
3.1.2 Polymer Blends 24	*3.2.10 Joining and Welding* 33
3.1.3 Additives 25	*3.2.11 Medical Grade Plastics* 33
3.1.3.1 Fillers, Reinforcement, Composites 25	**3.3 Common Medical Device Polymers** 34
3.1.3.2 Release Agents 26	*3.3.1 Polyethylene* 34
3.1.3.3 Slip Additives/Internal Lubricants 26	*3.3.2 Polypropylene* 35
3.1.3.4 Catalysts 27	*3.3.3 Polystyrene* 36
3.1.3.5 Impact Modifiers and Tougheners 27	*3.3.4 Polyester* 36
3.1.3.6 Radiation Stabilizers 28	*3.3.5 Polyester (PLA and Other Biosorbable Plastics)* 37
3.1.3.7 Optical Brighteners 28	*3.3.6 Polycarbonate* 38
3.1.3.8 Plasticizers 28	*3.3.7 Polyvinyl Chloride* 40
3.1.3.9 Pigments, Extenders, Dyes, Mica 28	*3.3.8 Polyethersulfone* 41
3.1.3.10 Coupling Agents 28	*3.3.9 Polyacrylate (Acrylic, PMMA)* 41
3.1.3.11 Thermal Stabilizers 28	*3.3.10 Hydrogel (Acrylate)* 42
3.1.3.12 Antistats 29	*3.3.11 Polysulfone* 42
3.2 Medical Devices—Material Selection Process 29	*3.3.12 Polyetheretherketone* 43
3.2.1 Physical and Mechanical Properties 29	*3.3.13 Thermoplastic Elastomers (TPE, TPU)* 44
3.2.2 Thermal Properties 31	*3.3.14 Thermoset Elastomers—Silicone* 46
3.2.3 Electrical Properties 31	*3.3.15 Poly-p-xylylene (Parylene)* 47
3.2.4 Chemical Resistance 31	*3.3.16 Fluoropolymers* 47
	3.4 Summary 49
	References 52

Medical devices range from simple devices, to test equipment, to implants. Plastics are used more and more in these devices, for weight, cost, and performance purposes. Examples of medical devices include surgical instruments, catheters, coronary stents, pacemakers, magnetic resonance imaging (MRI) machines, X-ray machines, prosthetic limbs, artificial hips/knees, surgical gloves, and bandages.

This chapter will discuss plastics used in the construction of medical devices in three sections. The first section will review the general composition of plastic materials which will include the materials added to the basic polymers. The second section will discuss many factors that contribute to the plastic selection. The final section will review the chemistry, the response to sterilization processes, and the application of most common plastic materials in medical products.

3.1 Plastic Compositions

The basic components of plastic and elastomer materials are polymers. The word polymer is derived from the Greek term for "many parts." Polymers are large molecules comprised of many repeat units, called monomers, that have been chemically bonded into long chains. There are thousands of commercially available polymers that are the basis of plastics. While some plastics are neat polymers, more often than not they are formulated products containing a blend of ingredients each added for a purpose.

3.1.1 Polymer Properties

For any given polymer type, there can be hundreds of grades manufactured by multiple resin manufacturers with distinctly different properties. Some of these grades include variations of the basic polymer: its size or its structure. Other variations are the added ingredients (or additives) which may be incorporated to modify performance, appearance, or other purposes. Variations in the polymer structure are discussed in the next section.

3.1.1.1 Linear, Branched, and Cross-linked Polymers

Some polymers are linear, a long chain of connected monomers. Polyethylene, polyvinyl chloride (PVC), Nylon 66, and polymethyl methacrylate (PMMA) are some linear commercial examples found in this chapter. Branched polymers can be visualized as a linear polymer with side chains of the same polymer attached to the main chain. While the branches may themselves be further branched, the secondary branches do not connect to another polymer chain. The ends of the branches are not connected to any other chemical structure. Special types of branched polymers include star polymers, comb polymers, brush polymers, dendronized polymers [1], ladders, and dendrimers. Cross-linked polymers, sometimes called network polymers, are characterized by connection of different chains. The branches are essentially connected to different polymer chains

on the ends. These three polymer structures are shown in Figure 3.1.

3.1.1.2 Isomers

Isomers (from Greek isomerès, isos = "equal," méros = "part") are compounds with the same molecular formula but a different arrangement of atoms. There are many kinds of isomers and the properties can differ widely or almost not at all.

Structural Isomers

Structural isomers have the atoms arranged in a completely different order as shown in Figure 3.2. Here both polymer repeating groups have the same formula, $-C_4H_8-$, but the atoms are arranged differently. The properties of structural isomers may be very different from each other.

Often the repeating group in a polymer has exactly the same formula, but the repeating group is flipped over as shown in Figure 3.3. If one views the repeating group as having a head and a tail, then the different ways to connect neighboring repeating units is head–tail, head–head, and tail–tail.

Geometric Isomers

When there is a carbon–carbon double bond in a molecule, there may also be two ways to arrange the groups attached to the double bonds. This is

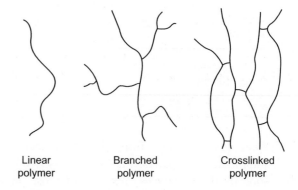

Figure 3.1 Linear, branched, and cross-linked polymers.

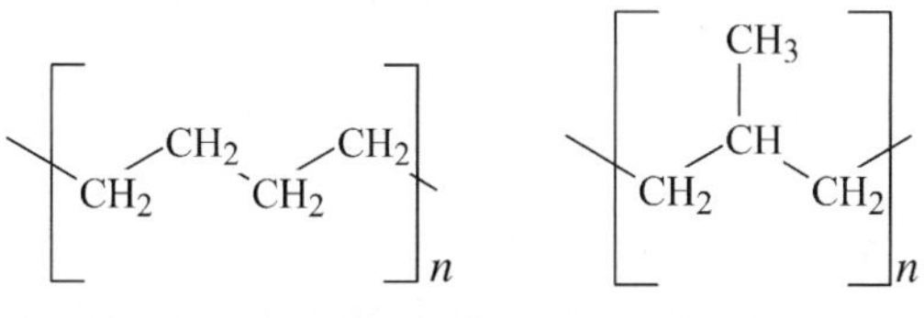

Figure 3.2 Structural isomers.

best seen in side-by-side structures as shown in Figure 3.4.

These structures are called *geometric isomers* which owe their existence to hindered rotation about double bonds. If the substituents are on the same side of the double bond, then the isomer is referred to as *cis-* (Latin: on this side). If the substituents are on the opposite side of the double bond, these are referred to as *trans-* (Latin: across).

Stereoisomers—Syndiotactic, Isotactic, Atactic

Stereoisomerism occurs when two or more molecules have identical molecular formula and the same structural formula (i.e., the atoms are arranged in the same order). However, they differ in their two or three dimensional (spatial) arrangements of their bonds. This means distinct spatial arrangements of the atoms—even though they are bonded in the same order. The concept would best be understood by an example.

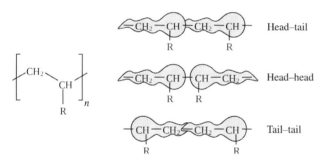

Figure 3.3 Head to tail isomers [2].

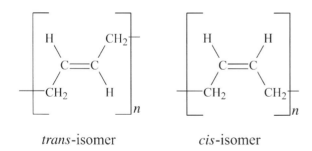

Figure 3.4 *cis-* and *trans-*isomers.

Polypropylenes (PPs) all have the same simplified structural polymer formula of polypropene as shown in Figure 3.5.

There are, however, subtle differences in the ways the polypropene structure can be arranged. Figure 3.6 shows a longer structure of polypropene, one that also shows some three-dimensional structure. This structure shows how some bonds (the dotted lines) are behind the plane of the paper while others stick out of the paper (the ones on the ends of the little triangular wedges). In this structure, some of the $-CH_3$ groups are presented above the paper plane and others are behind the paper plane. This is called *atactic* polypropene.

Atactic polypropene has at random about 50% of hydrogen/methyl groups in the front and the back of the C—C—C chain viewing plane. This form of polypropene is amorphous (noncrystalline) and has an irregular structure due to the random arrangement of the methyl groups attached to the main carbon—carbon chain. It tends to be softer and more flexible than the other forms of this polymer which are described next.

In *isotactic* polypropene, all the methyl groups are positioned in front of the C—C—C chain viewing plane and all of the hydrogen atoms are at back, as shown in Figure 3.7. This stereoregular structure maximizes the intermolecular contacts and thus increases the intermolecular forces as compared to the atactic form. This regular structure is much stronger (than the atactic form) and is used in sheet and film form for packaging and carpet fibers.

Syndiotactic polypropene has a regular alternation of 50% of hydrogen/methyl groups in front/

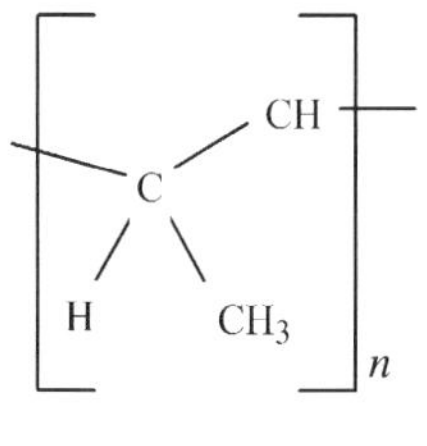

Figure 3.5 The structure of polypropene.

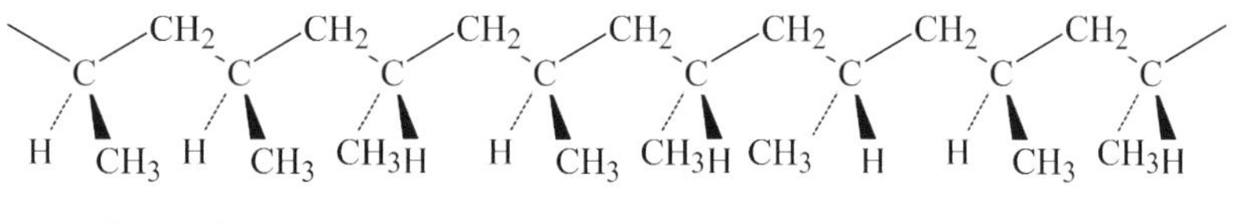

Figure 3.6 The structure of atactic polypropene.

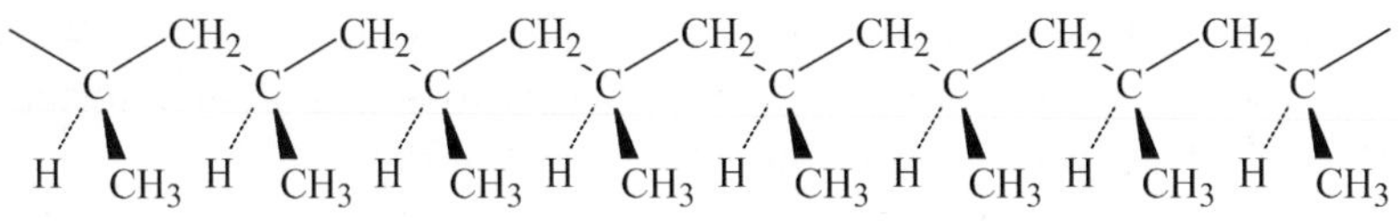

Figure 3.7 The structure of isotactic polypropene.

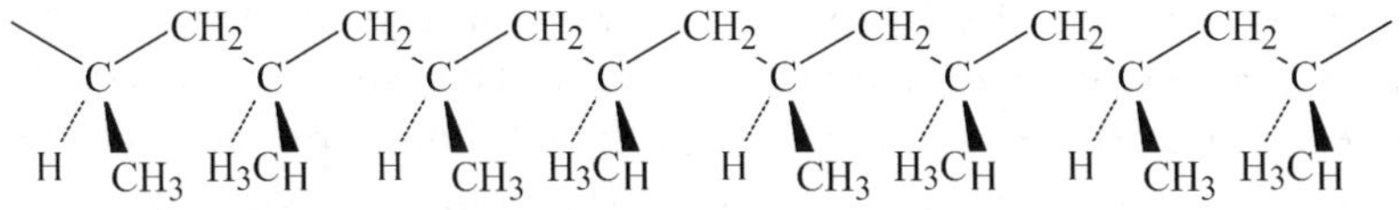

Figure 3.8 The structure of syndiotactic polypropene.

back of the C—C—C chain viewing plane as shown in Figure 3.8. Its properties are similar to isotactic polypropene rather than the atactic form, i.e., the regular polymer structure produces stronger intermolecular forces and a more crystalline form than the atactic polypropene.

3.1.1.3 Molecular Weight

A polymer's molecular weight is the sum of the atomic weights of individual atoms that comprise a molecule. It indicates the *average* length of the bulk resin's polymer chains. All polymer molecules of a particular grade do not have the exact same molecular weight. There is a range or distribution of molecular weights. Another common means of expressing the length of a polymer chain is the *degree of polymerization*; this quantifies the average number of monomers incorporated into the polymer chain. The average molecular weight can be determined by several means, but this subject is beyond the scope of this book. Low molecular weight polyethylene chains have backbones as small as 1000 carbon atoms long. Ultrahigh molecular weight polyethylene (UHMWPE) chains can have 500,000 carbon atoms along their length.

Many plastics are available in a variety of chain lengths or different molecular weight grades. These resins can also be classified indirectly by a viscosity value or by a proxy parameter called *melt flow rate*, rather than molecular weight. Within a resin family, such as polycarbonate (PC), higher molecular weight grades have higher melt viscosities. For example, in the viscosity test for PC, the melt flow rate ranges from approximately 4 g/10 min for the highest molecular weight, standard grades to more than 60 g/10 min for lowest molecular weight, high-flow, specialty grades.

Molecular weight of the polymers that are used in medical plastics affects a number of their properties. While it is not always possible to quantify the molecular weights of plastics, as mentioned previously, higher flowing plastics of a given series of products generally have lower molecular weights.

3.1.2 Polymer Blends

Polymers can often be blended. Occasionally, blended polymers have properties that exceed those of either of the constituents. For instance, blends of PC resin and PET polyester originally created to improve the chemical resistance of the PC actually have fatigue resistance and low-temperature impact resistance superior to either of the individual polymers.

Sometimes a material is needed that has some of the properties of one polymer and some of the properties of another. Instead of going back into the lab and trying to synthesize a brand-new polymer with all the desired properties, two polymers can be melted together to form a blend that possesses some of the properties of each constituent.

Two polymers that do actually mix well are polystyrene and polyphenylene oxide. Other examples of polymer pairs that form blends include:

- Polyethylene terephthalate (PET) with polybutylene terephthalate (PBT)
- PMMA with polyvinylidene fluoride.

Phase-separated mixtures are obtained when one tries to mix most polymers. But strangely enough, the phase-separated materials also turn out to be sometimes useful. They are called immiscible blends.

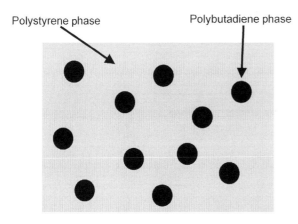

Figure 3.9 An immiscible blend of polystyrene and polybutadiene.

Polystyrene and polybutadiene are immiscible. When polystyrene is mixed with a small amount of polybutadiene, the two polymers do not blend. Polybutadiene separates from the polystyrene into little spherical blobs. If this mixture is viewed under a high-power microscope, it resembles the picture shown in Figure 3.9.

Multiphase polymer blends are of major economic importance in the polymer industry. The most common examples involve the impact modification of a thermoplastic by the microdispersion of a rubber into a brittle polymer matrix. Most commercial blends consist of two polymers combined with small amounts of a third compatibilizing polymer which typically consists of a block or graft copolymer. Multiphase polymer blends are often easier to process than a single polymer with similar properties.

Blending two or more polymers offers yet another method of tailoring resins to a specific application. Because blends are only physical mixtures, the resulting polymer usually has physical and mechanical properties that lie somewhere between the values of its constituent materials. Additional information on the subject of polymer blends is available in the literature [3–5].

3.1.3 Additives

The properties of neat polymers are often ideal neither for production nor for the end use. When this is the case, additives are added to the polymer to improve the performance shortfall. The additives can also improve the processing of polymers in addition to modifying its properties.

Additives encompass a wide range of substances that aid processing or add value to the final product [6,7]. Found in virtually all plastics, most additives are incorporated into a resin family by the supplier as part of a proprietary package. For example, you can choose standard PC resin grades with additives for improved internal mold release, ultraviolet (UV) stabilization, and flame retardance; or nylon grades with additives to improve impact performance.

Additives often determine the success or failure of a resin or system in a particular application. Many common additives are discussed in the following sections. Except for reinforcement fillers, most additives are added in very small amounts.

3.1.3.1 Fillers, Reinforcement, Composites

Reinforcing fillers can be added in large amounts. Some plastics may contain as much as 60% reinforcing fillers. Often, fibrous materials, such as glass or carbon, are added to resins to create reinforced grades with enhanced physical or mechanical properties. For example, adding 30% short glass fibers by weight to Nylon 6 improves creep resistance and increases stiffness by 300%. These glass-reinforced plastics usually suffer some loss of impact strength and ultimate elongation, and are more prone to warping because of the relatively large difference in mold shrinkage between the flow and cross flow directions.

Plastics with non-fibrous fillers such as glass spheres or mineral powders generally exhibit higher stiffness characteristics than unfilled resins, but not as high as fiber-reinforced grades. Resins with particulate fillers are less likely to warp and show a decrease in mold shrinkage. Particulate fillers typically reduce shrinkage by a percentage value roughly equal to the volume percentage of filler in the polymer, an advantage in tight tolerance molding.

Often reinforced plastics are called *composites*. The plastic/polymer material containing the reinforcement is referred to as the matrix. One can envision a number of ways different reinforcing materials might be arranged in a composite. Many of these arrangements are shown in Figure 3.10.

Particulates, in the form of pigments, may be added to impart color. Occasionally particulates, called *extenders*, are added to reduce the amount of

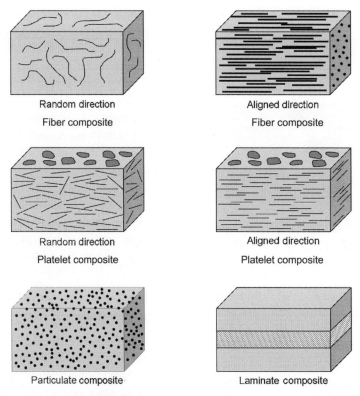

Figure 3.10 Several types of composite materials.

relatively expensive polymer used which reduces the overall cost.

Platelet additives may impart color and luster, metallic appearance, or a pearlescent effect, but they also can strongly affect permeation properties. Most of these additives have little or no permeation through themselves, so when a film contains particulate additives, the permeating molecule must follow a path around the particulate additive as shown in Figure 3.11. This is called a *tortuous path effect*.

3.1.3.2 Release Agents

External release agents are lubricants, liquids, or powders, which coat a mold cavity to facilitate part removal. Internal release agents, which are part of the plastic formulation, can accomplish the same purpose. The identities of the release agents are rarely disclosed, but frequently they are fine fluoropolymer powders (called micropowders), silicone resins, or waxes.

3.1.3.3 Slip Additives/Internal Lubricants

When polymeric films slide over each other, they encounter a resistance that is quantified in terms of the coefficient of friction (COF). Plastic films with high COF tend to stick together instead of sliding over one another. Sticking makes the handling, use, and conversion of films difficult. To overcome sticking, slip agents are added.

Slip additives are divided into two migrating and non-migrating types. Migrating slip additives are the most common class and they are used above their solubility limit in the polymer. These types of additives are molecules comprised of two distinct parts, typically pictured as a head and tail as shown in Figure 3.12. One part of the molecule, usually the head, is designed to be soluble in the polymer (particularly when it is molten during processing) making up the plastic. The other part, the tail, is insoluble. As the plastic cools and solidifies from its molten state, these molecules migrate to the surface, where the insoluble end "sticks out" reducing the COF. This process is shown in Figure 3.12. These additives are typically fatty acid amides.

Some common non-migrating slip additives are *dusted* on plastic surfaces. These include:

- PTFE (polytetrafluoroethylene) in micropowder form imparts the lowest COF of any internal

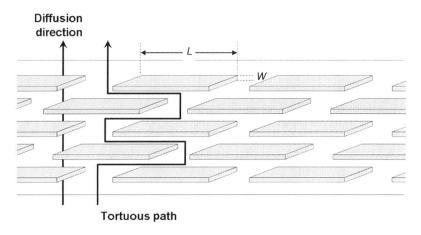

Figure 3.11 Tortuous path of permeant molecule through a particulate containing film.

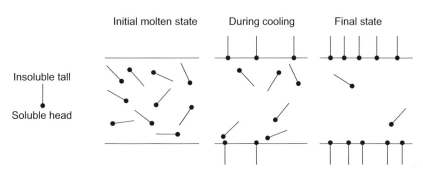

Figure 3.12 Mode of action of a typical migrating slip additive.

lubricant. Manufacturers and suppliers are many, including DuPont™, Zonyl®, and 3 M Dyneon™.

- Molybdenum disulfide, commonly called "*moly*," is a solid lubricant often used in bearing applications.
- Graphite is a solid lubricant used like molybdenum disulfide.

3.1.3.4 Catalysts

Catalysts, substances that initiate or change the rate of a chemical reaction, do not undergo a permanent change in composition or become part of the molecular structure of the final product. Occasionally they are used to describe a setting agent, hardener, curing agent, promoter, etc., and they are added in minute quantities, typically less than 1% usually to thermosetting plastics.

3.1.3.5 Impact Modifiers and Tougheners

Many plastics do not have sufficient impact resistance for the use for which they are intended. Rather than changing to a different type of plastic, they can be impact-modified in order to fulfill the performance in use requirements. Addition of modifiers called *impact modifiers* or *tougheners* significantly improves impact resistance. This is one of the most important additives. There are many suppliers and chemical types of these modifiers.

General-purpose impact modification is considered a low level of impact modification. It improves room temperature impact strength but does not take into account any requirements for low-temperature (<0°C) impact strength. For most of these types of applications, only low levels of impact modifier is required (<10%).

Low-temperature impact strength is required for applications that require a certain level of low-temperature flexibility and resistance to breakage. For example, this is the case for many applications in the appliances. For this purpose, modifier levels between 5% and 15% of mostly reactive modifiers are required. Reactive modifiers can bond chemically to the base polymer.

Super tough impact strength may be required for applications in which a part must not fail even if it is struck at low temperatures ($-30°C$ to $-40°C$) under high speed. This requirement can only be fulfilled with high levels (20–25%) of reactive impact modifier with low glass transition temperature.

3.1.3.6 Radiation Stabilizers

Radiation stabilizers, also referred to in the art as "antirads," may be used to mitigate the detrimental effects of the gamma ray dose on plastics generally. Stabilizers like antioxidants and free radical scavengers can prevent degradation and cross-linking. In general, polymers that contain aromatic ring structures are more resistant to radiation effects compared to aliphatic polymers.

UV stabilizers: Another way plastics may degrade is by exposure to UV light. UV radiation can initiate oxidation in air. Plastics which are used outdoors or exposed to lamps emitting UV radiation are subject to photooxidative degradation. UV stabilizers are used to prevent and retard photooxidation. Pigments and dyes may also be used in applications not requiring transparency. Photooxidative degradation starts at the exposed surface and propagates throughout the material. Many UV stabilizers, like phenolics, hindered amine light stabilizers, and phosphates, may offer some protection against gamma and electron beam radiation.

3.1.3.7 Optical Brighteners

Many polymers have a slight yellowish color. They can be modified to appear whiter and brighter by increasing reflected bluish light (in the range of 400–600 nm). One way to accomplish this is by incorporating an additive that absorbs in the UV range but reemits the energy at higher wavelength in the visible range. This effect is called *fluorescence* and these types of additives are called optical brighteners or fluorescent whitening agents.

3.1.3.8 Plasticizers

Plasticizers are added to enhance and maintain flexibility in a plastic. Various phthalates are commonly used for this purpose. Since they are small molecules, they may extract or leach out of the plastic causing a loss of flexibility with time. Just as deliberately added, small molecules may leach out, and small molecules from the environment may be absorbed by the plastic and act like a plasticizer. The absorption of water by nylons (polyamides) is an example of this phenomenon.

3.1.3.9 Pigments, Extenders, Dyes, Mica

Pigments are added to impart color to a plastic, but they may also affect the physical properties. Extenders are usually cheap materials added to reduce the cost of a plastic resins. Dyes are colorants that are chemically different to pigments. Mica is a special pigment added to impact sparkle or metallic appearance.

3.1.3.10 Coupling Agents

The purpose of adding fillers is either to lower the cost of the polymer, make it tougher or stiffer, or make it flame retardant so that it does not burn when it is ignited. Often the addition of the filler will reduce the elongation at break, the flexibility, and in many cases the toughness of the polymer because the fillers are added at very high levels. One reason for the degradation of properties is that the fillers are not compatible with the polymers, thus form stress rises centers. The addition of coupling agents can improve the compatibility of the filler with the polymer. As a result, the polymer will like the filler more, the filler will adhere better to the polymer matrix, and the properties of the final mixture (e.g., elongation, flexibility) will be enhanced.

3.1.3.11 Thermal Stabilizers

One of the limiting factors in the use of plastics at high temperatures is their tendency not only to become softer but also to thermally degrade. Thermal degradation can present an upper limit to the service temperature of plastics. Thermal degradation can occur at temperatures much lower than those at which mechanical failure is likely to occur. Plastics can be protected from thermal degradation by incorporating stabilizers into them.

3.1.3.12 Antistats

Antistatic additives are capable of modifying properties of plastics in such a way that they become antistatic, conductive, and/or improve electromagnetic interference shielding (EMI). Carbon fibers, conductive carbon powders, and other electrically conductive materials are used for this purpose.

When two (organic) substrates rub against one other, electrostatic charges can build up. This is known as tribocharging. Electrostatic charges can impact plastic parts in several ways; one of the most annoying being the attraction of dust particles. One way to counter this effect is to use antistats (or antistatic additives). This effect is principally a surface effect, although one potential counter measure (conductive fillers) converts it into a bulk effect.

Tools that decrease electrostatic charges and hence increase the conductivity of an organic substrate can be classified as:

- external antistat (surface effect);
- conductive filler (bulk and surface effect);
- internal antistat (surface effect).

An external antistat is applied via a carrier medium to the surface of the plastic part. The same considerations and limitations apply as with non-migrating slip additives. Conductive filler is incorporated into the organic substrates and builds up a conductive network on a molecular level. While both approaches are used in organic substrates, they are not the most common.

An internal antistat is compounded into the organic substrate and migrates to the plastic part surface. The same principle considerations apply as for migrating slip additives (see Figure 3.12).

The need to protect sensitive electronic components and computer boards from electrostatic discharge during handling, shipping, and assembly has provided the driving force for development of a different class of antistatic packaging materials. These are sophisticated laminates with very thin metalized films.

There are other additives used in plastics, but the ones discussed above are the most common.

3.2 Medical Devices—Material Selection Process

In the United States, medical devices, whether they contain plastics or not, are regulated by the Food and Drug Administration (FDA). Devices are classified into three classes: Class I, Class II, and Class III depending upon their risk and criticality. Table 3.1 provides a few examples of devices of each FDA class.

The United States Pharmacopoeia (USP) further classifies medical devices as given in Table 3.2.

Each device class requires a different level of regulation and compliance. Certifying compliance can be a complex and expensive process.

When choosing a plastic for a medical device, design considerations are important. Materials selection, production process selection, and part geometry are interdependent. Usage conditions such as temperature, chemical contact and resistance, and applied stresses during use, are considered. Also, very important for medical devices is sterilization method compatibility including consideration of single vs. repeat sterilization. A summary of many of these considerations follows.

Table 3.1 Examples of Medical Devices Associated with FDA Device Class

Class I devices	Tongue depressors
	Bandages
	Gloves
	Bedpans
	Simple surgical devices
Class II devices	Wheelchairs
	X-ray machines
	MRI machines
	Surgical needles
	Catheters
	Diagnostic equipment
Class III devices	Heart valves
	Stents
	Implanted pacemakers
	Silicone implants
	Hip and bone implants

3.2.1 Physical and Mechanical Properties

Physical properties are important; one must know the dimensions, size, and weight requirements for the part or product. If used by a surgeon,

Table 3.2 USP Classification of Medical Devices

Device Category	Contact	Exposure Time	USP Class
Surface device	Skin	Limited	USP Class I
		Prolonged	USP Class I
		Permanent	USP Class I
Mucosal surfaces	Limited	USP Class I	
		Prolonged	USP Class III
		Permanent	USP Class V
	Breached or compromised surfaces	Limited	USP Class III
		Prolonged	USP Class V
		Permanent	USP Class VI
External communicating devices	Blood path indirect	Limited	USP Class IV
		Prolonged	USP Class V
		Permanent	USP Class VI
	Tissue/bone/dentin communicating	Limited	USP Class IV
		Prolonged	USP Class VI
		Permanent	USP Class VI
	Circulating blood	Limited	USP Class IV
		Prolonged	USP Class VI
		Permanent	USP Class VI
Implant devices	Implant devices	Permanent	Class VI

it must be light enough to handle precisely. The design engineer must consider the loads, stresses, and impact that the product might see during its use. Other physical properties can be important including transparency/opacity, color (some items might use color to aid in identification), aesthetics, water absorption, lubricity, and wear resistance. Important mechanical properties are tensile strength, tensile elongation, tensile modulus, impact resistance (all for toughness), and flexural modulus. Details on the importance of these properties and their measurement are available in the literature [8].

3.2.2 Thermal Properties

Thermal effects must be evaluated both during the production and use of the part or product. Molding temperatures seen during part production are typically much higher than end-use temperatures. Plastic material properties at melting temperatures, sterilization temperatures, and environmental conditions that include both temperature and humidity need to be characterized. Thermal properties of interest include melting point, processing temperatures, heat deflection (or distortion) temperature under load, glass transition temperature, continuous use temperature, and thermal conductivity.

3.2.3 Electrical Properties

Electrical and computer technology is an important part of modern medical treatments, so electrical properties such as conductivity and insulation properties must be considered. Some materials may need to dissipate accumulated static charge, whereas other materials might need electrical insulation properties. Electrical properties to consider are surface and volume conductivity or resistivity, dielectric strength, and comparative tracking index (CTI).

3.2.4 Chemical Resistance

Many medical devices may require chemical resistance to various types of oils, greases, processing aids, disinfectant, bleaches, and other hospital chemicals. Chemical resistance must be considered for the product during production, use and cleaning, sterilizing or disinfecting.

3.2.5 Sterilization Capability

Many reusable, disposable, implant, and packaging materials will need to be sterilized by various methods like steam, dry heat, ethylene oxide (EtO), electron beam, and gamma radiation. They must be able to withstand these conditions and still maintain their properties for the intended use. Of particular importance is hydrolytic stability for steam sterilization, thermal resistance to steam and autoclave conditions, chemical resistance to EtO, and resistance to high-energy radiation including electron beam, gamma, and UV. This is the subject of a reference work by this author [9].

Examples of the effect of sterilization processes on plastics properties are found in Figures 3.13–3.15.

3.2.6 Long-Term Durability

Devices may need to perform for a long period of time under various environmental and thermal conditions. Materials must be selected to meet these long-term aging needs. Instruments must have good ergonomics and functionality. Identification methods like the use of color are also gaining importance. Drug-delivery products comprise needles, tubing, bags, manifolds, Y-sites, clips, and connectors. These are mainly disposable products. Apart from cost, these parts must have excellent chemical and/or lipid

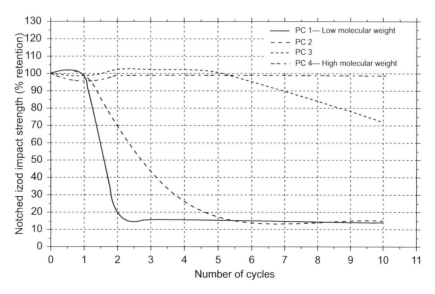

Figure 3.13 The effect of steam sterilization on the impact strength of PCs [10].

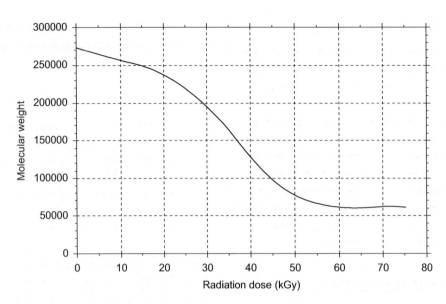

Figure 3.14 The effect of electron beam sterilization on the molecular weight of polylactic acid (PLA).

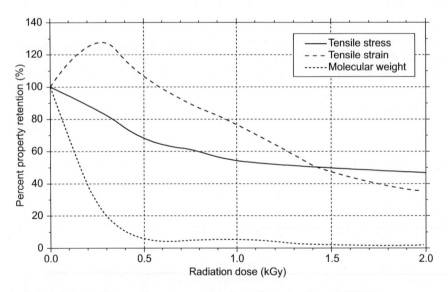

Figure 3.15 Effect of gamma sterilization on some retention of properties of PTFE.

resistance, flexibility, transparency and clarity, sterilization resistance, toughness, tear and burst strength, softness, and no leachables and extractables (discussed in the next section). End-of-life and disposal requirements are also important. Endoscopy is one area that uses a lot of electronics and ancillary products like cameras, light sources, monitors, and recording equipment. Electric, power, and thermal management is very important, including material durability and toughness. Infection control products and devices include gloves, masks, drapes, and gowns. Apart from fit and comfort, materials for these products must be nonirritating, chemically resistant, and stain resistant.

3.2.7 Leachables and Extractables

An important criterion for the use of plastics in medical device applications is quantifying the type and amount and identifying the material that is leached out or extracted from the plastic when in contact with chemicals, reagents, or bodily fluids during the end use. *Extractables* and *leachables* are compounds that can be extracted from the elastomeric or plastic components, or coatings. This is commonly considered for containers and medical devices that come into contact with solvents such as alcohol at various temperatures of use and storage. The difference between extractables and leachables is slight; leachables is generally a more aggressive exposure that is meant to indicate a worst-case scenario.

Both extractables and leachables are affected by the type and amount of additives in the formulation of the plastic. They include plasticizers, antioxidants, stabilizers, pigments, lubricants, vulcanizers, catalysts, residual monomers and oligomers, residual solvents, and contaminants.

The extracts or leachants are often used for the further biological tests. *Cytotoxicity* is the assessment of the (toxic) effect of chemicals on cells. *Sensitization* tests determine the allergic or hyper sensitivity reactions of skin and tissues when exposed to materials or their extracts for prolonged periods of time. *Irritation* tests determine whether the part, material, or extract causes local irritation on skin or mucous membranes via exposure through skin, eye, or mucosa. *Acute system toxicity* testing evaluates whether the extracts cause toxicity effects on various systems of the body when injected into the animal. *Subchronic toxicity* testing is used for all implants. The extract is injected intraperitoneally (in the abdomen walls) or intravenously (in the veins) and evaluated for system toxicity effects. *Genotoxicity* testing evaluates the genetic damage caused by the extracts. *Hemocompatibility* evaluates the compatibility of materials and their extracts with blood and blood components.

3.2.8 Supplemental Tests

Additional tests are occasionally required that may include:

- Carcinogenesis—Long-term tests for implants to test for formation of cancerous cells.
- Reproductive—Long-term test on the effects of the materials and extracts on the reproductive system.
- Biodegradation—Long-term evaluation of material degradation in the body.

3.2.9 Shelf Life and Aging

Accurate prediction of medical product shelf-life performance is critical. Fortunately, the majority of medical products are constructed from a limited number of polymers that have been well characterized in terms of change in their properties over extended-use periods. A procedure known as the simplified protocol for accelerated aging (also called the "10-degree rule") is used. When applied to well-characterized polymer systems over moderate temperature ranges, the test results obtained can be within the required degree of accuracy [11].

3.2.10 Joining and Welding

Medical devices may have complex shapes that cannot be molded directly. In these cases, the plastic parts made need to be separately made and joined together with adhesives or by welding. A number of techniques are used for welding, including:

- Hot gas welding
- Speed tip welding
- Extrusion welding
- Contact welding
- Hot plate welding
- High-frequency welding
- Injection welding
- Ultrasonic welding
- Friction welding
- Spin welding
- Laser welding
- Solvent welding.

Changes in the plastics from welding processes must be considered as well as introduction of adhesives and the chemicals used in them.

3.2.11 Medical Grade Plastics

The effort to evaluate many of these factors can be reduced by using medical grades of the plastics of interest. The manufacturers of these plastics may have already had a significant number of the studies done thereby reducing the time and cost of commercialization.

3.3 Common Medical Device Polymers

This section covers many of the common plastics that are used in various medical devices. It is primarily focused on the polymers and has a chemistry focus. Included for each polymer are chemical structures, some sterilization guidance, and some example uses.

3.3.1 Polyethylene

Polyethylene can be made in a number of ways. The way it is produced can affect its physical properties. It can also have very small amounts of comonomers, which will alter its structure and properties.

The basic types or classifications of polyethylene, according the ASTM D1248, are:

- Ultra-low-density polyethylene (ULDPE), polymers with densities ranging from 0.890 to 0.905 g/cm^3, contains comonomer.
- Very-low-density polyethylene (VLDPE), polymers with densities ranging from 0.905 to 0.915 g/cm^3, contains comonomer.
- Linear low-density polyethylene (LLDPE), polymers with densities ranging from 0.915 to 0.935 g/cm^3, contains comonomer.
- Low-density polyethylene (LDPE), polymers with densities ranging from about 0.915 to 0.935 g/m^3.
- Medium density polyethylene (MDPE), polymers with densities ranging from 0.926 to 0.940 g/cm^3, may or may not contain comonomer.
- High-density polyethylene (HDPE), polymers with densities ranging from 0.940 to 0.970 g/cm^3, may or may not contain comonomer.

Figure 3.16 shows the differences graphically. The differences in the branches in terms of number and length affect the density and melting points of some of the types.

Branching affects the crystallinity. A diagram of a representation of the crystal structure of polyethylene is shown in Figure 3.17. One can imagine how branching in the polymer chain can disrupt the crystalline regions. The crystalline regions are the

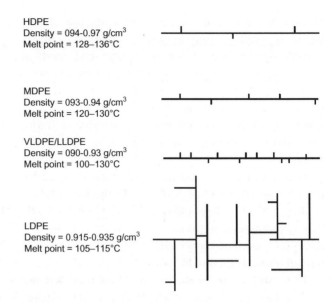

Figure 3.16 Graphical depictions of polyethylene types.

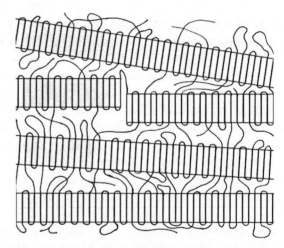

Figure 3.17 Graphical diagram of polyethylene crystal structure.

highly ordered areas in the shaded rectangles of Figure 3.17. A high degree of branching would reduce the size of the crystalline regions, which leads to lower crystallinity.

Sterilization:

The low heat deflection temperatures of polyethylene plastics (30–50°C) make them unsuitable for steam and autoclave sterilization. The plastics would bend, warp, and deform under the temperatures (100–130°C) used in these sterilization methods. EtO, gamma radiation, and e-beam sterilization methods are suitable.

EtO has no effect on the properties of HDPE. Polyethylene will oxidize or cross-link under high-energy radiation and needs to be stabilized to reduce it. In some cases, UHMWPE is deliberately cross-linked with high-energy radiation to improve the wear behavior in the knee and hip implants. Radiation doses of 50–100 kGy are used for cross-linking and standard doses of 25–40 kGy (in an inert atmosphere) are used to sterilize the UHMWPE parts.

Applications and uses: Containers, packaging films, pouches, lidstock, breather patches, and headers for bags. UHMWPE is used as the wear-bearing surface of hip and knee arthroplasty and total joint replacement.

3.3.2 Polypropylene

The three main types of PP are generally available:

1. *Homopolymers* are made in a single reactor with propylene and catalyst. It is the stiffest of the three propylene types and has the highest tensile strength at yield. In the natural state (no colorant added), it is translucent and has excellent see-through or contact clarity with liquids. In comparison to the other two types, it has less impact resistance, especially below 0°C.

2. *Random copolymers* (homophasic copolymer) are made in a single reactor with a small amount of ethylene (<5%) added which disrupts the crystallinity of the polymer allowing this type to be the clearest. It is also the most flexible with the lowest tensile strength of the three. It has better room temperature impact than homopolymer but shares the same relatively poor impact resistance at low temperatures.

3. *Impact copolymers* (heterophasic copolymer), also known as block copolymers, are made in a two reactor system where the homopolymer matrix is made in the first reactor and then transferred to the second reactor where ethylene and propylene are polymerized to create ethylene propylene rubber (EPR) in the form of microscopic nodules dispersed in the homopolymer matrix phase. These nodules impart impact resistance both at ambient and cold temperatures to the compound. This type has intermediate stiffness and tensile strength and is quite cloudy. In general, the more ethylene monomer added, the greater the impact resistance with correspondingly lower stiffness and tensile strength.

Oriented and multilayered films of PP are also common.

Sterilization resistance: The use of PP films in radiation-sterilized applications is somewhat limited. The high ratio of film surface area to mass, combined with the sensitivity of irradiated PP to oxygen-promoted degradation, causes them to be severely embrittled after normal sterilizing doses of radiation. Even resin formulations which yield highly radiation-resistant injection molded devices are badly degraded after irradiation in thin film form. Special formulations of medical PP are coming to market specifically to overcome this disadvantage. Blends of PP and metallocene-catalyzed, ethylene-based plastomers are particularly suited to the construction of highly radiation-resistant, thin-gauge medical device packages.

Gamma radiation resistance: Basell offers several grades which are specially formulated to minimize the effects after typical radiation sterilization dosages of up to 5 megarads, as tested by Basell protocol. Catastrophic failures have been reported in gamma-sterilized PP materials that experienced shelf-life storage. This was a result of long-term degradation. "Long-lived free radicals trapped in the crystalline domains migrated toward the crystalline/amorphous interface combining with available oxygen to form peroxy and hydroperoxy radicals that initiated degradation near the interface. As enough tie molecules between crystallites were cut through the chain scission process, significant reduction of PP's elongation could occur which would lead to catastrophic failures" [12].

PP materials that are adequately stabilized can survive the radiation stabilization process with enough antioxidant remaining to protect the sterilized product from further degradation. The stability of sterilized PP depends on the supplier stabilizer system, and the stability of a radiation-sterilized PP can be simply and rapidly determined by oxygen induction testing (OIT) [13].

Autoclave sterilization: PP has a melting temperature high enough for autoclave application.

Applications and uses:

- Homopolymer: Thermoforming, slit film and oriented fibers, high clarity, syringes, and closures, sutures, drapes, and gowns.
- Random copolymer: Food, household chemicals, beauty aid products, clear containers, and hot fill applications.
- Impact copolymers: Film, sheet, profiles, high-pressure resistance, medical trays, and thin-wall parts.

3.3.3 Polystyrene

Polystyrene is the simplest plastic based on styrene. Its structure is shown in Figure 3.18. Pure solid polystyrene is a colorless, hard plastic with limited flexibility. Polystyrene can be transparent or can be made in various colors. It is economical and is used for producing plastic model assembly kits, plastic cutlery, CD "jewel" cases, and many other common objects where a fairly rigid, economical plastic is desired. There are numerous medical applications.

Three general polystyrene types are:

1. General purpose or crystal (PS or GPPS)
2. High impact (HIPS)
3. Syndiotactic (SPS).

Sterilization:
Polystyrene is not recommended for steam and autoclave sterilization. Its low heat distortion temperature will cause the parts to warp and disfigure. Polystyrene can be sterilized with EtO.

EtO resistance: Polystyrene resins retain their properties after exposure to one normal EtO sterilization cycle. Excessive or multiple exposures to EtO sterilization are not recommended because EtO can cause embrittlement and stress cracking of the polymer [13].

Gamma and electron beam resistance: Polystyrene is very stable to gamma radiation and electron beam due to its high aromatic content. Color changes are seen after e-beam sterilization [14].

UV light sterilization resistance: Styron is resistant to sterilization by UV light. This technology is based on a short wavelength of 254 nm during which the part-to-lamp distance is controlled [15].

Applications and uses:

- *General purpose*: Diagnostic instruments and disposable laboratory ware, Petri dishes, tissue culture components, flasks, and pipettes.
- *Oriented*: Oriented polystyrene films can be printed and laminated to foams for food service plates and trays offering improved esthetics. The films can also be used as a laminate to polystyrene sheet for a high-gloss shine.
- *High impact*: Laboratory ware and other medical devices.

3.3.4 Polyester

Polyesters are formed by a condensation reaction that is very similar to the reaction used to make polyamide or nylons. A diacid and dialcohol are reacted to form the polyester with the elimination of water as shown in Figure 3.19.

While the actual commercial route to making the polyesters may be more involved, the end result is the same polymeric structure. The diacid is usually aromatic. Polyester resins can be formulated to be brittle and hard, tough and resilient, or soft and

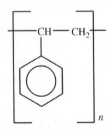

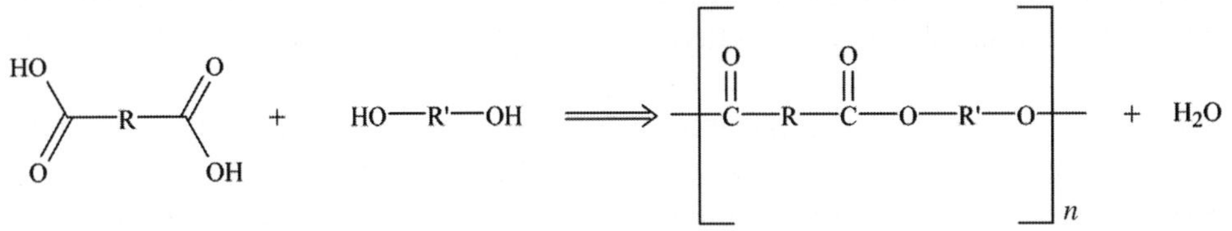

Figure 3.18 Chemical structure of polystyrene.

Figure 3.19 Chemical structure of polyester.

flexible. In combination with reinforcements such as glass fibers, they offer outstanding strength, a high strength-to-weight ratio, chemical resistance, and other excellent mechanical properties. The three dominant materials in this plastics family are PC, PET, and PBT. Liquid crystal polymers are also considered to be polyesters. Thermoplastic polyesters are similar in properties to Nylon 6 and Nylon 66, but have lower water absorption and higher dimensional stability than the nylons.

Sterilization:

EtO Sterilization:

Polyesters generally can be sterilized with EtO. Due to their low hydrolytic stability (i.e., the polymer chains can be cleaved by hydrolysis) and low glass transition temperatures, steam and higher heat autoclave sterilizations are not recommended. All polyesters based on terephthalic acid contain aromatic groups and hence can be sterilized with gamma and e-beam radiation.

Gamma radiation resistance: Ticona Vectra® liquid crystalline polymers (LCPs) have excellent resistance to gamma radiation.

Steam sterilization resistance: Ticona Vectra® LCP has good resistance to hydrolysis. Prolonged exposure to hot water and steam at high temperatures (121°C, 2 bar up to 1000 h) leads to hydrolytic degradation however. The glass-fiber-reinforced grades exhibit a more severe decline in mechanical properties, as do many other glass-fiber-reinforced polymers, owing to capillary action at the glass-fiber/polymer interface (wick effect). Ticona Vectra® A625 has particularly good resistance to hydrolysis. Under selected test conditions, virtually no change in tensile strength or elastic modulus occurred after 1000 h.

PBT can be sterilized by gamma ray or dry heat, up to about 180°C.

Applications and uses:

Liquid crystalline polymer: Sterilizable trays, dental tools, and surgical instruments, surgical device control cables, surgical tubing, cannulae, films.

PBT: Packaging, syringe pump component, dental instruments, miniature scalpel blade holders, melt blown for liquid filtration applications, high-temperature caps.

3.3.5 Polyester (PLA and Other Biosorbable Plastics)

Bioresorbable polymer implants are rapidly growing alternatives to traditional implants in many applications. These implants are only required to serve for a certain time period ranging from weeks to months. PLA is derived from renewable resources, such as corn starch or sugarcanes. PLA polymers are considered biodegradable and compostable. PLA is a thermoplastic, high-strength, high-modulus polymer that can be made from annually renewable sources to yield articles for use in either the industrial packaging field or the biocompatible/bioabsorbable medical device market. Bacterial fermentation is used to make lactic acid, which is then converted to the lactide dimer to remove the water molecule which would otherwise limit the ability to make high molecular weight polymer. The lactide dimer, after the water is removed, can be polymerized without the production of the water. This process is shown in Figure 3.20.

The dimer can be isolated into three forms: the optically active L-lactide, the optically active D-lactide, and the optically inactive DL mixture DL-lactide. These stereoisomer structures are shown in Figure 3.21. The enantiomeric ratio of the dimer can be controlled. Fermentation-derived lactic acid is 95% L-isomer.

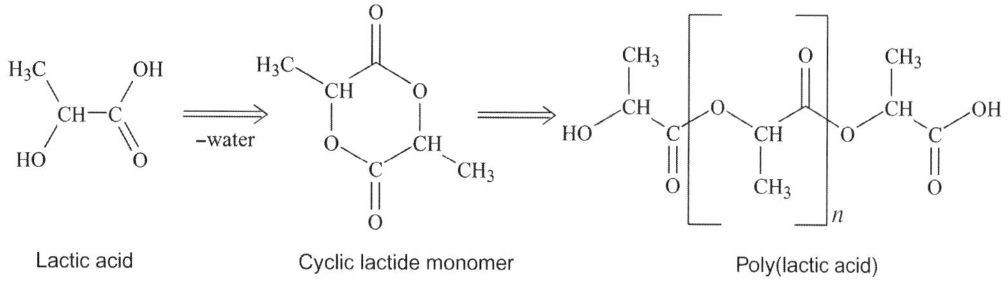

Figure 3.20 Conversion of lactic acid to PLA.

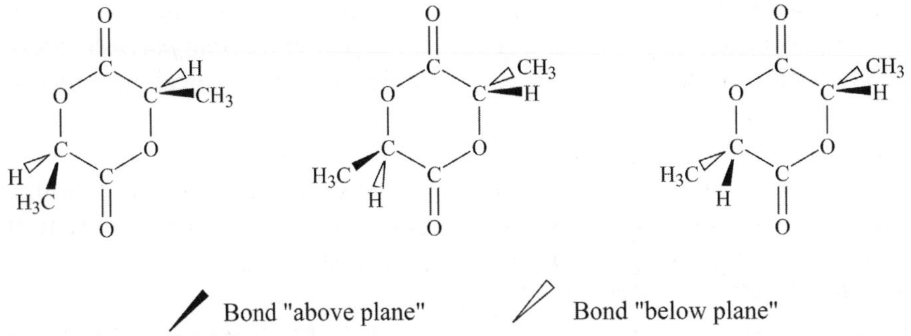

Figure 3.21 Stereoisomeric structures of the lactide dimer.

Polyhydroxyalkanoates (PHAs) are naturally produced and include poly-3-hydroxybutyrate (PHB or PH3B), polyhydroxyvalerate (PHV), and polyhydroxyhexanoate (PHH). A PHA copolymer called PHBV (poly(3-hydroxybutyrate-co-3-hydroxyvalerate)) is less stiff and tougher, and it may be used as packaging material. Chemical structures of some of these polymers are shown in Figure 3.22.

Sterilization:

Autoclave and *dry heat* is usually performed at temperatures equal to or higher than 121°C. PLA, PGA, and PLGA implants are susceptible to hydrolysis and their deformation at higher temperatures therefore precludes the use of these sterilization methods.

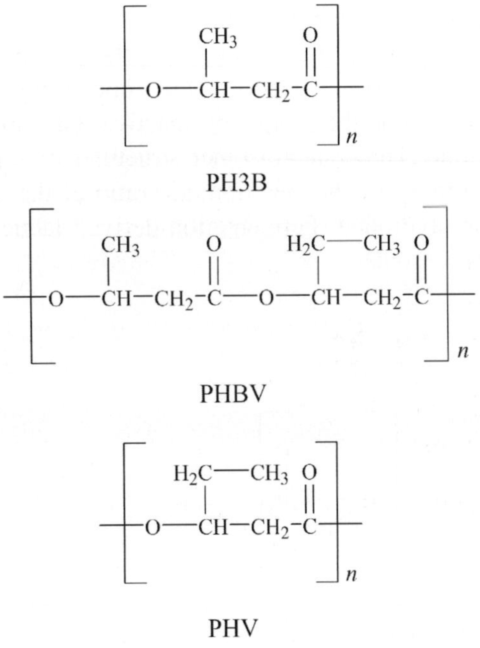

EtO sterilization: EtO is chemically highly reactive and acts as a plasticizer for PLA, PGA, and PLGA, which can lead to changes in the polymer structure. EtO sterilization is performed at temperatures of 50–60°C, which can lead to molecular weight loss. Therefore, EtO sterilization is not suggested.

Radiation sterilization: For the radiation sterilization of bioresorbable polymers, temperature and dose conditions need to be closely controlled to avoid significant degradation. Gamma sterilization at dry ice temperatures is preferred.

Applications and uses: Commercially available biodegradable devices are employed in sutures, orthopedic fixation devices, dental implants, ligature clips, tissue staples, and skin covering devices; stents, dialysis media, and drug-delivery devices. It is also being evaluated as a material for tissue engineering.

3.3.6 Polycarbonate

PC is a type of polyester but is being discussed separately. Theoretically, PC is formed from the reaction of bis-phenol A and carbonic acid. The structures of these two monomers are shown in Figure 3.23.

Commercially, different routes are used (different monomers), but the PC polymer of the structure shown in Figure 3.24 is the result.

PC performance properties include:

- Very impact resistant, is virtually unbreakable and remains tough at low temperatures
- "Clear as glass" clarity
- High heat resistance
- Dimensional stability
- Resistant to UV light, allowing exterior use
- Flame retardant properties.

Figure 3.22 Structures of several PHAs.

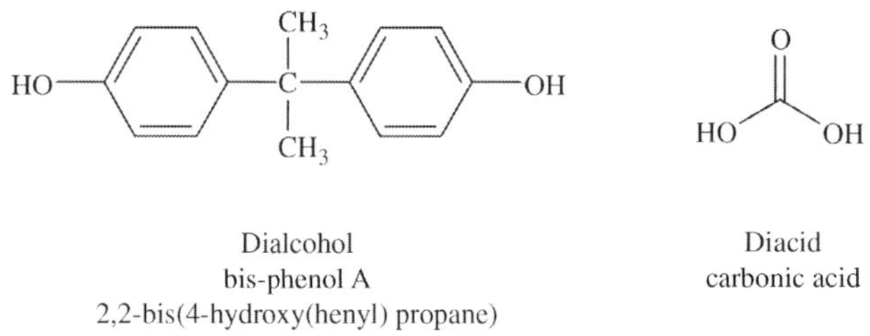

Figure 3.23 Chemical structures of monomers used to make PC polyester.

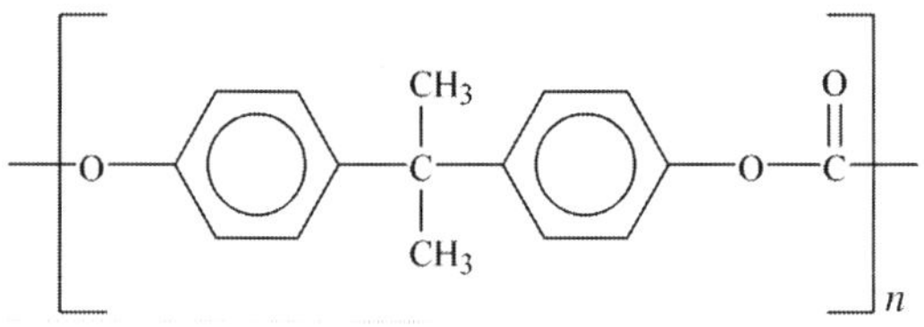

Figure 3.24 Chemical structure of PC polyester.

Typical application requirements include:

- Optical clarity: transparent and colorable
- Durability/impact resistance
- Ductility to withstand impact of rigorous use
- Biocompatible tested grades
- Sterilizable: gamma, EtO; limited autoclave
- Dimensional stability
- Ultrasonic weldable; bondable

Sterilization:
PCs can be sterilized by high-energy gamma and e-beam radiation but must be stabilized to prevent polymer degradation and discoloration.

Gamma radiation resistance: PC is much more resistant to gamma irradiation than most polymers. The primary effect of gamma irradiation on PC is chain scission (chain breakage). Fortunately, the high chain stiffness of PC makes it very difficult for the two ends of the chain to move apart. Therefore, many of the broken chains will recombine. In addition, the aromatic nature of the PC gives it other opportunities to absorb the energy from the gamma photon, rather than just breaking the polymer chain. From a retention of mechanical properties point of view, PC has always been considered one of the most resistant materials for gamma irradiation [16]. Assuming that 28 kGy (2.8 megarads) of energy is required to sterilize PC, the resin can be sterilized 10–20 times before any appreciable reduction in mechanical strength occurs. PC does, however, become progressively more yellow with each sterilization. Special stabilizers can make them less susceptible to color changes.

EtO resistance: The properties of polystyrene resins are unchanged to 50 EtO sterilization cycles [17]. The temperature during sterilization should not exceed 65°C. Tests have shown that repeated sterilization can cause slight brittleness combined with crack formation. The impact strength of test specimens treated with pure EtO at 55°C for 50 cycles of 6 h each is unchanged in comparison with the starting level despite slight crack formation.

Steam resistance: After one to three autoclave cycles (Hi-Vac at 132°C), PC resins have limited utility [18]. Makrolon® DP 1-1262 and Makrolon® Rx-1805 can be sterilized by employing superheated steam (121°C) [18,19]. To prevent deformation of the molded parts, the sterilization temperature should not exceed 125°C. Care must also be taken to ensure that Makrolon parts are not damaged by substances added to the boiler feed water, such as alkaline corrosion inhibitors, and that the article is positioned in such a way that no condensation can accumulate inside it. As a rule, it is possible to sterilize molded parts made of Makrolon many times before gradual chemical decomposition reduces the mechanical strength to a level where it is no longer adequate for certain applications. Sterilization tests on test specimens have shown that even after 100 cycles of 30 min each at 120–125°C, the part still retains comparatively good impact strength. This also generally applies even if the material exhibits hairline cracks and the molded part appears slightly milky as a result of the high stresses imposed on the material by repeated sterilization.

Sterilization with peracetic acid: Makrolon can be sterilized with 2% concentration peracetic acid without suffering damage.

Sterilization with hot air: Sterilization with hot air plays only a minor role for molded parts in Makrolon, since temperatures of 180–200°C are generally used to save time. No problems are to be expected with molded parts of Makrolon up to a hot air temperature of 135°C.

Applications and uses: Medical apparatus (sterilizable), reservoirs, high-pressure syringes, artery cannulas, stopcocks, luers, centrifugal force separators, blood filter housings, dialyzer housings; glucose meters, pumps, insulin pens; surgical device handles and housings.

3.3.7 Polyvinyl Chloride

PVC is a flexible or rigid material that is chemically nonreactive. Rigid PVC is easily machined, heat formed, welded, and even solvent cemented. PVC can also be machined using standard metal working tools and finished to close tolerances and finishes without great difficulty. PVC resins are normally mixed with other additives such as impact modifiers and stabilizers, providing hundreds of PVC-based materials with a variety of engineering properties.

There are three broad classifications for rigid PVC compounds: Type I, Type II, and CPVC. Type II differs from Type I due to greater impact values, but lower chemical resistance. CPVC has greater high temperature resistance. These materials are considered "unplasticized," because they are less flexible than the plasticized formulations. PVC has a broad range of applications, from high-volume construction-related products to simple electric wire insulation and coatings.

PVC is the most widely used plastic resin in medical devices. Approximately 25% of all plastic medical products are made of PVC, according to most market estimates. The main reason is the resin's low cost, ease of processing, and the ability to tailor its properties to a wide range of applications. The following is a more thorough list of reasons for the popularity of PVC in medical devices:

- Used successfully for over 50 years in various medical devices with no known adverse or toxic effects.
- Plasticized PVC has good clarity and transparency retention so that tubes and other products allow for continual monitoring of fluid flow.
- PVC can be manufactured in a range of flexibilities and its resistance to kinking in tubing reduces the risk of fluid flow being interrupted.
- PVC can be used in a wide range of temperatures, and it retains its flexibility, strength, and durability at low temperatures.
- PVC formulations exhibit excellent strength and toughness.
- PVC exhibits very good chemical resistance and stability and is also biocompatible for applications in blood bags and drug delivery.
- Plasticized PVC maintains its product integrity under various sterilization environments like steam, radiation, and EtO.
- PVC can be easily welded to various other plastics by a wide range of methods.
- Its relatively lower cost and high-performance value maintains its position as the number one plastic used in medical devices.
- PVC has safety and cost advantages for a wide variety of medical applications, especially for single-use disposable devices.

A large number of plasticizers have been used with PVC to reduce rigidity, the most common family being the phthalates, especially, di(2-ethylhexyl) phthalate (DEHP). It is sometimes called dioctyl phthalate and abbreviated DOP. These plasticizers are incorporated in amounts ranging from 40% to 65%. There are many other plasticizers used in medical applications.

Heat stabilizers are typically used in medical grade PVC, to protect it against not only the high temperatures the resin might see during processing, but also the high heat it may encounter in storage or autoclaving. Barium–zinc additives are very effective heat stabilizers for PVC but are restricted for medical applications in some countries. Alternatives like calcium–zinc formulations are often used to stabilize medical-grade PVC. Heat stabilizers trap the hydrogen chloride that is generated when PVC decomposes at high temperatures. This prevents discoloration and degradation. Rigid PVC may contain up to 15% by weight of thermal stabilizers. Another additive, Tinuvin®–P, 2-(2H-benzotriazol-2-yl)-*p*-cresol, is used to provide stability from exposure to UV light.

Sterilization:

Gamma radiation resistance: Gamma-ray sterilization generally uses an energy dose of about 2.5 megarads. Sterilization at excessive dosage rates or with excessive sterilization times can result in discoloration or odor. Rigid PVC suffers more severe adverse effects than flexible PVC when inappropriate procedures of this type are used. Specific gamma radiation-resistant PVC blends are commercially available [20]. PVC degrades by chain scission when exposed to high-energy radiation causing degradation or the radicals can react with oxygen to form oxidized products leading to discoloration.

EtO resistance: EtO sterilization is recommended for PVC. When choosing EtO gas sterilization, a 7- to 14-day quarantine period is necessary to assure that there is no EtO residue [10]. Sterilization using EtO gas is a method which has proven particularly useful for PVC products having a large number of cavities or capillaries [10].

Autoclave sterilization: Steam sterilization in autoclaves is conducted at temperatures from 121°C to 134°C. The temperature used is above the glass transition temperature of PVC. Rigid unplasticized PVC is unsuitable for use in steam and autoclave sterilizations as the material and parts will warp and distort when exposed to that temperature range. The temperature range poses no problem for flexible PVC, which is a rubbery material. Plasticized, flexible PVC can be sterilized using steam or autoclave. Low-temperature steam sterilization (conducted at 60–80°C) can be used for both rigid and flexible PVC.

Low-temperature plasma sterilization: PVC products can also be sterilized using newly developed low-temperature plasma technology (Sterrad® plasma sterilization) [10].

Applications and uses:

- Rigid PVC: luer connectors and Y-sites.
- Flexible PVC: secondary packaging, blister packs, solution containers, fluid transport tubes, drip chambers, diaphragms, pull rings, oxygen facemasks, and gloves.

3.3.8 Polyethersulfone

Polyethersulfone (PES) is an amorphous polymer and a high-temperature engineering thermoplastic. Even though PES has high-temperature performance, it can be processed on conventional plastics processing equipment. Its chemical structure is shown in Figure 3.25. PES has an outstanding ability to withstand exposure to elevated temperatures in air and water for prolonged periods.

Because PES is amorphous, mold shrinkage is low and is suitable for applications requiring close tolerances and little dimensional change over a wide temperature range. Its properties include:

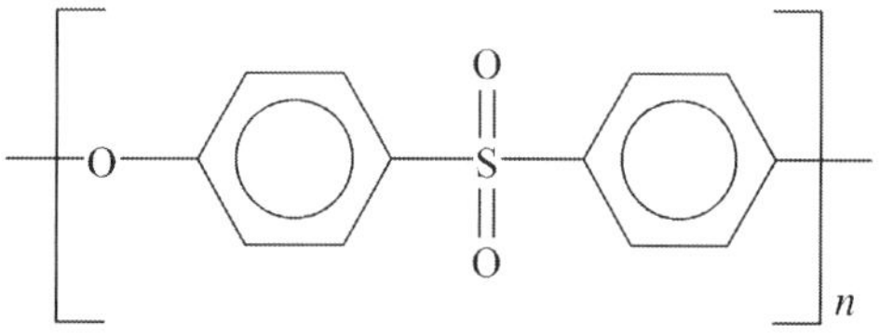

Figure 3.25 Structure of PES.

- Excellent thermal resistance—T_g 224°C
- Outstanding mechanical, electrical, flame, and chemical resistance
- Very good hydrolytic and sterilization resistance
- Good optical clarity

Sterilization:

General sterilization resistance: PES withstands cold sterilants, disinfectants, and germicides.

Gamma and electron beam radiation resistance: PES offers very high resistance to gamma radiation over the entire range of service temperatures. PES products exposed to high-energy radiation suffer a noticeable decrease in tensile strength at yield and a significant decrease in ultimate elongation. Gassing is very slight; transmittance for gamma rays is very high.

Autoclave or steam sterilization resistance: PES parts can be repeatedly sterilized in superheated steam. After more than 100 sterilization cycles, samples remain transparent and largely retain their high level of mechanical properties. PES absorbs more water and is thus suitable only for steam sterilization without a vacuum phase. In order to avoid environmental stress cracking, the level of molded in stress in parts should be as low as possible.

Applications: Medical equipment that requires repeated sterilization; fluid handling couplings/fittings.

3.3.9 Polyacrylate (Acrylic, PMMA)

While a large number of acrylic polymers are manufactured, PMMA is by far the most common. The structure of PMMA is shown in Figure 3.26. Nearly everyone has heard of Plexiglas®. PMMA has two very distinct properties that set the products apart from others. First, it is optically clear and colorless. It has a light transmission of 92%. The 4%

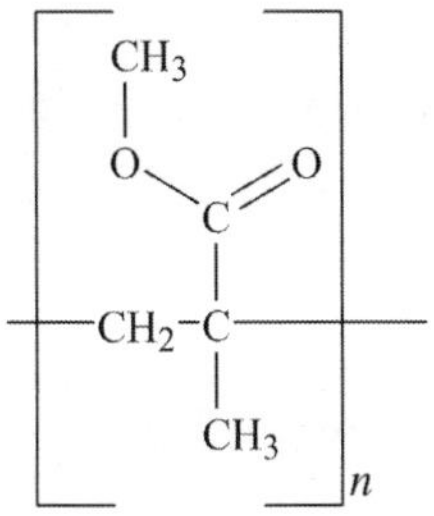

Figure 3.26 Structure of PMMA.

reflection loss at each surface is unavoidable. Second, its surface is extremely hard. They are also highly weather resistant.

PMMA films show very good abrasion resistance, weather resistance (with a UV absorber), and are absolutely colorless.

Acrylic resins are available as homopolymer (primarily PMMA), copolymer, and terpolymer. Each of these is discussed separately in the following sections.

Sterilization resistance: Wet EtO and steam sterilization methods are not recommended for acrylic [21].

Gamma radiation resistance: Plexiglas SG-7 exposed to 5.0 megarads of gamma radiation experiences virtually no yellowing or discoloration. Properties such as impact, tensile, and flexural strength, modulus of elasticity, and percent elongation are constant [22]. Gamma sterilization has a tendency to yellow most acrylics. This yellowing is often temporary and recovery can be complete, with the parts retaining their original integrity. The higher the radiation dosage, the greater the yellowing, and the longer the required recovery time. Current techniques have cut recovery time to a week for some grades [22].

E-beam radiation resistance: Plexiglas maintains constant impact, tensile, and flexural strength, modulus of elasticity, and percent elongation properties [23].

EtO resistance: Acrylics and impact-modified acrylics are compatible with EtO gas and can be EtO sterilized without adversely affecting the medical device.

Applications and uses: Clear, disposable plastics—only glass transmits light as well; chest drainage units, medical spikes, breathing apparatus accessories, urological accessories, Y-sites, check valves, filter housings, IV adaptors, IV pump housings, medical cassettes, blood handling components, and catheter accessories.

3.3.10 Hydrogel (Acrylate)

Hydrogel is a special acrylic polymer or blend of acrylic and silicone polymers that is used in contact lenses. The acrylic is made from monomers that have hydroxyl (—OH) groups on them that "like" water. One such hydrophilic polymer is poly (hydroxyl ethyl acrylate) (or PHEA) or poly (hydroxyl ethyl methacrylate) (or PHEMA). Blends of a hydrophobic silicone with a hydrophilic PHEMA produce a lens material that has improved oxygen transmissibility.

The oxygen transmission is the difference between silicone hydrogel lenses and conventional hydrogel lenses.

Hydrogels used in dressings are also an important component in many different types of wound care. The hydrogel dressing is designed to hold moisture in the surface of the wound, providing the improved environment for both cleaning the wound, and allowing the body to rid itself of necrotic tissue. The moisture in the wound is also essential in pain management for the patient, and these dressings are very soothing and cooling.

Sterilization: Hydrogel contact lenses are generally chemically sterilized by soaking in solutions designed for that purpose.

Applications and uses: Soft contact lenses, wound dressings, drug delivery.

3.3.11 Polysulfone

Polysulfone (PSU) is a rigid, strong, tough, high-temperature amorphous thermoplastic. The structure of PSU is shown in Figure 3.27.

Its properties are:

- High thermal stability
- High toughness and strength
- Good environmental stress crack resistance
- Inherent fire resistance
- Transparency.

General sterilization resistance: PSU maintains a high enough glass transition temperature to withstand different sterilization techniques including steam, EtO, and gamma and electron beam radiation.

Gamma and electron beam radiation resistance: PSUs are highly resistant to degradation by gamma

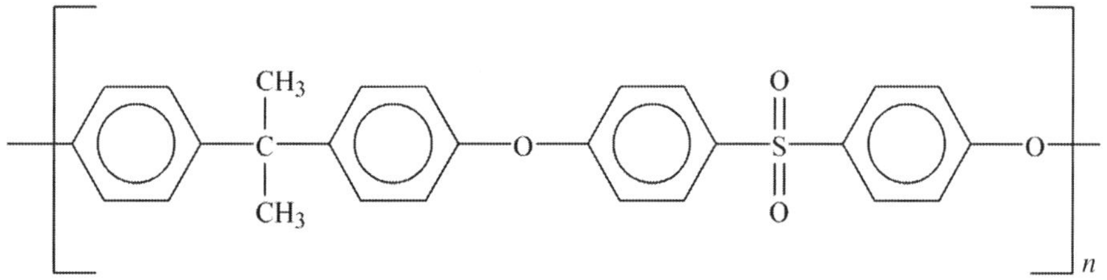

Figure 3.27 Structure of PSU.

or electron beam radiation. There is no evidence of change in mechanical properties after irradiation at 2.5, 4, or 6 megarads. Tensile strength, elongation, modulus, and notched Izod impact values remain essentially unchanged. There is no significant change in chemical resistance following irradiation. PSU discolors during irradiation; the level of discoloration increases with the radiation dosage.

EtO resistance: MPU couplings can be EtO sterilized up to five cycles.

Autoclave or steam sterilization resistance: PSU can withstand greater than 1000 autoclave cycles at 140°C with no significant change in mechanical properties. Transparent PSU will retain its clarity during extended service life. PSU parts can be repeatedly sterilized in superheated steam. After more than 100 sterilization cycles, samples remain transparent and largely retain their high level of mechanical properties. MPU couplings can be autoclave sterilized at 121°C (270°F) for 60 min. The maximum number of cycles recommended is 25.

Dry heat sterilization: Products made from PSU can be dry heat sterilized at 140°C; recommended exposure is 6 h in dry 125°C heat.

Chemical sterilants: PSU performs well, retaining its strength in a wide variety of aqueous disinfectants including buffered glutaraldehyde, phenol, quaternary ammonium, iodophor and formaldehyde types, and detergent germicide.

Applications: Membranes and fluid handling applications and MPU couplings.

3.3.12 Polyetheretherketone

Polyetheretherketones (PEEK) are also referred to as polyarylketones. The most common structure is given in Figure 3.28.

PEEK is a thermoplastic with extraordinary mechanical properties. The Young's modulus of elasticity is 3.6 GPa and its tensile strength is 170 MPa. PEEK is partially crystalline, melts at around 350°C,

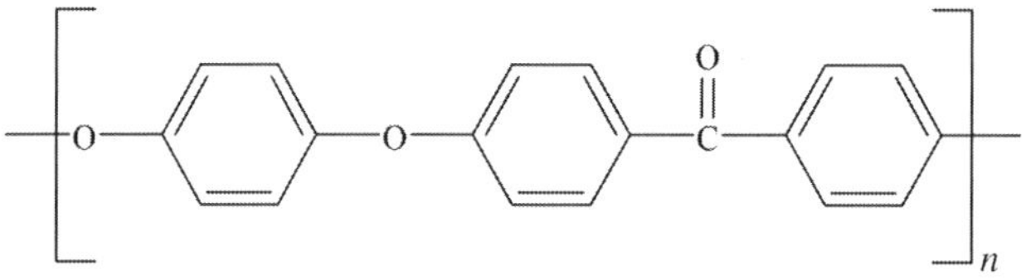

Figure 3.28 Structure of PEEK.

and is highly resistant to thermal degradation. The material is also resistant to both organic and aqueous environments, and is used in bearings, piston parts, pumps, compressor plate valves, and cable insulation applications. It is one of the few plastics compatible with ultrahigh vacuum applications. In summary, the properties of PEEK include:

- Outstanding chemical resistance
- Outstanding wear resistance
- Outstanding resistance to hydrolysis
- Excellent mechanical properties
- Outstanding thermal properties
- Very good dielectric strength, volume resistivity, tracking resistance
- Excellent radiation resistance

Gamma radiation resistance: Victrex® PEEK shows excellent resistance to hard (gamma) irradiation, absorbing over 1000 megarads of radiation without suffering significant damage and showing no embrittlement of the polymer. It is believed that PEEK will resist dose levels of well over 10,000 megarads of particle (alpha or beta) irradiation without significant degradation of properties. Fiber-reinforced grades are expected to show even better performance than this.

EtO resistance: PEEK polymers can be sterilized by EtO methods.

Steam sterilization resistance: PEEK maintains high mechanical strength, stress cracking resistance, and hydrolytic stability in the presence of pressurized steam (200°C, 14 bar), dry heat (170–180°C), hot water, solvents, and chemicals. PEEK can withstand high temperatures and pressures for extended periods of time.

Applications and uses: Reusable medical components including dental syringes and keyhole surgery devices, catheters, disposable surgical instruments.

3.3.13 Thermoplastic Elastomers (TPE, TPU)

An elastomer is a polymer with the property of "elasticity," generally having notably low Young's modulus and high yield strain compared with other materials [23]. The term is often used interchangeably with the term rubber. Elastomers are amorphous polymers existing above their glass transition temperature, so that considerable segmental motion is possible, so it is expected that they would also be very permeable. At ambient temperatures, rubbers are thus relatively soft and deformable. Their primary uses are for seals, adhesives, and molded flexible parts. Elastomers may be thermosets (requiring vulcanization, a form of cross-linking) or thermoplastic, called thermoplastic elastomer or TPE.

TPEs have two big advantages over the conventional thermoset (vulcanized) elastomers. Those are ease and speed of processing. Other advantages of TPEs are the ability to recycle scrap, lower energy costs for processing, and the availability of standard, uniform grades (not generally available in thermosets).

TPEs are molded or extruded on standard plastics-processing equipment in considerably shorter cycle times than those required for compression or transfer molding of conventional rubbers. They are made by copolymerizing two or more monomers, using either the block or graft polymerization techniques. One of the monomers provides the hard, or crystalline, polymer segment that functions as a thermally stable component; the other monomer develops the soft or amorphous segment, which contributes the elastomeric or rubbery characteristic. This is shown in Figure 3.29 in which the hard crystalline parts of the molecule are the thick lined segments of the polymer chain. As shown, the hard segments can be aligned together forming crystalline regions.

Physical and chemical properties can be controlled by varying the ratio of the monomers and the length of the hard and soft segments. Block

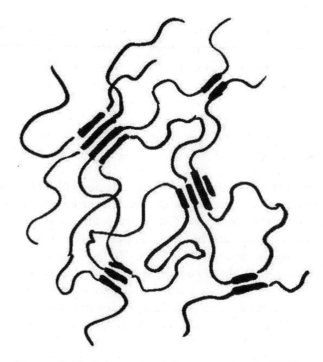

Figure 3.29 Schematic of the structure of a TPE.

techniques create long-chain molecules that have various or alternating hard and soft segments. Graft polymerization methods involve attaching one polymer chain to another as a branch. The properties that are affected by each phase can be generalized.

"Hard phase"—plastic properties:

1. Processing temperatures
2. Continuous use temperature
3. Tensile strength
4. Tear strength
5. Chemical and fluid resistance
6. Adhesion to inks, adhesives, and overmolding substrates.

"Soft phase"—elastomeric properties:

1. Lower service temperature limits
2. Hardness
3. Flexibility
4. Compression set and tensile set.

ISO 18064 [8] sets a standard nomenclature system for TPEs. Those having a prefix TP shall be followed by a letter representing each category of TPEs.

The categories are outlined below:

1. TPA—polyamide TPE, comprising a block copolymer of alternating hard and soft segments with amide chemical linkages in the hard blocks and ether and/or ester linkages in the soft blocks.
2. TPC—copolyester TPE, consisting of a block copolymer of alternating hard segments and soft segments, the chemical linkages in the main chain being ester and/or ether.
3. TPO—olefinic TPE, consisting of a blend of a polyolefin and a conventional rubber, the rubber phase in the blend having little or no cross-linking.
4. TPS—styrenic TPE, consisting of at least a triblock copolymer of styrene and a specific diene, where the two end blocks (hard blocks) are polystyrene and the internal block (soft block or blocks) is a polydiene or hydrogenated polydiene.
5. TPU—urethane TPE, consisting of a block copolymer of alternating hard and soft segments with urethane chemical linkages in the hard blocks and ether, ester or carbonate linkages or mixtures of them in the soft blocks.
6. TPV—thermoplastic rubber vulcanizate consisting of a blend of a thermoplastic material and a conventional rubber in which the rubber has been cross-linked by the process of dynamic vulcanization during the blending and mixing step.
7. TPZ—unclassified TPE comprising any composition or structure other than those grouped in TPA, TPC, TPO, TPS, TPU, and TPV.

Urethanes are a reaction product of a diisocyanate and long and short chain polyether, polyester, or caprolactone glycols. The polyols and the short chain diols react with the diisocyanates to form linear polyurethane molecules. This combination of diisocyanate and short chain diol produces the rigid or hard segment. The polyols form the flexible or soft segment of the final molecule. Figure 3.30 shows the molecular structure in schematic form.

The properties of the resin depend on the nature of the raw materials, the reaction conditions, and the ratio of the starting raw materials. The polyols used have a significant influence on certain properties of the thermoplastic polyurethane. Polyether and polyester polyols are both used to produce many products.

The polyester-based TPUs have the following characteristic features:

- Good oil/solvent resistance
- Good UV resistance
- Abrasion resistance
- Good heat resistance
- Mechanical properties.

The polyether-based TPUs have the following characteristic features:

- Fungus resistance
- Low-temperature flexibility
- Excellent hydrolytic stability
- Acid/base resistance.

In addition to the basic components described above, most resin formulations contain additives to facilitate production and processability.

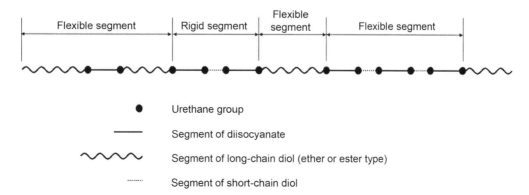

Figure 3.30 Molecular structure of a thermoplastic polyurethane elastomer.

The polyether types are slightly more expensive and have better hydrolytic stability and low-temperature flexibility than the polyester types.

Gamma radiation resistance: The physical properties of transparent rigid thermoplastic polyurethanes are not significantly affected by exposure to a maximum of 10 megarads of gamma radiation. Discoloration is dramatic upon exposure to gamma radiation. Yellowness index increases from 6.3 before exposure to 77.6 after exposure. The discoloration is permanent with minimal bleach-back.

EtO resistance: Transparent and opaque rigid thermoplastic polyurethanes are compatible with multiple cycles of EtO sterilization. They generally retain tensile strength and Izod impact properties after exposure to five cycles of EtO gas. Less than 300 ppm residual EtO was present on the first day following exposure with continued degassing over time.

Applications and uses: Catheters, valves, needleless syringes, surgical instruments, wound dressing and tape, shunts, drug patches, medical bags, and tubing.

3.3.14 Thermoset Elastomers—Silicone

One of the most important thermoset elastomers is silicone, also known as siloxane, polyorganosiloxane, or polysiloxane. Silicone rubber is a semi-organic synthetic. Its polymer backbone structure consists of a chain of silicon and oxygen atoms rather than carbon and hydrogen atoms, as in the case with other types of rubber. The molecular structure of silicone rubber results in a very flexible—but weak—chain. Silicones are very stable at low and high temperatures. Although fillers may improve properties somewhat, tear and tensile strengths remain relatively low. Figure 3.31 shows four of the primary groups that make up a typical polysiloxane. To simplify the discussion of polysiloxane composition, the monomers are identified by letters:

"M" stands for Me_3SiO
"D" for Me_2SiO_2
"T" for $MeSiO_3$
"Q" for SiO_4
"P" for replace Me with phenyl side groups
"V" for replace Me with vinyl side groups (typically <1%)
"F" for replace Me with fluorine.

Some common abbreviations for the polymers include MQ, VMQ, PMQ, PVMQ, PDMS poly(1-trimethylsilyl-1-propyne) or PTMSP.

Because silicones, in general, are temperature and moisture resistant, they are typically not affected by most sterilization methods. The most common sterilization methods used for medical devices that contain silicone include dry heat, steam autoclaving, EtO, gamma radiation, and electron beam (e-beam) radiation.

Dry heat or steam autoclaving will most likely have little effect on silicone's physical properties because of its moisture and heat resistance. The drawback to heat sterilization of silicone materials is that the high heat may cause the silicone to expand which must be taken into consideration how the device is configured and packaged.

EtO sterilization: Silicones generally have a high permeability to EtO molecules allowing the EtO to diffuse through the polymer network, inducing sterilization throughout the polymer matrix. The only precaution is to ensure that all of the EtO has been removed from the silicone device before it is used, which usually takes 24 h.

Gamma and electron beam sterilization: Radiation is known to induce changes in the molecular architecture of silicone rubber, increasing its molecular weight and decreasing elasticity.

Applications and uses: prostheses, artificial organs, facial reconstruction, catheters, artificial skin, contact lenses, drug-delivery systems, contact lenses.

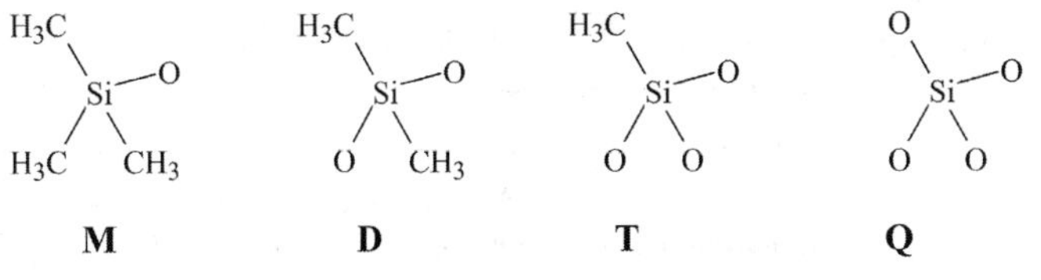

Figure 3.31 Structure of groups that make up polysiloxanes.

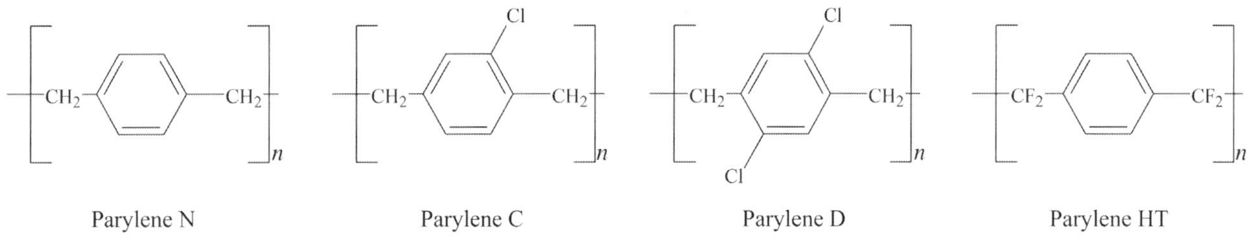

Figure 3.32 Structures of the Parylene polymer molecules.

3.3.15 Poly-p-xylylene (Parylene)

Parylene is the generic name for members of a series of polymers. The basic member of the series, called Parylene N, is poly-para-xylylene, a completely linear, highly crystalline material. The structures of four Parylene types are shown in Figure 3.32.

Parylene polymers are not manufactured and sold directly. They are deposited from the vapor phase by a process which in some respects resembles vacuum metalizing. The Parylenes are formed at a pressure of about 0.1 torr from a reactive dimer in the gaseous or vapor state. Unlike vacuum metalizing, the deposition is not line of sight, and all sides of an object to be encapsulated are uniformly impinged by the gaseous monomer. Due to the uniqueness of the vapor phase deposition, the Parylene polymers can be formed as structurally continuous films from as thin as a fraction of a micrometer to as thick as several millimeters.

The first step is the vaporization of the solid dimer at approximately 150°C. The second step is the quantitative cleavage (pyrolysis) of the dimer vapor at the two methylene—methylene bonds at about 680°C to yield the stable monomeric diradical, para-xylylene. Finally, the monomeric vapor enters the room temperature deposition chamber where it spontaneously polymerizes on the substrate. The substrate temperature never rises more than a few degrees above ambient.

Parylene is used as a coating on medical devices ranging from silicone tubes to advanced coronary stents, synthetic rubber products ranging from medical grade silicone rubber to EPDM (ethylene propylene diene monomer rubber).

The manufacturer of coating equipment and starting materials is Para Tech Coating, Inc. They also offer coating services.

Sterilization:

Parylene coatings respond to these sterilization methods in a variety of ways (see summary of responses in Table 3.3). With regard to tensile properties, Parylene N and C were largely unaffected by any of these sterilization techniques. Only steam appears to have had any effect, causing an annealing impact on samples coated with Parylene C, seen as an increase in film crystallinity with a slight change in the tensile properties. Similarly, the tensile modulus property of Parylene N exhibited a minor change.

H_2O_2 *plasma sterilization* treatment appeared to alter dielectric strength, with a minimal change in Parylene C, and no change in Parylene N.

Applications and uses: Needles, prosthetic devices, implantable components, catheter, electrodes, stents, epidural probes, cannulae assemblies.

3.3.16 Fluoropolymers

PTFE polymer is an example of a linear fluoropolymer. Its structure in simplistic form is shown in Figure 3.33.

Formed by the polymerization of tetrafluoroethylene (TFE), the ($-CF_2-CF_2-$) groups repeat many thousands of times. The fundamental properties of fluoropolymers evolve from the atomic structure of fluorine and carbon and their covalent bonding in specific chemical structures. The backbone is formed of carbon—carbon bonds and the pendant groups are carbon—fluorine bonds. Both are extremely strong bonds. The basic properties of PTFE stem from these two very strong chemical bonds. The size of the fluorine atom allows the formation of a uniform and continuous covering around the carbon—carbon bonds and protects them from chemical attack, thus imparting chemical resistance and stability to the molecule. PTFE is rated for use up to (260°C). PTFE does not dissolve in any known solvent. The fluorine sheath is also responsible for the low surface energy (18 dynes/cm) and low COF (0.05—0.8, static) of PTFE. Another attribute of the uniform fluorine sheath is the electrical inertness (or non-polarity) of the PTFE molecule. Electrical fields impart only slight polarization in

Table 3.3 Effects of Various Sterilization Methods on Parylene [24]

Sterilization Method	Parylene N					Parylene C			
	Dielectric Strength	WVT	Tensile Strength	Tensile Modulus	COF	Dielectric Strength	WVT	Tensile Strength	Tensile Modulus	COF
Steam	None	Δ43%	None	Δ12%	Δ38%	None	Δ5*	Δ17%	Δ9%	None
EtO	None	Δ21%	None	None	Δ33%	None	8%	None	None	None
E-beam	NA	None	None	None	None	NA	None	None	None	None
H₂O₂ plasma	None	None	None	None	Δ48%	Δ9%	None	None	None	Δ188%
Gamma	None	None	None	None	None	None	Δ5%	None	None	None

*5% values are not likely to be statistically significant. NA = not applicable; COF = coefficient of friction; WVT = water vapor transmission.

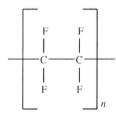

Figure 3.33 Chemical structure of PTFE.

this molecule, so volume and surface resistivities are high.

The PTFE molecule is simple and is quite ordered. PTFE can align itself with other molecules or other portions of the same molecule. Disordered regions are called *amorphous* regions. This is important because polymers with high crystallinity require more energy to melt. In other words, they have higher melting points. When this happens it forms what is called a crystalline region. Crystalline polymers have a substantial fraction of their mass in the form of parallel, closely packed molecules. High molecular weight PTFE resins have high crystallinity and therefore high melting points, typically as high as 320–342°C (608–648°F). The crystallinity of as-polymerized PTFE is typically 92–98%. Further, the viscosity in the molten state (called melt creep viscosity) is so high that high molecular weight PTFE particles do not flow even at temperatures above its melting point. They sinter much like powdered metals; they stick to each other at the contact points and combine into larger particles.

PTFE is called a *homopolymer*, a polymer made from a single monomer. Recently many PTFE manufacturers have added minute amounts of other monomers to their PTFE polymerizations to produce alternate grades of PTFE designed for specific applications. Fluoropolymer manufacturers continue to call these grades modified homopolymer at below 1% by weight of comonomer. These modified granular PTFE materials retain the exceptional chemical, thermal, antistick, and low-friction properties of conventional PTFE resin, but offer some improvements:

- Weldability
- Improved permeation resistance
- Less creep
- Smoother, less porous surfaces
- Better high-voltage insulation

The copolymers described in the next sections contain significantly more of the non-TFE monomers.

Sterilization:

Exposure to high-energy (ionizing) radiation, regardless of the source, degrades PTFE by breaking down the molecules and reducing its molecular weight, resulting in a marked decrease in melt viscosity. As in thermal degradation, radiation stability of PTFE is much better under vacuum compared to air.

Applications and uses: fittings, valves, pumps, tubing.

Expanded PTFE[25]:

One of the most unique and remarkable developments in the processing of homofluoropolymers is the expansion of the polymeric matrix without the use of soluble fillers, foaming agents, or chemical additives. This invention constitutes the physical inducement of billions of small pores in the structure of an article of PTFE resulting in new properties and significant savings in material consumption. W.L. Gore and Associates invented this technology in the early 1970s. The trademark Gore-Tex® is well known in lightweight waterproof and breathable fabrics, microfiltration membranes, medical implants, microwave carriers, industrial sealants, and high tensile fabrics.

Applications and uses: microfiltration membranes, medical implants.

Fluorocoatings:

Fluorocoatings are used in medical devices. They often provide dry lubrication, insulation, and nonstick properties. Coatings are used on catheter guide wires and on metered dose inhaler canisters and valves.

3.4 Summary

There are many more polymers used in medical device applications than those listed in this chapter and more are being developed and used all the time. There are also dozens of other ways to sterilize than the ones mentioned. Table 3.4 provides a basic summary of the performance of a wide range of polymers used in plastics when sterilized by the most common methods.

Table 3.4 Sterilization Matrix of Plastics [26]

Polymer	Polymer Abbreviation	Steam	Dry Heat	Ethylene Oxide	Gamma Radiation	Electron Beam
Polyolefins						
High-density polyethylene	HDPE	Poor	Poor	Good	Good	Good
Low-density polyethylene	LDPE	Poor	Poor	Good	Good	Good
Ultrahigh molecular weight polyethylene	UHMWPE	Poor	Poor	Good	Good	Good
Polypropylene[a]	PP	Good	Fair	Good	Fair	Fair
Polypropylene copolymers		Good	Fair	Good	Fair	Fair
Cyclo olefin copolymer	COC	Fair	Fair	Good	Good	Good
Polyvinyl chloride plasticized[a,b]	PVC	Fair	Fair	Good	Good	Good
Polyvinyl chloride unplasticized[a,b]	PVC	Poor	Poor	Good	Fair	Fair
Polystyrene/styrenics						
Polystyrene	PS	Poor	Poor	Good	Good	Good
Acrylonitrile butadiene styrene copolymer (Abs)	ABS	Poor	Poor	Good	Good	Good
Styrene–acrylonitrile copolymer (San)	SAN	Poor	Poor	Good	Good	Good
Acrylonitrile styrene acrylate	ASA	Poor	Poor	Good	Good	Good
Methacrylate acrylonitrile butadiene styrene copolymer	MABS	Poor	Poor	Good	Good	Good
Styrene–butadiene copolymer	SBC	Poor	Poor	Good	Good	Good
Acrylics[a,b]		Poor	Poor	Good	Good	Good
Polycarbonates[a,b]		Fair	Fair	Good	Good	Good
High heat polycarbonates		Good	Good	Good	Good	Good
Polyurethanes		Poor	Poor	Good	Good	Good
Acetals	POM	Good	Good	Good	Poor	Poor
Polyamides						
Nylon 6, Nylon 66	PA6, PA66	Fair	Fair	Good	Fair	Fair
Aromatic		Good	Good	Good	Good	Good
Nylon 12, 6/12	PA12	Poor	Poor	Good	Fair	Fair

(*Continued*)

Table 3.4 Sterilization Matrix of Plastics [26]—*Cont'd*

Polymer	Polymer Abbreviation	Steam	Dry Heat	Ethylene Oxide	Gamma Radiation	Electron Beam
Polyesters						
Poly butylene terephthalate	PBT	Fair	Fair	Good	Good	Good
Poly ethylene terephthalate	PET	Poor	Poor	Good	Good	Good
Copolyesters		Poor	Poor	Good	Good	Good
High-temperature thermoplastics						
Polysulfones	PSU	Good	Good	Good	Good	Good
Polyphenylene sulfide	PPS	Good	Good	Good	Good	Good
Liquid crystalline polymer	LCP	Good	Good	Good	Good	Good
Polyetherimide	PEI	Fair	Fair	Good	Good	Good
Polyamide–imide	PAI	Fair	Fair	Good	Good	Good
Polyetheretherketone	PEEK	Good	Good	Good	Good	Good
Fluoropolymers						
Polytetrafluoroethylene[a]	PTFE	Fair	Fair	Good	Poor	Poor
Fluorinated ethylene propylene	FEP	Good	Good	Good	Fair	Fair
Perfluoro alkoxy	PFA	Good	Good	Good	Good	Good
Ethylene chlorotrifluoroethylene	ECTFE	Good	Good	Good	Good	Good
Ethylene tetrafluoroethylene	ETFE	Good	Good	Good	Good	Good
Polyvinyl fluoride	PVF	Good	Good	Good	Good	Good
Polyvinylidene difluoride	PVF2	Good	Good	Good	Good	Good
Elastomers						
Silicones		Good	Good	Good	Good	Good
Urethane thermoplastic elastomer	TPU	Poor	Fair	Good	Good	Good
Copolyester thermoplastic elastomer	TPC	Poor	Good	Good	Good	Good
Polyamide thermoplastic elastomer	TPA	Poor	Poor	Good	Good	Good
Styrenic thermoplastic elastomer	TPS	Poor	Poor	Good	Good	Good
Olefinic thermoplastic elastomer	TPO	Poor	Fair	Good	Good	Good

(*Continued*)

Table 3.4 Sterilization Matrix of Plastics [26]—Cont'd

Polymer	Polymer Abbreviation	Steam	Dry Heat	Ethylene Oxide	Gamma Radiation	Electron Beam
Biopolymers						
PLLA	PLLA	Fair	Good	Good	Good	Good
Polylactic acid	PLA	Poor	Fair	Good	Good	Good
Polyhydroxybutyrate	PHB	Poor	Poor	Good	Fair	Fair
Polyglycolic acid	PGA	Good	Good	Good	Good	Good
Poly(lactic-co-glycolic acid)	PLGA	Poor	Poor	Good	Fair	Fair
Polycaprolactone	PCL	Fair	Good	Good	Good	Good

[a]Radiation stable grades should be considered for gamma and e-beam radiation sterilization.
[b]PVC, acrylics, PC—require corrective tint to compensate for discoloration.

References

[1] Available from: http://en.wikipedia.org/wiki/Dendronized_polymers.

[2] This is a file from the Wikimedia Commons which is a freely licensed media file repository.

[3] Utracki LA. Polymer blends handbook, vols. 12. Springer-Verlag; 2002.

[4] Utracki LA. Commercial polymer blends. Springer-Verlag; 1998.

[5] Utracki LA. Encyclopaedic dictionary of commercial polymer blends. ChemTec Publishing; 1994.

[6] Flick EW. Plastics additives—an industrial guide. 2nd ed. William Andrew Publishing/Noyes; 1993.

[7] Pritchard G. Plastics additives—an A-Z reference. Springer-Verlag; 1998.

[8] International Standard ISO 18064 Thermoplastic Elastomers—Nomenclature and Abbreviated Terms, First Edition 2003-09-01 (Reference Number ISO 18064:2003(E)).

[9] McKeen LW. The effect of sterilization on plastics and elastomers. William Andrew Publishing; 2012.

[10] Selecting Materials for Medical Products: From PVC to Metallocene Polyolefins, Medical Device & Diagnostic Industry, 1996.

[11] Karl J. Hemmerich, General Aging Theory and Simplified Protocol for Accelerated Aging of Medical Devices, MDDI Medical Device and Diagnostic Industry News Products and Suppliers, 1998.

[12] Shang S, Ling MTK, Westphal SP, Woo L. Baxter healthcare radiation sterilization compatibility of medical packaging materials, vol. 3. Antec; 1997.

[13] Technical library, general purpose polystyrene resins. The Dow Chemical Company; 1995–2004.

[14] Hermanson NJ. EtO and gamma sterilization from standard tests to medical devices, 1997.

[15] Hermanson NJ, Steffens JF. The physical and visual property changes in thermoplastic resins after exposure to high energy sterilization—gamma versus electron beam. ANTEC 1993, conference proceedings. Society of Plastics Engineers; 1993.

[16] Lexan GR Resin Gamma Resistant Product Information Book, supplier marketing literature (NBM-110), General Electric Company.

[17] Sterilization Comparison, supplier marketing literature ACB/3/93, GE Plastics, 1993.

[18] McIlvaine JE. The Effect of Gamma Sterilization on Glass-Reinforced and Lubricated Thermoplastics, Medical Plastics and Biomaterials Magazine, January 1977.

[19] Fluoropolymer Tubing, Teleflex Medical, 2003.

[20] Bruder, Axel, PVC—The Material for Medical Products (translated), Swiss Plastics No. 4, 1999 and Swiss Chem No. 5, 1999.

[21] Whitaker WA. Acrylic Polymers: A Clear Focus, January 1996.

[22] Plexiglas Acrylic Resin from AtoHaas Clearly The Best, supplier marketing literature (PL-1700b), AtoHaas, 1993.

[23] McKeen LW. The effect of temperature and other factors on plastics. Plastics Design Library, William Andrew Publishing; 2008.

[24] Wolgemuth L. Assessing the effects of sterilization methods on parylene coatings. Medical Device & Diagnostic Industry; 2002.

[25] Ebnesajjad S. Fluoroplastics, volume 1—non-melt processible fluoroplastics. William Andrew Publishing/Plastics Design Library; 2000.

[26] Sastri V. Plastics in medical devices. Elsevier Inc.; 2010.

4 Polymeric Biomaterials

Wei He and Roberto Benson

OUTLINE

4.1 Introduction 55
4.2 Polymeric Biomaterials in Ophthalmology 56
   4.2.1 Polymeric Contact Lens 56
   4.2.2 Polymeric Intraocular Lens 58
   4.2.3 Polymeric Artificial Cornea 58
4.3 Polymeric Biomaterials in Orthopedics 60
   4.3.1 Polyethylene 60
   4.3.2 Polyacrylates 61
   4.3.3 Natural Polymers 61
4.4 Polymeric Biomaterials in Cardiovascular Diseases 62
   4.4.1 Polyurethanes 62
   4.4.2 Polyethylene Terephthalate 63
   4.4.3 Expanded PTFE 63
4.5 Polymeric Biomaterials for Wound Closure 64
4.6 Polymeric Biomaterials in Extracorporeal Artificial Organs 66
4.7 Polymeric Biomaterials for Nerve Regeneration 67
4.8 Conclusions and Future Outlook 68
References 69

Biomaterials are an indispensable element in improving human health and quality of life. Applications of biomaterials include diagnostics (gene arrays and biosensors), medical supplies (blood bags and surgical tools), therapeutic treatments (medical implants and devices), and emerging regenerative medicine (tissue-engineered skin and cartilage). Polymers, being organic, offer a versatility that is unmatched by metals and ceramics. The wide spectrum of physical, mechanical, and chemical properties provided by polymers has fueled the extensive research, development, and applications of polymeric biomaterials. The significance of polymers as biomaterials is reflected in the market size of medical polymers, estimated to be approximately $1 billion. Many of these polymers were initially developed as plastics, elastomers, and fibers for nonmedical industrial applications, but were later developed as biomedical-specific materials. With rapid growth in modern biology and interdisciplinary collaborative efforts, polymeric biomaterials are being fashioned into bioactive and biomimetic materials, with excellent biocompatibility.

4.1 Introduction

Biomaterials is an exciting and highly multidisciplinary field. These materials have matured into an indispensable element in improving human health and quality of life in the modern era. Applications of biomaterials range from diagnostics such as gene arrays and biosensors, to medical supplies such as blood bags and surgical tools, to therapeutic treatments such as medical implants and devices, to emerging regenerative medicine involving tissue-engineered skin and cartilage, etc. A general classification divides biomaterials into three main categories: metals, ceramics, and polymers. Polymers, being organic in nature, offer a versatility that is unmatched by metals and ceramics. The wide spectrum of physical, mechanical, and chemical properties that polymers can provide has fueled the extensive research, development, and applications of polymeric biomaterials. Furthermore, the significance of polymers in the field of biomaterials is clearly reflected in the staggering market size of medical polymers, estimated to be roughly $1 billion with yearly growth of 10–20% [1].

This chapter provides a brief overview of several medical applications that polymers have made seminal contributions to over the years. Many of the polymers discussed here are initially developed as plastics, elastomers, and fibers for nonmedical industrial applications. They were "borrowed" by the surgeons post-World War II to address medical problems. Since then, they have led to the development of biomedical-specific materials. Currently, with the rapid growth in modern biology and collaborative effort, cross-discipline work involving materials science, engineering, chemistry, biology, and medicine, is resulting in polymeric biomaterials that are bioactive, biomimetic, and, most importantly, have excellent biocompatibility. Examples of this newer generation of polymeric biomaterials are also included in this chapter.

4.2 Polymeric Biomaterials in Ophthalmology

Ophthalmology focuses on the diseases of the eye, which is a complex and vital organ for daily life. Application of biomaterials in ophthalmology can be dated back to the mid-nineteenth century, when Adolf Fick successfully invented the glass contact lens. Since then, a wide variety of ophthalmological biomaterials have been developed and some are finding overwhelming success in clinical applications. Applications of biomaterials in ophthalmology include contact lenses [2], intraocular lenses (IOLs) [3], artificial orbital walls [4], artificial corneas [5], artificial lacrimal ducts [6], glaucoma filtration implants [7], viscoelastic replacements [8], drug delivery systems [9], scleral buckles [10], retinal tacks and adhesives [11], and ocular endotamponades [12]. Although ceramics and metals have also been used in ophthalmology, modern ophthalmic implants are mainly made of polymers. The focus of this section will be on polymers used for contact lens, IOL, and artificial corneas.

4.2.1 Polymeric Contact Lens

A contact lens is an optical device placed on the cornea of the eye for corrective, therapeutic, or cosmetic effects. It is estimated that there are approximately 125 million contact lens wearers worldwide. A myriad of principle properties have been sought in high performance contact lens materials, including (1) good transmission of visible light; (2) high oxygen permeability; (3) tear-film wettability; (4) resistance to deposition of components from tear-film, such as lipid, protein, and mucus; (5) ion permeability; (6) chemical stability; (7) good thermal conductivity; and (8) amenability to manufacture [13]. A wide variety of polymers have been used in contact lenses, and their modulus of elasticity defines contact lenses to be either hard or soft. Structures of the various monomers commonly used in contact lenses are shown in Figure 4.1. The first generation of polymeric contact lenses was made of poly(methyl methacrylate) (PMMA), a polymer commercially known as Plexiglas® and a classical example of hard or rigid lens material. PMMA can be prepared using bulk free radical polymerization and lathed into lens shape. It has excellent optical properties such as index of refraction with greater clarity than glass, remarkable durability, and good resistance against deposition of components from the tear-film due to its hydrophobicity. However, major drawbacks such as lack of oxygen permeability and tendency to change the shape of the eye have limited the usage of PMMA contact lenses. In order to improve the permeability of oxygen, rigid gas-permeable (RGP) contact lenses were developed in the late 1970s. Materials used for RGP contact lenses are typically copolymers of methyl methacrylate (MMA) with a monomer that imparts high oxygen permeability, e.g., methacryloxypropyl tris(trimethylsiloxy silane) (TRIS), hexafluoroisopropyl methacrylate (HFIM), and 2,2,2-trifluoroethyl methacrylate (TFEMA). The incorporation of highly hydrophobic siloxane into the copolymer reduces the lens wettability, which leads to undesired increase of lipid deposition. Therefore, hydrophilic monomers, such as methacrylic acid (MAA), 2-hydroxyethyl methacrylate (HEMA), or N-vinyl-2-pyrrolidone (NVP), are commonly used as wetting agents in RGP lens formulation to compensate for reduction in wettability.

Soft contact lenses emerged in the 1960s when Otto Wichterle developed poly(2-hydroxyethyl methacrylate) (PHEMA) [14] and forever changed the contact lens industry. Generally, soft contact lenses are made from hydrogel, a cross-linked network capable of retaining a significant amount of water. The first PHEMA soft lens contained 40% water of hydration. Despite its improvement in wearer comfort over rigid lens, the low oxygen

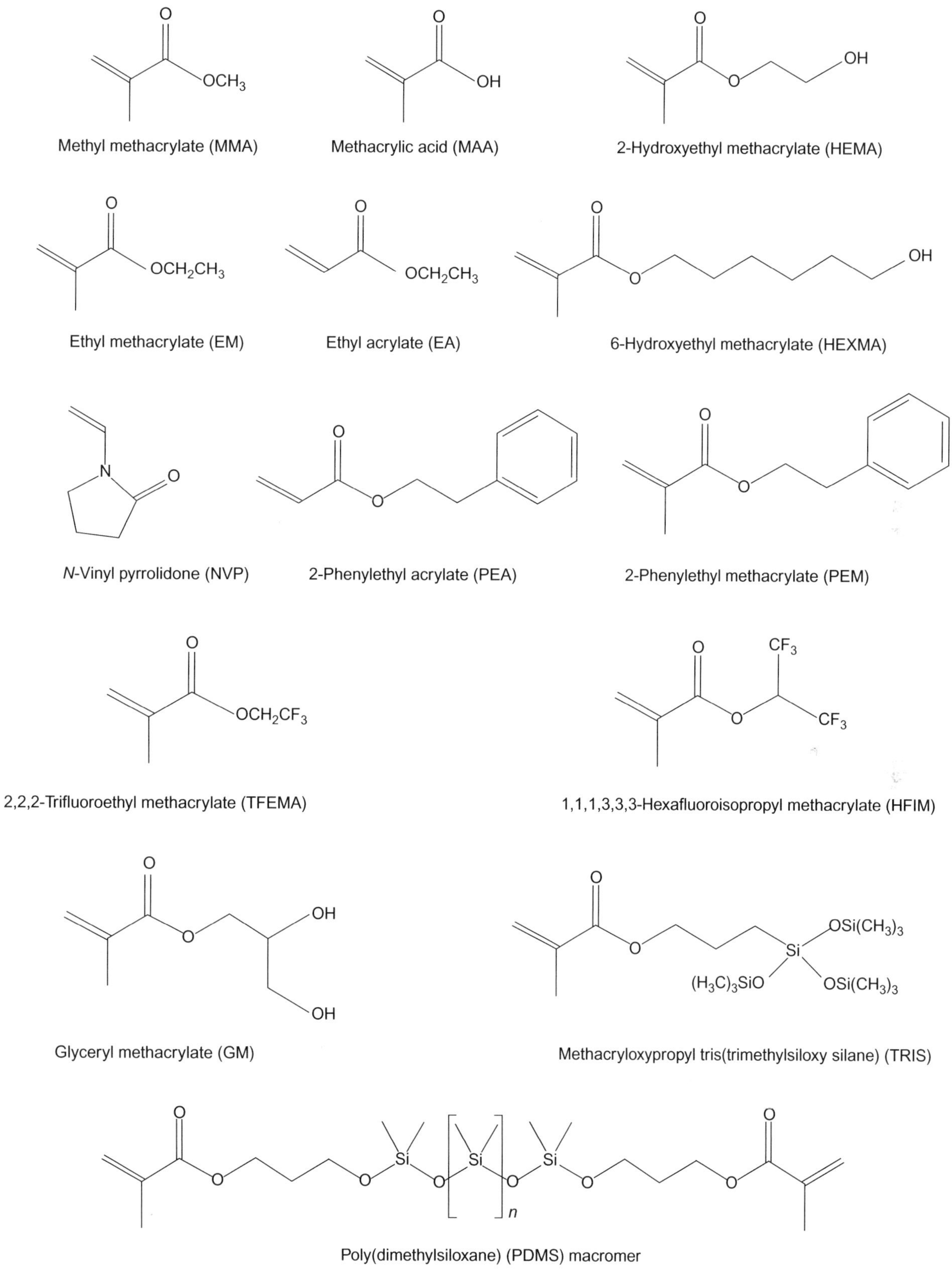

Figure 4.1 Chemical structures of common monomers used in contact lenses and intraocular lenses.

permeability of PHEMA was interfering with the normal corneal metabolism. Since the extent of hydration directly affects the permeability of oxygen, hydrogels with high water content ($>50\%$) have been developed by copolymerizing HEMA with highly hydrophilic monomers such as NVP, MAA, and glyceryl methacrylate (GMA). A drawback associated with increased hydrophilicity is the higher protein binding to the lens, which could cause discomfort and complications such as increased bacterial adhesion [15]. High water content hydrogels also tend to cause corneal desiccation. In the quest for high oxygen permeability, researchers have developed a new type of siloxane-containing hydrogels for soft contact lenses. It is well known that due to the bulkiness of the siloxane groups ($-Si(CH_3)_2-O-$) and the chain mobility, siloxane-containing materials typically have high diffusivity of oxygen. On the other hand, siloxane materials are highly hydrophobic and, therefore, prone to lipid deposition and are less comfortable with rubbery-like behavior. To offset these shortcomings, functionalized siloxane macromer (shown in Figure 4.1) was copolymerized with hydrophilic monomers (e.g., NVP and HEMA) into hydrogels that offer sufficiently high oxygen transmission required by the cornea as well as the softness for comfortable extended wear. Currently, commercialized siloxane hydrogel contact lenses include Focus® Night & Day™ (lotrafilcon A by CIBA Vision Corp.) and PureVision™ (balafilcon A by Bausch and Lomb). It is worth noting that the presence of siloxane moieties on the surface of these hydrogels demands further treatments in order for the lens to be tolerated on the eye. Examples of surface treatment for siloxane hydrogels include radiofrequency glow discharge (RFGD) [16] and graft polymerization of hydrophilic monomers (e.g., acrylamide [17]) on the lens surface to improve surface hydrophilicity.

4.2.2 Polymeric Intraocular Lens

IOLs are commonly used to replace natural lenses and provide clear optical imaging for patients undergoing cataract surgery. IOL is a major area in ocular biomaterials research for its critical role in treating cataract-induced blindness, which was predicted to reach 40 million cases by the year 2020 [18]. IOL also holds a special place in the biomaterials history, where its invention was originated from Sir Harold Ridley's accurate observations of the biological reaction to accidentally implanted pieces of canopy in a World War II pilot's eyes. Since the canopy material, PMMA, was well tolerated by the eye, Ridley was inspired to use the material to invent the first biocompatible IOL, and it is well recognized as a pioneering breakthrough in biomaterial science. The key material requirements for IOLs include the optical property, i.e., able to maintain a clear path for optical imaging and the long-term biocompatibility as the implant is intended to reside in the eye permanently. PMMA dominated the IOL market for 40 years before other materials emerged. Despite its excellent optical properties and relative tolerance by the eye, PMMA still induces damage to the tissues around the IOL implant. Of primary concern are the injury of the corneal endothelium associated with the lens rigidity, and the accumulation of inflammatory cells to the IOL surface, which can lead to complications such as iris adhesion to the IOL, uveitis, and loss of vision [19]. Such issues have led to newer IOL designs and materials selection. In contrast to the original hard and bulky PMMA IOL, common IOLs nowadays are featured as soft and foldable.

The most widely used foldable IOL, AcrySof®, is fabricated from a copolymer of phenylethyl acrylate and phenylethyl methacrylate with a cross-linking reagent and a UV-absorbing chromophore. Its improved optical property, i.e., higher refractive index ($n = 1.55$) compared to PMMA ($n = 1.49$), allows a thinner IOL configuration. The mechanical characteristic of the copolymer results in a slow and better controlled unfolding of the IOL, which contributes to the significant reduction in posterior capsular opacification (PCO). Other materials used in foldable IOL fabrication include silicone elastomers, hydrophilic acrylics (with water content higher than 18%), and collagen copolymers (Table 4.1). Although hydrophilic acrylic IOLs have shown good uveal biocompatibility due to the reduction in protein adsorption and macrophage adhesion, they tend to present higher rate of PCO and cause anterior capsular opacification, which has reduced their application in the market [22–25].

4.2.3 Polymeric Artificial Cornea

The cornea is a transparent tissue situated at the front of the eye. It is the main element in the ocular

Table 4.1 Examples of Biomaterials for IOLs

Manufacturer	Lens Type	Material	Refractive Index
Advanced Medical Optics	Rigid	PMMA	1.49
ALCON	ACRYSOF® foldable	PEA/PEMA	1.55
Bausch & Lomb	Hydroview® foldable	HEMA/HEXMA	1.47
Calhoun Vision	Multifocal foldable	PDMS	1.41
STAAR Surgical	Collamer® foldable	Collagen/HEMA	1.45

(Modified from Lloyd and Patel [20,21])

optical system, and plays various roles from refracting light onto the retina to form an image, to acting as a protective barrier for the delicate internal eye tissue. Damage to the cornea can result in loss of vision, which accounts for the second most common cause of blindness worldwide after cataract [26]. The most widely accepted treatment of corneal blindness is transplantation of human donor corneas. However, limitations in the availability of donor cornea tissues have called for design and development of artificial cornea substitutes. Artificial corneas, also known as keratoprostheses, come in a variety of forms, from fully synthetic to tissue-engineered. The focus of this discussion will be on polymer-based synthetic keratoprostheses. Several excellent comprehensive reviews on artificial corneas are available for further reading [27–29].

The cornea tissue is complex, avascular, highly innervated, and immune privileged. It is arranged in three major cellular layers: an outer stratified epithelium, an inner single-layered endothelium, and sandwiched in between a stromal compartment, which is responsible for the optical properties of the cornea. Although it is challenging to duplicate the complex structure of the natural cornea, it is possible to construct an artificial cornea that can simulate the physical features of the natural cornea and restore some functional level of vision. An ideal artificial cornea should meet the following specific requirements: (1) transparent with a smooth anterior surface of appropriate curvature, (2) suitable refractive index, (3) flexible and sufficient tensile strength for surgical handling, (4) ability to heal with the host cornea, (5) ability to promote and sustain the growth of epithelium over the anterior surface of the artificial cornea, (6) ability to avoid the formation of a retrocorneal fibroblastic membrane, and (7) biocompatibility [30]. Early generations of artificial corneas were made from a number of different hydrophobic polymers, such as PMMA, nylon, poly(tetrafluoroethylene) (PTFE), polyurethane (PU), and poly(ethylene terephthalate) (Dacron®) [20,31–33]. The design evolved from one material button-like full piece to the more widely used "core-and-skirt" configuration, where the core is made from transparent material with good optical properties and the skirt is made either from the same or different material to ensure host integration. Among these polymers, PMMA is arguably the most extensively used due to its remarkable optical properties, as discussed in the above IOL section. Even though the application of PMMA in artificial cornea continues, the associated complications such as retroprosthetic membrane formation, glaucoma, extrusion, endophthalmitis, and rejection [34–36] have led to the development of soft, hydrogel-based artificial corneas. Most of the research has been directed toward HEMA-based hydrogel. An interesting observation with HEMA is that when the monomer is polymerized with the presence of 40% or less of water, it forms a homogeneous transparent hydrogel; when the water content is higher, phase separation occurs during polymerization, and the resulting hydrogel is heterogeneous and opaque. Taking advantage of such characteristics, the first "core-and-skirt" hydrogel-based artificial cornea was created using HEMA, and the device is commercially known as AlphaCor [37]. The core is the transparent, lower water content PHEMA, and the skirt is the phase-separated, macroporous opaque PHEMA. Even though PHEMA is considered a hydrophilic polymer, its water content remains far below the water level found in the natural cornea (78%). Such high water content is essential for the stability and survival of the epithelium as it facilitates nutrient diffusion. In order to increase the water content of the artificial cornea, various strategies have been explored. Examples include copolymerization of HEMA with an ionic acrylate MAA [38], and hydrogels made from homopolymer of poly(vinyl alcohol) (PVA), which can contain over 80% water at equilibrium [39,40]. Several groups have also reported making biomimetic hydrogels for artificial corneas. As the extracellular matrix of the cornea is dominated by type I collagen, it has been used in the preparation of a copolymeric hydrogel based on N-isopropylacrylamide (NIPAAm), acrylic acid, N-acryloxysuccinimide, and collagen [41]. The engineered hydrogel is essentially a network comprising of collagen cross-linked to the copolymers of acrylic acid and NIPAAm using the succinimide pendant groups. This material has demonstrated the biomechanical properties and the required optical clarity to be used for corneal transplantation. *In vivo* animal studies have shown successful regeneration of host corneal epithelium, stroma, and nerves [41]. Clinical trials are currently underway to evaluate this material for therapeutic use in humans.

Interpenetrating polymer networks (IPNs) have also been used for artificial cornea applications. IPN represents a mixture of polymer networks where one polymer is cross-linked in the presence of another polymer network to form a mesh of two different polymers. The major advantage with IPN is that it combines the beneficial properties of both polymers into the final material. Early application of IPNs in artificial corneas was at the connection between the optical core and the peripheral skirt, where an interdiffusion zone of IPN provides a permanent and reliable union of the PHEMA sponge skirt with the PHEMA core [42]. More recent efforts focus on incorporating IPNs in the entire artificial cornea construct. One design is based on IPNs of poly(dimethylsiloxane) (PDMS) and PNIPAAm [43], where the mechanical strength, transparency, and oxygen permeability of PDMS is combined with the hydrophilicity and nutrient permeability of PNIPAAm to form a functional artificial cornea. Another example is IPN of a neutral cross-linked poly(ethylene glycol) (PEG) and a charged, loosely cross-linked polyacrylic acid (PAA) [44,45]. Such IPN has displayed optical transparency with good mechanical properties and glucose diffusion coefficients comparable to that of the natural cornea [46]. Although most of the artificial corneas have shown satisfying biocompatibility in animal models, it is critical to ensure that the materials are nontoxic, nonimmunogenic, and nonmutagenic, and do not result in corneal opacification.

4.3 Polymeric Biomaterials in Orthopedics

Traditionally, orthopedic biomaterials are mainly metallic, largely due to the close property resemblance to that of bone tissue such as high strength, hardness, and fracture toughness. Polymers have also been used in orthopedics over the years, and they are receiving increasing interest for bone tissue engineering. Historically, the use of polymers in orthopedics for the most part is reserved for those capable of performing well for fixation of structural devices and under cyclic load-bearing conditions such as in knee and hip arthroplasty. Despite hundreds of orthopedics applications available in the market, they are dominated by only a few types of polymers, including ultrahigh-molecular-weight polyethylene (UHMWPE) and PMMA.

4.3.1 Polyethylene

UHMWPE is a linear polyethylene with molecular weight usually between 2 and 6 million. The fracture toughness, low friction coefficient, high impact strength, and low density of UHMWPE have made it a popular choice as the articulating surfaces of joint replacements, such as hip, knee, ankle, and shoulder. Although UHMWPE possesses numerous attractive bulk and surface properties, these properties can be compromised by the presence of long-term radicals in the bulk resulting from the ionizing radiation employed in the sterilization process [47]. These radicals can interact with oxygen, leading to the generation of oxygen containing functional groups and deterioration of the surface and bulk properties, particularly the rate of production of particles during the wear process. An overproduction of wear debris has been linked to the inflammatory reaction in the tissues adjacent to the implant. This adverse tissue response will lead to granulomatous lesions, osteolysis, bone resorption, and implant failure [48]. In an effort to overcome the oxidation, a number of additives, such as antioxidant α-tocoferol and vitamin C, are currently used to retard oxidation and enhance surface properties [49]. UHMWPE has been considered the weak link in any total joint replacement because of the wear issue. To improve wear resistance, highly cross-linked UHMWPE has been produced and used in joint replacement. Cross-linking is achieved by irradiating UHMWPE with electron beam or gamma irradiation, followed by a melting step to eliminate the free radicals produced during irradiation. Currently, there is a debate on cross-linking and the clinical performance of UHMWPE. Those in favor have shown evidence of the efficacy of highly cross-linked UHMWPE in reducing the wear in total joint arthroplasties and the associated peri-prosthetic osteolysis [50]. The opposition states that improvement of wear resistance by cross-linking is at the expense of reduction in the static mechanical properties, such as tensile and yield strength as well as fatigue crack propagation resistance, which could affect the implant longevity, especially in total knee arthroplasty [51]. Complete data regarding the ultimate long-term performance of highly cross-linked UHMWPE will help settle the scientific debate.

4.3.2 Polyacrylates

Application of PMMA as fixative for bone was first demonstrated by Charnley [52]. The PMMA bone cement is composed of the liquid monomer MMA, a partially polymerized PMMA powder, an initiator (commonly used dibenzoyl peroxide), an activator (N,N-dimethyl-p-toluidine), a radiopacifier (visible to X-rays) such as barium sulfate or zirconium oxide, and a copolymer to influence the mixing and handling of the cement [53]. In some cases, an antibiotic (e.g., gentamicin) is included in the formulation to minimize infection during implantation. The polymerization is initiated by the interaction between the activator and the initiator, yielding a free radical that reacts with the monomer. The solidified polymer is able to secure a firm fixation of the prosthesis in the bones. Although acrylic bone cements are widely used in orthopedics, several drawbacks are related with their use. The residual monomer could leak into the body and cause fat embolism [54]. The exothermic nature of the polymerization process can be a potential cause for necrosis of the surrounding tissue. The most critical drawback is aseptic loosening, i.e., loosening of the implant within the cement. The cause of aseptic loosening could be mechanical and/or biochemical. Mechanically, cyclic loading of the implant could lead to fatigue fracture of the cement [55]. Biochemically, wear debris of the polyethylene component could migrate to the bone–cement interface and trigger inflammatory response, leading to osteolysis and weakening the implant interface [56]. In order to improve upon PMMA fixation, a possible strategy is to avoid cement fracture by increasing the mechanical strength of the cement. Researchers have developed bone cement with higher bonding strength and compressive modulus than conventional PMMA, using a bisphenol-A-glycidyl dimethacrylate (Bis-GMA)-based resin impregnated with bioactive glass ceramics [57,58]. Another approach takes advantage of composites by reinforcing PMMA with hydroxyapatite (HA) [59] and bioactive glass [60], which combines strength and elasticity with bioactivity.

The other acrylate bone cement is based on polyethylmethacrylate (PEMA) and n-butylmethacrylate (n-BMA) monomer [61]. Comparing to PMMA cement, less heat is produced during polymerization of the PEMA-n-BMA cement, and the polymer has a relatively low modulus and high ductility to reduce the issue of fracture. The biocompatibility of the PEMA-n-BMA cement has been excellent [62]. But these bone cements have been found to be susceptible to creep. To improve creep resistance, bioactive HA particles were incorporated [63]. Although HA improved bioactivity and creep behavior of the cement, the cement failed at lower number of cycles.

4.3.3 Natural Polymers

Natural polymers are finding increasing applications in the area of bone replacement and hard tissue augmentation. Ideally, materials used for such purpose should be biocompatible; able to mimic the three-dimensional characteristics, physical, and mechanical nature of the bone and hard tissue; able to support appropriate cellular functions; and able to be replaced gradually by the regenerating new tissue. A variety of natural polymers have been used, including extracellular matrix proteins such as collagen [64]; polysaccharides such as chitosan [65], alginate [66], starch [67], and cellulose [68]; as well as glycosaminoglycans such as hyaluronic acid [69]. Some of the natural polymers can provide a template for biomimetic apatite formation, which is highly desirable to induce rapid bone colonization. Recent studies by Hutchens *et al.* [70] revealed the formation and characterization of bacterial cellulose/hydroxyapatite composites with the potential for bone replacement. Both degradable and nondegradable bacterial cellulose were used to form the composite. The hydroxyapatite present in the composite has ordered nanometer needle-like particles with nonstoichiometric composition similar to that observed in human bone. The combined bioactivity and biocompatibility substantiates the potential of this composite for orthopedic application.

4.4 Polymeric Biomaterials in Cardiovascular Diseases

Biomaterials have played a vital role in the treatment of cardiovascular diseases; examples of applications include heart valve prostheses, vascular grafts, stents, indwelling catheters, ventricular assist devices, total implantable artificial hearts, pacemakers, automatic internal cardioverter defibrillators, intra-aortic balloon pumps, etc. A key requirement for materials in cardiovascular applications, particularly blood-contacting devices, is blood compatibility, i.e., nonthrombogenic. Additional requirements include mechanical and surface properties that are application-specific. Surveying the field of polymers used in cardiovascular applications reveals that PUs, polyethylene terephthalate (PET), and expanded PTFE (ePTFE) are the most commonly used. This section will review each of the three polymers followed by a brief introduction of other emerging polymers for use in the cardiovascular area.

4.4.1 Polyurethanes

PUs are among the most commonly selected biomedical polymers for blood-contacting medical devices. They can be found in hemodialysis bloodlines, catheters, stents, insulation for pacemaker leads, heart valves, vascular grafts and patches, left ventricular assist devices (LVADs), etc. PUs are characterized as segmented block copolymers with a wide range of mechanical and blood contact properties, simply by varying the type and/or molecular weight of the soft segment and coupling agents.

The urethane linkage, $-NH-C(=O)-O-$, in biomedical PUs can be formed through a two-step process. The initial step is a reaction involving the end-capping of the macrodiol soft segments (e.g., polyether, polyester, polycarbonate, and polysiloxane) with diisocyanate to form a prepolymer. The second reaction is the coupling of the prepolymer with a low-molecular-weight chain extender—generally a diol or a diamine [71]. The hard segment usually refers to the combination of the chain extender and the diisocyanate components.

Due to the chemical incompatibility between the soft and hard segments, the morphology of PUs consists of hard segments aggregation to form domains that are dispersed in a matrix formed by the soft segments [72,73]. Such unique morphology is responsible for the exceptional mechanical properties and biocompatibility of the biomedical PUs. For example, depending on the relative molecular weights and amounts of the hard and soft segments, the obtained PU can be elastomeric or rigid. The mechanical properties of PU can also be tailored by changing the chemical nature of the chain extender. Generally, PUs prepared with aliphatic chain extender are softer than those with aromatic chain extender. Biocompatibility of PU is also closely related to the chemical nature of the chain extender and the soft segment. Early studies by Lyman *et al.* [74] showed that changes in the molecular weight of the polypropylene soft segments affected protein adsorption. Lysine diisocyanate and hexamethylene diisocyanate are preferred over aromatic diisocyanates in the synthesis of biodegradable PUs, partly because of the putative carcinogenic nature of aromatic diisocyanates [75]. Recent studies have reported using natural polymers, such as chitin [76] and chitosan [77] as chain extender to improve the biocompatibility of PUs.

Biostability has been and continues to be a main research focus of PUs. Depending on the intended medical applications, the desired biostability of PUs varies. For example, PUs used as a pacemaker lead covering should have superior long-term stability, whereas PUs used as a scaffold to build engineered tissue construct for the replacement of diseased cardiovascular tissues should be biodegradable. The challenge to maintain long-term *in vivo* biostability of PUs lies in the fact that biodegradation of PUs is a complicated and multifactor-mediated process. Mechanisms responsible for PU biodegradation include (1) hydrolysis,

(2) oxidative degradation, metal or cell catalyzed, (3) enzymatic degradation, (4) surface cracking, (5) environmental stress cracking, and (6) calcification [75]. It is well known that PUs containing polyester soft segments have poor hydrolytic stability, and PUs with polyether soft segments are prone to oxidative degradation. Guided with valuable information collected from extensive investigation of molecular pathways leading to the biodegradation of PUs, more bioresistant PUs have been designed over the years. These strategies include using polycarbonate macrodiols [78,79], polyether macrodiols with larger hydrocarbon segments between ether groups [80], and siloxane-based macrodiols [81–83]. On the other end of the spectrum, bioresorbable PUs are attracting increasing attention as elastomeric tissue engineering scaffolds. For this class of PUs, soft segments such as polylactide or polyglycolide, polycaprolactone, and polyethylene oxide are most commonly used [84]. Furthermore, degradation is engineered into the hard segments. Enzyme-sensitive linkages have been incorporated into the hard segment, leading to specific enzymatic degradation in contrast to nonspecific hydrolytic degradation [85–87]. Another interesting addition to the hard segments is bioactive molecule such as antimicrobial drug [88]. Polymer degradation will thus lead to free drug release, making this class of PUs very attractive for biomedical applications.

4.4.2 Polyethylene Terephthalate

PET is a member of the engineering polyester family. It is a semicrystalline polymer with industrial applications as synthetic fibers and beverage and food containers. In the medical field, PET is widely used as prosthetic vascular grafts, sutures, and wound dressings in either fiber or fabric form (commercially known as Dacron®). Despite the presence of hydrolytically cleavable ester linkage, PET is relatively stable *in vivo* largely due to the high crystallinity and hydrophobicity. It is one of the two standard biomaterials of prosthetic vascular grafts used clinically. It is widely used for larger vessel (diameter >6 mm) applications. PET for vascular applications can be prepared either woven or knitted, which will determine the porosity and mechanical property of the graft. Generally, a woven finish has less porosity than a knitted graft, therefore, reducing the chance of transmural blood extravasation. Dacron® vascular graft is strong and stiff, much less compliant than natural arteries [89]. Such compliance mismatch has been considered the cause of patency loss of the graft over a long time frame (>6 months) [90]. The other major complication related to the PET graft is its thrombogenicity. When the graft comes in contact with blood, plasma protein is adsorbed to the luminal and capsular surfaces, leading to thrombus formation and inflammatory response. Various strategies have been explored to make the graft surface thrombo-resistant, including passivating the surface with albumin [91], coating with fluoropolymer [92], coating with hydrophilic polymer [93], covalent or ionic binding of the anticoagulant heparin–albumin [94–96], covalent linkage of antithrombotic agent thrombomodulin [97], etc. Although some improvement has been reported in terms of acute thrombosis, there is still a long way to go to achieve satisfying long-term functionality of PET-based vascular grafts.

4.4.3 Expanded PTFE

ePTFE, commercially also known as Gore-Tex®, is one of the two standard biomaterials of prosthetic vascular grafts used clinically. Besides vascular uses, ePTFE is also used as patches for soft tissue regeneration, such as hernia repair, and surgical sutures. It is produced by a series of extrusion, stretching, and heating processes to create a microporous material with pore size ranging from 30 to about 100 μm. Similar to PET, ePTFE is highly crystalline, hydrophobic, and highly stable. It has an extremely low coefficient of friction, making it easy for handling. Its tensile strength and tensile modulus are lower than those of PET. Even though the compliance of ePTFE grafts is relatively lower than that of PET grafts, it is still too high compared to natural arteries. Generally, ePTFE is the choice over PET to bypass smaller vessels. However, it still faces a patency issue. Femoropopliteal reconstruction using ePTFE has a 5-year patency rate of 40–50%, compared to the 70–80% achieved by using autogenous vein grafts [98]. Similar to PET, the cause of low patency is the thrombogenicity of the material. It has been reported that the graft fails to develop a full coverage of endothelial cells on the lumen side of the graft [99,100]. To address this issue, one approach is to increase the porosity to promote tissue ingrowth. But it requires a careful balance to prevent leakage of blood elements as mentioned earlier. Other approaches focus on reducing surface thrombogenicity, including carbon coating to increase surface electronegativity [101], attachment of anticoagulant or antithrombotic agents [102,103], and impregnation with fibrin glue to deliver growth factors that can promote endothelialization [104,105]. The actual benefits of these treatments are yet to be determined through longer-term *in vivo* investigations.

The challenge posed by small diameter vascular repair has spurred research for alternative biomaterials that would match or surpass the autograft. A notable effort is to build a tissue-engineered graft *ex vivo* using a synthetic biodegradable scaffold. Conceptually, such graft will have mechanical properties closely mimicking those of the native tissues without the concern of chronic inflammatory responses commonly induced by the presence of synthetic materials. Till date, a wide variety of biodegradable polymers have been used to build such constructs, including poly(α-hydroxyesters); poly(glycolic acid) (PGA); poly(lactic acid) (PLA); and their copolymers poly(lactic-*co*-glycolic acid) (PLGA), polycaprolactone, polyanhydride, polyhydroxyalkanoate, and polypeptide. Several excellent reviews are available discussing the current status of materials as scaffolding for vascular tissue engineering [106–108].

The other cardiovascular application in which polymers are poised to make a significant impact is biodegradable stents. Current stents are mainly made of metallic materials, such as stainless steel, cobalt–chromium, or Nitinol. However, long-term complications associated with metal stents have prompted research of fully degradable replacement. Several key requirements have to be satisfied by the polymeric stent, with the top two being mechanical properties and degradation characteristics. In terms of degradation, the products of degradation should be biocompatible, and the degradation process should not compromise the structural integrity of the device up to 6 months [90]. As for mechanical properties, the polymer should withstand the deployment and the blood vessel contractions. Both requirements are challenging, but with a good appreciation of the underlying biology and the versatility of polymer structure–property relationship, newer materials are likely to emerge in the near future. For example, researchers are imparting degradation and shape memory capabilities into polymers that can self-expand and degrade over time [109,110].

4.5 Polymeric Biomaterials for Wound Closure

Surgical wounds can be closed by various means, including sutures [111], adhesives [111], tapes [111], staples [111], and laser tissue welding [112]. Among these methods, sutures are the most frequently used. The sutures are sterile filaments used to approximate and maintain tissue until the healing has provided the wound with appropriate strength to withstand mechanical stresses. Sutures can be classified based on the origin of the materials as natural or synthetic; performance of the materials as absorbable or nonabsorbable; and physical configurations as monofilament, multifilament, braided, or twisted. In general, polymers selected for sutures should elicit minimal adverse biological response in addition to having fiber-forming rheological properties. The sutures must have minimum tissue drag, good strength retention, and knot security. To improve the lubricity and reduce tissue drag, coatings such as tetrafluoroethylene and silicones are normally applied to the suture. The following sections will discuss some of the common nonabsorbable and absorbable polymeric sutures currently commercially available.

In general, nonabsorbable sutures can retain their tensile strength longer than 2 months [113]. The synthetic polymers used to make nondegradable sutures include polypropylene (PP), polyamides, polyesters such as PET and polybutylene terephthalate (PBT), and polyether–ester based on poly(tetramethylene glycol), 1,4-butanediol, and dimethyl terephthalic acid [114]. The base polymer and filament configurations for common nonabsorbable sutures are summarized in Table 4.2.

The PP monofilament sutures are made from isotactic polypropylene [115]. During preparation, the PP monofilament is subjected to a series of post-spinning operations including annealing, designed to increase crystallinity [116]. Although PP sutures are highly resistant to hydrolytic degradation, it can undergo thermo-oxidative degradation [117]. PP sutures are usually sterilized by ethylene oxide or autoclave due to their susceptibility to ionizing radiation such as γ-radiation from cobalt-60 source

Table 4.2 A List of Commercially Available Nonabsorbable Suture Materials

Generic Name	Polymer	Configuration	Trade Name
Polyamide	Nylon-6, nylon-6,6	Monofilament	Dermalon
		Multifilament, braided	Nurolon
		Multifilament, braided and silicone coating	
Polypropylene	PP	Monofilament	Prolene
		Monofilament	Surgipro
Polyethylene	Polyethylene	Monofilament	Dermalene
Polyester	PET	Braided	Dacron
		Braided with silicone coating	Ti-Cron
		Braided with polybutylate coating	Ethibond
		Braided with PTFE coating	Polydek

that is normally used for radiation sterilization. In terms of performance, PP sutures cause one of the lowest tissue responses.

Polyamide sutures are commonly made out of nylon-6 and nylon-6,6. Nylon-6 is synthesized by ring-opening polymerization of caprolactam, while nylon-6,6 is prepared by condensation polymerization of adipic acid and hexamethylene diamine. These polyamide sutures are processed into monofilament, braided multifilament, and core−sheath configurations. The braided multifilament nylon sutures are often coated (e.g., silicone coating) to reduce tissue drag. The observed decrease in strength retention over time is associated with the susceptibility of the amide bond to hydrolytic degradation in the nylon structure. The tensile strength of nylon sutures decreases at a yearly rate of approximately 15−25% [118]. The tissue reaction to nylon sutures appears to be independent of configuration, with both braided and monofilament eliciting low reactivity.

The need to suture very delicate and complicated tissues have led to the development and use of sutures based on fluoropolymers such as PTFE and polyvinylidene fluoride (PVDF), and copolymers of PVDF and hexafluoropropylene (HFP) [119]. PTFE is a stable ($T_m = 327°C$) semicrystalline linear polymer. ePTFE sutures are highly crystalline microporous fibers prepared by wet spinning an aqueous mixture of PTFE powder and cellulose xanthate. The morphology of ePTFE fibers consists of nodules connected by thin crystalline fibers that control tensile strength. The mechanical properties, biological response, and handling can be directly correlated with the porosity of the PTFE fibers [120]. The bending stiffness of ePTFE sutures is low due to the microporous structure [121], but the porous structure also contributes to the decrease in strength. PVDF is also highly crystalline ($T_m = 175°C$). Sutures prepared from PVDF exhibit good creep resistance and tensile strength retention. Morphological studies have demonstrated high surface stability, i.e., no visible signs of bulk or surface fracture [122]. PVDF sutures are susceptible to thermo-oxidative degradation, but can be readily sterilized with γ-radiation. PVDF elicits moderate tissue and cell response—a behavior similar to PP sutures. Sutures derived from copolymers of PVDF and HFP were originally designed to combine the beneficial handling properties and biological response of PVDF and PP into one material. In addition, PVDF/HFP sutures were also designed to emulate the durability of polyester sutures. The tensile strength, size, biological response, and handling of the PVDF/HFP sutures can be tailored by manipulating the copolymer compositions. The major target areas for usage of PVDF/HFP sutures are wound closure during cardiovascular, neurological, and ophthalmic surgeries [119]. These PVDF/HFP sutures are normally used as uncoated monofilaments.

Among the most commonly used polyester-based nonabsorbable sutures are PET and PBT. In addition, there are polyester-based sutures made from copolymers of poly(tetramethylene ether terephthalate) and poly(tetramethylene terephthalate) called polyetheresters. PET is synthesized by condensation polymerization of ethylene glycol and terephthalic acid. PET is a polymer with a melting temperature of approximately 265°C. The thermal stability of PET enables melt spinning to form monofilament fibers with variable profiles. During processing, the fibers are subjected to hot drawing that enhances molecular orientation, crystallinity, and tensile strength. The PET sutures are commercially available as coated or uncoated monofilament or braided multifilament configurations. The surface treatments of PET sutures include coatings of PTFE and silicone. PET sutures are very stable in the biological environment with no evidence of hydrolytic degradation. The strength retention of PET sutures remains for an extended period of time. The tissue response to PET sutures is dependent on the configuration with braided multifilament and monofilament having moderate and low tissue reactivity, respectively. Compared to PET, PBT sutures are generally less brittle and stiff, due to the longer aliphatic segment in the polymer structure. Polybutester sutures are obtained from block copolymers of PBT and poly(tetramethylene ether) glycol terephthalate (PTMG). In the copolymer, the PBT is the hard segment and PTMG is the flexible segment. Chemical incompatibility between the hard PBT and soft PTMG blocks renders these copolymers elastomeric. Such unique mechanical behavior makes the polybutester sutures ideal for wounds prone to edema formation.

The synthetic absorbable sutures are made from polymers capable of degradation in the biological environment without adverse effects. One overall advantage of absorbable sutures is the elimination of clinical visits for their removal. These sutures are either homopolymers or copolymers based on degradable polymeric units such as polyglycolic acid, polylactic acid, or poly-p-dioxanone.

Polyglycolic acid (PGA) can be synthesized by condensation or ring-opening polymerization. Sutures based on PGA were the first absorbable sutures made [123]. PGA sutures are commercially available coated or uncoated in a braided configuration. Glycolide has been copolymerized with lactic acid, trimethylene carbonate, and ε-caprolactone [119]. Glycolic acid was copolymerized with L- or DL-lactic acid to form random copolymer. The performance of the glycolide-L-lactide sutures is dependent on composition. The initial tensile strength and retention through the healing process of the glycolide-L-lactide sutured wound is directly dependent on the concentration of the crystallizable glycolide monomers [124]. Copolymers based on the DL-lactide do not exhibit the same composition dependence as observed for the L-lactide copolymers [119]. Glycolide has been copolymerized with trimethylene carbonate to form a triblock copolymer where the middle block is a random copolymer of glycolide and trimethylene carbonate and the terminal blocks based on glycolide. These sutures are available as uncoated monofilaments. The copolymerization of glycolide and ε-caprolactone leads to formation of segmented copolymers. In these copolymers, the glycolide and ε-caprolactone form the soft and hard segments, respectively.

Poly-p-dioxanone (PDS) is synthesized by ring-opening polymerization of 1,4-dioxanone-2,5-dione. The monofilament sutures are produced by melt spinning. The fibers are subjected to a drawing process to improve tensile strength and performance. Recently, attempts have been made to copolymerize PDS with PGA and PLLA to produce sutures with different properties [125].

Current research focus in wound closure suture is to incorporate extra functionality to the suture besides closing the wound. These efforts include to control wound infection by developing antimicrobial sutures, and to accelerate the wound healing process by using bioactive material such as chitin, or to deliver therapeutics that can impact the wound healing response.

4.6 Polymeric Biomaterials in Extracorporeal Artificial Organs

Extracorporeal artificial organs provide mass-transfer operations to support failing or impaired organ systems [126]. Common examples include kidney substitute, hemodialysis, cardiopulmonary bypass (CPB), apheresis therapy, peritoneal dialysis, lung substitute and assist, and plasma separation. A critical component involved in the extracorporeal artificial organ is the membrane that serves to separate the undesired substance from the blood or plasma. Ideally, materials used as the membrane in these particular applications should have appropriate cellular and molecular permeability, as well as blood compatibility (i.e., hemocompatibility). Over the years, both natural and synthetic polymers have been used as membrane materials.

The most widely used natural membrane is cellulosic. Taking hemodialysis as an example, early applications of cellulose membrane in the dialyzer used regenerated cellulose, i.e., unsubstituted with rich hydroxyl groups along the repeating saccharide units. Studies have found that regenerated cellulose has poor hemocompatibility. It activates the complement system, which leads to inflammation and other serious immune responses. The complement activation has been attributed to the high concentration of hydroxyl groups on the membrane rendering it nucleophilic and susceptible to protein deposition, particularly C3b. Such observation spurred later research of using substituted cellulose for dialysis membrane, examples include cellulose acetate and cellulose triacetate, where in both cases a fraction of the hydroxyl groups are replaced with acetate functionality. These modified cellulose materials greatly limit complement activation by eliminating the active surface sites for complement protein interaction. Besides chemically blocking complement interaction, approaches using steric hindrance effect have also been explored. A bulky chemical group such as benzyl substitution group or tertiary amine group has been used to replace the hydroxyl group to sterically minimize the complement protein interaction with the membrane [127,128].

Current dialysis membranes are mostly made from synthetic polymers, including polysulfone, polyethersulfone, polyacrylonitrile, PMMA, polyamide, and polypropylene hollow fibers. Compared with natural cellulosic membrane, synthetic membranes are less prone to complement activation. The reason behind the improved complement compatibility is the diminished level of surface nucleophiles for C3b deposition. Furthermore, some of the synthetic membranes are rich in negative charges on the surface, which can absorb the activated cationic complement peptide (e.g., C5a) and minimize the subsequent cascade of inflammation. Synthetic membranes generally have significantly larger pore sizes and higher hydraulic permeability than cellulosic membranes [129]. Therefore, synthetic membranes are the choice for high-flux applications. The larger pore size also allows for removal of middle molecules with molecular weight between 500 and 2000 Da, which have been deemed bioactive and may have a potential biological impact [130]. The hydrophobic nature of most synthetic membranes contributes to the adsorptive capacity toward noxious compounds such as interleukin-1, tumor necrosis factor, interleukin-6, and β_2-microglobulin [131]. PMMA and polyacrylonitrile usually exhibit the most pronounced adsorption capacity. Regardless of their origin, the membranes have been used either in hollow-fiber design, which is most common, or as sheet films in parallel-plate design.

4.7 Polymeric Biomaterials for Nerve Regeneration

Repair of the damaged nerves presents enormous challenge due to the physiology complexity of the nervous system. Even though progress has been made over the past decades, it is still not possible to fully repair the damage so that lost functions of the nervous systems can be restored. The nervous system is generally classified into the central nervous system (CNS) and the peripheral nervous system (PNS). Various strategies have been explored for nerve repair in both the CNS and the PNS, including guidance conduits, scaffolds with cell transplantation, and delivery of therapeutics. This section will mainly focus on polymers used in the nerve guidance conduit approach.

It has been widely accepted that physical guidance of axons, the long processes extending from the neuron cell body and conducting electrical signals, plays a critical role in nerve repair. The nerve guidance conduit is designed to (1) direct the outgrowth of axons from the proximal nerve end bridging across the lesion, (2) provide a channel for the diffusion of biomolecules secreted by the injured nerve ends, and (3) reduce the scar tissue invasion to the regeneration zone [132]. To fulfill these functions, an ideal nerve guidance conduit should be semipermeable with oriented topographical features inside the conduit, supportive of electrical activity, able to deliver bioactive factors, and able to support cell adhesion and migration. The versatility of polymers makes them the top choice in engineering of nerve guidance conduits. Early research has used nondegradable synthetic polymers including silicone [133] and ePTFE [134]. Although silicone nerve guidance conduits have shown success in bridging gaps up to 10 mm, they have failed to support regeneration across larger defects. Therefore, effort has been shifted to develop biodegradable guidance conduits. The advantage of using a degradable material lies in the fact that long-term complications such as fibrotic reaction and nerve compression can be minimized. The degradation characteristics of the material should meet the following requirements: (1) the degradation profile should match with the axonal outgrowth profile, so that the guidance conduit will maintain sufficient mechanical support during the regeneration process and (2) the degradation product(s) should induce minimum to zero tissue reaction. A series of degradable polymers have been used, including biodegradable poly(esters) such as PGA [135], PLA [136], PLGA [137], and poly(caprolactones) [138]; polyphosphazenes [139]; polyurethanes [140]; and poly (3-hydroxybutyrate) [141].

Since the emergence of studies showing that electrical charge affects neurite extension *in vitro* [142,143] and improves nerve regeneration *in vivo* [144], polymers that can provide electrical stimulus have been included in guidance conduit development. These polymers include piezoelectric polymers such as PVDF and its copolymer [144], and conducting polymers like polypyrrole and its biologically modified derivatives [143,145]. Other electroactive polymers, such as polyaniline, may also provide support for nerve growth, as studies have shown encouraging results with cardiac myoblast cells [146].

Nerve guidance conduits can be hollow or filled with matrix to support axonal elongation. A popular filler choice is natural polymeric gel. Ideally, the gel should be soft with mechanical properties matching those of the nervous tissue, porous to allow axonal ingrowth, biodegradable, and biocompatible. A number of natural polymers have been investigated, including agarose [147], chitosan [148], methylcellulose [149], hyaluronic acid [150], alginate [151], fibrin gels [152], collagen [153], keratin [154], and self-assembling peptide scaffolds [155]. Agarose is a thermally reversible polysaccharide hydrogel. Its gelling temperature can be modified by changing the functional groups attached to the sugar residues. It can also be functionalized with various biological motifs, such as laminin-derived peptide sequences RGD, YIGSR, and IKVAV, to enhance neurite extension [156]. Fibrin is a natural wound-healing matrix that can be found in the early stages of regeneration. It is formed from the blood coagulation cascade to restore hemostasis and initiate tissue repair. Using fibrin gels as the filler can closely mimic the natural matrix formed in the guidance conduit bridging short nerve gaps, where a fibrin cable is usually formed from the exuding serum by the damaged blood vessels in the nerve ends [157]. Peptide sequences have also been cross-linked into the filling fibrin matrix to further induce neurite extension [158]. In addition to gel filler, longitudinal filaments, either synthetic or natural, have been used in the conduit to align the growing axons in the direction of regeneration. Materials used in filament preparation include polyamide, catgut, polydioxanone, polyglactin, poly(acrylonitrile-*co*-methylacrylate), collagen, PLA, PGA, etc. [159–162].

Recently, materials research on nerve guidance conduits has been taken to a new level, where the old paradigm of passive material has shifted to new bioactive material design. Chemical messengers such as neurotransmitters have been polymerized into the polymer backbone to impart neuroactivity for the resulting biomaterial [163]. The first example of this new class of polymer is dopamine polymerized with a diglycidyl ester to form a biodegradable material that has shown vigorous neurite outgrowth *in vitro* and good tissue compatibility *in vivo*. Another example of new bioactive polymer is polysialic acid and its hydrogel. Polysialic acid is a dynamically regulated posttranslational modification of the neural cell adhesion molecule [164]. It has been shown to significantly improve cell adhesion and viability *in vitro*. With the increasing understanding of the biology behind nerve regeneration, it is expected that more bioactive materials will be developed in the future to achieve timely functional recovery from nerve damage.

4.8 Conclusions and Future Outlook

Polymers have made significant impact on biomedical research and medical practice, and will continue to be the major workforce for biomaterials in the twenty-first century. The polymeric biomaterials and their applications presented here are only the tip of an iceberg. With the growing understanding of the biological response to existing biomaterials and a better grasp of human organ composition, function, biomechanics, and disease etiology, chemists and polymer scientists should continue working collaboratively with biologists, physicians, and engineers to develop tailor-made polymers for biomedical applications. In contrast to the old inert synthetic polymers, bioactive, biomimetic, and smart polymers will be at center stage. Furthermore, as the interactions of the biological system with polymers occur at the interface, surface-related research will continue to thrive, especially surface characterization and surface modification. One can be hopeful to foresee a better management of diseases with the help of a new generation of biomaterials, and a seamless integration of the biomaterials into the body.

References

[1] Reisch MS. Medical polymers renaissance. Chem Eng News 2007;85:14−7.

[2] Mann I. A brief review of contact lens work. Trans Ophthalmol Soc Aust 1939;1:107−15.

[3] Schillinger RJ, Shearer RV, Levy OR. Animal experiments with a new type of intraocular acrylic lens. Arch Ophthalmol 1958;59:423−34.

[4] Perry AC. Advances in enucleation. Ophthalmol Clin North Am 1991;4:173−82.

[5] Flowers CW, McDonnell PJ. Mechanical methods in refractive corneal surgery. Curr Opin Ophthalmol 1994;5:81−9.

[6] Migliori ME, Putterman AM. Silicone intubation for the treatment of congenital lacrimal duct obstruction − successful results removing the tubes after 6 weeks. Ophthalmology 1988;95:792−5.

[7] Molteno ACB. New implant for drainage in glaucoma, animal trial. Brit J Ophthalmol 1969;53:161−8.

[8] Liesegang TJ. Viscoelastic substances in ophthalmology. Surv Ophthalmol 1990;34:268−93.

[9] Bawa R, Nandu M. Physicochemical considerations in the development of an ocular polymeric drug delivery system. Biomaterials 1990;11:724−8.

[10] Schepens CL, Acosta F. Scleral implants: an historical perspective. Surv Ophthalmol 1991;35:447−53.

[11] Gilbert CE. Adhesives in retinal-detachment surgery. Br J Ophthalmol 1991;75:309−10.

[12] Jonas JB, Knorr HL, Rank RM, Budde WM. Intraocular pressure and silicone oil endotamponade. J Glaucoma 2001;10:102−8.

[13] Mc Glinchey SM, McCoy CP, Gorman SP, Jones DS. Key biological issues in contact lens development. Expert Rev Med Devices 2008;5:581−90.

[14] Wichterle O, Lim D. Hydrophilic gels for biological use. Nature 1960;185:117−8.

[15] Taylor RL, Willcox MD, Williams TJ, Verran J. Modulation of bacterial adhesion to hydrogel contact lenses by albumin. Optom Vis Sci 1998;75:23−9.

[16] Hesby RM, Haganma CR, Standford CM. Effects of radiofrequency glow discharge on impression material surface wettability. J Prosthet Dent 1997;77:414−22.

[17] Okada T, Ikada Y. Modification of silicone surface by graft polymerization of acrylamide with corona discharge. Makromol Chem 1991;192:1705−13.

[18] Brian G, Taylor H. Cataract blindness: challenges for the 21st century. Bull World Health Organ 2001;79(3):249−56.

[19] Obstbaum AS. Biologic relationship between poly-(methyl methacrylate) intraocular lenses and uveal tissue. J Cataract Refract Surg 1992;18:219−31.

[20] Lloyd AW, Faragher RGA, Denyer SP. Ocular biomaterials and implants. Biomaterials 2001;22:769−85.

[21] Patel AS. Intraocular lens implants: a scientific perspective. In: Ratner BD, Hoffman AS, Schoen FJ, Lemons JE, editors. Biomaterials science: an introduction to materials in medicine. San Diego, CA: Elsevier; 2004. Chapter 7.11.

[22] Koch MU, Kalicharan D, Vanderwant JJL. Lens epithelial cell formation related to hydrogel foldable intraocular lenses. J Cataract Refract Surg 1999;25:1637−40.

[23] Werner L. Biocompatibility of intraocular lens materials. Curr Opin Ophthalmol 2008;19:41−9.

[24] Werner L, Apple DJ, Kaskaloglu M, Pandey SK. Dense opacification of the optical component of a hydrophilic acrylic intraocular lens: a clinicopathologic analysis of 9 explanted lenses. J Cataract Refract Surg 2001;27:1485−92.

[25] Izak AM, Werner L, Pardey SK, Apple DJ. Calcification of modern foldable hydrogel

[25] intraocular lens designs. Eye 2003;17: 393–406.
[26] Whitcher JP, Srinivasan M, Upadhyay MP. Corneal blindness: a global perspective. Bull World Health Organ 2001;79:214–21.
[27] Myung D, Duhamel PE, Cochran JR, Noolandi J, Ta CN, Frank CW. Development of hydrogel-based keratoprostheses: a materials perspective. Biotechnol Prog 2008;24: 735–41.
[28] M. Griffith, W.B. Jackson, N. Lagali, K. Merrett, F. Li, P. Fagerholm, Artificial corneas: a regenerative medicine approach, Eye (in press).
[29] Sheardown H, Griffith M. Regenerative medicine in the cornea. In: Atala A, Lanza R, Thompson J, Nerem R, editors. Principles of regenerative medicine. Boston: Elsevier; 2008. p. 1060–71.
[30] Chirila TV, Hichs CR, Dalton PD, Vijayasekaran S, Lou X, Hong Y, et al. Artificial cornea. Prog Polym Sci 1998;23:447–73.
[31] Caldwell DR. The soft keratoprosthesis. Trans Am Ophthalmol Soc 1997;95:751–802.
[32] Pintucci S, Pintucci F, Caiazza S, Cecconi M. The Dacron felt colonizable keratoprosthesis, after 15 years. Eur J Ophthalmol 1996;6: 125–30.
[33] Barber JC. Keratoprosthesis: past and present. Int Ophthalmol Clin 1988;28:103–9.
[34] Yaghouti F, Dohlman CH. Innovations in keratoprosthesis, proved and unproved. Int Ophthalmol Clin 1999;39:27–36.
[35] Khan BE, Dudenhoefer J, Dohlman CH. Keratoprosthesis, an update. Curr Opin Ophthalmol 2001;12:282–7.
[36] Nouri M, Terada H, Alfonso EC, Foster CS, Durand ML, Dohlman CH. Endophthalmitis after keratoprosthesis, incidence, bacterial causes risk factors. Arch Ophthalmol 2001; 11:484–9.
[37] Chirila TV. An overview of the development of artificial corneas with porous skirts and the use of PHEMA for such an application. Biomaterials 2001;22:3311–7.
[38] Jacob JT, Wallace C, Bi J. Characterization of corneal epithelial cell adhesion on novel hydrogels. Invest Ophthalmol Vis Sci 2004; 45:U564.
[39] Peppas NA, Merrill EW. Development of semicrystalline poly(vinyl alcohol) hydrogels for biomedical applications. J Biomed Mater Res 1977;11:423–34.
[40] Miyashita H, Shimmura S, Kobayashi H, Taguchi T, Asano-Kato N, Uchino Y, et al. Collagen-immobilized poly(vinyl alcohol) as an artificial cornea scaffold that supports a stratified corneal epithelium. J Biomed Mater Res 2005;76B:56–63.
[41] Li F, Carlsson D, Lohmann C, Suuronen E, Vascotto S, Kobuch K, et al. Cellular and nerve regeneration within a biosynthetic extracellular matrix for corneal transplantation. Proc Natl Acad Sci USA 2003;100:15346–51.
[42] Chirila TV, Vijayasekaran S, Horne R, Chen YC, Dalton PD, Constable IJ, et al. Interpenetrating polymer network (IPN) as a permanent joint between the elements of a new type of artificial cornea. J Biomed Mater Res 1994;28:745–53.
[43] Liu L, Sheardown H. Sheardown Glucose permeable poly(dimethyl siloxane) poly (N-isopropylacrylamide) interpenetrating networks as ophthalmic biomaterials. Biomaterials 2005;26:233–44.
[44] Myung D, Koh W, Ko J, Hu Y, Carrasco M, Noolandi J, et al. Biomimetic strain hardening in interpenetrating polymer network hydrogels. Polymer 2007;48:5376–87.
[45] Myung D, Koh W, Bakri A, Zhang F, Marshall A, Ko J, et al. Design and fabrication of an artificial cornea based on a photo-lithographically patterned hydrogel construct. Biomed Microdev 2007;9:911–22.
[46] Myung D, Farooqui N, Waters D, Schaber S, Koh W, Carrasco M, et al. Glucose-permeable interpenetrating polymer network hydrogels for corneal implant applications, a pilot study. Curr Eye Res 2008;9:29–43.
[47] Premnath V, Harris WH, Jasty M, Merrill EW. Gamma sterilization of UHMWPE articular implants: an analysis of the oxidation problem. Biomaterials 1996;17:1741–53.
[48] Maloney WJ, Smith RL. Periprosthetic osteolysis in total hip arthroplasty: the role of particulate debris. J Bone Joint Surg 1995; 77A:1448–61.
[49] Tomita N, Kitakura T, Onmori N, Ikada Y, Aoyama E. Prevention of fatigue cracks in ultrahigh molecular weight polyethylene joint components by the addition of vitamin E. J Biomed Mater Res 1999;48:474–8.

[50] Jasty M, Rubash HE, Muratoglu O. Highly cross-linked polyethylene: the debate is over—in the affirmative. J Arthroplasty 2005; 20:55–8.

[51] Ries MD. Highly cross-linked polyethylene: the debate is over—in opposition. J Arthroplasty 2005;20:55–8.

[52] Charnley J. The bonding of prosthesis to bone by cement. J Bone Joint Surg 1964;46: 518–29.

[53] Navarro M, Michiardi A, Castano O, Planell JA. Biomaterials in orthopaedics. J R Soc Interface 2008;5:1137–58.

[54] Koessler MJ, Pitto RP. Fat and bone marrow embolism in total hip arthroplasty. Acta Orthop Belg 2001;67:97–109.

[55] Maloney WJ, Jasty M, Rosenberg A, Harris WH. Bone lysis in well-fixed cemented femoral components. J Bone Joint Surg Br 1990; 72:966–70.

[56] Freeman MA, Bradley GW, Revell PA. Observations upon the interface between bone and polymethylmethacrylate cement. J Bone Joint Surg Br 1982;64:489–93.

[57] Kawanabe K, Tamura J, Yamamuro T, Nakamura T, Kokubo T, Yoshihara S. New bioactive bone cement consisting of bis-GMA resin and bioactive glass powder. J Appl Biomater 1993;4:135–41.

[58] Tamura J, Kitsugi T, Iida H, Fujita H, Nakamura T, Kokubo T, et al. Bone bonding ability of bioactive cements. Clin Orthop 1997;343:183–91.

[59] Dalby MJ, Disilvio L, Harper EJ, Bonfield W. In vitro evaluation of a new polymethylmethacrylate cement reinforced with hydroxyapatite. J Mater Sci Mater Med 1999;10:793–6.

[60] Heikkila JT, Aho AJ, Kangasniemi I, Yli-Urpo A. Polymethylmethacrylate composites: disturbed bone formation at the surface of bioactive glass and hydroxyapatite. Biomaterials 1996;17:1755–60.

[61] Weightman B, Freeman MAR, Revell PA, Braden M, Alberkttsson BEJ, Carlson LV. The mechanical properties of cement and loosening of the femoral component of hip replacements. J Bone Joint Surg 1987;69B: 558–64.

[62] Revell P, Braden M, Weightman B, Freeman M. Experimental studies of the biological response to a new bone cement: II soft tissue reactions in the rat. Clin Mater 1992; 10:233–8.

[63] Harper EJ, Behiri JC, Bonfield W. Flexural and fatigue properties of a bone cement based upon polyethylmethacrylate and hydroxyapatite. J Mater Sci Mater Med 1995; 6:799–803.

[64] Uemura T, Dong J, Wang Y, Kojima H, Saito T, Iejima M, et al. Tateishi, transplantation of cultured bone cells using combinations of scaffolds and culture techniques. Biomaterials 2003;24:2277–86.

[65] Jiang T, Abdel-Fattah WI, Laurencin CT. In vitro evaluation of chitosan/poly(lactic acid-glycolic acid) sintered microsphere scaffolds for bone tissue engineering. Biomaterials 2006;27:4894–903.

[66] Fragonas E, Valente M, Pozzi-Mucelli M, Toffanin R, Rizzo R, Silvestri F, et al. Articular cartilage repair in rabbits by using suspensions of allogenic chondrocytes in alginate. Biomaterials 2000;21:795–801.

[67] Ongpipattanakul B, Nguyen T, Zioncheck TF, Wong R, Osaka G, DeGuzman L, et al. Development of tricalcium phosphate/amylopectin paste combined with recombinant human transforming growth factor beta 1 as a bone defect filler. J Biomed Mater Res 1997; 36:295–305.

[68] Dias GJ, Peplow PV, Teixeira F. Osseous regeneration in the presence of oxidized cellulose and collagen. J Mater Sci Mater Med 2003;14:739–45.

[69] Vögelin E, Jones NF, Huang JI, Brekke JH, Lieberrman JR. Healing of a critical-sized defect in the rat femur with use of a vascularized periosteal flap, a biodegradable matrix, and bone morphogenetic protein. J Bone Joint Surg Am 2005;87:1323–31.

[70] Hutchens SA, Benson RS, Evans BR, O'Neill HM, Rawn CJ. Biomimetic synthesis of calcium-deficient hydroxyapatite in a natural hydrogel. Biomaterials 2006;27:4661–70.

[71] Lyman DJ. Polyurethanes. 1. The solution polymerization of diisocyanates with ethylene glycol. J Polym Sci 1960;45:49–59.

[72] Blackwell J, Gardner KH. Structure of the hard segments in polyurethane elastomers. Polymer 1979;20:13–7.

[73] Blackwell J, Lee CD. Hard-segment polymorphism in MDI diol-based polyurethane

elastomers. J Polym Sci Polym Phys 1984; 22:759–72.

[74] Lyman DJ, Brash JL, Chaikin SW, Klein KG, Carini M. Effects of chemical structure and surface properties of synthetic polymers on coagulation of blood. 2. Protein and platelet interaction with polymer surfaces. Trans Am Soc Artif Int Org 1968;14:250–5.

[75] Santerre JP, Woodhouse K, Laroche G, Labow RS. Understanding the biodegradation of polyurethanes: from classical implants to tissue engineering materials. Biomaterials 2005;26:7457–70.

[76] Zia KM, Barikani M, Bhatti IA, Zuber M, Bhatti HN. Synthesis and characterization of novel, biodegradable, thermally stable chitin-based polyurethane elastomers. J Appl Polym Sci 2008;110:769–76.

[77] Xu D, Meng Z, Han M, Xi K, Jia X, Yu X, et al. Novel blood-compatible waterborne polyurethane using chitosan as an extender. J Appl Polym Sci 2008;109:240–6.

[78] Szycher M, Poirier VL, Dempsey DJ. Development of an aliphatic biomedical grade polyurethane elastomer. J Elastom Plast 1982; 15:81–95.

[79] Pinchuk L. A review of the biostability and carcinogenicity of polyurethanes in medicine and the new generation of "biostable" polyurethanes. J Biomater Sci Polym Ed 1994; 6:225–67.

[80] Gunatillake PA, Meijs GF, Rizzardo E, Chatelier RC, McCarthy SJ, Brandwood A, et al. Polyurethane elastomers based on a novel macrodiols and MDI: synthesis, mechanical properties and resistance to hydrolysis and oxidation. J Appl Polym Sci 1992;46:319–28.

[81] P.A. Gunatillake, G.F. Meijs, S.J. McCarthy, Polysiloxane-containing polyurethane elastomeric compositions, International Patent Application PCT/AU97/00619, 1996.

[82] Thakahara A, Hergenrother RW, Coury AJ, Cooper SL. Effect of soft segment chemistry on the biostability of segmented polyurethanes. I. In vitro oxidation. J Biomed Mater Res 1991;25:341–56.

[83] Thakahara A, Hergenrother RW, Coury AJ, Cooper SL. Effect of soft segment chemistry on the biostability of segmented polyurethanes. II. In vitro hydrolytic stability. J Biomed Mater Res 1992;26:801–18.

[84] Guelcher SA. Biodegradable polyurethanes: synthesis and applications in regenerative medicine. Tissue Eng PT B Rev 2008; 14:3–17.

[85] Skarja GA, Woodhouse KA. Structure-property relationships of degradable polyurethane elastomers containing an amino acid-based chain extender. J Appl Polym Sci 2000;75:1522–34.

[86] Skarja GA, Woodhouse KA. In vitro degradation and erosion of degradable, segments polyurethanes containing an amino acid-based chain extender. J Biomater Sci Polym Ed 2001;12:851–73.

[87] Guan J, Wagner WR. Synthesis, characterization and cytocompatibility of polyurethane-urea elastomers with designed elastase sensitivity. Biomacromolecules 2005;6: 2833–42.

[88] Woo GLY, Mittelman MW, Santerre JP. Synthesis and characterization of a novel biodegradable antimicrobial polymer. Biomaterials 2000;21:1235–46.

[89] Seifalian AM, Giudiceandrea A, Schmitz-Rixen T, Hamilton G. Noncompliance: the silent acceptance of a villain. In: Zille P, Greisler HP, editors. Tissue engineering of vascular prosthetic grafts. Georgetown: Landes; 1999. Chapter 2.

[90] Venkatraman S, Boey F, Lao LL. Implanted cardiovascular polymers: natural, synthetic and bio-inspired. Prog Polym Sci 2008;33: 853–74.

[91] Rumisek J, Wade C, Kaplan K, Okerberg C, Corley J, Barry M, et al. The influence of early surface thromboreactivity on long-term arterial graft patency. Surgery 1989;105: 654–61.

[92] Eiderg JP, Roder O, Stahl-Madsen M, Eldrup N, Qvarfordt P, Laursen A, et al. Fluropolymer-coated Dacron graft versus PTFE grafts for femorofemoral crossover by pass. Eur J Vasc Endovasc Surg 2006;32: 431–8.

[93] San Román J, Buján J, Bellón JM, Gallardo A, Escudero MC, Jorge E, et al. Experimental study of the antithrombogenic behavior of Dacron vascular grafts coated with hydrophilic acrylic copolymers bearing salicylic acid residues. J Biomed Mater Res 1996;32: 19–27.

[94] Kottke-Marchant K, Anderson J, Umemura Y, Marchant R. Effect of albumin coating on the in vitro blood compatibility of Dacron arterial prostheses. Biomaterials 1989;10:147−55.

[95] Merhi Y, Roy R, Guidoin R, Hebert J, Mourad W, Slimane SB. Cellular reactions to polyester arterial prostheses impregnated with cross-linked albumin: in vivo studies in mice. Biomaterials 1989;10:56−8.

[96] Parsson H, Jundzill W, Johansson K, Jonung T, Norgren L. Healing characteristics of polymer-coated or collagen-treated Dacron grafts: an experimental porcine study. Cardiovasc Surg 1994;2:242−8.

[97] Kishida A, Ueno Y, Fukudome N, Yashima E, Maruyama I, Akashi M. Immobilization of human thrombomodulin onto poly(ether urethane urea) for developing antithrombogenic blood-contacting materials. Biomaterials 1994;15:848−52.

[98] Veith FJ, Gupta SK, Ascer E, White-Flores S, Samson RH, Scher LA, et al. Bergan, six-year prospective multicenter randomized comparison of autologous saphenous vein and expanded polytetrafluoroethylene grafts in infringuinal arterial reconstruction. J Vasc Surg 1986;3:104−14.

[99] Clowes AW, Gown AM, Hanson SR, Reidy MA. Mechanisms of arterial graft failure. 1. Role of cellular proliferation in early healing of PTFE prostheses. Am J Pathol 1985;118:43−54.

[100] Bellon JM, Bujan J, Contreras LA, Hernando A, Jurado F. Similarity in behavior of polytetrafluoroethylene (ePTFE) prostheses implanted into different interfaces. J Biomed Mater Res 1996;31:1−9.

[101] Akers DL, Du YH, Kempscinski RF. The effect of carbon coating and porosity on early patency of expanded polytetrafluoroethylene grafts: an experimental study. J Vasc Surg 1993;18:10−5.

[102] Walpoth BH, Rogulenko R, Tikhvinskaia E, Gogolewski S, Schaffner T, Hess OM, et al. Improvement of patency rate in heparin-coated small synthetic vascular grafts. Circulation 1998;98:II319−23.

[103] Fisher JL, Thomson RC, Moore JW, Begovac PC. Functional parameters of thromboresistant heparinized e-PTFE vascular grafts. Cardiovasc Pathol 2002;11:42.

[104] Greisler HP, Cziperle DJ, Kim DU, Garfield JD, Petsikas D, Murchan PM, et al. Enhanced endotheliazation of expanded polytetrafluoroethylene grafts by fibroblast growth factor type 1 pretreatment. Surgery 1992;112:244−54.

[105] Walpoth BH, Zammaretti P, Cikirikcioglu M, Khabiri E, Djebaili MK, Pache JC, et al. Enhanced thickening of expanded polytetrafluoroethylene grafts coated with fibrin or fibrin-releasing vascular endothelial growth factor in the pig carotid artery interposition model. J Thorac Cardiovasc Surg 2007;133:1163−70.

[106] Couet F, Rajan N, Mantovani D. Macromolecular biomaterials for scaffold-based vascular tissue engineering. Macromol Biosci 2007;7:701−18.

[107] Xue L, Greisler HP. Biomaterials in the development and future of vascular grafts. J Vasc Surg 2003;37:472−80.

[108] Rabkin E, Schoen FJ. Cardiovascular tissue engineering. Cardiovasc Pathol 2002;11:305−17.

[109] Chen MC, Tsai HW, Chang Y, Lai WY, Mi FL, Liu CT, et al. Rapidly self-expandable polymeric stents with a shape-memory property. Biomacromolecules 2007;8:2774−80.

[110] Wong YS, Xiong Y, Venkatraman SS, Boey FY. Shape memory in un-cross-linked biodegradable polymers. J Biomater Sci Polym Ed 2008;19:175−91.

[111] Reiter D. Methods and materials for wound closure. Otolaryngol Clin North Am 1995;28:1069−80.

[112] Drew DK, Supik L, Darrow CR, Price GF. Tissue repair using laser: a review. Orthopaedics 1993;16:581−7.

[113] Swanson NA, Tromovitch TA. Suture materials, 1980s: properties, uses, and abuses. Int J Dermatol 1982;21:373−8.

[114] Seyomour RB, Carraher CE, editors. Structure−property relationships in polymers. New York: Plenum Press; 1984.

[115] G.L. Listner, Polypropylene (PP) sutures, Patent 3 630 (1971) 205.

[116] Wishman M, Hagler GE. Polypropylene fibers. In: Lewin M, Pearce EM, editors. Handbook of fiber science and technology, vol. 4. New York: Marcel Dekker; 1985.

[117] Apple DJ, Mamalis N, Brady SE, Loftfield K, Kavka-Van Norman D, Olson RJ. Biocompatibility of implant materials: a review and scanning electron microscopic study. J Am Intraocul Implant Soc 1984;10:53–66.

[118] Chu CC. Chemical structure and manufacturing processes. In: Chu CC, von Fraunhofer J, Greisler HP, editors. Wound closure biomaterials and devices. Boca Raton, FL: CRC Press; 1997.

[119] Chu CC. Textile-based biomaterials for surgical applications. In: Dumitriu S, editor. Polymeric biomaterials. New York: Marcel Dekker; 2003.

[120] Chu CC, Kizil Z. Qualitative-evaluation of stiffness of commercial suture materials. Surg Gynecol Obstet 1989;168:233–8.

[121] Dang MC, Thacker JG, Hwang JCS, Rodeheaver GT, Melton SM, Edlich RF. Some biomechanical considerations of polytetrafluoroethylene sutures. Arch Surg 1990;125:647–50.

[122] Urban E, King MW, Guidoin R, Laroche G, Marois Y, Martin L, et al. Why make monofilament sutures out of polyvinylidene fluoride? ASAIO 1994;40:145–56.

[123] Frazza EJ, Schmitt EE. A new absorbable suture. J Biomed Mater Res 1971;5:43–58.

[124] Miller RA, Brady JM, Cutright DE. Degradation rates of oral resorbable implants (polylactates and polyglycolates): rate modification with changes in PLA/PGA copolymer ratios. J Biomed Mater Res 1977;11:711–9.

[125] Shalaby SW. Synthetic absorbable polyesters. In: Shalaby SW, editor. Biomedical polymers: designed to degrade systems. New York: Hanser Press; 1994.

[126] Malchesky PS. Extracorporeal artificial organs. In: Ratner BD, Hoffman AS, Schoen FJ, Lemons JE, editors. Biomaterials science: an introduction to materials in medicine. San Diego, CA: Elsevier; 2004. Chapter 7.6.

[127] Schaefer R, Horl W, Kokot K, Heidland A. Enhanced biocompatibility with a new cellulosic membrane: cuprophan vs hemophan. Blood Purif 1987;5:262–7.

[128] Bowry S, Rintelen T. Synthetically modified cellulose: a cellulosic hemodialysis membrane with minimized complement activation. ASAIO J 1998;44:M579–83.

[129] Clark WR, Hamburger RJ, Lysaght MJ. Effect of membrane composition and structure on solute removal and biocompatibility in hemodialysis. Kidney Int 1999;56: 2005–15.

[130] Vanholder R, De Smet R, Glorieux G, et al. Review on uremic toxins: classification, concentration, and interindividual variability. Kidney Int 2003;63:1934–43.

[131] Bouman CS, van Olden RW, Stoutenbeek CP. Cytokine filtration and adsorption during pre- and postdilution hemofiltration in four different membranes. Blood Purif 1998;16:261–8.

[132] Schmidt C, Leach JB. Neural tissue engineering: strategies for repair and regeneration. Annu Rev Biomed Eng 2003;5: 293–347.

[133] Dahlin L, Lundborg G. The use of silicone tubing in the late repair of the median and ulnar nerves in the forearm. J Hand Surg (Br) 2001;26:393–4.

[134] Vasconcelos BC, Gay-Escoda C. Facial nerve repair with expanded polytetrafluoroethylene and collagen conduits: an experimental study in the rabbit. J Oral Maxillofac Surg 2000;58:1257–62.

[135] Molander H, Olsson Y, Engkvist O, Bowald S, Eriksson I. Regeneration of peripheral nerve through a polyglactin tube. Muscle Nerve 1982;5:54–7.

[136] Evans GR, Brandt K, Widmer MS, Lu L, Meszlenyi RK, Gupta PK, et al. In vivo evaluation of poly(L-lactic acid) porous conduits for peripheral nerve regeneration. Biomaterials 1999;20:1109–15.

[137] Nyilas E, Chiu TH, Sidman RL, Henry EW, Brushart TM, Dikkes P, et al. Peripheral nerve repair with bioresorbable prosthesis. Trans Am Soc Artif Int Org 1983;29:307–13.

[138] Valero-Cabré A, Tsironis K, Skouras E, Perego G, Navarro X, Neiss WF. Superior muscle reinnervation after autologous nerve graft or poly-L-lactide-epsilon-caprolactone (PLC) tube implantation in comparison to silicone tube repair. J Neurosci Res 2001; 63:214–23.

[139] Nicoli Aldini N, Fini M, Rocca M, Giavaresi G, Giardino R. Guided regeneration with resorbable conduits in experimental peripheral nerve injuries. Int Orthop 2000;24: 121–5.

[140] Soldani G, Varelli G, Minnocci A, Dario P. Manufacturing and microscopical characterization of polyurethane nerve guidance channel featuring a highly smooth internal surface. Biomaterials 1998;19:1919–24.

[141] Young RC, Wiberg M, Terenghi G. Poly-3-hydroxybutyrate (PHB): a resorbable conduit for long-gap repair in peripheral nerves. Br J Plast Surg 2002;55:235–40.

[142] Valentini RF, Vargo TG, Gardella Jr. JA, Aebischer P. Electrically charged polymeric substrates enhance nerve fiber outgrowth in vitro. Biomaterials 1992;13:183–90.

[143] Schmidt CE, Shastri VR, Vacanti JP, Langer R. Stimulation of neurite outgrowth using an electrically conducting polymer. Proc Natl Acad Sci USA 1997;94:8948–53.

[144] Fine EG, Valentini RF, Bellamkonda R, Aebischer P. Improved nerve regeneration through piezoelectric vinylidenefluoride-trifluoroethylene copolymer guidance channels. Biomaterials 1991;12:775–80.

[145] Collier JH, Camp JP, Hudson TW, Schmidt CE. Synthesis and characterization of polypyrrole-hyaluronic acid composite biomaterials for tissue engineering applications. J Biomed Mater Res 2000;50:574–84.

[146] Bidez III PR, Li S, Macdiarmid AG, Venancio EC, Wei Y, Lelkes PI. Polyaniline, an electroactive polymer, supports adhesion and proliferation of cardiac myoblasts. J Biomater Sci Polym Ed 2006;17:199–212.

[147] Balgude AP, Yu X, Szymanski A, Bellamkonda RV. Agarose gel stiffness determines rate of DRG neurite extension in 3D cultures. Biomaterials 2001;22:1077–84.

[148] Haipeng G, Yinghui Z, Jianchun L, Yandao G, Nanming Z, Xiufang Z. Studies on nerve cell affinity of chitosan-derived materials. J Biomed Mater Res 2000;52:285–95.

[149] Wells MR, Kraus K, Batter DK, Blunt DG, Weremowitz J, Lynch SE, et al. Gel matrix vehicles for growth factor application in nerve gap injuries repaired with tubes: a comparison of biomatrix, collagen, and methylcellulose. Exp Neurol 1997;146:395–402.

[150] Seckel BR, Jones D, Hekimian KJ, Wang KK, Chakalis DP, Costas PD. Hyaluronic acid through a new injectable nerve guide delivery system enhances peripheral nerve regeneration in the rat. J Neurosci Res 1995;40:318–24.

[151] Hashimoto T, Suzuki Y, Kitada M, Kataoka K, Wu S, Suzuki K, et al. Peripheral nerve regeneration through alginate gel: analysis of early outgrowth and late increase in diameter of regenerating axons. Exp Brain Res 2002;146:356–68.

[152] Herbert CB, Nagaswami C, Bittner GD, Hubbell JA, Weisel JW. Effects of fibrin micromorphology on neurite growth from dorsal root ganglia cultures in three-dimensional fibrin gels. J Biomed Mater Res 1998;40:551–9.

[153] Satou T, Nishida S, Hiruma S, Tanji K, Takahashi M, Fujita S, et al. A morphological study on the effects of collagen gel matrix on regeneration of severed rat sciatic nerve in silicone tubes. Acta Pathol Jpn 1986;36:199–208.

[154] Sierpinski P, Garrett J, Ma J, Apel P, Klorig D, Smith T, et al. The use of keratin biomaterials derived from human hair for the promotion of rapid regeneration of peripheral nerves. Biomaterials 2008;29:118–28.

[155] Holmes TC, de Lacalle S, Su X, Liu G, Rich A, Zhang S. Extensive neurite outgrowth and active synapse formation on self-assembling peptide scaffolds. Proc Natl Acad Sci USA 2000;97:6728–33.

[156] Yu X, Dillon GP, Bellamkonda RV. Tissue-engineered scaffolds are effective alternatives to autografts for bridging peripheral nerve gaps. Tissue Eng 1999;9:421–30.

[157] Williams LR, Varon S. Modification of fibrin matrix formation in situ enhances nerve regeneration in silicone chambers. J Comp Neurol 1985;231:209–20.

[158] Schense JC, Hubbell JA. Cross-linking exogenous bifunctional peptides into fibrin gels with factor XIIIa. Bioconjug Chem 1999;10:75–81.

[159] Chen MB, Zhang F, Lineaweaver WC. Luminal fillers in nerve conduits for peripheral nerve repair. Ann Plast Surg 2006;57:462–71.

[160] Ngo TT, Waggoner PJ, Romero AA, Nelson KD, Eberhart RC, Smith GM. Poly(L-Lactide) microfilaments enhance peripheral

nerve regeneration across extended nerve lesions. J Neurosci Res 2003;72:227−38.

[161] Wang X, Hu W, Cao Y, Yao J, Wu J, Gu X. Dog sciatic nerve regeneration across a 30-mm defect bridged by a chitosan/PGA artificial nerve graft. Brain 2005;128:1897−910.

[162] Ceballos D, Navarro X, Dubey N, Wendelschafer-Crabb G, Kennedy WR, Tranquillo RT. Magnetically aligned collagen gel filling a collagen nerve guide improves peripheral nerve regeneration. Exp Neurol 1999;158:290−300.

[163] Gao J, Kim YM, Coe H, Zern B, Sheppard B, Wang Y. A neuroinductive biomaterial based on dopamine. Proc Natl Acad Sci USA 2006;103:16681−6.

[164] Haile Y, Haastert K, Cesnulevicius K, Stummeyer K, Timmer M, Berski S, et al. Culturing of glial and neuronal cells on polysialic acid. Biomaterials 2007;28:1163−73.

5 Biofilms, Biomaterials, and Device-Related Infections

Paul Stoodley, Luanne Hall-Stoodley, Bill Costerton, Patrick DeMeo, Mark Shirtliff, Ellen Gawalt and Sandeep Kathju

OUTLINE

5.1 Introduction	77
5.2 Bacterial Biofilms	78
5.2.1 What Are Biofilms, Where Are They Found, and Why Are They Problematic?	78
5.2.2 Adaptation of Biofilm Structure for Survival in Changing Environments	78
5.2.3 Resistance of Bacteria in Biofilms	79
5.3 Biofilm Microbiology and Infectious Disease	79
5.3.1 Bacterial Adhesion to Surfaces	79
5.3.2 Processes of Biofilm Formation	80
5.4 Device-Related Infection	81
5.4.1 Biofilm Formation by Staphylococci	82
5.4.2 Detecting Device-Related Infections	83
5.4.3 Nucleic Acid-Based Detection Methods	84
5.5 Clinical Examples of Biofilm Infections	85
5.5.1 Infection Related to Surgical Repair Materials	85
5.5.2 Bacterial Biofilms on Sutures	85
5.5.3 Bacterial Biofilms on Surgical Mesh	87
5.5.4 Bacterial Biofilms in Orthopedic Prosthetic Joint Infection	87
5.6 Prevention and Treatment	89
5.6.1 Biofilm-Resistant Biomaterials	89
5.6.2 Testing for Antibacterial and Antibiofilm Properties of Biomaterials	89
5.6.3 Potential Agents for the Control of Microbial Colonization of Biomaterials	91
5.6.4 Delivery of Biofilm Control Agents at Biomaterial Surfaces	92
5.6.5 The Bioelectric Effect as an Adjunct to Antibiotics	92
5.6.5.1 Biomaterials that Resist Bacterial Attachment and Biofilm Formation	93
5.7 Conclusions	94
References	94

5.1 Introduction

The initial design criteria in the choice of indwelling materials for medical and dental purposes may be pragmatic, and based on the necessary mechanical properties required to fashion a functional device. Orthopedic implants require strong materials for weight-bearing, and articulating surfaces such as joints require durability and resistance to wear. Stents and shunts require flexibility and patency, and sutures require a high tensile strength yet also must be flexible enough for intricate manipulation. As the devices became more sophisticated and developments in materials science provided more options for manufacture, implants are being used more frequently and with longer anticipated lifetimes. Concurrently, the design process increasingly incorporated biocompatibility and comfort into the design criteria. However, with longer lifetimes, the more frequent use of invasive surgical procedures involving indwelling devices and biologically-friendly materials, there has been a rise in the number of incidences of device-related infection. Urinary catheters have been estimated to account for 30% of all nosocomial infections [1]. Between 66 and 88% of these occur after urinary catheterization [2]. It is also reported that almost 100% of catheterized patients develop an infection in an openly draining indwelling catheter which has been in place for four days or more [2]. For some procedures, such as orthopedic joint arthroplasties, the diagnosed surgical site infection rates are relatively low (between 1% and 2%; [3]); however, the increasing number of patients undergoing joint-replacement surgery translates to large numbers of patients afflicted with the consequences of complicating infections per year. Furthermore, infection of artificial joints can be devastating, since oral or IV antibiotic therapy frequently fails to resolve the infection, with the only remaining course of action being surgical debridement or partial or total revision. These two examples, the first with very high numbers of patients but of lesser severity in terms of impact to the individual, and the second, low numbers but severe patient impact, reflect the incentive to pursue a third design criteria—that of infection resistance—into materials and devices [4]. In the following sections we will discuss the role of bacterial biofilms in infection, and the growing literature highlighting biofilms as an important cause of device-related infection.

5.2 Bacterial Biofilms

5.2.1 What Are Biofilms, Where Are They Found, and Why Are They Problematic?

Bacterial biofilms are communities of bacteria which attach and subsequently grow on surfaces of abiotic materials, as well as host tissues [5,6] (Figure 5.1). The bacteria embed themselves in a highly hydrated protective matrix termed "extracellular polymeric substance" (or sometimes slime) (EPS) [7]. Biofilm development is an ancient adaptation of prokaryotes which is believed to have facilitated survival in hostile environments, and allowing colonization of new niches by active dispersal mechanisms [8–12].

Bacteria in biofilms also demonstrate coordinated behavior that culminates in the development of complex three-dimensional structures comprised of functionally heterogeneous bacterial communities on virtually all surfaces. Phenotypic heterogeneity and localized specialization in biofilms can be seen by differential expression of pili, fimbriae, flagella [13], carbohydrate [14], adhesins [15,16], and genes associated with dormancy [17,18] and antibiotic resistance [19]. Biofilm bacteria coordinate their behavior by cell–cell communication using

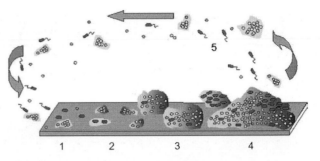

Figure 5.1 Key processes in biofilm development based on the conceptual model described by Stoodley *et al.* [5]. For illustrative purposes this schematic shows a mixed biofilm consisting of rods capable of swimming motility (i.e., *P. aeruginosa* shown in red) and two types of non-motile cocci (i.e., *S. aureus* and *S. epidermidis* shown in green and yellow). The EPS slime matrix surrounding the cells is shown in green. (1) Initial attachment of single cells and clumps of detached biofilm bacteria. (2) Production of EPS to more firmly adhere cells to the surface. (3) Early development of biofilm clusters by clonal expansion (can be mixed or single species colonies). (4) Mature biofilm when the biofilm is in (pseudo) steady-state. (5) Dispersion of single cells by motility-driven swarming dispersion (*P. aeruginosa*) and the sloughing of biofilms clusters containing cells and EPS.

secreted chemical signals which allow the bacteria to sense and respond to their environment by assessing cell density or environmental cues, resulting in modification of gene expression. This ability to adapt to and modify micro-niches at a surface interface allows bacteria in biofilms to facilitate survival at a population level.

5.2.2 Adaptation of Biofilm Structure for Survival in Changing Environments

Biofilms growing in highly varied environments from hot springs to urinary catheters appear to utilize similar strategies to attach and grow on surfaces, and can also show remarkable structural similarity suggesting a selective advantage that surface association offers. This suggests that structural specialization in different environments reflects an important survival strategy. For example, biofilm growth under high fluid shear often exhibits filamentous streamers, while biofilms grown in low shear environments form towers or mound-like structures which vary according to different nutrient conditions or mass transfer-determined localized growth patterns. These observations suggest that bacteria in biofilms can rapidly adapt to their local environment, to an extent not possible with multicellular eukaryotic organisms [7,20].

5.2.3 Resistance of Bacteria in Biofilms

Numerous studies document that bacteria in biofilms are more resistant to environmental stresses, such as dehydration, metals toxicity, and UV light exposure, than free floating or planktonic, bacteria. These strategies which have evolved for survival in the natural environment appear to be readily adapted to facilitate survival against human attempts to eradicate them with modern materials, antibiotics, and antimicrobials. The exact nature of the resistance is not fully understood, but the most commonly considered mechanisms are: (1) bacteria in the interior of the biofilm enter a dormant-like state [21], possibly induced by nutrient depletion caused by consumption by bacteria on the periphery of the biofilm cell clusters [22]; (2) reaction of the antimicrobial agent with the extracellular polymeric slime (EPS) matrix (binding and/or degradation) [23]; and (3) the development of resistant populations, such as slow growing small colony variants or "persister" cells which occur at greater frequency and in higher numbers in biofilm populations than in planktonic populations [24].

The first and second mechanisms have been referred to as "tolerance" rather than "resistance," the latter of which is usually associated with a genetic basis [25]. In addition to providing a nidus for bacterial biofilm formation, foreign materials also suppress the efficacy of phagocytic clearance. The EPS matrix of carbohydrates, proteins, and extracellular bacterial DNA (eDNA) provides structural integrity, as well as protecting the bacterial cells within from phagocytic attack [26–28]; although *in vitro* experiments suggest that the degree of protection also depends on the species and age of the biofilm [29]. The EPS also reduces the ability of IgG human antibodies to penetrate the biofilm [30,31]. Therefore, biofilm formation also appears to be a mechanism which helps bacteria to evade host immunity. Indeed, many diseases associated with biofilms (infection of the cystic fibrosis (CF) lung, otitis media, gingivitis) are also associated with chronic inflammation. Mounting evidence suggests that the "inappropriate" inflammatory response to biofilms often fails to eradicate the biofilm, and may in fact contribute to the pathology pathogenesis by degrading host tissue, which in turn provides nutrients to the bacteria.

5.3 Biofilm Microbiology and Infectious Disease

Many of the concepts and techniques that have served microbiologists well in the understanding, diagnosis, and treatment of many acute epidemic bacterial diseases, are being re-evaluated with respect to device-related and other biofilm-associated infections. This section on biofilm microbiology will focus on how biofilm bacteria differ from their planktonic counterparts, and the importance of using appropriate biofilm *in vitro* assays to assess the potential bacterial colonization of biomaterials *in vivo*.

5.3.1 Bacterial Adhesion to Surfaces

Derjaguin, Landau, Verwey, and Overbeek (DLVO) theory is often applied to the study of bacterial adhesion to surfaces [32]. This classic concept of colloid behavior characterizes a planktonic bacterial cell as a smooth particle that interacts with a surface in a manner based on the charges on both surfaces, which overcome the basic repulsion of individual particles. However, direct observations of the surfaces of planktonic bacteria using electron microscopy have demonstrated that these surfaces are not smooth [33]. In addition to protein appendages (i.e., flagella and pili) projecting as much as 2–6 μm from the cell, the entire surface of bacterial planktonic cells is covered by a structured matrix of hydrophobic exopolysaccharide (EPS) fibers and protein. The external glycocalyx of planktonic cells is anchored to the polysaccharide O antigen fibers that project from the lipopolysaccharide (LPS) of the outer membrane of gram-negative cells, and to the polysaccharide teichoic acid fibers that project from the cell wall of gram-positive cells. Elegant freeze-substitution microscopy preparations have shown that the actual surface of planktonic bacterial cells capable of interacting with a surface to be colonized consists of a 0.2–0.4 μm thick layer of protein and polysaccharide fibers. Thus, the planktonic bacterial cell is not a smooth-surfaced colloid particle, and the actual interaction of these cells with surfaces is based on the bridging of bacterial fibers with fibers adsorbed to the surface being colonized. Therefore, DLVO theory has a limited application in the study of bacterial adhesion.

Moreover, the reliance on bacteria isolated from the system of interest, but subcultured repeatedly in rich media, also does not serve us well in biofilm studies relevant to medical devices. This method, which dates from the 19th century, may select for strains of bacteria that exhibit rapid planktonic growth on rich media, since slow-growing strains might not be cultured or overgrown, and strongly adherent bacteria may not be readily transferred. Such strains may lack many surface structures that would be necessary for their survival in the real world on a surface where they are challenged by antibacterial agents, nutrient limitation, competing bacteria or host defenses. However, these laboratory-adapted strains used in studies of bacterial adhesion to biomaterials may be physically closer to the smooth-surfaced colloidal particles suggested in DLVO theory, potentially confounding data designed to further the understanding of device-related infections [33]. This may help to explain why many novel biomaterials perform less successfully *in vitro* when tested with clinical isolates, and further highlights the necessity of using clinical strains in biomaterials testing. However, there are also challenges with using clinical isolates. Techniques such as rapid genomic sequencing [34] and multi-locus strain typing (MLST) [35] have revealed an enormous amount of genomic and phenotypic diversity between strains of the same species, and indeed biofilms appear to accelerate the generation of variants [36,37]. Thus, data generated from any one clinical isolate might, like reference strains, also not be generalizable. Thus, ideally, anti-biofilm assays should be conducted with reference strains to allow benchmark comparisons between studies in different laboratories, as well as at least two or three low-passage clinical isolates.

Many researchers in the biomaterials field have intuitively speculated that a few key surface characteristics can inhibit (or favor) bacterial adhesion, and surfaces engineered with various combinations of these characteristics have been tried in the search for colonization-resistant biomaterials. Bacteria adhere equally well to very hydrophobic (e.g., Teflon™) and to very hydrophilic (e.g., PVC) surfaces, can colonize smooth surfaces as well as rough surfaces [38,39], and can colonize surfaces in relatively high physiologically-relevant shear flows [26]. Indeed, Bos et al. have reported that hydrophobicity had little correlation with initial attachment of various bacterial strains to surfaces, but was correlated with attachment strength [40]. Thus, currently, while there is no perfect biocompatible biomaterial surface which also inherently resists bacterial colonization, more sophisticated non-fouling surfaces which incorporate designer antimicrobial peptides to target and kill bacteria [41] or zwitterionic surfaces which are generally resistant to protein adhesion [42] show potential for this application.

5.3.2 Processes of Biofilm Formation

When planktonic cells adhere to a surface, they exhibit behaviors that have been divided into "reversible" and "irreversible" patterns [43]. Motile organisms (e.g., *P. aeruginosa*) may use their flagella for initial attachment, followed by type IV pili for twitching motility that allow them to form elaborate structures [13]. However, surface appendages and motility are not required for biofilm formation, staphylococci and streptococci are both capable of forming biofilms *in vitro* and *in vivo*, although in these cases it is assumed that biofilm structures develop from clonal growth. Movies showing the attachment of various biofilm bacteria are available on the Center for Biofilm Engineering (CBE) web site (www.erc.montana.edu). Such movies show that many cells that adhere to surfaces may also quickly detach, before they make the phenotypic switch to initiate irreversible attachment and subsequent biofilm formation.

When a bacterial cell colonizes a surface, the pattern of gene expression is profoundly different from the previous planktonic phenotype, resulting in a distinct biofilm phenotype that may differ by as much as 70% in the proteins expressed [44]. Among the first genes that are upregulated in adherent cells are those involved in the production of molecules associated with the EPS that forms the biofilm matrix and anchors the cell irreversibly to the surface. In mucoid *P. aeruginosa*, the upregulation of *algC*, which is a part of the alginate synthesis pathway, occurs within 18 minutes of initial cell adhesion [45], and there is a secretion of bacterial biofilm matrix material by these cells within 30 minutes. Once attached, cells which have triggered the conversion to the biofilm phenotype and the formation of a multicellular community on the colonized surface begin to accrete larger numbers of cells through growth. As they increase in numbers and produce more EPS matrix material, the attached cells form microcolonies which constitute approximately 10% of the volume, with the EPS matrix occupying approximately 90% of the biofilm. Recent data suggest that the structure of the EPS is much more sophisticated than previously thought, with confocal and SEM (scanning electron microscope) images showing features such as "honeycombs" and 3D networks in *P. aeruginosa* and staphylococcal biofilms grown *in vitro* [46]. Borlee et al. [47] have found evidence for secreted proteins which specifically cross-link extracellular polysaccharides, suggesting a possible mechanism for extracellular remodeling of the EPS.

The microcolonies can assume tower-like, frond, and mushroom-like structures in many natural and cultured biofilms, but other morphologies may be dictated by individual species characteristics, and by nutrient availability. As the biofilm matures and undergoes more phenotypic changes, the processes of growth and recruitment are balanced by detachment of planktonic cells from the sessile community and sloughing of larger pieces of biofilm. *In vitro* studies suggest that biofilms reach a mature thickness and a stable community structure within a week or two of their initiation of colonization [5]. Numerous *in vitro* studies show that both gram-negative and gram-positive pathogens are clearly capable of forming extensive biofilms on commonly used medical materials, including devices themselves, such as surgical sutures and meshes [48], and orthopedic implants and catheters [49,50].

5.4 Device-Related Infection

Although biofilm formation may be an ancient adaptation of prokaryotic life, the full impact of biofilms on human health is only now being realized, through one of the fastest technologically advancing fields—the development of medical devices, which are all susceptible to colonization with microorganisms growing in biofilms.

Medical and surgical practices rely on an increasing array of biomedical implants, and tens of millions are implanted each year. Intravenous catheters, prosthetic heart valves, joint prostheses, peritoneal dialysis catheters, cardiac pacemakers, cerebrospinal fluid shunts, and endotracheal tubes certainly save millions of lives, but all carry the risk of surface-associated infections. Device-related infections were among the first clinical problems to be identified as having a bacterial biofilm etiology. Biofilms associated with medical devices were first noted in the literature in the early 1980s, although Bayston and Penny published a report in 1972 that correlated *Staphylococcus mucoidy* as a possible factor in the colonization of Holter shunts [51]. Electron microscopy revealed bacteria deposited on the surface of indwelling devices such as intravenous catheters and a cardiac pacemaker lead [38]. However, the relationship between medical devices and infection is arguably best established for catheters [52]. Many types of catheters and fluid management devices, such as central venous catheters, dialysis catheters, ventilators, neurosurgical shunts, and drains are also commonly associated with infection [53].

Implant infections are common occurrences, with rates estimated between 4–5% for orthopedic implants and 7% for cardiovascular implants [54,55]. Due to the increasing use of these interventions, infections affect millions of patients per year, making device related infections a serious clinical problem that is being addressed from many perspectives.

There is a clear correlation between implanted devices and risk of infection, which may not be surprising since any time the protective skin barrier is breached, the possibility for introduction of bacteria to normally sterile sites exists. A 1979 study by Fitzgerald [56], and discussed in Subbiahdoss et al. [57], reported that during surgery a wound was exposed to approximately 270 bacterial-carrying particles per cm^2 per hour. No doubt with improved operating room (OR) facilities, such as laminar flow air handling and the implementation of more rigorous practices aimed at reducing the rates of nosocomial infections, this rate will have decreased. Nevertheless, the study illustrates that possible airborne contamination can occur within the "sterile field." Possibly of greater concern is the introduction of skin pathogens during the procedure. Higher rates of infection associated with more heavily microbially-colonized anatomical sites (such as the groin or armpit), suggest that transmission from the skin, despite disinfection of the skin, is an important route of transmission. Even devices which are not transdermal or surgically implanted, such as urinary catheters, are associated with a high risk for infection, in part due to the fact that these devices are placed in patients who are already immunocompromised, and it is likely that many catheters are being placed in an already infected site.

In the controlled condition of a hospital the device be implanted is sterile immediately out of the packaging. However, once it is exposed there is potential for the implant to be contaminated with bacteria that might also have inadvertently enter the wound during surgery. The probability of infection has been related to the relative time taken to colonize the artificial surface by host cells or infectious microorganisms. This was termed "The race to the surface" by Gristina et al. [58], who hypothesized that if a surface was colonized with host cells before a biofilm could become established, the probability of subsequent infection was low, even if bacteria were introduced during the procedure. Subbiahdoss et al. [57] experimentally demonstrated the importance of the "race to the surface" by showing that the successful colonization of a glass substratum by osteosarcoma cells was negatively influenced by preseeded *S. epidermidis* cells on the surface. Whether this observation is generalizable to the *in vivo* situation remains to be verified.

Although device-related infections are initially localized to the site where the device is inserted, these infections are often chronic in nature and can be a source of periodic acute sepsis. The direct link between the presence of a foreign body and bacterial sepsis in hemodialysis catheters is illustrated in a study by Feely [59]. In a group of hemodialysis patients with a history of recurrent bacteremia, the rate of catheter-related bacteremia went down from 9.13 per 1000 catheter days to 1.04 after catheter-lock solutions (CLS) were instigated. When CLS was discontinued, the rate rose back up to 7.94 per 1000. Catheter lock is a technique whereby a controlled volume of antibiotic solution is introduced into a catheter so as to fill the catheter, but is not allowed to enter the bloodstream. Thus, much higher concentrations of antibiotics can be applied directly to the catheter than would otherwise be tolerated systemically. This study clearly implicates the foreign body as harboring the source of infection.

The organisms most frequently observed with medical devices are the staphylococci, both the coagulase negative staphylococci (particularly *Staphylococcus epidermidis*) and *S. aureus* followed by *P. aeruginosa* and other opportunistic bacteria that survive in the environment. Biofilm formation on medical implants, most notably by *S. epidermidis*, has led to the characterization of a new infectious disease: "chronic polymer-associated infection" [60,61]. *S. epidermidis*, a common colonizer of the skin, is therefore frequently found in wounds and implants. It was not considered even an opportunistic pathogen until device-related infections became problematic [62]. Biofilm formation therefore can be considered a virulence factor in the context of device-related infections—a bacterial strategy that contributes to its ability to cause and maintain an infection.

5.4.1 Biofilm Formation by Staphylococci

Staphylococci are particularly problematic in biofilm-associated infections with surgical site infection of deep tissue implants. This is partly due to the propensity of these organisms to form biofilms, and the increasing spread of multi drug-resistant methicillin-resistant *S. aureus* (MRSA) and *S. epidermidis* (MRSE). Biofilm formation is characterized by two stages with staphylococci: (1) adhesion to a solid surface; and (2) growth-dependent cell accumulation resulting in multiple cell layers in microcolonies. In *S. epidermidis*, the cell–cell layer aggregation is specifically linked with a β-1,6-linked glycosaminoglycan polysaccharide complex know as polysaccharide intercellular adhesin (PIA) [63]. Proteins involved in the synthesis of this matrix polysaccharide are regulated by the *ica* gene locus in *S. epidermidis* [64,65] which is conserved among phyologenetically related staphylococci. However, PIA and *ica* are not absolutely required for biofilm formation, since mutants lacking the *ica* locus have been isolated which can still form biofilms, suggesting complex, redundant mechanisms for biofilm development. For example, an *S. epidermidis* transposon mutant, unable to form biofilms on polystyrene, formed biofilms on glass, suggesting that bacterial adhesion mechanisms vary according to the substratum [64].

A further level of complexity comes from the numerous environmental factors that can affect biofilm formation. For example, biofilm formation in *S. epidermidis* is strongly influenced by sugar substrate, oleic acid, antibiotic treatment, oxygen levels, iron, osmolarity, temperature, and ethanol stress [61]. Also, the initial adhesion stage alone is multifactorial, depending on the physio-chemical properties of the biomedical polymer material, and the nature of the bacterial cell surface. Bacterial surface proteins contribute significantly to adhesion, and several key proteins have been identified that play a role in staphylococcal biofilm formation. In *S. aureus*, teichoic acid lacking D-alanine (dltA) resulted in a change in surface charge that affected several characteristics, including biofilm formation [66]. Interestingly, dltA mutants were defective in the ability to attach to polystyrene and glass. While consistent with charge equilibrium of surface interactions, the biofilm defect was re-established by the addition of magnesium ions. Other researchers found that *S. epidermidis* biofilm formation was enhanced by Mg^{2+} and inhibited by EDTA [67]. Another surface protein in *S. aureus*, the biofilm-associated protein or bap, was shown to contribute to biofilm formation on microtiter plates, but more importantly showed increased pathogenesis in a mouse foreign-body infection model [68].

5.4.2 Detecting Device-Related Infections

Biofilm-associated infections are often difficult to detect using conventional culturing methods [69], and many of the clinical studies which conclude that biofilms were present on a medical device rely on indirect evidence such as the recovery of bacteria removed using sonication [70–72] or the culture of strains positive for slime production or biofilm formation [73]. Arguably, at the present time microscopic examination of the devices and associated tissue themselves, are still the only way to definitively demonstrate the presence of biofilm [6,38]. Confocal microscopy has an advantage over electron microscopy, in that it can be performed on fully hydrated specimens using water immersion objectives, which, in itself, demonstrates firm attachment of the bacteria to the surface, and is also compatible with a wide range of specific fluorescent staining techniques, including antibody labeling and fluorescent *in situ* hybridization (FISH), to identify bacterial species, or membrane integrity-based nucleic acid viability staining methods to detect live and dead bacteria. Figure 5.2 shows an example of predominantly staphylococcal biofilm growing on a surgical screw.

Bacteria can also be identified through the detection of their DNA. First, a specimen or swab is digested to release any bacterial DNA. Next the polymerase chain reaction (PCR) is used to amplify specifically targeted fragments of DNA. In some cases the targets are specifically designed for a certain species, genus or strain. In other cases sections of universal genes, such as 16s ribosomal DNA (rDNA), are amplified using primers to highly conserved regions while the sequencing of the variable region between the primers can identify the bacteria.

While PCR-based 16S rDNA detection methods appear to be much more accurate than conventional clinical culture, which has increasingly been shown to produce high levels of false negatives in chronic biofilm-associated infections, PCR for targeted genes does not differentiate between biofilm and planktonic infections. PCR has also been criticized for being too sensitive, and producing false positives from contaminants which are not clinically relevant. However, the visual demonstration of clusters of bacteria firmly attached to devices demonstrates a "growth-in-place" process, which is unlikely to have resulted from contamination during the relatively short period of the surgery. Therefore, confocal microscopy, PCR, and reverse transcriptase PCR (RT-PCR) have been used in combination to provide strong evidence for the presence of active bacterial biofilms on various implant materials [74–77] as well as host tissue [78–81]. However, a drawback of confocal microscopy-based diagnosis of biofilm is that it requires highly specialized equipment and training, along with laborious searching for clusters of bacteria with dimensions as low as 10s to 100s of microns on implants that might have large areas with convoluted surfaces.

While confocal microscopy might be useful to validate more rapid methods which are conducive to standardization in the setting of a clinical laboratory, it will require refinement of the existing technology before it can be used as a routine diagnostic tool. Ideally, the diagnosis of a biofilm infection would be made prior to surgery. One approach is to devise enzyme-linked immunosorbent array (ELISA) type assays to detect biofilm specific proteins through a simple blood test [82]. Another approach is to

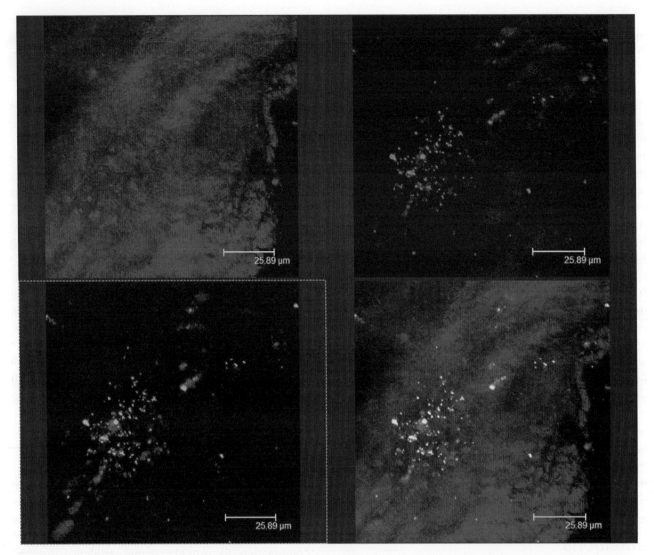

Figure 5.2 Biofilm attached to orthopedic screws from a non-union fracture case. The surface of the screw and associated invested tissue are blue and imaged by reflected confocal microscopy. Staphylococci were stained red by fluorescence *in situ* hybridization (FISH) using the Sau probe. General bacteria were stained green with the Eub338 probe. The overlay (bottom left) shows that the biofilm consisted primarily of staphylococci with occasional other types of cocci. Scale bar = 25 μm.

develop medical imaging techniques, such as X-ray computed tomography (CT) scan or magnetic resonance imaging (MRI) scans, so that biofilms can be visualized in place. However, the small size of the biofilm, and the lack of contrast between biofilm and host tissue, makes imaging a challenge. In diagnostic imaging for cancer detection contrast agents are used which help distinguish the malignant cells from the healthy tissue. The importance of more effectively treating cancer through early detection has led to much research and development in the imaging of ever smaller tumors, and it is possible that techniques developed in oncology could be utilized for detection of biofilms. Imaging is not only useful for diagnostics, but also has the added advantage in that it can be invaluable in monitoring and planning surgical intervention.

5.4.3 Nucleic Acid-Based Detection Methods

PCR-based detection techniques generally fall into one of two categories. One approach is targeted PCR in which genus, species or strain-specific primers or combinations of primers are used to detect pathogens of interest. However, this approach does not provide any information regarding the presence or absence of non-targeted bacteria. A second approach is a "finger-printing method," by which primers are used to amplify universal DNA sequences (16S rDNA is commonly used). The amplicon is separated out as bands on a gel by techniques such as denaturing gel gradient electrophoresis (DGGE) [83] or, after digestion using restriction enzymes, by restriction fragment length polymorphism (RFLP) [84]. The separation patterns can be used to identify specific species. However, in polymicrobial infections the many overlapping and complex patterns of bands can be difficult to resolve. A more specific approach is to sequence the various 16S amplimers from individual bacterial colonies in a clone library or directly by high-throughput sequencing techniques, such as 454 pyrosequencing [85,86]. Individual species can be identified by comparing the cloned sequences with database sequences, using tools such as the Basic Local Alignment Search Tool (BLAST). The drawback of these approaches is that they are relatively time consuming, either in the preparation of the library or the data analysis, and are not yet conducive for utility where a rapid diagnosis is needed. An alternative approach is the combination of PCR with ion spray mass spectroscopy to precisely weigh each complementary strand of the amplimer. Bacterial species can be identified by mass due to differences in the nucleotide ratios. Multiple sets of primers are used to amplify sequences from genes which are universal to bacteria (i.e., 16S and 23s rDNA), and genes or alleles specific to certain species or strain [87]. More targeted primer sets can be designed to identify site-specific pathogens or the presence of the bacterial virulence genes, such as *mecA* which is responsible for methicillin resistance in *S. aureus* (MRSA) [77,88]. primer sets could be designed to detect genes associated with biofilm formation, such as the *ica* operon which regulates EPS production in staphylococci.

5.5 Clinical Examples of Biofilm Infections

5.5.1 Infection Related to Surgical Repair Materials

Surgical repair materials, such as staples, sutures, and meshes, have also been identified as possible foci of infection in such diverse anatomic sites and procedures as abdominal wall repair and ocular and dental procedures [48,74,89,90]. The implication of the foreign body as a causative factor of infection is supported in a study by Wissing et al. [91], who reported that the late post-operative incidence of suture sinus development associated with fascia repair after midline laparotomy was significantly greater with nonabsorbable sutures (nylon) than with absorbable sutures (polyglactin or polydioxanone). There was a direct relationship between material absorption time and incidence of sinus formation, which was 3–4% for polyglactin, which is fully absorbed after 70 days, 11% for polydioxanone, which is fully absorbed after 180 days, and 23% for nylon, which is permanent. This study nicely illustrates the compromise that has to be made between functionality of the material and the risk of infection, since there was an inverse relationship between the incident rate of incisional herniation and suture absorption time caused by the loss of tensile strength during the absorption process.

5.5.2 Bacterial Biofilms on Sutures

Bacterial adherence to, and colonization of, suture material has been of interest to the surgical community for decades. Thirty years ago Osterberg and Blomstedt observed that multifilament "capillary" suture material recovered from *S. aureus*-inoculated tissues in a rat model harbored substantially greater quantities of bacteria than "non-capillary" suture [92]. Their conclusion was that: "in the case of the capillary suture material, the bacteria would tend to be protected through their enclosure in the interstices of the material." In a subsequent study, Osterberg further commented that "bacteria which are enclosed in the interstices of multifilament suture material, and protected from the phagocytic activity of leukocytes, can sustain and prolong an infection" [93]. These prescient early observations concur well with our present understanding of bacterial biofilm formation and persistence, but suture material as a host for pathogenic biofilm in patients has thus far been only occasionally examined (principally in the ophthalmologic literature). We have reported several cases where biofilm was documented on clinical specimens of explanted permanent suture material, with resolution of the infection on removal of the offending suture substratum [94,95] (Figure 5.3). Multiple studies have noted that "suture sinuses" are associated with nonabsorbable suture materials, presumably due to resident biofilm, although direct evidence was lacking [96,97].

Prevention of infectious complications by modifying the suture material itself has recently become an area of intense interest. A number of studies have focused on suture materials coated with the antimicrobial agent triclosan. *In vitro* and *in vivo* animal experiments have shown that coated polyglactin 910 suture (braided) can significantly decrease the number of viable bacteria recovered from inoculated suture material versus a non-coated control [90,98]. Similar antimicrobial activity has also been reported with the addition of triclosan to poliglecaprone 25 [99] and polidioxanone [100] suture. Early clinical experience has also been promising: use of triclosan-coated polyglactin 910 suture versus uncoated polidioxanone suture in

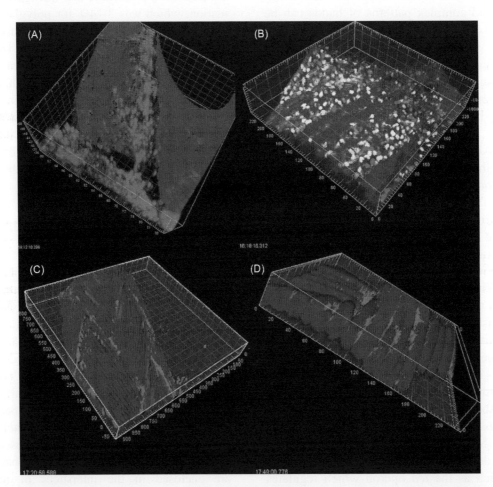

Figure 5.3 Biofilm infected sutures. (A) Ti-cron braided polyester suture used for hernia repair following open gastric bypass surgery removed from a chronic draining wound was found to have a biofilm formed from live cocci (stained green with the BacLight™ Live/Dead® kit). Diffuse green staining (arrow) is suggestive of eDNA in the biofilm slime matrix. The individual filaments of the suture are shown by autofluorescence (blue). Biofilm was particularly noted in the crevices formed from the braiding. Scale bar = 4 μm. (B) The same suture as in "A" but at a location a few mm away. In this location there were many inflammatory cells indicated by nuclear morphology (nuclei stained yellow and red). Scale bar = 20 μm. (C) *In vitro* biofilm grown on braided sutures from a clinical MRSA (stained green with the Live/Dead® kit) isolated from a patient with an infected surgical repair mesh. Similar to the *ex vivo* image the biofilm preferentially grew in the protected crevices between individual filaments in the braid. Scale bar = 50 μm. (D) Higher magnification confocal image of the suture at a different location. Scale bar = 20 μm.

2088 patients undergoing midline laparotomy resulted in a significantly reduced reported incidence of wound infection [101].

5.5.3 Bacterial Biofilms on Surgical Mesh

Surgical mesh implants are routinely used to address the clinical problem of hernia. These implants typically restore structural domain to the abdominal/pelvic wall and prevent extrusion of visceral contents. Multiple complications have been associated with the use of surgical mesh, including infection, extrusion, and erosion into subjacent structures (i.e., development of enterocutaneous fistula). Not infrequently, surgical mesh implants must be removed, often due to infectious complications, and recently an entirely new "current procedural terminology" code (11008) describing the explantation of abdominal wall mesh due to chronic and necrotizing infection has been recognized.

Multiple studies have examined the morphological and surface characteristics of various available meshes, and have documented the ability of both gram-negative and gram-positive organisms to form biofilms on these materials [102,103]. The hydrophobicity of the mesh surface, as well as the presence of numerous niches (or pockets) in multifilament mesh configurations, appear to correlate with the extent of biofilm formation *in vitro* [102]. We have been able to demonstrate biofilms present on clinical specimens of explanted mesh from patients with a variety of clinical presentations (Stoodley et al., manuscript in preparation).

A similar approach to modifying mesh materials (as has been done with suture) may prove beneficial to reducing the infectious complications noted with surgical mesh, but these studies are in their infancy. Monofilament polypropylene mesh modified with a coating to release nitric oxide in bactericidal quantities was found to significantly inhibit biofilm from multiple organisms *in vitro*, but had little effect in an *in vivo* animal model [104]. Clinically, acellular dermal grafts composed entirely of organic materials and therefore presumably less susceptible to the establishment of persistent biofilms, have recently gained popularity as alternatives to mesh reconstruction in abdominal wall surgery.

5.5.4 Bacterial Biofilms in Orthopedic Prosthetic Joint Infection

Orthopedic implant infections differ clinically from the previous infections described, for several reasons. First, although they are chronic and persistent like all biofilm infections, they often develop months or years after the implant. Second, these infections are often difficult to detect in orthopedic implants via routine examination or culturing, thereby delaying diagnosis and treatment. Third, unlike the catheter lock solution treatment, there is no easy way to deliver high doses of antibiotics to the site. Therefore, orthopedic infections often require repeated antibiotic applications to resolve the infection, which increases the risk of the development of antibiotic resistance. Finally, treatment of chronic infections that fail to resolve with conventional antibiotic treatment may require sustained high dose antibiotic therapy, removal of the implant, and replacement of the orthopedic implant, resulting in pain and discomfort, immobility, and excessive costs to the patient and healthcare facility. The failure of antibiotics to effectively and fully treat these infections suggests that other strategies are necessary; approaches to resolve these problems range from enhancing hospital sterility protocols to the investigation of active release [54], non-adhesive or bactericidal coatings [105–107]. Despite researchers' best efforts, often the only treatment for intractable implant infections is revision surgery, requiring removal of the infected implant and placement of a new one. However, secondary (revisional) total hip replacements have a higher infection rate (3.2%), and secondary total knee replacements exhibit a remarkable 5.6% re-infection rate. To compound the problem, in revision surgery a larger implant must be used, since bone is destroyed during the original implantation and subsequent explantation. This process may require splintering the surrounding bone, along with substantial soft tissue resection and debridement. The patient is then confined to absolute bed rest and continuous intravenous antibiotic therapy for several weeks. If the revisional surgery fails, limb amputation may occur. The number of total hip and knee replacements within the United States surpassed 1,000,000 in 2009 (http://www.cdc.gov/nchs/fastats/insurg.htm), and is expected to increase dramatically over the next several decades due to specific risk factors within the US population that include obesity, sports injuries, and longer lifespan. In addition to the physical and emotional costs, the financial cost of revisions is high, with explant surgery, post-procedural medical treatment, and re-implantational surgery exceeding $500,000 per patient. Conservative estimates put the current costs of revisional therapy in excess of two billion dollars annually.

Addressing this objective, the 2004 Association of Bone and Joint Surgeons Musculoskeletal Infection Workshop [108] suggested that orthopedic materials designed to prevent bacterial biofilm formation would be a relevant clinical strategy for reducing orthopedic device infections. Therefore, the investigation of antimicrobial surfaces that inhibit or retard biofilm development represents a significant new direction in the antimicrobial arsenal against bacterial biofilm formation and implant infections. These antimicrobial surfaces fall into two broad categories: (1) those surfaces that are made of materials that resist bacterial attachment; and (2) those materials that are impregnated or coated with antimicrobial compounds, which upon diffusion from the surface inhibit or abrogate bacterial growth at the implant site. This direction of research is at an early stage, and represents an important part of the unmet need of the pharmaceutical therapeutic market, but most saliently, the proven effectiveness of orthopedic materials specifically designed to resist bacterial colonization and biofilm formation would result in a significant advance in patient care.

Total joint replacement (TJR) is one of the most common and successful surgical procedures in orthopedics. The majority of patients undergoing TJR benefit from marked improvements in their pain, functional status, and overall quality of life [109]. Infection following primary TJR is uncommon, occurring with a prevalence of $\sim 1-3\%$, but it can be a debilitating complication of TJR surgery. Infection following revision arthroplasty is significantly higher, approaching 10% [110]. In the US, revisions are usually in two stages with a period of time between removal of the old hardware and replacement of the new which allows resolution of the infection. However, the fact that infection rates in revised cases are higher than for primary surgeries suggests that, although the symptoms might have resolved, the bacterial source of the underlying infection might not have been fully eradicated. The treatment of an infected joint prosthesis is both complicated and expensive. Diagnosis can itself be problematic, and the necessary intervention may vary depending on the clinical picture; e.g., acute post-operative infections may be initially managed with operative debridement, intravenous antibiotics, and retention of the implant, whereas late chronic infections will likely ultimately require more extensive surgery, typically in multiple stages. Even with aggressive measures there is a $\sim 10\%$ rate of failure to eradicate the infection, and the patient may proceed to resection of the arthroplasty, arthrodesis, or even amputation, in each case with significantly greater morbidity [110].

Although the concept of biofilm as a relevant physiological factor in prosthetic joint infections has gained some currency, there are actually few examples of experimentally imaged bacteria in biofilm configuration from any orthopedic implanted material. Gristina and Costerton first found bacteria in biofilms on orthopedic explants by scanning electron micrography [111]. Confocal microscopy has visualized biofilm on the surface of an explanted hip prosthesis, and the microscopic identification of clusters of bacteria consistent with biofilms were present in sonicate from infected explanted prostheses, where the sonication was used to dislodge any extant attached biofilm [112]. We have documented bacterial biofilm in the aspirate, on tissue, and on bone cement originally impregnated with gentamicin in a patient with a chronic infection after total elbow arthroplasty [75]. The majority of reports imputing biofilms on orthopedic prostheses and surfaces, however, have been in *in vitro* systems, and a major argument for biofilm involvement in chronic orthopedic prosthetic joint infections remains the highly suggestive clinical features demonstrated by such infections, supported by our general understanding of the bacterial propensity to occupy available abiotic surfaces.

Nethertheless, surgeons and investigators have become increasingly interested in adjuvant techniques and technologies that minimize the risk of prosthetic joint infection, possibly by preventing adherence to and colonization of the implant in the first place. Orthopedic surgeons already routinely use antibiotic-loaded bone cement in surgery, and the use of other antibiotic-supplemented materials is under active investigation. Direct covalent attachment of an antibiotic moiety (vancomycin) to a titanium surface has been shown to inhibit both *S. aureus* and *S. epidermidis* colonization of the modified implant material *in vitro*, despite repeated challenges and over prolonged incubation times [113]. The use of vancomycin-modified titanium implants in a rat model similarly showed evidence of reduced bacterial adherence [114]. An alternative approach to direct modification that would still provide high local concentrations of antibiosis to an implant surface is the deployment of antibiotic-loaded conforming films or sheaths for orthopedic prostheses [115].

5.6 Prevention and Treatment

5.6.1 Biofilm-Resistant Biomaterials

In previous sections we have discussed biofilm-related complications associated with considerable morbidity and mortality. Here we will discuss some of the new agents and strategies that may give more effective control over the colonization of biomaterials, and the incidence of device-related infections. Finally, we will discuss new methods for the release/delivery of these agents at the surfaces of biomaterials. But first we discuss the evaluation of novel surfaces for resistance to bacterial adhesion, and the formation of bacterial biofilms.

5.6.2 Testing for Antibacterial and Antibiofilm Properties of Biomaterials

There are serious concerns with the utility and information content of some of the methods used to assess the biofilm resistance of biomaterials; namely, if a biomaterial gives a positive zone of inhibition test, what does this mean? Fundamentally, this widely-used test indicates that the biomaterial contained an antibacterial agent, which was released in the moist environment of the surface of an agar plate, was still active, and the agent could prevent the planktonic bacteria deposited on the agar from growing. The major parameter operative in the test is the diffusion of the antibacterial agent through the agar or in the fluid on the agar surface, as well as the effectiveness of the agent. A very potent agent may produce a small or no zone of inhibition, if it is not released or moves slowly through agar, and a less potent agent may produce a large zone if it diffuse rapidly through agar. Shake flask test such as the ASTM E2149-10 tests, in which candidate biomaterials are suspended in a growth medium that is simultaneously inoculated with planktonic bacteria, are equally naïve. If the biomaterials release enough of an antibacterial agent in the first few minutes of the test, all of the planktonic cells in the inoculum will be killed, resulting in a situation where there are no organisms left to colonize the biomaterial. So, an antibiotic-releasing biomaterial that releases all of its antibacterial agents in a few minutes may emerge from this test as a favorable candidate, although this may not reflect a physiologically relevant timescale over which the biomaterial is expected to perform. Generally, tests are conducted over a few hours in rich medium, in an essentially "closed" system, while *in vitro* the biomaterials might be expected to perform over days, or even years, in open systems where leached active agents can diffuse away. Therefore, such conventional tests are largely inappropriate, and may lead to the development of biomaterials that fail in biofilm resistance in animal and clinical trials.

More appropriate tests are ones that mimic the conditions in the systems in which the biomaterial is targeted for use. If the biomaterial will be subjected to flow or fluid exchange, the test should include these parameters. If the biomaterial will be used in a body fluid, such as blood or urine, an accurate simulation of that fluid should be used in the test, and the bacteria supplying the challenge should be adapted to the fluid. One of the pitfalls of laboratory testing is to base a culture medium on the relevant physiological chemistry, but then to add rich components, such as yeast or amino acid extracts, to stimulate growth to allow for rapid testing, typically over a 24-hour period or less. The concept is valid, that is, to accelerate natural processes; however, as discussed earlier, a rich medium and much higher concentrations of bacteria than might be physiologically relevant might also unintentionally interfere with surface chemistry and product efficacy.

Flow cells are useful for quantifying the rates of bacterial attachment and biofilm formation under a defined fluid shear stress, because they allow direct observation of the surface which can be monitored continuously. Confocal microscopy is particularly suited for biofilm assays since it allows the examination of living hydrated preparations, microbial cells that adhere to the biomaterial surface can be easily visualized (Figure 5.4). If the adherent cells survive, they will initiate biofilm formation, and the adherent cells will gradually form matrix-enclosed structured biofilm cell clusters (Figure 5.4, bottom panel), within which the cells will be separated by EPS. The formation of biofilms requires that the adherent cells must be alive, so the observation of live biofilm on surfaces that make antibacterial and antibiofilm claims could have unfortunate clinical consequences [116].

Optimally the preference is for biomaterials which inherently resist attachment or kill colonizing bacteria, and do not retain these dead cells on the surface, i.e., prevention rather than treatment. For this reason, one of several available live/dead probes to ascertain the viability of adherent bacterial cells on biomaterials can be used. The Molecular Probes® BacLight™ Live/Dead® kit has become a standard research method for distinguishing live cells on the basis of membrane integrity; live cells stain green while dead cells stain red. In practical terms, biomaterials set up in flow cells can be exposed to realistic fluid shear containing potentially pathogenic bacteria, and the colonization of its surface can be monitored by confocal microscopy.

Although direct observation is still the "gold standard" to test the resistance of biomaterials to bacterial colonization, confocal microscopes are complex and relatively expensive. Alternatively, sessile biofilm bacteria can be removed from colonized surfaces and enumerated by standard microbiological techniques; commonly referred to as "scraping and plating." The theory behind the technique is that it first removes all biofilm from a surface, then completely breaks up the clumps of bacteria into single unassociated cells, and finally spreads various dilutions of the cells on the surface of an agar plate so that each cell gives rise to one colony when the plate is incubated. Although this technique can drastically underestimate the actual surface cell concentration (usually expressed as colony forming units/cm^2, CFU/cm^2), microscopy can be used to validate the removal and homogenization steps which can be major sources of error. First, some cells may be left on the surface by the removal method, whether it is physical scraping, sonication or another method. Second, the removed biofilm must be completely homogenized to break up clumps of bacteria to ensure that each living bacterium gives rise to one colony on the agar plate. This step is usually achieved by vortexing, sonicating or use of a homogenizer. Sonication may kill some cells, so it is therefore important to calibrate the sonication time for each type of biofilm until microscopy shows that the resultant

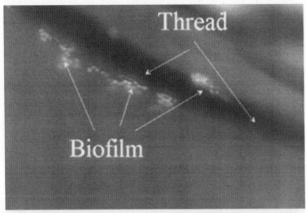

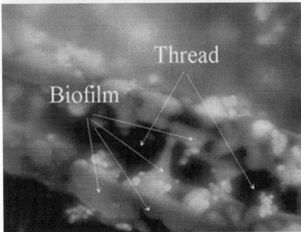

Figure 5.4 Confocal microscope images of unfixed biofilms formed on individual fibers of the cloth-like material used to form the sewing cuffs of mechanical heart valves. The biofilms formed when fibers of a silver-coated medical device were exposed to planktonic cells of *Staphylococcus epidermidis*, in a flow cell [116] after 24 (top panel) and 48 hours (bottom panel). Staining with the Live/Dead® BacLight™ probe showed that many cells were live (green) in marked contrast to dead cells (red). After 48 hours distinct biofilm cell clusters had formed on the fibers. Diffuse staining between and around the individual cells with the green nucleic acid stain Syto9 is associated with staining of the eDNA in the EPS slime matrix.

suspension is mostly single cells, and most of these cells are alive.

When scraping and plating are used without such validation, this method can yield data that are up to 4 logs lower than the bacterial numbers seen by direct microscopy. However, the scrape and plate method can yield accurate and consistent *in vitro* data when it is properly calibrated by microscopy, and the first biofilm method using this enumeration technique was ASTM Method E 2196-02. Darla Goeres and Marty Hamilton at the Center for Biofilm Engineering were instrumental in developing this method, and have been actively involved in developing other statistically robust experimental methods for biofilm evaluation which undoubtedly will form the basis for standard testing and claims substantiation in the anti-infective biomaterials industry. More rapid approaches include the development of conventional multi-well plates or biofilm-specific devices, used in combination with a plate reader to estimate biofilm biomass by general stains such as crystal violet staining or live/dead ratios.

5.6.3 Potential Agents for the Control of Microbial Colonization of Biomaterials

The strategy most commonly used in current antibacterial biomaterials is the incorporation of conventional antibiotics into the material, with the objective of killing incoming planktonic cells before they can adhere and initiate biofilm formation at the implant site [54]. The release strategy has been used for years to infuse bone cements with gentamicin, and is actively pursued with researchers showing that release of NO, antibiotics, antibodies, and silver ion (Ag^+) from polymers and hydroxapatite materials reduce bacterial growth on plates in culture [107,117,118]. This approach shows promise, and is being actively pursued. However, one problem is that these coatings are not synthetically flexible or covalently adhered to the surface, leading to bursts of antimicrobial activity and localized toxicity stemming from the introduction of non-resorbable coatings into the body [107].

The quandary of balancing antimicrobial efficacy against the danger of promoting bacterial resistance does not affect the large cohort of bacterial manipulation molecules that is currently moving briskly toward the biomaterials market. Some of these biofilm control molecules are specifically targeted to interfere with the bacteria's own developmental signaling pathways to affect both biofilm formation and detachment. The theory is that by influencing natural signaling processes, bacteria can be manipulated not to form biofilms or to detach by triggering a dispersal event, thus reducing the likelihood of inducing defense responses or the generation of resistant mutants. Natural antibiofilm strategies developed by marine seaweeds, which use furanones to interfere with natural biofilm signaling pathways show promise since these defense strategies have been presumably developed over millions of years of coevolution, yet still remain effective [119]. The pivotal concept is that bacteria in contact with a biomaterial would be prevented from forming a biofilm on its surface, would be "locked" in the planktonic phenotype, and would be subsequently killed by host defenses (antibodies and activated leukocytes) and any antibiotics that might be present. The best described signal pathways are the acetyl homoserine lactone (AHL) systems of some gram-negative species [120], and the autoinducer two (AI2) signaling peptides in both gram-negative and gram-positive species [121]. Of relevance to the design of biomaterials which utilize signal blocking is the finding that the effect of AI2 on biofilm is concentration dependent [122], and while very low, μM concentrations added exogenously inhibited biofilm formation, higher concentrations showed no effect or actually stimulated biofilm formation.

A third class of signaling molecule which controls biofilm formation in staphylococci is RNAIII-inhibiting peptide (RIP) which targets the RNAIII-activating protein (RAP), and has been shown to prevent infection on implant materials in rats [123]. When specific antibiotics were administered to these test animals, while the challenging bacteria were locked in the planktonic phenotype, no live cells could be recovered from the biomaterial surfaces of the surrounding tissues. More recently, attention has been focused on the secondary messenger cyclic-di-GMP, which is not secreted into the surrounding medium but is intracellular [124]. Cyclic di-GMP is influenced by nitric oxide, but as with AI2, concentration is important. At higher concentrations, NO is toxic to the cells, but at nM levels appears to act as a dispersal signal [10], thus highlighting the importance of precisely controlling the concentration to achieve the desired effect, perhaps a difficult challenge in an *in vivo* setting. Another potential biofilm dispersal signal is the fatty acid signal *cis*-2-decenoic acid, which is produced by *P. aeruginosa* (and possibly other species) and has been shown to be active *in vitro* against a broad range of organisms, over a wide range of concentrations [11]. Such a signal makes a good candidate for antibiofilm biomaterials. However, while existence of a "universal" biofilm prevention or dispersal signal is attractive, the reality might be elusive. From an evolutionary perspective it seems unlikely that a diverse multitude of bacteria would so easily give up control of their biofilm development to a single molecule produced by competing species [125].

5.6.4 Delivery of Biofilm Control Agents at Biomaterial Surfaces

Killing the planktonic bacteria before they have time to initiate biofilm formation is the objective of many research programs, and this can be accomplished by three general strategies:

1. Systemic antibiotic therapy that produces bactericidal concentrations in the body fluids in the operative field;
2. Release of antibiotics and other bacterial manipulation molecules from the biomaterials to produce sustained effective concentrations of the agent in the immediate vicinity of the device;
3. Irrigation and other techniques that deliver antibiotics to the biomaterial surface after the device is installed, but before the operative wound is closed.

Many surgeons use systemic antibiotic therapy in the perioperative timeframe, and most also use this strategy in subsequent operations (including dental procedures) if a device has recently been installed and might not be fully epithelialized. The simplest manifestation of the antibiotic-releasing biomaterial strategy is a class of materials that can be "loaded," such as a sponge, by soaking them in a solution of the antibiotic in question immediately before the device is installed. In the case of filler or adhesive materials, such as poly-methylmethacrylate (PMMA), an active agent can be directly mixed prior to polymerization in the OR. Whenever a molecule is loaded into or onto a polymer there will be an immediate initial burst of diffusion in the early timeframe, followed by a tapering off over time as the concentration in this reservoir is depleted. These biomaterials are useful, but the low-level release of the agent for months or years after this effective timeframe cannot be controlled. This produces a prolonged period in which the agent is present at a sublethal concentration, near the device and sometimes in the whole body, and raises the specter of the development of acquired antibiotic resistance in many potentially dangerous bacterial species. Recently, several papers have even shown that subinhibitory concentrations of antibiotic may actually induce biofilm formation [126].

There is a similar problem with antibiotic impregnated coatings, since usually these coatings are not synthetically flexible or covalently adhered to the surface, leading to bursts of antimicrobial activity, and possibly localized toxicity stemming from the introduction of non-resorbable coatings into the body. The controlled release of active agents is one of the most problematic aspects of devices which rely on this technology for infection protection. One solution is to engineer surfaces to release active agents "on demand." Biomaterials can be coated with a molecular "skin," a self-assembled surface layer, that completely contains molecules loaded into an underlying plastic and can be temporarily deranged (by ultrasonic energy) to yield a controlled release [127]. Such a coating has been used to deliver insulin, as well as ciprofloxacin in controlled pulses in the laboratory [128]. High concentrations of these agents could be released at the surfaces of medical devices perioperatively or at any preliminary signs of device-related infection.

5.6.5 The Bioelectric Effect as an Adjunct to Antibiotics

Coatings which release antibiotics at the site of potential infection have the advantage over systemically administered antibiotics, in that they can achieve much higher local concentrations and avoid toxicity effects, since the overall amount of antibiotic can be relatively small. However, due to difficulties with the controlled release and surfaces which are challenging to modify, it is desirable to be able to sensitize bacteria to conventional antibiotics. As discussed previously, one approach is to use signals in an attempt to induce a planktonic phenotype through cell signaling. Another promising area is to achieve planktonic-like antibiotic sensitivity by applying low voltage electrical fields [129]. The so called "bioelectric effect" has recently shown promise at treating *S. epidermidis* chronic foreign-body osteomyelitis in a rabbit model [130]; however, the same group also reports that the efficacy is dependant on the pathogen and the class of antibiotic [131].

5.6.5.1 Biomaterials that Resist Bacterial Attachment and Biofilm Formation

An alternative approach to killing posited by the Association of Bone and Joint Surgeons Musculoskeletal Infection Workshop is to design coatings for implant surfaces that resist bacterial attachment. Most of the work in the literature has focused on the model systems of self-assembled monolayers (SAMs) on gold or polymeric coatings [132,133]. SAMs have many advantages as a flexible platform over macromolecules (Figure 5.5). One major advantage of SAMs is their ease in engineering interfacial structures at the molecular level, due to the fact that they form defined structures on the surface and therefore present functional tail groups in a consistent, active manner [134–136]. They are also synthetically flexible, which allows for the modification of the tail group for prevention of non-specific adsorption of cells. However, the SAM technology developed in model systems is not necessarily directly transferable to metal oxide systems used in biomaterials, and coating the surface with gold is not always practical. Alkanethiols form SAMs on gold and other noble metals, such as silver or copper, but not on oxide surfaces, such as those used in biomaterials [137]. Functional groups can be immobilized through basic organic chemistry at the tail groups of the monolayer or by synthesizing molecules with functional tail groups and forming a mixed SAM that includes multiple functionalities. Delivering multiple, active groups in a single polymeric coating is synthetically challenging [138]. Polymeric coatings that are peptidomimetic have been successful in the laboratory at resisting bacteria adhesion, and could also be used as platforms for further functionalization [106,136,139]. As a result, new chemistry for non-specific bacterial resistance on metal oxide surfaces must be developed that is appropriate for orthopedic implant materials.

The underlying mechanism by which SAMs render surfaces inert is under study. Many tail groups have been employed to render gold surfaces inert to protein and non-specific cellular adhesion. SAMs techniques are also being applied to more relevant metals used in surgery. The technique has been used to tether gentamicin and vancomycin to 316L stainless steel, which retarded biofilm formation for up to 48 hours [140]. While oligo-ethylene glycol has been the standard by which inert surfaces are measured, and is the only SAM system used to mitigate bacterial adhesion, other groups such as mannitol, maltose, taurin [141], and tertiary amine oxides have rendered gold surfaces inert to protein and cellular adhesion. A survey of literature suggests that formation of an inert surface utilizing self-assembled monolayers is a combination of many parameters including substrate wettability, tail functionality, lateral packing density, conformational flexibility of the molecule, structure of water on the surface, and kosmotropicity (the degree to which solutes stabilize water-to-water interactions, and hence affect molecular interactions) [141]. The underlying reason for their inert effect on surfaces

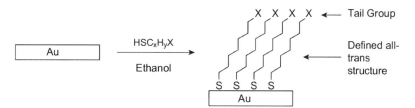

Figure 5.5 Self-assembled monolayers form spontaneously on a surface placed in a solution. They consist of organic monomers with reactive head groups and exposed tail groups. Tail groups can be designed to accomplish a task, such as cell resistance, or to participate in chemical reaction for further functionalization of the surface. SAMs on gold form defined structures in which all of the carbon–carbon bonds are oriented "trans" to one another (at an angle of 109.5°). These monolayers are considered ordered.

may be due to their ability to order surrounding water molecules, excluding them from the surface and rendering the surface inert to protein adsorption. However, the molecular basis for the resistance of some surfaces continues to be debated, in part due to conflicting data in the literature, with some favoring the hydrophobic effect as the driving force [142], while others disagree. Due to the large interdependent, complex interactions between cells and organically modified surfaces, the understanding and harnessing of the phenomenon of controlling adhesion on oxide surfaces has been difficult.

Biomimicry or bioinspiration is another approach used by engineers in the design of inherently non-fouling surfaces [125]. Nano-textured patterns found on the skins of sharks have been found to resist initial bacterial attachment in laboratory experiments. It is thought that this approach, originally designed as a control for marine biofouling [143], might be utilized for medical devices [144], illustrating the importance of interdisciplinary collaboration and thinking in the area of biomaterials design. A similar approach was used in the development of the natural and synthetic furanone cell signal blockers, which were first discovered to play a role in the resistance of red algae to marine biofouling, and are now being developed for infection protection of medical devices [119].

5.7 Conclusions

Undoubtedly, medical devices will be increasingly used in patient management, whether temporarily or intermittently for fluids exchange, as in the case of catheters, or as permanent implants to repair loss of function, as is the case for orthopedic joints and cardiovascular stents. What is also ensured is that as more devices are used bacteria will take advantage of an access site into the body and with the convenience of an abiotic surface to colonize the spread of antibiotic resistant strains may likely increase. For permanent implants, overall rates of infection may drop as data show that there is an inverse correlation with surgical-site infection and numbers of procedures performed per institution and surgeon. However, the overall number of patients with surgical-site infections will inevitably rise, as more and more people undergo such surgeries, whether out of absolute necessity or to improve quality of life. To a certain extent, infection associated with permanent implants can be minimized through the controlled environment of the OR and the ever-increasing experience of the surgeon. Infections associated with catheters might present a greater challenge, since they require frequent manipulations and are usually managed in less controlled environments.

A challenge to biomaterials engineers and surface scientists is to design and develop materials for the manufacture of devices which are functional, biocompatible, resistant to infection, and do not add to the development of resistant strains. While 100% biofilm-proof surfaces may be a long way off, we at least now know our enemy much more intimately than even less than a decade ago. Observational studies of biofilms have begun to reveal the true complexities and coordination that pathogenic bacteria are capable of, and molecular techniques are revealing the mechanisms of biofilm development and dispersal, as well as revealing the full extent of diversity of biofilm populations, including the genetic and phenotypic divergence that develops in biofilms formed from a single strain in only a matter of hours to days. The challenge is formidable, but the rewards are great, with the potential to improve the quality of life of millions of people. To quote from *The Art of War* written by Sun Tzu in the 6th century: "So it is said that if you know your enemies and know yourself, you can win a hundred battles without a single loss. If you only know yourself, but not your opponent, you may win or may lose. If you know neither yourself nor your enemy, you will always endanger yourself." With our current understanding of biofilms we are only just beginning to know the enemy with respect to device-related biofilm infections. Even if the "biofilm-proof" surface proves elusive, the challenge is to effectively utilize what we have learned about biofilm biology to engineer playing fields which tip the balance for the race to the surface in favor of ourselves and away from the bacteria.

References

[1] Gould CV, Umscheid CA, Agarwal RK, Kuntz G, Pegues DA. Guideline for prevention of catheter-associated urinary tract infections 2009. Infect Control Hosp Epidemiol 2010;31 (4):319–26.

[2] Wong ES. Guideline for prevention of catheter-associated urinary tract infections. Am J Infect Control 1983;11(1):28–36.

[3] Hsieh PH, Lee MS, Hsu KY, Chang YH, Shih HN, et al. Gram-negative prosthetic joint infections: Risk factors and outcome of treatment. Clin Infect Dis 2009;49(7):1036–43.

[4] Maki DG, Tambyah PA. Engineering out the risk for infection with urinary catheters. Emerg Infect Dis 2001;7(2):342–7.

[5] Stoodley P, Sauer K, Davies DG, Costerton JW. Biofilms as complex differentiated communities. Annu Rev Microbiol 2002; 56:187–209.

[6] Hall-Stoodley L, Stoodley P. Evolving concepts in biofilm infections. Cell Microbiol 2009;11(7):1034–43.

[7] Donlan RM, Costerton JW. Biofilms: Survival mechanisms of clinically relevant microorganisms. Clin Microbiol Rev 2002;15(2):167–93.

[8] Hall-Stoodley L, Stoodley P. Biofilm formation and dispersal and the transmission of human pathogens. Trends Microbiol 2005;13(1):7–10.

[9] Purevdorj-Gage B, Costerton WJ, Stoodley P. Phenotypic differentiation and seeding dispersal in non-mucoid and mucoid *Pseudomonas aeruginosa* biofilms. Microbiology 2005;151(Pt 5):1569–76.

[10] Barraud N, Schleheck D, Klebensberger J, Webb JS, Hassett DJ, et al. Nitric oxide signaling in *Pseudomonas aeruginosa* biofilms mediates phosphodiesterase activity, decreased cyclic di-GMP levels, and enhanced dispersal. J Bacteriol 2009;191(23):7333–42.

[11] Davies DG, Marques CN. A fatty acid messenger is responsible for inducing dispersion in microbial biofilms. J Bacteriol 2009;191(5):1393–403.

[12] Kaplan JB. Biofilm dispersal: Mechanisms, clinical implications, and potential therapeutic uses. J Dent Res 2010;89(3):205–18.

[13] Barken KB, Pamp SJ, Yang L, Gjermansen M, Bertrand JJ, et al. Roles of type IV pili, flagellum-mediated motility and extracellular DNA in the formation of mature multicellular structures in *Pseudomonas aeruginosa* biofilms. Environ Microbiol 2008;10(9):2331–43.

[14] Vuong C, Kocianova S, Voyich JM, Yao Y, Fischer ER, et al. A crucial role for exopolysaccharide modification in bacterial biofilm formation, immune evasion, and virulence. J Biol Chem 2004;279(52):54881–6.

[15] Hendrickx AP, van Luit-Asbroek M, Schapendonk CM, van Wamel WJ, Braat JC, et al. SgrA, a nidogen-binding LPXTG surface adhesin implicated in biofilm formation, and EcbA, a collagen binding MSCRAMM are two novel adhesins of hospital-acquired *Enterococcus faecium*. Infect Immun 2009;77(11):5097–106.

[16] Vergara-Irigaray M, Valle J, Merino N, Latasa C, Garcia B, et al. Relevant role of fibronectin-binding proteins in *Staphylococcus aureus* biofilm-associated foreign-body infections. Infect Immun 2009;77(9):3978–91.

[17] Stewart PS, Franklin MJ. Physiological heterogeneity in biofilms. Nat Rev Microbiol 2008;6(3):199–210.

[18] Perez-Osorio AC, Williamson KS, Franklin MJ. Heterogeneous rpoS and rhlR mRNA levels and 16 S rRNA/rDNA ratios within *Pseudomonas aeruginosa* biofilms, sampled by laser capture microdissection. J Bacteriol 2010;192(12):2991–3000.

[19] Bagge N, Schuster M, Hentzer M, Ciofu O, Givskov M, et al. *Pseudomonas aeruginosa* biofilms exposed to imipenem exhibit changes in global gene expression and beta-lactamase and alginate production. Antimicrob Agents Chemother 2004;48(4):1175–87.

[20] Hall-Stoodley L, Costerton JW, Stoodley P. Bacterial biofilms: From the natural environment to infectious diseases. Nat Rev Microbiol 2004;2(2):95–108.

[21] Klapper I, Gilbert P, Ayati BP, Dockery J, Stewart PS. Senescence can explain microbial persistence. Microbiology 2007;153(Pt 11):3623–30.

[22] Fux CA, Wilson S, Stoodley P. Detachment characteristics and oxacillin resistance of *Staphyloccocus aureus* biofilm emboli in an *in vitro* catheter infection model. J Bacteriol 2004;186(14):4486–91.

[23] Anderl JN, Franklin MJ, Stewart PS. Role of antibiotic penetration limitation in *Klebsiella pneumoniae* biofilm resistance to ampicillin and ciprofloxacin. Antimicrob Agents Chemother 2000;44(7):1818–24.

[24] Lewis K. Persister cells and the riddle of biofilm survival. Biochemistry (Mosc) 2005;70(2):267–74.

[25] Harrison JJ, Ceri H, Turner RJ. Multimetal resistance and tolerance in microbial biofilms. Nat Rev Microbiol 2007;5(12):928–38.

[26] Leid JG, Shirtliff ME, Costerton JW, Stoodley P. Human leukocytes adhere to, penetrate, and respond to *Staphylococcus aureus* biofilms. Infect Immun 2002;70(11):6339–45.

[27] Jesaitis AJ, Franklin MJ, Berglund D, Sasaki M, Lord CI, et al. Compromised host defense on *Pseudomonas aeruginosa* biofilms: Characterization of neutrophil and biofilm interactions. J Immunol 2003;171(8):4329–39.

[28] Bjarnsholt TPO, Jensen M, Burmolle M, Hentzer JA, Haagensen HP, et al. *Pseudomonas aeruginosa* tolerance to tobramycin, hydrogen peroxide and polymorphonuclear leukocytes is quorum-sensing dependent. Microbiology 2005;151(Pt2):373–83.

[29] Guenther F, Stroh P, Wagner C, Obst U, Hansch GM. Phagocytosis of staphylococci biofilms by polymorphonuclear neutrophils: *S. aureus* and *S. epidermidis* differ with regard to their susceptibility towards the host defense. Int J Artif Organs 2009;32(9):565–73.

[30] deBeer D, Stoodley P, Lewandowski Z. Measurement of local diffusion coefficients in biofilms by micro-injection and confocal microscopy. Biotechnol Bioeng 1997;53(2):151–8.

[31] Bryers JD, Drummond F. Local macromolecule diffusion coefficients in structurally non-uniform bacterial biofilms using fluorescence recovery after photobleaching (FRAP). Biotechnol Bioeng 1998;60(4):462–73.

[32] van Loosdrecht MC, Norde W, Zehnder AJ. Physical chemical description of bacterial adhesion. J Biomater Appl 1990;5(2):91–106.

[33] Fux CA, Shirtliff M, Stoodley P, Costerton JW. Can laboratory reference strains mirror "real-world" pathogenesis? Trends Microbiol 2005;13(2):58–63.

[34] Hiller NL, Janto B, Hogg JS, Boissy R, Yu S, et al. Comparative genomic analyses of seventeen *Streptococcus pneumoniae* strains: Insights into the pneumococcal supragenome. J Bacteriol 2007;189(22):8186–95.

[35] Jefferies JM, Smith A, Clarke SC, Dowson C, Mitchell TJ. Genetic analysis of diverse disease-causing pneumococci indicates high levels of diversity within serotypes and capsule switching. J Clin Microbiol 2004;42(12):5681–8.

[36] Webb JS, Lau M, Kjelleberg S. Bacteriophage and phenotypic variation in *Pseudomonas aeruginosa* biofilm development. J Bacteriol 2004;186(23):8066–73.

[37] Starkey M, Hickman JH, Ma L, Zhang N, De Long S, et al. *Pseudomonas aeruginosa* rugose small-colony variants have adaptations that likely promote persistence in the cystic fibrosis lung. J Bacteriol 2009;191(11):3492–503.

[38] Marrie TJ, Nelligan J, Costerton JW. A scanning and transmission electron microscopic study of an infected endocardial pacemaker lead. Circulation 1982;66(6):1339–41.

[39] Sottile FD, Marrie TJ, Prough DS, Hobgood CD, Gower DJ, et al. Nosocomial pulmonary infection: Possible etiologic significance of bacterial adhesion to endotracheal tubes. Crit Care Med 1986;14(4):265–70.

[40] Bos R, van der Mei HC, Busscher HJ. Physico-chemistry of initial microbial adhesive interactions: Its mechanisms and methods for study. FEMS Microbiol Rev 1999;23(2):179–230.

[41] Loose C, Jensen K, Rigoutsos I, Stephanopoulos G. A linguistic model for the rational design of antimicrobial peptides. Nature 2006;443(7113):867–9.

[42] Cheng G, Zhang Z, Chen S, Bryers JD, Jiang S. Inhibition of bacterial adhesion and biofilm formation on zwitterionic surfaces. Biomaterials 2007;28(29):4192–9.

[43] Marshall KC, Stout R, Mitchell R. Selective sorption of bacteria from seawater. Can J Microbiol 1971;17(11):1413–6.

[44] Sauer K, Camper AK. Characterization of phenotypic changes in *Pseudomonas putida* in response to surface-associated growth. J Bacteriol 2001;183(22):6579–89.

[45] Davies DG, Geesey GG. Regulation of the alginate biosynthesis gene algC in *Pseudomonas aeruginosa* during biofilm development in continuous culture. Appl Environ Microbiol 1995;61(3):860–7.

[46] Schaudinn C, Stoodley P, Kainović A, O'Keeffe T, Costerton JW, et al. Bacterial biofilms, other structures seen as mainstream concepts. Microbe 2007;2(5):231–7.

[47] Borlee BR, Goldman AD, Murakami K, Samudrala R, Wozniak DJ, et al. *Pseudomonas aeruginosa* uses a cyclic-di-GMP-regulated adhesin to reinforce the biofilm extracellular matrix. Mol Microbiol 2010;75(4):827–42.

[48] Engelsman AF, van der Mei HC, Ploeg RJ, Busscher HJ. The phenomenon of infection with abdominal wall reconstruction. Biomaterials 2007;28(14):2314–27.

[49] Jacobsen SM, Stickler DJ, Mobley HL, Shirtliff ME. Complicated catheter-associated urinary tract infections due to *Escherichia coli* and *Proteus mirabilis*. Clin Microbiol Rev 2008;21(1):26–59.

[50] Machado JD, Suen VM, Figueiredo JF, Marchini JS. Biofilms, infection, and parenteral nutrition therapy. J Parenter Enteral Nutr 2009;33(4):397–403.

[51] Bayston R, Penny SR. Excessive production of mucoid substance in staphylococcus SIIA: A possible factor in colonisation of Holter shunts. Dev Med Child Neurol Suppl 1972;27:25–8.

[52] O'Grady NP, Alexander M, Dellinger EP, Gerberding JL, Heard SO, et al. Guidelines for the prevention of intravascular catheter-related infections. Centers for Disease Control and Prevention. MMWR Recomm Rep 2002;51(RR-10):1–29.

[53] Rolighed T, Moser C, Hall-Stoodley L, Stoodley P. The role of bacterial biofilms in infections of Catheters and Shunts. In: Bjarnsholt T, Jensen PO, Moser C, Hoeby N, editors. Biofilm infections. New York, NY: Springer; 2010.

[54] Campoccia D, Montanaro L, Arciola CR. The significance of infection related to orthopedic devices and issues of antibiotic resistance. Biomaterials 2006;27(11):2331–9.

[55] Hetrick EM, Schoenfisch MH. Reducing implant-related infections: Active release strategies. Chem Soc Rev 2006;35(9):780–9.

[56] Fitzgerald Jr. RH. Microbiologic environment of the conventional operating room. Arch Surg 1979;114(7):772–5.

[57] Subbiahdoss G, Kuijer R, Grijpma DW, van der Mei HC, Busscher HJ. Microbial biofilm growth vs. tissue integration: "The race for the surface" experimentally studied. Acta Biomater 2009;5(5):1399–404.

[58] Gristina AG, Naylor P, Myrvik Q. Infections from biomaterials and implants: A race for the surface. Med Prog Technol 1988;14(3–4):205–24.

[59] Feely T, Copley A, Bleyer AJ. Catheter lock solutions to prevent bloodstream infections in high-risk hemodialysis patients. Am J Nephrol 2007;27(1):24–9.

[60] von Eiff C, Heilmann C, Herrmann M, Peters G. Basic aspects of the pathogenesis of staphylococcal polymer-associated infections. Infection 1999;27(Suppl. 1):S7–10.

[61] Gotz F. *Staphylococcus* and biofilms. Mol Microbiol 2002;43(6):1367–78.

[62] Otto M. *Staphylococcus epidermidis*: The "accidental" pathogen. Nat Rev Microbiol 2009;7(8):555–67.

[63] Mack D, Fischer W, Krokotsch A, Leopold K, Hartmann R, et al. The intercellular adhesin involved in biofilm accumulation of *Staphylococcus epidermidis* is a linear beta-1,6-linked glucosaminoglycan: Purification and structural analysis. J Bacteriol 1996;178(1):175–83.

[64] Heilmann C, Hussain M, Peters G, Gotz F. Evidence for autolysin-mediated primary attachment of *Staphylococcus epidermidis* to a polystyrene surface. Mol Microbiol 1997;24(5):1013–24.

[65] Chang YM, Jeng WY, Ko TP, Yeh YJ, Chen CK, et al. Structural study of TcaR and its complexes with multiple antibiotics from *Staphylococcus epidermidis*. Proc Natl Acad Sci USA 2010;107(19):8617–22.

[66] Gross M, Cramton SE, Gotz F, Peschel A. Key role of teichoic acid net charge in *Staphylococcus aureus* colonization of artificial surfaces. Infect Immun 2001;69(5):3423–6.

[67] Dunne Jr. WM, Burd EM. The effects of magnesium, calcium, EDTA, and pH on the *in vitro* adhesion of *Staphylococcus epidermidis* to plastic. Microbiol Immunol 1992;36(10):1019–27.

[68] Cucarella C, Tormo MA, Knecht E, Amorena B, Lasa I, et al. Expression of the biofilm-associated protein interferes with host protein receptors of *Staphylococcus aureus* and alters the infective process. Infect Immun 2002;70(6):3180–6.

[69] Parsek MR, Singh PK. Bacterial biofilms: An emerging link to disease pathogenesis. Annu Rev Microbiol 2003;57:677−701.

[70] Tunney MM, Patrick S, Gorman SP, Nixon JR, Anderson N, et al. Improved detection of infection in hip replacements. A currently underestimated problem. J Bone Joint Surg Br 1998;80(4):568−72.

[71] Trampuz A, Widmer AF. Infections associated with orthopedic implants. Curr Opin Infect Dis 2006;19(4):349−56.

[72] Bjerkan G, Witso E, Bergh K. Sonication is superior to scraping for retrieval of bacteria in biofilm on titanium and steel surfaces *in vitro*. Acta Orthop 2009;80(2):245−50.

[73] Arciola CR, Campoccia D, Baldassarri L, Donati ME, Pirini V, et al. Detection of biofilm formation in *Staphylococcus epidermidis* from implant infections. Comparison of a PCR-method that recognizes the presence of *ica* genes with two classic phenotypic methods. J Biomed Mater Res A 2006;76(2):425−30.

[74] Nucci C, Artini M, Pasmore M, Missiroli F, Costerton JW, et al. A microbiological and confocal microscopy study documenting a slime-producing *Staphylococcus epidermidis* isolated from a nylon corneal suture of a patient with antibiotic-resistant endophthalmitis. Graefes Arch Clin Exp Ophthalmol 2005;243(9):951−4.

[75] Stoodley P, Nistico L, Johnson S, Lasko LA, Baratz M, et al. Direct demonstration of viable *Staphylococcus aureus* biofilms in an infected total joint arthroplasty. A case report. J Bone Joint Surg Am 2008;90(8):1751−8.

[76] Stoodley P, Braxton EE, Nistico L, Hall-Stoodley L, Johnson S, et al. Direct demonstration of a *Staphylococcus* biofilm in an external ventricular drain in a patient with a history of recurrent ventriculoperitoneal shunt failure. Pediatric Neurosurgery 2010;46(2):127−32.

[77] Stoodley P, Conti S, DeMeo PJ, Nistico L, Melton-Kreft R, Johnson S, et al. Characterization of a mixed MRSA/MRSE biofilm in an explanted total ankle arthroplasty. FEMS IMM 2011;62(1):66−74.

[78] Hall-Stoodley L, Hu FZ, Gieseke A, Nistico L, Nguyen D, et al. Direct detection of bacterial biofilms on the middle-ear mucosa of children with chronic otitis media. JAMA 2006;296(2):202−11.

[79] James GA, Swogger E, Wolcott R, Pulcini E, Secor P, et al. Biofilms in chronic wounds. Wound Repair Regeno 2008;16(1):37−44.

[80] Schlafer S, Nordhoff M, Wyss C, Strub S, Hubner J, et al. Involvement of *Guggenheimella bovis* in digital dermatitis lesions of dairy cows. Vet Microbiol 2008;128(1−2):118−25.

[81] Bjarnsholt T, Tolker-Nielsen T, Givskov M, Janssen M, Christensen LH. Detection of bacteria by fluorescence *in situ* hybridization in culture-negative soft tissue filler lesions. Dermatol Surg 2009;35(Suppl. 2):1620−4.

[82] Brady RA, Leid JG, Kofonow J, Costerton JW, Shirtliff ME. Immunoglobulins to surface-associated biofilm immunogens provide a novel means of visualization of methicillin-resistant *Staphylococcus aureus* biofilms. Appl Environ Microbiol 2007;73(20):6612−9.

[83] Li Y, Ku CY, Xu J, Saxena D, Caufield PW. Survey of oral microbial diversity using PCR-based denaturing gradient gel electrophoresis. J Dent Res 2005;84(6):559−64.

[84] Dempsey KE, Riggio MP, Lennon A, Hannah VE, Ramage G, et al. Identification of bacteria on the surface of clinically infected and non-infected prosthetic hip joints removed during revision arthroplasties by 16S rRNA gene sequencing and by microbiological culture. Arthritis Res Ther 2007;9(3):R46.

[85] Hamady M, Walker JJ, Harris JK, Gold NJ, Knight R. Error-correcting barcoded primers for pyrosequencing hundreds of samples in multiplex. Nat Methods 2008;5(3):235−7.

[86] McKenna P, Hoffmann C, Minkah N, Aye PP, Lackner A, et al. The macaque gut microbiome in health, lentiviral infection, and chronic enterocolitis. PLoS Pathog 2008;4(2):e20.

[87] Ecker DJ, Sampath R, Massire C, Blyn LB, Hall TA, et al. Ibis T5000: A universal biosensor approach for microbiology. Nat Rev Microbiol 2008;6(7):553−8.

[88] Costerton JW, Post JC, Ehrlich GD, Hu FZ, Kreft R, Nistico L, et al. New methods for the detection of orthopaedic and other biofilm infections. FEMS Immuno Microbiol 2011;61(2):133−40.

[89] Otten JE, Wiedmann-Al-Ahmad M, Jahnke H, Pelz K. Bacterial colonization on different suture materials: A potential risk for intraoral dentoalveolar surgery. J Biomed Mater Res B Appl Biomater 2005;74(1):627–35.

[90] Edmiston CE, Seabrook GR, Goheen MP, Krepel CJ, Johnson CP, et al. Bacterial adherence to surgical sutures: Can antibacterial-coated sutures reduce the risk of microbial contamination?. J Am Coll Surg 2006;203(4):481–9.

[91] Wissing J, van Vroonhoven TJ, Schattenkerk ME, Veen HF, Ponsen RJ, et al. Fascia closure after midline laparotomy: Results of a randomized trial. Br J Surg 1987;74(8):738–41.

[92] Osterberg B, Blomstedt B. Effect of suture materials on bacterial survival in infected wounds. An experimental study. Acta Chir Scand 1979;145(7):431–4.

[93] Osterberg B. Influence of capillary multifilament sutures on the antibacterial action of inflammatory cells in infected wounds. Acta Chir Scand 1983;149(8):751–7.

[94] Kathju S, Nistico L, Hall-Stoodley L, Post JC, Ehrlich GD, et al. Chronic surgical site infection due to suture-associated polymicrobial biofilm. Surg Infect (Larchmt) 2009;10(5):457–61.

[95] Kathju S, Lasko LA, Nistico L, Colella JJ, Stoodley P. Cutaneous fistula from the gastric remnant resulting from a chronic suture-associated biofilm infection. Obes Surg 2010;20(2):251–6.

[96] Hodgson NC, Malthaner RA, Ostbye T. The search for an ideal method of abdominal fascial closure: A meta-analysis. Ann Surg 2000;231(3):436–42.

[97] van't Riet M, Steyerberg EW, Nellensteyn J, Bonjer HJ, Jeekel J. Meta-analysis of techniques for closure of midline abdominal incisions. Br J Surg 2002;89(11):1350–6.

[98] Storch ML, Rothenburger SJ, Jacinto G. Experimental efficacy study of coated VICRYL plus antibacterial suture in guinea pigs challenged with *Staphylococcus aureus*. Surg Infect (Larchmt) 2004;5(3):281–8.

[99] Ming X, Nichols M, Rothenburger S. *In vivo* antibacterial efficacy of MONOCRYL plus antibacterial suture (Poliglecaprone 25 with triclosan). Surg Infect (Larchmt) 2007;8(2):209–14.

[100] Ming X, Rothenburger S, Nichols MM. *In vivo* and *in vitro* antibacterial efficacy of PDS plus (polidioxanone with triclosan) suture. Surg Infect (Larchmt) 2008;9(4):451–7.

[101] Justinger C, Moussavian MR, Schlueter C, Kopp B, Kollmar O, et al. Antibacterial [corrected] coating of abdominal closure sutures and wound infection. Surgery 2009;145(3):330–4.

[102] Engelsman AF, van der Mei HC, Busscher HJ, Ploeg RJ. Morphological aspects of surgical meshes as a risk factor for bacterial colonization. Br J Surg 2008;95(8):1051–9.

[103] Aydinuraz K, Agalar C, Agalar F, Ceken S, Duruyurek N, et al. *In vitro* S. epidermidis and S. aureus adherence to composite and lightweight polypropylene grafts. J Surg Res 2009;157(1):e79–86.

[104] Engelsman AF, Krom BP, Busscher HJ, van Dam GM, Ploeg RJ, et al. Antimicrobial effects of an NO-releasing poly(ethylene vinylacetate) coating on soft-tissue implants *in vitro* and in a murine model. Acta Biomater 2009;5(6):1905–10.

[105] Senaratne W, Andruzzi L, Ober CK. Self-assembled monolayers and polymer brushes in biotechnology: Current applications and future perspectives. Biomacromolecules 2005;6(5):2427–48.

[106] Khoo X, Hamilton P, O'Toole GA, Snyder BD, Kenan DJ, et al. Directed assembly of PEGylated-peptide coatings for infection-resistant titanium metal. J Am Chem Soc 2009;131(31):10992–7.

[107] Zhao L, Chu PK, Zhang Y, Wu Z. Antibacterial coatings on titanium implants. J Biomed Mater Res B Appl Biomater 2009;91(1):470–80.

[108] Hanssen AD, Patel R, Osmon DR. Editorial comment. Clin Orthop Relat Res 2005;437:2.

[109] NIH. NIH Consensus statement on total knee replacement NIH. NIH Consens State Sci Statements 2003;20(1):1–34.

[110] Cui Q, Mihalko WM, Shields JS, Ries M, Saleh KJ. Antibiotic-impregnated cement spacers for the treatment of infection associated with total hip or knee arthroplasty. J Bone Joint Surg Am 2007;89(4):871–82.

[111] Gristina AG, Costerton JW. Bacterial adherence to biomaterials and tissue. The

significance of its role in clinical sepsis. J Bone Joint Surg Am 1985;67(2):264–73.

[112] Neut D, van Horn JR, van Kooten TG, van der Mei HC, Busscher HJ. Detection of biomaterial-associated infections in orthopaedic joint implants. Clin Orthop Relat Res 2003;413:261–8.

[113] Antoci Jr. V, King SB, Jose B, Parvizi J, Zeiger AR, et al. Vancomycin covalently bonded to titanium alloy prevents bacterial colonization. J Orthop Res 2007;25(7):858–66.

[114] Antoci Jr. V, Adams CS, Hickok NJ, Shapiro IM, Parvizi J. Vancomycin bound to Ti rods reduces periprosthetic infection: Preliminary study. Clin Orthop Relat Res 2007;461:88–95.

[115] Aviv M, Berdicevsky I, Zilberman M. Gentamicin-loaded bioresorbable films for prevention of bacterial infections associated with orthopedic implants. J Biomed Mater Res A 2007;83(1):10–9.

[116] Cook G, Costerton JW, Darouiche RO. Direct confocal microscopy studies of the bacterial colonization *in vitro* of a silver-coated heart valve sewing cuff. Int J Antimicrob Agents 2000;13(3):169–73.

[117] Nablo BJ, Rothrock AR, Schoenfisch MH. Nitric oxide-releasing sol-gels as antibacterial coatings for orthopedic implants. Biomaterials 2005;26(8):917–24.

[118] Hetrick EM, Shin JH, Paul HS, Schoenfisch MH. Anti-biofilm efficacy of nitric oxide-releasing silica nanoparticles. Biomaterials 2009;30(14):2782–9.

[119] de Nys R, Givskov M, Kumar N, Kjelleberg S, Steinberg PD. Furanones. Prog Mol Subcell Biol 2006;42:55–86.

[120] Davies DG, Parsek MR, Pearson JP, Iglewski BH, Costerton JW, et al. The involvement of cell-to-cell signals in the development of a bacterial biofilm. Science 1998;280(5361):295–8.

[121] Camilli A, Bassler BL. Bacterial small-molecule signaling pathways. Science 2006;311(5764):1113–6.

[122] Rickard AH, Palmer Jr. RJ, Blehert DS, Campagna SR, Semmelhack MF, et al. Autoinducer 2: A concentration-dependent signal for mutualistic bacterial biofilm growth. Mol Microbiol 2006;60(6):1446–56.

[123] Kiran MD, Giacometti A, Cirioni O, Balaban N. Suppression of biofilm related, device-associated infections by staphylococcal quorum sensing inhibitors. Int J Artif Organs 2008;31(9):761–70.

[124] Hengge R. Principles of c-di-GMP signalling in bacteria. Nat Rev Microbiol 2009;7(4):263–73.

[125] Salta M, Wharton JA, Stoodley P, Dennington SP, Goodes LR, et al. Designing biomimetic antifouling surfaces. Phil Trans A, Royal Society 2010;368(1929):4729–54.

[126] Hoffman LR, D'Argenio DA, MacCoss MJ, Zhang Z, Jones RA, et al. Aminoglycoside antibiotics induce bacterial biofilm formation. Nature 2005;436(7054):1171–5.

[127] Kwok CS, Mourad PD, Crum LA, Ratner BD. Self-assembled molecular structures as ultrasonically-responsive barrier membranes for pulsatile drug delivery. J Biomed Mater Res 2001;57(2):151–64.

[128] Norris P, Noble M, Francolini I, Vinogradov AM, Stewart PS, et al. Ultrasonically controlled release of ciprofloxacin from self-assembled coatings on poly(2-hydroxyethyl methacrylate) hydrogels for *Pseudomonas aeruginosa* biofilm prevention. Antimicrob Agents Chemother 2005;49(10):4272–9.

[129] Khoury AE, Lam K, Ellis B, Costerton JW. Prevention and control of bacterial infections associated with medical devices. ASAIO J 1992;38(3):M174–8.

[130] Del Pozo JL, Rouse MS, Euba G, Kang CI, Mandrekar JN, et al. The electricidal effect is active in an experimental model of *Staphylococcus* epidermidis chronic foreign body osteomyelitis. Antimicrob Agents Chemother 2009;53(10):4064–8.

[131] Del Pozo JL, Rouse MS, Mandrekar JN, Sampedro MF, Steckelberg JM, et al. Effect of electrical current on the activities of antimicrobial agents against *Pseudomonas aeruginosa, Staphylococcus aureus*, and *Staphylococcus epidermidis* biofilms. Antimicrob Agents Chemother 2009;53(1):35–40.

[132] Vaudaux PE, Lew DP, Waldvogel FA. Host factors predisposing to and influencing therapy of foreign body infections. In: Bisno AL, Waldvogel FA, editors. Infections Associated With Indwelling Medical Devices.

Washington, DC: American Society for Microbiology; 1994. p. 1–29.
[133] Sampedro MF, Patel R. Infections associated with long-term prosthetic devices. Infect Dis Clin North Am 2007;21(3):785–819.
[134] Laibinis PE, Hickman JJ, Wrighton MS, Whitesides GM. Orthogonal self-assembled monolayers: Alkanethiols on gold and alkane carboxylic acids on alumina. Science 1989;245(4920):845–7.
[135] Hederos M, Konradsson P, Liedberg B. Synthesis and self-assembly of galactose-terminated alkanethiols and their ability to resist proteins. Langmuir 2005;21(7):2971–80.
[136] Jiang W, Zhitenev N, Bao Z, Meng H, Abusch-Magder D, et al. Structure and bonding issues at the interface between gold and self-assembled conjugated dithiol monolayers. Langmuir 2005;21(19):8751–7.
[137] Ostuni E, Chapman RG, Liang MN, Meluleni G, Pier G, et al. Self-assembled monolayers that resist the adsorption of proteins and the adhesion of bacterial and mammalian cells. Langmuir 2001;17(20):6336–43.
[138] Kang SM, Rho J, Choi IS, Messersmith PB, Lee H. Norepinephrine: Material-independent, multifunctional surface modification reagent. J Am Chem Soc 2009;131(37):13224–5.
[139] Statz AR, Meagher RJ, Barron AE, Messersmith PB. New peptidomimetic polymers for antifouling surfaces. J Am Chem Soc 2005;127(22):7972–3.
[140] Kruszewski KM, Nistico L, Longwell MJ, Hynes MJ, Maurer JA, Hall-Stoodley L, et al. Reducing Staphylococcus aureus biofilm formation on stainless steel 316L using functionalized self-assembled monolayers. Mater Sci Eng C Mater Biol Appl 2013;33(4):2059–69.
[141] Espeland EM, Wetzel RG. Complexation, stabilization, and UV photolysis of extracellular and surface-bound glucosidase and alkaline phosphatase: Implications for biofilm microbiota. Microb Ecol 2001;42(4):572–85.
[142] Dibdin GH, Assinder SJ, Nichols WW, Lambert PA. Mathematical model of beta-lactam penetration into a biofilm of *Pseudomonas aeruginosa* while undergoing simultaneous inactivation by released beta-lactamases. J Antimicrob Chemother 1996;38(5):757–69.
[143] Schumacher JF, Carman ML, Estes TG, Feinberg AW, Wilson LH, et al. Engineered antifouling microtopographies: Effect of feature size, geometry, and roughness on settlement of zoospores of the green alga Ulva. Biofouling 2007;23(1–2):55–62.
[144] Chung KK, Schumacher JF, Sampson EM, Burne RA, Antonelli PJ, et al. Impact of engineered surface microtopography on biofilm formation of *Staphylococcus aureus*. Biointerphases 2007;2(2):89–94.

6 Adhesives for Medical and Dental Applications

Sina Ebnesajjad
President, FluoroConsultants Group, LLC

OUTLINE

6.1 Introduction	103
6.2 Natural Adhesives	104
6.3 Synthetic and Semisynthetic Adhesives	104
6.4 Cyanoacrylic Adhesives	104
6.4.1 Medical Grade Cyanoacrylate Adhesives	107
6.4.2 Commercial Grades of Cyanoacrylate Tissue Adhesives	109
6.5 Test Methods to Characterize Strength of Tissue Adhesives	110
6.6 Medical and Dental Applications of Adhesives	111
6.6.1 Adhesives for Skin Closure	112
6.6.2 Case Studies of Tissue Adhesives	112
6.6.2.1 Comparison of Effects of Suture and Tissue Adhesive on Bacterial Counts	112
6.6.2.2 Sutureless Anastomoses of Small and Medium Vessels	114
6.6.2.3 Tissue Adhesive as Dressing after Open Pediatric Urological Procedures	114
6.6.2.4 Tissue Adhesive Applications in Gastrointestinal Endoscopic Procedures	115
6.6.2.5 Tissue Adhesives in Topical Skin Wounds	116
6.6.2.6 Tissue Adhesive for Closure of Hernia Incisions	116
6.6.2.7 Use of Tissue Adhesive for Skin Closure in Plastic Surgery	119
6.7 Bone Adhesives	119
6.8 Dental Applications of Adhesives	119
6.8.1 Methacrylic Acid	121
6.8.2 Methyl Methacrylate	122
6.8.3 Hydroxy Ethyl Methacrylate	123
6.8.4 4-Methacryloyloxyethyl Trimellitic Acid	123
6.8.5 4-Acryloyloxyethyl Trimellitate Anhydride	123
6.8.6 10-Methacryloyloxydecyl Dihydrogen Phosphate	123
6.8.7 Other Monomers	124
References	124

This chapter focuses on adhesives used in direct physiological contact in dental and medical procedures. Activity in both areas has been quite extensive outside the United States for decades. In contrast, adhesive use in medical devices, patches, and plasters has been ongoing in the United States for a long time. In the case of medical devices, adhesion is concerned with the joining of materials such as plastics, elastomers, textiles, metals, and ceramics, which are examined in other chapters of the present volume and are covered in various references [1–6], The coverage of this chapter is devoted to applications where adhesives are in direct contact with tissues and other live organs.

6.1 Introduction

The use of adhesives in medicine and dentistry is often critical and functional and with little visibility to patients. Infant immunization, flu shots, restorative dental fillings, blood transfusions, heart bypass surgery, urological surgery, anesthetic administration, intravenous drug delivery, and numerous other medical procedures would not be possible today if not for advanced adhesives. The modern adhesives are used to assemble thousands of medical devices around the world, or they are used in direct physiological interactive modes [7].

There are different types of commercially available tissue adhesives, classified into three categories: natural or biological, synthetic and semisynthetic, and biomimetic adhesives. The biological tissue adhesives such as fibrin glues and collagen are quite effective in select applications. Their drawbacks are high cost and limited availability. Biomimetic adhesives are based on adhesion of algae to wet surface and the Gecko's ability "to stick" its paws to surfaces [8].

6.2 Natural Adhesives

Surgical adhesives and sealants based on natural polymers, cross-linked via biochemical reactions, offer in general a more biocompatible alternative to synthetic glues. The main biological adhesives are based on fibrin and collagen. Gelatin and polysaccharide-based adhesives are newer adhesive classes which have attracted attention and research. Fibrin sealants are made from a number of components produced from pooled human plasma that enables the adhesive to mimic the final stages of blood clotting. The most basic fibrin sealants consist of combinations of thrombin and fibrinogen. Collagen-based adhesives adsorb blood and coagulation products on their fibers, trapping them in the interstices and adhering well to the wound. This biopolymer also induces platelet adhesion and aggregation, and activates coagulation factors [9].

6.3 Synthetic and Semisynthetic Adhesives

Semisynthetic and synthetic surgical adhesives include gelatine–resorcinol–formaldehyde (GRF), urethane prepolymers, and cyanoacrylates. These adhesives have some shortcomings such as low bioabsortion and metabolic rates, cytotoxicity (low biocompatibility), low adherence to wet surfaces and chronic inflammation induced by the release of formaldehyde from GRF, and cyanoacrylate polymers and aromatic diamine from aromatic polyurethanes [10].

6.4 Cyanoacrylic Adhesives

These so-called *wonder* adhesives are marginally thermosetting materials and were first introduced commercially by Eastman Chemicals. They form strong thermosetting bonds between many materials without heat or an added catalyst. They are particularly useful in bonding metal to nonmetal. Lap-shear strengths of 13.7 MPa have been reported. However, the resistance capability of these adhesives to moisture is still somewhat low [11]. These materials set very quickly when squeezed out to thin film between many types of adherends.

A cyanoacrylate adhesive is a relatively rapid curing adhesive also from the acrylic family tree, but has a completely different cure system. Cyanoacrylate monomer (Figure 6.1) is made from

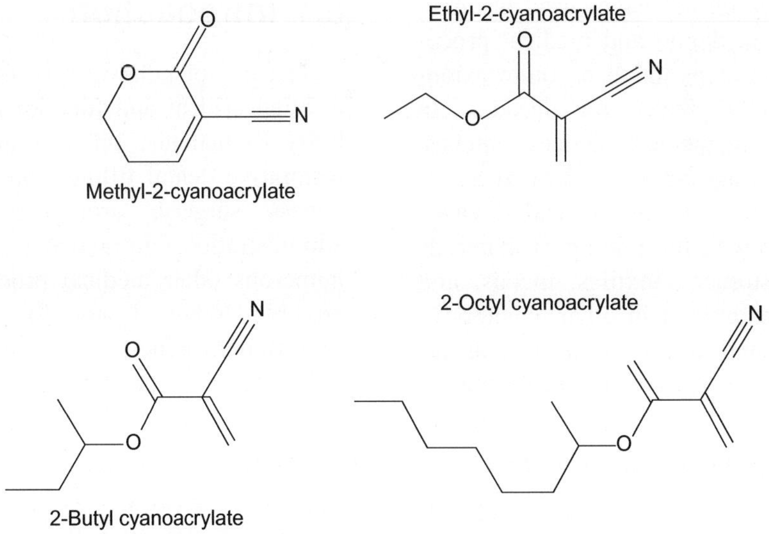

Figure 6.1 Structures of some cyanoacrylate monomers.

a complex chemical process. The monomer produces a very reactive polymerization. The reaction or polymerization process is stabilized and the monomer is kept in the liquid state by the addition of a small amount of an acid stabilizer material [12].

When a drop of cyanoacrylate adhesive is put on the surface of a part, the acid stabilizer molecules react with the water molecules present on the surface of the part from the relative humidity in the air. The reaction of the water and acid causes the acid stabilizer to be neutralized. The cyanoacrylate molecules then react with each other and form polymer chains without cross-linking [12].

Cyanoacrylate adhesives undergo anionic polymerization in the presence of a weak base, such as water, and are stabilized through the addition of a weak acid. The stabilizer is usually in the form of a weak acidic gas such as SO_2, NO, or BF_3. An essential function of the stabilizer is to prevent polymerization in the container, which is usually made of polyethylene. When the adhesive contacts a slightly alkaline surface, trace amounts of adsorbed water or hydroxide ions (OH^-) that are present on the substrate's surface neutralize the acidic stabilizer in the adhesive, resulting in rapid polymerization as shown in Figure 6.2.

The amount of stabilizer molecules in cyanoacrylate is very small—measured in parts per million—and very little moisture molecules are required to cause rapid polymerization. Cyanoacrylates begin to form polymer chains immediately on contact with the water vapor on the surface of the part. If parts are moved during initial contact, the polymerization process and polymer chains are stopped. The process must start again at a new catalyzed site [12].

Cyanoacrylates are very rapid in curing and provide high bond strengths on plastic and rubber materials. These adhesives are versatile which renders them highly useful in all industries. Some of the larger application areas are in electronics for printed circuit board wires and components, and in medical technology for disposable plastic medical devices. Other applications include toy, small and large appliance, automotive, and cosmetic packaging. Applications exist in all industries for repair of all rubber and plastic parts as well as some metal parts. The consumer market is a large volume user of cyanoacrylate adhesives for repairing everything in the home from wallpaper tears to broken toys to torn and false fingernails.

Cyanoacrylate adhesive can be made from different acrylate monomers, such as methyl, ethyl, butyl, and isopropyl. These molecules differ in size and adhesives made from them exhibit different physical properties. Methyl is the smallest molecule and seems to work best on metal and rubber parts, whereas ethyl works best on plastic parts. Many modifications can be made to the monomers to alter or improve their properties as adhesives. They can be toughened with rubber or formulated to have low odor, resistance to thermal cycling, or less sensitivity to surface conditions, which tend to stabilize the adhesive and slow down the cure [12].

As with other acrylics, the monomers are liquids of low viscosity that polymerize very easily in the presence of a slightly basic surface containing adsorbed water. Polymerization is ionic. The resulting polymers have different properties, depending on the alkyl group. The methyl ester (methyl-2-cyanoacrylate) is the most commonly used compound. This material is formulated with a thickener (to prevent starved joints from being formed) and a plasticizer to make it more resistant to shock loading. The thickener can be a polymer of the same

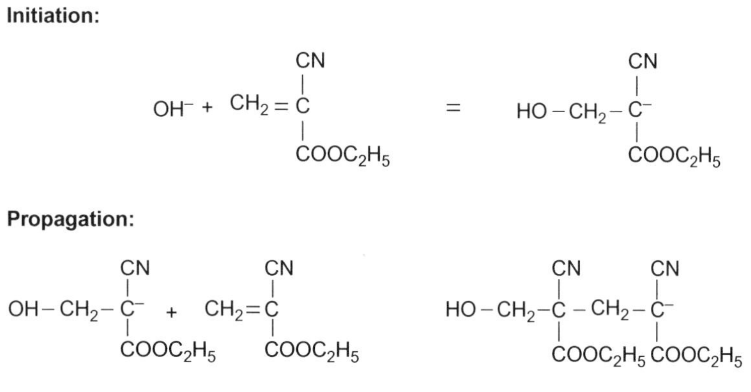

Initiation:

$$OH^- + CH_2=C(CN)(COOC_2H_5) \ = \ HO-CH_2-C^-(CN)(COOC_2H_5)$$

Propagation:

$$OH-CH_2-C^-(CN)(COOC_2H_5) + CH_2=C(CN)(COOC_2H_5) \ \rightarrow \ HO-CH_2-C(CN)(COOC_2H_5)-CH_2-C^-(CN)(COOC_2H_5)$$

Figure 6.2 Polymerization reaction of cyanoacrylate adhesives [13].

monomer. An essential feature is a stabilizer to prevent polymerization in the adhesive container, which is usually made of polyethylene [14].

The polymerization of cyanoacrylates is inhibited by low pH (high acidity), thus it does not proceed satisfactorily on acid surfaces such as wood. The suggested incorporation of poly-N-vinyl pyridine or polyethyleneamine, or even simple amines, presumably serves the dual purpose of thickening the liquid and increasing the pH.

Adhesives based on higher homologs than the methyl form have been in use for a number of years. These include the ethyl, propyl, and butyl esters of cyanoacrylic acid. Moisture resistance of the methyl-2-cyanoacrylate is only fair. Ethyl cyanoacrylate has been shown to form stronger bonds than the methyl form between several different types of plastic surfaces. The higher homologs, however, generally do not form bonds as strongly as the methyl form. The most important step in the successful application of a cyanoacrylate adhesive is the application of a thin adhesive film between two well-mated surfaces. The thinner the film is, the faster the rate of bond formation, and the higher the bond strength. Bond strength is dependent on proper surface preparation.

In general, aging properties of the cyanoacrylates are good. Rubber-to-rubber and rubber-to-metal bonds typically have endured outdoor weathering for over 7 years. These bonds have also passed stringent water-immersion and salt-spray tests. Plastic-to-plastic and plastic-to-rubber bonds have aged satisfactorily for 3–5 years. Metal-to-metal bonds generally age rather poorly, except under special conditions where the minimal glue line is exposed to moisture. Solvent resistance is also generally satisfactory. Dilute alkaline solutions weaken the bond considerably, while dilute acid solutions weaken it to a lesser degree. Impact resistance is generally poor because of the thin, inflexible bond.

This is especially true with two rigid substrates, such as metals. The methyl cyanoacrylate bond melts at approximately 165°C. Prolonged exposure to temperatures in this range results in a gradual but permanent breakdown of the bond. Generally, the upper temperature limit for continuous exposure is about 77°C. At low temperatures, bonds remain intact at least down to −54°C. Grades of cyanoacrylates with specialized improved properties are available. For example, one grade has improved heat resistance to 246°C, high viscosity, and very fast setting ability [15].

Among the advantages of the cyanoacrylates are the following (see also Table 6.1):

- Very fast bond formation
- High bond strength with thin glue line
- No added catalyst or mixing needed
- No solvent to evaporate during bond formation
- Contact pressure is usually sufficient
- Very low shrinkage
- Economical because of minute quantities needed, although relatively expensive.

Table 6.1 Benefits and Limitation of Cyanoacrylate Adhesives [13]

Benefits	Limitations
• Excellent adhesion to a wide variety of substrates	• Blooming/frosting
• Substrate variety	• Difficult to cure fillet or exposed liquid adhesive without activator
• Simple cure mechanism	• Limited gap cure
• Rapid strength development	• Stress cracking could occur to some plastics
• High strength possible on polyolefins and fluorocarbons using primers	• Soluble in polar solvents
• Available in USP Class VI compliant formulations	• Thermal and chemical stability not as good as with certain other structural adhesives
• High shear strength	• Unmodified formulations have low peel **and** impact strengths
• No measuring or mixing required	• Relatively high materials cost
	• Pungent odor associated with early formulations

The Loctite Corporation offers a rubber-toughened cyanoacrylate adhesive, such as 380 Black Max®, which is reported to achieve improved strength, resiliency, and fast fixturing at the expense of a rather limited shelf life (about 4 months) [16]. This adhesive cures to fixturing strength in 2 min in the case of most substrates. It reaches to 80% strength in 24 h and to full strength in 72 h (Table 6.2). On aluminum, its average strength is 16.6 MPa after full room temperature cure, vs. 6.2 MPa for a typical epoxy adhesive and 3.8 MPa for "instant" adhesives. After 240 h of tensile-shear thermal-cycling tests, this adhesive improved its strength to 21.3 MPa for "instant" adhesive. Loctite claims that this adhesive is consistently 20 times stronger than epoxies on aluminum, 10 times stronger on neoprene, 4 times stronger on steel, and 2 times stronger on epoxy/glass after the tests. This adhesive is designed for assembly-line cure (Table 6.3) [17].

6.4.1 Medical Grade Cyanoacrylate Adhesives

Butyl cyanoacrylate is an intermediate-length cyanoacrylate (Figure 6.1) adhesive that was the first product to be broadly used for closing cutaneous wounds. This compound has been approved for use in Europe and Canada as Histoacryl® Blue (trademark of Aesculap, Inc.) and GluStitch® (trademark of GluStitch, Inc.) for nearly 40 years. It had not been approved by the US Food and Drug Administration (FDA) for use in the United States for a long time. In Europe, Canada, and Japan, it

Table 6.2 Typical Performance of Cured Loctite 380 Cyanoacrylate Adhesive [16]

Adhesive properties		
After 24 h at 22°C		
Lap shear strength, ISO 4587		
Steel (grit-blasted)	N/mm² (psi)	26 (3,770)
Aluminum (etched)	N/mm² (psi)	18 (2,610)
ABS	N/mm² (psi)	>6 (>870)
PVC	N/mm² (psi)	>4 (>580)
Polycarbonate	N/mm² (psi)	>5 (>725)
Phenolic	N/mm² (psi)	10 (1,450)
Neoprene	N/mm² (psi)	>10 (>1,450)
Nitrile	N/mm² (psi)	>10 (>1,450)
Tensile strength, ISO 6922		
Steel (grit-blasted)	N/mm² (psi)	18.5 (2700)
After 48 h at 22°C		
Lap shear strength, ISO 4587		
Steel (grit-blasted)	N/mm² (psi)	≥17.2^{LMS} (≥2,495)
Cured for 24 h at 22°C, followed by 24 h at 121°C, tested at 121°C		
Lap shear strength, ISO 4587		
Steel (grit-blasted)	N/mm² (psi)	≥6.9^{LMS} (≥1,000)
Cured for 24 h at 22°C, followed by 24 h at 121°C, tested at 22°C		
Lap shear strength, ISO 4587		
Steel (grit-blasted)	N/mm² (psi)	≥19.3^{LMS} (≥2,800)

LMS, Loctite material specification.

Table 6.3 Bond Strength of Methyl or Ethyl Cyanoacrylate Adhesive as a Function of Substrate and Time [13]

Joint Substrates	Age of Bond	Shear Strength, psi
Steel–steel	10 min	1920
	48 h	3300
Aluminum–aluminum	10 min	1480
	48 h	2270
Butyl rubber–butyl rubber	10 min	150[a]
SBR rubber–SBR rubber	10 min	130
Neoprene–neoprene	10 min	100[a]
SBR rubber–phenolic	10 min	110[a]
Phenolic–phenolic	10 min	930[a]
	48 h	940[a]
Phenolic–aluminum	10 min	650
	48 h	920[a]
Aluminum–nylon	10 min	500
	48 h	950
Nylon–nylon	10 min	330
	48 h	600
Acrylic–acrylic	10 min	810[a]
	48 h	790[a]
ABS–ABS	10 min	640[a]
	48 h	710[a]
Polystyrene–polystyrene	10 min	330[a]
Polycarbonate–polycarbonate	10 min	790
	48 h	950[a]
Polyester glass–polyester glass	10 min	680

[a]Substrate failure.

has been used for middle ear procedures, to close cerebrospinal leaks, to repair incisions and lacerations, and to affix skin since the 1970s [18–24].

Short-chain cyanoacrylates (methyl, ethyl) are toxic to tissue; this is not the case with butyl cyanoacrylate when applied topically. In an experimental model of incision wound healing in hamsters, butyl cyanoacrylate resulted in less inflammation than 4.0 silk sutures on histologic assessment [19]. Randomized clinical trials were conducted in a study of just under 100 patients with facial lacerations suitable for tissue adhesive closure. The patients underwent closure using either butyl cyanoacrylate or octyl-2-cyanoacrylate (2-OCA), and results failed to reveal a difference in cosmetic result after 3 months. The ratings were from photographs by a plastic surgeon using a visual analog scale [25]. A toxic reaction was prevented by taking precaution to prevent the adhesive from being trapped in the wound itself might cause [26]. Because of these concerns, n-butylcyanoacrylate has been recently approved by FDA for use in the United States. In 2010, B. Braun manufactured Histoacryl that consists of n-butyl-2 cyanoacrylate. This sterile, liquid topical skin adhesive is available in two formulations: Histoacryl and Histoacryl Blue [27].

2-OCA has a longer chain than butyl cyanoacrylate. It was approved by the FDA for use in the United States in August 1998 for certain types of laceration. Its applications have been expanded and are now marketed as Dermabond® (a trademark of Ethicon, Inc., a Johnson & Johnson Company) topical skin adhesive for closure of lacerations and incisions in place of sutures or staples. Later on, a 2-OCA formulated for greater flexibility, Liquid Bandage, was approved for use in the over-the-counter market in the United States for the treatment of minor cuts and abrasions [28].

The longer side chain gives 2-OCA several potential advantages over shorter chain cyanoacrylates. 2-OCA, for instance, produces a stronger bond and is more flexible than butyl cyanoacrylate. It has four times higher volumetric break strength than butyl cyanoacrylate [29]. The increased strength and flexibility and reduced risk of tissue toxicity, 2-OCA is now widely used in the United States for closure of wounds. It is currently one of the best selling bandage brands in the United States.

Here is an excerpt of a 2004 but useful review of the tissue adhesives by Singer and Thode [30]: "Octylcyanoacrylate is a medical grade topical tissue adhesive that has been approved for closing surgical incisions and traumatic lacerations. We reviewed animal and human studies that evaluated its use for a variety of surgical indications and specialties. We also performed a metaanalysis of all clinical trials using octylcyanoacrylate. Data sources: Animal and human studies published in peer-reviewed articles as well as published abstracts. A search of Medline was performed using the MESH terms: tissue adhesives, cyanoacrylates, and octylcyanoacrylate. The current review and metaanalysis demonstrate that octylcyanoacrylate can be used successfully in a wide variety of clinical and surgical settings for multiple types of wounds covering most of the surface of the human body. Prior knowledge of the limitations and technical aspects specific to wound closure with octylcyanoacrylate as well as appropriate wound selection and preparation will help ensure optimal results."

6.4.2 Commercial Grades of Cyanoacrylate Tissue Adhesives

Some of the manufacturers of cyanoacrylate tissue adhesives are listed below:

Company Name: AESCULAP, Inc.
Address: 3773 CORPORATE PKWY
Center Valley, PA 18034
Product: TISSUE ADHESIVE
Proprietary Device Name: HISTOACRYL® & HISTOACRYL BLUE® TOPICAL SKIN ADHESIVE
Web site: www.aesculapusa.com

Company Name: CLOSURE MEDICAL CORP.
Address: 5250 GREENS DAIRY RD.
Raleigh, NC 27616
Product: TOPICAL TISSUE ADHESIVE
Proprietary Device Name: DERMABOND® TOPICAL SKIN ADHESIVE
Website: www.closuremed.com

Company Name: ETHICON, INC.
Address: Route 22 West
Somerville, NJ 08876
Product: TISSUE ADHESIVE
Proprietary Device Name: DERMABOND® TOPICAL SKIN ADHESIVE
Website: www.impactfs.com

Company Name: GEM S. r. l.
Address: Via dei Campi, 2—PO Box 427
Viareggio, LU, 55049, ITALY
Product: TISSUE ADHESIVE
Proprietary Device Name: Glubran2®
Website: www.gemitaly.it/web/en/glubran2.html

Company Name: HENKEL IRELAND LIMITED
ELECTRONIC AND BIOMEDICAL FACILITY
Address: Whitestown, Dublin, 24 EI
Product: TISSUE ADHESIVE
Proprietary Device Name: INDERMIL® TISSUE ADHESIVE
Website: www.henkel.com/cps/rde/xchg/henkel_com/hs.xsl/indermil-17865.htm?automaticTransfer = 3

Company Name: MEDISAV SERVICES, INC.
Address: 56 ELSON ST., #B
Markham, Ontario, L3S 1Y7 CA
Product: TISSUE ADHESIVE FOR REPAIR OF MINOR CUTS & LACERATIONS
Proprietary Device Name: EPIDERMGLU®
Website: http://www.ethicon.com

Company Name: PRAXIS, LLC.
Address: 1110 WASHINGTON ST.
Holliston, MA 01746
Product: TISSUE ADHESIVE
Proprietary Device Name: PRAXI STAT®
Website:

Company Name: SKINSTITCH CORP.
Address: 89 OLD RIVER RD.
P.O. BOX 179
Massena, NY 13662
Product: TISSUE ADHESIVE FOR REPAIR OF MINOR CUTS & LACERATIONS
Proprietary Device Name: SKINSTITCH™
Website: www.skinstitch.com

Cyanoacrylate tissue adhesives can be used vice sutures in a number of surgical procedures contributing to make the recovery easier and more comfortable [31]. They include:

1. OB/GYN surgeries, such as C-sections where excellent cosmetic outcomes are desired [32], as well as the ability for new mothers to shower immediately and move about without the discomfort of staples or sutures [33].
2. General surgeries, such as many abdominal surgeries, back surgeries, and routine surgeries of the face, neck, arms, and legs [34].
3. Cardiovascular surgeries that may involve incisions in the arm or leg as well as the chest [34].
4. Cosmetic surgery, particularly facial incisions, on areas such as the eyelid and the nose where suture removal can be painful. No stitches means no "suture marks" [35].
5. Sports surgery, involving lacerations that may need immediate attention, to help players to return to the game [36].

Dermabond (2-octylcyanoacrylate by Ethicon, a Johnson & Johnson Company), the latest in cyanoacrylate technology, has less toxicity and almost four times the strength of N-butyl-2-cyanoacrylate. Special plasticizers have been added to the formula to provide flexibility. It is marketed to replace sutures that are 5-0 or smaller in diameter for incision or laceration repair. Patients, especially children, readily accept the idea of being "glued" over traditional methods of repair [37]. This adhesive reaches maximum bonding strength within 2.5 min and is equivalent in strength to healed tissue at 7 days post-repair [38].

Dermabond (2-octylcyanoacrylate) has been found to create [39] a microbial barrier over the wound and protect against the penetration of the following bacteria, commonly associated with surgical site infections:

Staphylococcus aureus (S. aureus)

Staphylococcus epidermidis

Enterococcus faecium

Escherichia coli (E. coli)

Pseudomonas aeruginosa.

Dermabond adhesives [39]:

1. Provide the strength of healed tissue at 7 days in less than 3 min.

2. Offer three-dimensional strength that is at least three times stronger than *n*-butyl cyanoacrylate, another leading type of adhesive.
3. Help protect and seal out bacteria that can lead to infection.
4. Promote a moist wound-healing environment that has been shown to speed the rate of epithelialization.
5. Cause less pain and relieve anxiety over sutures, particularly important for pediatric patients; have been found to be as safe and effective as conventional sutures with equivalent cosmetic results.
6. Save valuable clinical time in that they can be applied more quickly than sutures, eliminating the need for the following process:
   a. Injecting a local anesthetic into the wound
   b. Waiting for the anesthetic to numb the area
   c. Closing the wound with sutures
   d. Placing a dressing over the wound.
7. Slough off naturally over time (usually 5–10 days), eliminating the need for a follow-up visit to remove stitches.

6.5 Test Methods to Characterize Strength of Tissue Adhesives

The following four test methods are used [40] to provide a means for comparison of the adhesive strengths of tissue adhesives for use as surgical adhesives or sealants on soft tissue. These or equivalent methods may be used in support of the bench testing outlined above:

ASTM F2255-05 Standard Test Method for Strength Properties of Tissue Adhesives in Lap-Shear by Tension Loading

ASTM F2256-05 Standard Test Method for Strength Properties of Tissue Adhesives in T-Peel by Tension Loading

ASTM F2258-05 Standard Test Method for Strength Properties of Tissue Adhesives in Tension

ASTM F2458-05 Standard Test Method for Wound Closure Strength in Tissue Adhesives and Sealants.

6.6 Medical and Dental Applications of Adhesives

The use of adhesives in medical applications has been restricted, for some time, to the manufacture of self-adhesive bandages (plasters, self-adhesive strips of fabric, etc.). The first pressure sensitive adhesives used for this were based on natural rubber, decades ago. This first usage was later partially superseded by synthetic rubbers (e.g., polyisoprene, polyisobutylene). In the mid-twentieth century, pressure sensitive adhesives based on polyacrylic acid esters gained significance in general use and in the composition of bandage materials [41].

Today, adhesives are used in various areas of medicine, replacing traditional methods with "friendlier" processes. Often, stitches can be avoided by applying special cyanoacrylate adhesives to quickly close skin wounds. An advantage of this method is that the whole wound can be covered, thereby largely suppressing secondary bleeding and the risk of infection. Cyanoacrylic acid butyl ester is normally preferred over the methyl and ethyl esters because it cures more slowly and the polymerization produces less heat. Cyanoacrylic also causes less tissue irritation. By and large, this adhesive is only used for relatively small wounds, and it is occasionally used in vascular surgery.

Consider the transdermal patches where the drug delivery mechanism to the bloodstream is through the skin: adhesives enable a more efficient method of drug delivery, rather than prescribing a high-ingestion dosage (which is subsequently flushed out of the body by the liver). Transdermal patch technology is highly effective because the adhesive that sticks the patch to the skin—made of products of chemistry like acrylic, acrylic-rubber hybrid, polyisobutylene, and styrenic rubber solution—actually controls the rate at which the drug enters the body. This mechanism ensures that the drug dosage is continuously and evenly administered throughout the day, without the spikes and falls associated with medicines administered orally [41].

The applications of these patches are numerous, including smoke cessation and hormone replacement, and cardiovascular aid, such as nitroglycerin delivery, is commonplace. New transdermal patches hit the market every day, with more items like pain cessation becoming a reality. Other innovative products, such as foot care and cosmetic patches, and nasal dilator strips, have hit the market in recent years. Their existence is possible because of the unique functional properties of the pressure sensitive adhesives integral to the product [41].

One of the newest bio-adhesives on the market enables drugs to be delivered through the inside of the mouth, nasal passages, and other mucus membranes, rather than only being administered through skin. The newest bio-adhesives adhere extremely well to the soft, wet mucus membranes of the body because the adhesives are made from starch-poly acrylic acid blends, which then completely erode and disappear. Drug makers are able to put their medicine into tablet, film, or powder form, and the patient is able to attach the product directly to a mucus membrane, providing a means for controlled delivery of drugs to specific areas of the body or systemically (throughout the body) [41].

Fibrin, which is made from fibrinogen, a soluble protein recovered from blood, is a key sealing agent in heart surgery. It has a hemostatic effect, meaning that it is an antihemorrhagic agent: a substance that promotes hemostasis, the halting of blood flow. Fibrin is much gentler on the body tissues when compared to cyanoacrylates. The disadvantage of fibrin is that before use it must undergo a special treatment in order to prevent microbial infection.

The use of methacrylate-based adhesives has been a great success in orthopedics for the purpose of anchoring hip socket implants to the bone. There are currently no other types of adhesive used for this application. The adhesive products comprise (a) a powder component (a mixture of polymethyl methacrylate (PMMA) and a polymerization initiator) and (b) a liquid component (whose main components are methyl methacrylate (MMA) and a polymerization accelerator). In spite of considerable stress that these adhesives exert on bone and tissue due to intense heat development, hip and knee implants anchored using this adhesive are in 90% of cases functional for 15 years [41].

In dentistry, restorative fillings based on UV curing acrylates have largely replaced traditional filling materials such as amalgams. The products have a long pot life or *open time* (the period during which they can be used after mixing) and bond in just a minute or so when exposed to UV light.

There are numerous orthodontic appliances or devices that are used to correct dental conditions in minor and adult patients. Most of these appliances involve use of adhesives. The advent of adhesive dentistry and direct bonding of orthodontic brackets is a dramatic event that has changed the course of clinical orthodontics. Product development and technological advances have occurred quite rapidly. This rapidity has, at times, complicated the decision-making process for practitioners [42].

6.6.1 Adhesives for Skin Closure

This section reviews the use of adhesives as an alternative to stitches. The key advantage of supplanting stitches with an adhesive is that the adhesive overlays the entire wound as a continuum. The global coverage prevents secondary bleeding and reduces the risk of infection by creating a temporary barrier while healing takes place. Other advantages of gluing the skin are that it is quick, saves surgery time, is inexpensive, does not have stitch removal, and is waterproof. The disadvantage of gluing is that doing so can be messy if applied incorrectly.

One of the adhesive options is copolymeric hydrogels, comprised [43] of aminated star polyethylene glycol and dextran aldehyde (PEG:dextran). These materials exhibit physicochemical properties that can be modified to achieve organ- and tissue-specific adhesion performance. The investigators reported that resistance to failure under specific loading conditions, as well as tissue response at the adhesive material–tissue interface, can be modulated through regulation of number and density of adhesive aldehyde groups.

There are two common adhesive choices: cyanoacrylic and methyl metacrylic. Cyanoacrylic acid butyl ester is usually preferred over the methyl and ethyl esters because of its slower cure (polymerization) rate. Consequently, the polymerization produces less heat; it also causes less tissue irritation. Cyanoacrylate glue is commonly used for approximation of skin after various surgical procedures [44], and is occasionally used to embolize blood vessels [45,46] and to occlude fistulas [47].

There is no need to apply a dressing to cover the wound after gluing the skin. Apart from eyes and mucous membranes, adhesive may be used to close various clean wounds of the skin, including to cover wounds of the face if there is no contraindication. However, glue application has some disadvantages: some glue applications are messy, may not hold oozing wound edges, and may stick to the instruments and gloves. Meticulous attention to different techniques in various situations may avoid most of the disadvantages. Gluing is common in surgery, but it is not formally taught. This illustrated chapter has been written to educate junior doctors without any practical experience in using tissue glue.

FDA approved cyanoacrylate adhesives are considered comparable to 5-0 sutures but are not recommended to be used alone in high tension areas.

6.6.2 Case Studies of Tissue Adhesives

In this section, examples of the use of tissue adhesives, namely cyanoacrylates, in the closure of different types of lacerations and surgical incisions are discussed. *In vitro* and *in vivo* animal and human studies have been conducted to assess the efficacy and outcome of tissue adhesives as compared to traditional stitching.

6.6.2.1 Comparison of Effects of Suture and Tissue Adhesive on Bacterial Counts

In this study [48], the effects of closing lacerations with suture or cyanoacrylate tissue adhesive on staphylococcal counts in inoculated guinea pig lacerations are investigated. Wounds closed with adhesive alone had lower counts than wounds containing suture material ($P < 0.05$). The results of a time-kill study were consistent with a bacteriostatic adhesive effect of the adhesive against *S. aureus*.

Another study used a well diffusion method to conclude that cyanoacrylate adhesive is bacteriostatic for gram-positive organisms [49]. It is also known that suture material increases the risk of wound sepsis by serving as an adherent foreign body [49,50]. In contrast, *Staphylococcus epidermidis* adheres to cyanoacrylate adhesive, which may thus promote wound infection [51]. The authors studied the difference in wound bacterial counts among the following wound closure methods (the terms are given in parentheses): use of a cyanoacrylate adhesive alone (glue), adhesive and subcutaneous suture (glue/SQ), skin suture alone (suture), and skin suture with subcutaneous suture (suture/SQ).

Four lacerations each, with a length of 3 cm, were made parallel to the spine to deep fascia. The lacerations were inoculated with *S. aureus* (ATCC 11632) and adjusted to a spectrophotometric absorbance of 0.138–0.139. Inocula were quantified at approximately 108 CFU/ml by standard microbiological methods. After inoculating the lacerations, the four wounds on each animal were approximated in one of four ways: (1) with Nexaband Liquid (*n*-butyl-2-cyanoacrylate and D and C violet number six dye) (glue), (2) with subcutaneous suture (i.e., intradermal stitches buried beneath the skin) followed by application of Nexaband Liquid (glue/SQ), (3) with simple skin suture (suture), or (4) with intradermal subcutaneous suture followed by simple skin suture (suture/SQ).

Table 6.4 summarizes the wound data. Any lacerations subject to protocol abrogations were excluded. Wound bacterial counts for glue were significantly lower than those for glue/SQ, suture, and suture/SQ. A time-kill study of Nexaband with *S. aureus* was also performed according to National Committee for Clinical Laboratory Standards guidelines [52]. Four drops of Nexaband, the approximate amount used to close each laceration, was suspended in Trypticase soy broth before vortexing. The results of the kill study are summarized in Figure 6.3. Broth containing cyanoacrylate exhibited bacterial growth levels significantly lower than those of the control.

The study concluded that contaminated wounds sealed with cyanoacrylate alone have appreciably lower staphylococcus counts than lacerations containing suture material. The presence of suture material in some wounds may be the reason for this effect. Bacteriostatic behavior of the products containing cyanoacrylate may also be at work. No study has, however, found any adhesive present in the wound after closure.

The microbiological permeability of cyanoacrylate compounds, using Liquiseal (MedLogic Global Ltd, Plymouth, UK) as an example, was studied [53] to verify its reported primary attribute as a compound that remains impervious to microorganisms and water for 1 week following application. The occlusive dressing used was OpSite (Smith & Nephew, London, UK), commonly used in surgical procedures. The methods used in the study are well established in the investigation of bacterial penetration through various materials [54]. The organisms selected were *S. aureus* and *E. coli*, both known to be common pathogens causing surgical site infections.

Table 6.4 Bacterial Counts for Contaminated Lacerations Treated with Tissue Adhesive and Suture[a][48]

Treatment Method	Mean Bacterial Count ± SD[b]	95% Confidence Interval
Glue	1.78 ± 1.9	0.5–3.06
Glue/SQ	4.42 ± 1.92	3.1–5.7
Suture	3.72 ± 1.4	2.83–4.62
Suture/SQ	4.58 ± 1.43	3.67–5.49

[a]*The adhesive used was n-butyl-2-cyanoacrylate tissue adhesive; skin sutures were done with monofilament nylon, and subcutaneous sutures were done with braided absorbable suture.*
[b]*Values are log10 conversions of CFU per gram of tissue.*

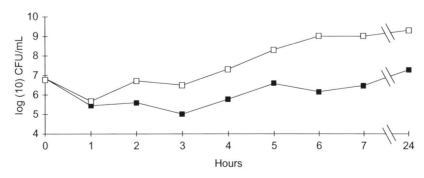

Figure 6.3 *S. aureus* kill curve [48].

This study [54] demonstrated that, as a barrier to microbiological penetration, cyanoacrylates are as effective as standard occlusive dressings. The limitations of the two types of dressing are similar; both have the potential to allow bacteria to travel around the edges of the dressing and potentially infect the wound. However, as suggested by Bady and Wongworawat, the adhesion that the cyanoacrylate compounds makes to the skin is effective in preventing the translocation of microorganisms across the skin [55].

6.6.2.2 Sutureless Anastomoses of Small and Medium Vessels

In a study in China [56], an animal model was used to assess the efficacy of sutureless anastomoses using tissue adhesives. The two cut ends of the rabbit common carotid artery were sutured by three stitches with a 1208 interval circumferentially. Then two optional threads were pulled horizontally and 0.1 ml cyanoacrylate adhesive was smeared on the attached surfaces of the two ends. The three stitches were removed after completion of anastomosis. The burst pressure of the anastomosis was measured and compared with that of a traditional sutured artery. The glued anastomosis was associated with a shorter completion time (8.25 ± 6.34 min vs. 20.67 ± 14.24 min, $P < 0.01$), less bleeding (3.17 ± 9.04 ml vs. 11.04 ± 16.28 ml, $P < 0.01$), and equivalent patency (93.8 vs. 87.5%, $P < 0.05$). The sutureless anastomosis was associated with less intimal thickening (decreased by 31.4, 24.5, 23.9, and 31.9%, $P < 0.01$ compared with the traditional suture group at 1, 2, 4, and 12 weeks, respectively). The study concluded that glued anastomoses provide an effective, simple, and feasible way for anastomosing small or medium caliber vessels. This technique can also reduce intimal injury (i.e., to the inner lining of the vessels).

Another paper [57] presents the results of an experimental study of small arterial anastomosis, combining suture with the cyanoacrylate tissue adhesive. At the distal end of the vessel, two parallel incisions were made, 180° apart from each other, and two sutures were placed passing from the proximal end to exit from the most distal part of the longitudinal incisions. The tissue adhesive was then applied to the proximal vessel, and the full-thickness vascular "lid" flap was closed over it on anterior and posterior surfaces. Eighty anastomoses were carried out at the left and the right femoral arteries of 40 Wistar rats. For all of the animals, conventional end-to-end anastomosis was carried out on the left side, and the lid technique was used on the right side. There was no statistically significant difference between the patency rates of the groups (two non-patent in control and two in the study group) ($P > 0.05$), whereas significantly reduced operation time (mean 16.2 and 10.7 min in control and study groups, respectively) ($P < 0.0001$) and bleeding time (median 1.5 and 0.5 min in control and study groups, respectively) ($P < 0.0001$) were documented in the study group. Histopathological evaluation of both the patent and non-patent vessels at day 21 revealed no signs of tissue toxicity or intraluminal adhesive leakage. In view of these data, the investigators concluded that using cyanoacrylate tissue adhesive provides an effective and simple method for end-to-end anastomosis of small-size arteries.

Akhtar [58] has put forth contradictory studies regarding the toxicity and long-term effects of cyanoacrylate. He cites that Barbalinardo et al. [59], who compared relative effectiveness of isobutyl 2-cyanoacrylate, fibrin adhesive, and oxidized regenerated cellulose, were determined by application of these hemostatic agents to sources of point bleeding. They found, in the meantime, that hemostasis was shorter in the cyanoacrylate group, but the reported inflammatory response that it induced, and its possible carcinogenicity, limited its availability for clinical use. Ellman et al. [60], also using oxidized cellulose (Surgicel) as control, assessed two formulations of a new cyanoacrylate compound. Long-term graft patency was assessed angiographically at 4, 6, and 18 months. Tissue reaction at 2 weeks, 1, 6, and 18 months was assessed grossly by vascular surgeons and microscopically by a blinded pathologist. There were no significant differences between groups with regard to graft patency. Histopathology showed mild to moderate tissue reaction at 2 weeks and 1 month in the cyanoacrylate groups compared with controls. Mild tissue reaction was seen at 6 and 18 months. Their conclusion was that the cyanoacrylate compound was an effective suture line sealant.

6.6.2.3 Tissue Adhesive as Dressing after Open Pediatric Urological Procedures [61]

In 2003, an effectiveness study of 2-OCA (Dermabond by Ethicon, Inc.) tissue adhesive as a sole dressing after open pediatric urological procedures. For a period of 6 months, February to August 2003, the investigators prospectively evaluated patients undergoing extragenital open and laparoscopic pediatric urological procedures at the Children's Hospital, University of Colorado School of Medicine in Denver, Colorado. All open incisions were closed in layers using a final layer of self-absorbing subcuticular stitches for the skin before applying Dermabond cyanoacrylate adhesive at the skin level alone. In laparoscopic cases, Dermabond alone was applied to the port sites (3 mm or less in diameter) and instrument sites without any sutures beneath the skin. No adjuvant occlusive dressings were applied to any of these wounds. All patients were allowed to bathe and return to normal lifestyle activities immediately postoperatively.

A total of 146 patients comprised the study with a total of 200 incisions (open 146, laparoscopy 54). Of these children, 103 who had had 142 incisions returned for follow-up visits during the period of study. Only one complication was identified. The subject, a 6-month old infant, presented with omental prolapse through the umbilical port (3 mm port) requiring urgent closure in the evening of surgery. There were no cases in which appreciable healing problems were identified by surgeon or parent examinations. No wound infection occurred. Dermabond alone provides a simple coverage for a vast range of pediatric urological surgical wounds. Immediate bathing and return to normal lifestyle activities do not seem to affect the wound healing adversely as long as a simple skin barrier is applied to the wound sites [61].

6.6.2.4 Tissue Adhesive Applications in Gastrointestinal Endoscopic Procedures [62]

This section is based on a 2006 review paper by Rayou and Thompson. Cyanoacrylates and other tissue adhesives can be applied locally for a variety of indications, including hemostatic, wound closure, and fistula repair. The main classes of tissue adhesives currently used in gastrointestinal (GI) endoscopy include cyanoacrylates, fibrin glues, and thrombin. The focus of this section is on applications of cyanoacrylates.

Gastric Variceal Bleeding

Injection therapy with cyanoacrylates is now the first line of endoscopic intervention for bleeding gastric varices as well as secondary prevention of gastric variceal bleeds outside of the United States [63].

In a randomized controlled trial of 59 patients, cyanoacrylate injection of bleeding gastric varices was reported to be more effective and safer than band ligation. Both initial hemostatic rate and rebleeding rates were lower in the cyanoacrylate group compared with the band ligation group. Initial hemostatic rates were 87% in the cyanoacrylate group compared with 45% in the band ligation group ($P = 0.03$); rebleeding rates in the cyanoacrylate group were 31% compared with 54% in the band ligation group ($P = 0.0005$). Treatment-induced ulcer bleeding occurred in two patients (7%) in the cyanoacrylate group and eight patients (28%) in the band ligation group ($P = 0.03$). The amount of blood transfusions required were also higher in the band ligation group than in the cyanoacrylate group (4.2 ± 1.3 vs. 2.6 ± 0.9 units, respectively) ($P < 0.01$) [64].

Esophageal Variceal Bleeding

Several randomized controlled studies have demonstrated that injection of cyanoacrylate is comparable to sclerotherapy in the endoscopic hemostasis of acute variceal bleeding and prevention of rebleeding [65–67].

Peptic Ulcer Bleeding

In a randomized controlled trial comparing injection of cyanoacrylate and hypertonic saline for bleeding gastroduodenal ulcers, initial hemostasis was similar in both groups and the rebleeding rate was lower after cyanoacrylate injection [68]. There are no studies comparing glue injection to a combination of injection and cautery or application of clips, which are considered more effective than saline injection alone for the treatment of bleeding ulcers.

Bleeding from Other Sources

Cyanoacrylate injection has been used successfully in the management of a few patients with Dieulafoy's lesions and bleeding tumors [69–70].

Closure of Fistula

Cyanoacrylates have been shown to be successful in the closure of pancreatic fistulas, biliary fistulas [71], and GI fistulas [72] (Seewald and coworkers reported successful closure of pancreatic fistulas in 8 of 12 patients using endoscopic injection of Histoacryl into the fistulous tract and endoscopic drainage) [73]. Seven of the eight successful patients required only one treatment over a median follow-up period of 21 months. Closure was temporary in two patients, unsuccessful in one patient, and there was one death within 24 h of treatment from pulmonary embolism.

Some complications have been described with the use of cyanoacrylates such as systemic inflammatory reaction to foreign body (pain and fever, local tissue necrosis) and inflammatory reaction to foreign body (mediastinitis, esophageal pleural fistula, duodenal ulcer perforation, pancreaticoduodenal necrosis, inflammatory pseudotumor of pancreatic tail) [74–78]. Other types of complications have also been reported [79–83].

6.6.2.5 Tissue Adhesives in Topical Skin Wounds [84]

There are over 7 million traumatic lacerations [85] in addition to tens of millions of surgical incisions. All require closure by surgeons, emergency physicians, and primary care practitioners [86]. These wounds and incisions have been traditionally closed with sutures, staples, or surgical tapes, and more recently tissue adhesives. An ideal wound closure device should be user friendly, quick, pain free and result in excellent cosmetics, without device removal requirement, and of course be cost-effective [87]. None of the current closure devices possess all of these requirements. Topical cyanoacrylate tissue adhesives, however, have a number of the characteristics of an ideal wound closure device.

Cyanoacrylate topical adhesives have some obvious advantages over sutures such as ease of use and pain-free application of the adhesive. Consequently, local anesthetics are unnecessary. In addition, because the cyanoacrylate adhesives slough off spontaneously within 5–10 days, no removal is required which is a procedure that may be painful and threatening, especially to children. Although the cost of the cyanoacrylate adhesives is higher than most sutures, a formal cost-effective analysis conducted several years ago that included the costs of the suture kits, suture removal kits, and dressing materials demonstrated that use of the adhesives actually reduces the costs [88]. The use of the topical cyanoacrylate adhesives also reduces the risks of needle sticks [89] and prevents the formation of suture marks on either side of the wound. Unlike suturing that has a learning curve of up to 2 years [90], proficiency at using the cyanoacrylate adhesives is rapidly attained [91]. They also have the potential to save operative time, especially with longer incisions and lacerations. In surveys, most surgical patients prefer topical adhesives to sutures or staples [92,93]. In contrast, in a study of 724 emergency department patients, of which two-thirds had a prior or current laceration, more patients preferred sutures to adhesives [53]. The surgical tapes offer many of the same advantages that the topical skin adhesives offer and are a reasonable alternative for closure of appropriate wounds [25,32]. The surgical tapes are easy to use, rapid, painless, and comfortable, do not require removal and are less costly than any of the wound closure devices. However, because of their low bursting strength and tendency to fall off, the use of surgical tapes is limited to simple very-low-tension wounds. Furthermore, the surgical tapes do not have microbial barrier properties. A summary of the advantages, disadvantages, and common indications for the various wound closure devices is presented in Table 6.5. A summary of potential pitfalls associated with the cyanoacrylates together with possible solutions is presented in Table 6.6.

6.6.2.6 Tissue Adhesive for Closure of Hernia Incisions

This study [94] intended to elucidate that suture-based permanent mesh fixation can be replaced by fixation with n-butyl-2-cyanoacrylate glue (Glubran® 2 by GEM S. r. l., Italy) for surgical repair of abdominal wall hernias. The aim of this study was to investigate in a rat animal model the efficacy of the use of a small amount of modified n-butyl-2-cyanoacrylate (Glubran 2) in abdominal mesh fixation as a feasible alternative to sutures and staples. Glubran 2 is a class III medical-surgical product (for internal and external surgical use) which has outstanding hemostatic and adhesive properties and, once set, produces an effective antiseptic barrier against infectious agents or pathogens commonly found in surgical settings. At the present, it is used in open and laparoscopic surgery, digestive tract endoscopy, interventional radiology, and vascular neuroradiology.

In 25 Wistar rats, two hernia defects (1.5 cm in diameter) per animal were created bilaterally in the midline of the abdominal wall. The peritoneum was spared. The lesions were left untreated for 10 days

Table 6.5 Comparison of the Wound Closure Devices [84]

	Sutures	Staple	Tapes	Adhesives
Advantages	Most meticulous approximation	Fast	Fast	Fast
	Great tensile strength	Good tensile strength	Simple	Simple
	Low dehiscence rate	Simple	Inexpensive	No risk of needle stick
	Time honored	Lower tissue reactivity	Minimal reactivity	No need for removal
		Lower risk of needle stick	No risk of needle stick	Microbial barrier
			No need for removal Comfortable	Occlusive dressing Comfortable
Disadvantages	Painful	Less meticulous approximation	Lowest tensile strength	Lower tensile strength than sutures
	Prolonged learning curve	Painful	Highest risk of dehiscence	Limited moisture resistance
	Require removal	Require removal	No moisture resistance	
	May leave suture marks			
	Risk of needle stick			
	Most reactive			
Indications	Most incisions and lacerations	Long linear incisions and lacerations	Linear low tension wounds and lacerations	Linear low tension wounds and lacerations
		Scalp wounds	Fragile skin (flaps and skin tears)	Fragile skin
			Wound support after suture/s taple removal	Under splints/casts
			Under splints/casts	
Contraindications	Infected or heavily contaminated wounds	Inadequate hemostasis	Inadequate hemostasis	Inadequate hemostasis
		Complex irregular wounds	High tension	High tension
			Hear bearing area Uncooperative patients Circumferential use around digits Proximity to moist areas	Hear bearing area Proximity to moist areas

Table 6.6 Potential Cyanoacrylate Pitfalls and Pearls [84]

Potential Pitfall	Pearl
Runoff	Position wound horizontally
	Apply small amount of adhesive
Spillage into eyes	Cover eyelids with ointment and moist gauze
	Place patient in Trendelenburg for wound above eye and reverse
	Trendelenburg for wounds below eye
	Apply small amount of adhesive
Burning sensation	Apply small amount of adhesive
	Avoid pooling of adhesive
	Spread out evenly
Wound dehiscence	Avoid in high tension wounds unless in conjunction with deep tension relieving sutures, surgical tapes, and immobilization
Wound infection	Use proper wound preparation
	Avoid in wounds with high risk of injection
Adherence to wound	Apply small amount of adhesive
	Horizontal positioning of wound
	Alternate the hand used to appose wound edges before complete polymerization
Introduction of adhesive into wound	Ensure meticulous wound apposition
	Avoid pressing down on wound with applicator (glide over wound surface)
	Remove adhesive by applying ointment
	Removal may be facilitated by using substance containing isopropyl merystate (such as silver sulfadiazine)

to achieve a chronic condition. Then the defects were covered with TiMESH extra light and fixed by 30 μL of Glubran 2 or traditional suture. The time points of sacrifice were 17 and 28 days, 3, 4, and 5 months. At autopsy, histology and immunohistochemistry were performed to evaluate the inflammatory response and the presence of apoptotic cells, respectively. Mesh fixation was excellent in all samples at each time point. At application sites, the inflammatory reaction was mild with a small number of macrophages and vascularized connective tissue presence around glue and mesh threads. Glue residues were observed in histologic sections at each time point. No presence of apoptotic cells was found. This study demonstrated that Glubran 2 can effectively replace traditional sutures in mesh fixation without affecting tissue healing and determining a physiological inflammatory reaction at the abdominal wall site.

In conclusion, on the basis of these experimental results, the use of a right amount of Glubran 2 can effectively replace traditional suture threads in fixing abdominal mesh, guaranteeing a long-term firm adhesion without increasing inflammation.

In another study [95], the investigators compared the skin adhesive 2-octylcyanoacrylate to subcuticular suture for closure of pediatric inguinal hernia incisions to determine if skin adhesive improves wound cosmesis, shortens skin closure time, and lowers operative costs. They prospectively randomized 134 children undergoing inguinal herniorrhaphy at the Children's Hospital of the University of Michigan to have skin closure with either skin adhesive ($n = 64$) or subcuticular closure ($n = 70$). Data collected included age, sex, weight, type of operation, total operative time, and skin closure time. Digital photographs of healing incisions were taken at the 6-week postoperative visit. The operating surgeon assessed cosmetic outcome of incisions using a previously validated visual analog scale, as well as an ordinate scale. A blinded assessment of cosmetic outcome was then performed by an independent surgeon comparing these photographs to the visual analog scale. Operating room time and resource use (i.e., costs) relative to the skin closure were assessed. Comparisons between groups were done using Student's t tests and χ^2 tests.

Children that enrolled in the study had a mean age of 3.7 ± 0.3 years and weighed 16 ± 0.8 kg. Patients were predominantly male (82%). Patients underwent one of three types of open hernia repair as follows: unilateral herniorrhaphy without peritoneoscopy ($n = 41$; 31%), unilateral herniorrhaphy with peritoneoscopy ($n = 55$; 41%), and bilateral herniorrhaphy ($n = 38$; 28%). Skin closure time was significantly shorter in the skin adhesive group (adhesive = 1.4 ± 0.8 min vs. suture = 2.4 ± 1.1 min; $P = 0.001$). Mean wound cosmesis scores based on the visual analog scale were similar between groups (adhesive = 78 ± 21; suture = 78 ± 18; $P = 0.50$). Material costs related to herniorrhaphy were higher for skin adhesive (adhesive = \$22.63 vs. suture = \$11.70; $P = 0.001$), whereas operating room time costs for adhesive skin closure were lower (adhesive = \$9.33 $\pm$ 5.33 vs. suture = \$16.00 $\pm$ 7.33; $P = 0.001$). Except for a 7% incidence of erythema in both groups, there were no complications encountered. In the meantime, the data from this trial suggest that skin adhesive wound closure in inguinal hernia repair is associated with a small reduction in operative time without effect upon total cost, complication rate, or cosmesis.

6.6.2.7 Use of Tissue Adhesive for Skin Closure in Plastic Surgery [96]

Abdominoplasty and mammoplasty are cosmetic surgeries that demand relatively more time for skin closure. Methods: Skin closure with 4.0 Mononylon (Ethicon) continuous subcuticular suture and with Dermabond (Ethicon) (octylcyanoacrylate) was compared among 37 patients who had undergone body contouring surgery (23 abdominoplasties and 14 mammoplasties). Each side of the scar, randomly selected, was closed either with adhesive or suture. The time required for skin closure and the aesthetic aspect of these scars were compared. Three observers evaluated the scars at 3, 6, and 12 months postoperatively using a categorical and a modified visual analog scale. Results: The average time for closure using suture was 7 min and 45 s for the abdominoplasty and 4 min and 25 s for the vertical incision of the mammoplasty. This was significantly different statistically, as compared with the 2 min required for polymerization of the skin adhesive. The mammoplasty and abdominoplasty scars showed no statistical difference at 3, 6, and 12 months according to both scales. Conclusions: The aesthetic aspects of the mammoplasty and abdominoplasty scars were similar on both sides at 3, 6, and 12 months. However, the adhesive allowed a shorter surgical time.

6.7 Bone Adhesives

One of the unmet clinical needs of orthopedic trauma surgeons is a "bone glue" or an adhesive to fix a broken bone instead of the conventional metal plates, nails, pins, and screws. Simplicity, quickness and preservation of joint function, especially when fixing fractures with many small fragments, are the main benefits of a bone adhesive. An additional benefit is elimination of a metal removal from fractures fixed solely with a biodegradable adhesive.

The development of bone adhesives has been under way since 1950s. It is still in relatively early stages and has not resulted in adhesives which meet the many requirements of a successful product (Table 6.7). There are a number of bone cements and bone void fillers on the marker though none claim any adhesive properties. Probably the best known of these products is PMMA bone cement that has long been used for the fixation of implants such as hip and knee replacements into bone. However, this material acts merely as a grout between the implant and bone and any attempts to use it to glue bones have generally been unsuccessful [97].

6.8 Dental Applications of Adhesives [98]

Dental adhesives are basically intended to provide retention to composite fillings or composite cements. A good adhesive not only should withstand

Table 6.7 Characteristics of a Successful Bone Adhesive [97]

Preferred
• High level of adhesion to bone, often in the presence of contaminants such as fats, proteins
• Bonds to wet surfaces/bond strength stable in wet environment
• Mechanical stability under tension, compression, shear
• Easy/quick to prepare and apply in operating room conditions
• Adequate working time for the surgeon to apply and form bond
• Rapid setting time (typically 1–10 min)
• Low exotherm on setting—no thermal necrosis
• Non-toxic and biocompatible (including any leachables, degradation products)
• Allows healing of the fracture
• Sterilisable
• Adequate shelf life
• Cost effective to use
• Commercially viable to manufacture
Desirable
• Adhesion to surgical alloys (e.g., stainless steel, Ti–6A1–4V, Co–Cr–Mo)
• Biodegradable in a controlled manner and timescale
• No special storage conditions (stable at room temperature)
• Ability to deliver drugs/bioactive agents, e.g., stimulate bone healing, prevent infection

mechanical forces, particularly shrinkage stress from the lining composite, but should be able to prevent leakage along the restoration's margins. Clinically, failure of restorations occurs more often due to inadequate sealing, with subsequent discoloration of the cavity margins, than due to loss of retention [99,100].

Capability of dental adhesives is dependent on two conditions. First, the adhesive must bond to enamel and dentin, and second, the adhesive adheres to the lining composite. The second condition has been shown to be due to a process of copolymerization of residual double bonds (–C=C–) in the oxygen inhibition layer. Bonding to enamel and dentin is believed to be by micromechanical adhesion as the main adhesion mechanism [101]. This takes place through an exchange process where inorganic tooth material is replaced by resin monomers that become interlocked in the retentions after polymerization [102,103]. Diffusion and capillarity are the primary mechanisms of micro-mechanical retention. Microscopically, this process is called "hybridization" [104]. Comprised of simple interlocking resin in etch-pits in enamel, entanglement of resin within the exposed collagen lattice occurs in dentin. Self-etch adhesives with a mild (relatively high) pH do not, however, completely expose collagen anymore. An additional mechanism of ionic bonding of acidic monomers and calcium in hydroxyapatite was established in 2004 [105] that might explain the successful clinical performance of some of these mild self-etch adhesives [106].

Some of the requirements of adhesive systems can be defined [98] using the knowledge of bonding mechanisms. Micromechanical interlocking occurs after consecutive demineralization, resin infiltration, and polymer setting. Consequently, adequately removing the smear layer together with demineralizing enamel and dentin to a small extent, good wetting, diffusion, penetration, and good polymerization of the resin components are all important. Chemical bonding can be achieved by adding specific monomers with affinity for hydroxyapatite. Finally, sufficient copolymerization between the adhesive and the lining composite will provide good adhesion to the composite.

Chemical composition of adhesives should be (is) selectively defined [98] such that the above mechanistic requirements may successfully be fulfilled. Even though dental adhesives can be classified into two main groups, i.e., etch and rinse (E&Rs) and self-etch adhesives (SEAs) (Figure 6.4), they all contain similar ingredients, irrespective of the number of bottles of which an adhesive consists. Nevertheless, the proportional composition differs between the different classes of adhesives. Traditionally, adhesives contain acrylic resin monomers, organic solvents, initiators and inhibitors, and sometimes filler particles. It is obvious that every component has a specific function. Good insights in the chemical properties of the adhesives' components are paramount to understand or even predict

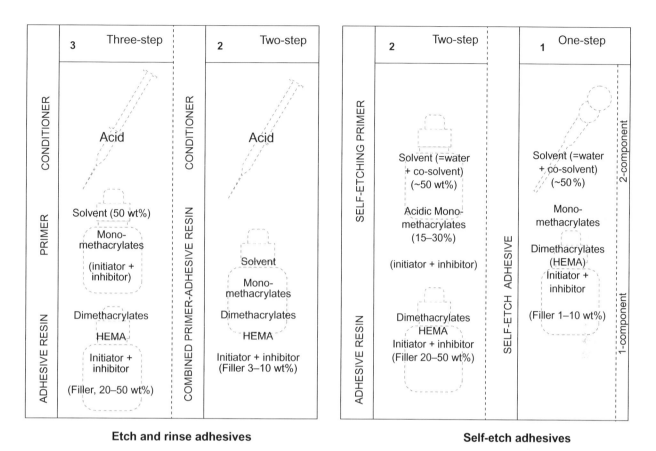

Figure 6.4 Classification of adhesives by Van Meerbeek et al. [101]. Adhesives' performance may differ significantly when the same components at different proportional amount of ingredients.

their behavior. Table 6.8 gives a list of the various ingredients of dental adhesives.

Resin monomers in dental adhesives play a similar role to those of composites. Just as in the composites, the cured resin in the adhesive forms a matrix which functions as a backbone providing structural continuity and thus physico-mechanical properties such as strength. Monomers are the most essential ingredient of the adhesive because they are the key constituents of adhesives. There are two classes of monomers: cross-linking and functional monomers. Typically, the functional monomers only have one polymerizable group while cross-linking monomers have two or more polymerizable groups such as vinyl linkages ($-C=C-$) [107]. Functional monomers, in addition to polymerizable group, exhibit a particular chemical group, which the functional species that embodies the monomer-specific functions imparted to the polymer.

Functional monomers form linear polymers upon polymerization contrary to the cross-linkers which supply the linkages for cross-linked polymers. Compared to linear polymers, the latter have proven to exhibit better mechanical strength, and cross-linking monomers are therefore important to the reinforcement of the adhesive resin [108–111]. Important characteristics of more common dental adhesive monomers are briefly covered in the followings sections [98].

6.8.1 Methacrylic Acid

Methacrylic acid (MA) is a strong irritant and corrosive because of its strongly acidity. It can also rapidly penetrate gloves and skin causing allergic reactions. This monomer is, therefore, seldom added to adhesives. It is, however, most likely to be present to different extents in the majority of adhesive resins, thanks to the hydrolysis of the ester group in

Table 6.8 Ingredients of Dental Adhesives [98]

Monomers
MAEPA: 2,4,6 trimethylphenyl 2-[4-(dihydroxyphosphoryl)-2-oxabutyl]acrylate
MAC-10: 11-methacryloyloxy-1,10-undecanedicarboxylic acid
10-MDP: 10-methacryloyloxydecyl dihydrogen phosphate
MDPB: methacryloyloxydodecylpyridinium bromide
4-META: 4-methacryloyloxyethyl trimellitate anhydride
4-MET: 4-methacryloyloxyethyl trimellitic acid
MMA: methyl methacrylate
MMEP: mono-2-methacryloyloxyethyl phthalate (sometimes also called PAMA: phthalic acid monomethacrylate)
5-NMSA (or MASA): *N*-methacryloyl-5-aminosalicylic acid
NPG-GMA: *N*-phenylglycine glycidyl methacrylate
NTG-GMA: *N*-tolylglycine glycidyl methacrylate or *N*-(2-hydroxy-3-((2-methyl-1-oxo-2-propenyl)oxy)propyl)-*N*-tolyl glycine
PEGDMA: polyethylene glycol dimethacrylate
PEM-F: pentamethacryloyloxyethylcyclohexaphosphazene monofluoride
PENTA: dipentaerythritol pentaacrylate monophosphate
Phenyl-P: 2-(methacryloyloxyethyl)phenyl hydrogen phosphate
PMDM: pyromellitic diethylmethacrylate or 2,5-dimethacryloyloxyethyloxycarbonyl-1,4-benzenedicarboxylic acid
PMGDM: pyromellitic glycerol dimethacrylate or 2,5-bis(1,3-dimethacryloyloxyprop-2-yloxycarbonyl)benzene-1,4-dicarboxylic acid
Pyro-EMA: tetramethacryloyloxyethyl pyrophosphate
TCB: butan-1,2,3,4-tetracarboxylic acid di-2-hydroxyethylmethacrylate ester
TEGDMA: triethylene glycol dimethacrylate
TMPTMA: trimethylolpropane trimethacrylate
UDMA: urethane dimethacrylate or 1,6-di(methacryloyloxyethylcarbamoyl)-3,30,5-trimethylhexaan
Initiators and inhibitors
BHT: butylhydroxytoluene or butylated hydroxytoluene or ,2,6-di-(tert-butyl)-4-methylphenol (inhibitor)
BPO: benzoylperoxide (redox initiator)
BS acid: benzenesulfinic acid sodium salt (redox initiator)
CQ: camphorquinone or camphoroquinone or 1.7.7-trimethylbicyclo-[2,2,1]-hepta-2,3-dione (photo-initiator)
DHEPT: *N,N*-di-(2-hydroxyethyl)-4-toluidine (co-initiator)
MEHQ: 4-methoxyphenol or monoethyl ether hydroquinone (inhibitor)
ODMAB: 2-(ethylhexyl)-4-(dimethylamino)benzoate (co-initiator)
TPO: Lucirin TPO, BASF (photo-initiator)
UV-9: 2-hydroxy-4-methoxybenzophenone (photo-initiator)
Fillers and silane coupling factors
Coupling factor A174: g-methacryloxypropyltrimethoxysilane
F-PRG: full reaction type pre-reacted glass-ionomer fillers
NaF: sodium fluoride
Na2SiF6: disodium hexafluorosilicate
POSS nano-particulates: polyhedral oligomer silsesquioxanes

other monomers as seen in Figure 6.5. Hydroxy ethyl methacrylate (HEMA) hydrolyzes and generates MA. Hydrolysis of methacrylate monomers is a problem associated with self-etching adhesives which routinely contain water and have fairly low pH, both of which result in easy hydrolysis [112].

6.8.2 Methyl Methacrylate

MMA, similar to MA, is one of the oldest monomers and is rarely sporadically added to adhesives because of the risk of allergic reactions [113]. It is no longer used for cosmetic applications because of

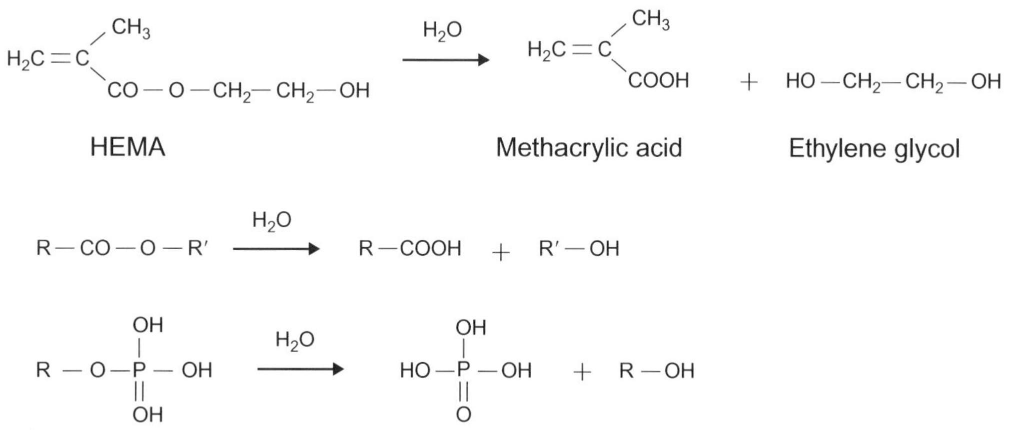

$$H_2C=C\overset{CH_3}{\underset{CO-O-CH_2-CH_2-OH}{}} \xrightarrow{H_2O} H_2C=C\overset{CH_3}{\underset{COOH}{}} + HO-CH_2-CH_2-OH$$

HEMA   Methacrylic acid   Ethylene glycol

$$R-CO-O-R' \xrightarrow{H_2O} R-COOH + R'-OH$$

$$R-O-\underset{OH}{\overset{OH}{\underset{\|}{P}}}-OH \xrightarrow{H_2O} HO-\underset{O}{\overset{OH}{\underset{\|}{P}}}-OH + R-OH$$

Figure 6.5 Hydrolysis of hydroxy ethyl methacrylate, an ester, and a phosphate [98].

a ban. Its role in adhesives is limited to dissolution of other monomers.

6.8.3 Hydroxy Ethyl Methacrylate

HEMA is a small monomer with widespread use, not only in dentistry but also in medical applications because of its relatively good biocompatibility [114] even though the uncured monomer is notorious for its high allergenic potential [115,116]. Unpolymerized HEMA appears as a fluid that is quite soluble in water, ethanol, and acetone. HEMA is purported to evaporate from the adhesive solutions, although only in small amounts [117]. A key characteristic of HEMA is its hydrophilicity. Even though this monomer cannot be used as a demineralizing agent, its hydrophilicity makes it an excellent adhesion-promoting monomer [118–122]. By enhancing wetting of dentin, HEMA significantly improves bond strengths [123,124]. In monomeric and polymerized states, HEMA will readily absorb water. Water uptake adversely influences the mechanical strength of its HEMA copolymers; high amounts of HEMA will result in flexible copolymers with inferior qualities. Homopolymer of HEMA is a flexible porous polymer [125,126]. As such, high concentrations of HEMA in an adhesive may have deteriorating effects on the mechanical properties of the resulting polymer.

6.8.4 4-Methacryloyloxyethyl Trimellitic Acid

4-Methacryloyloxyethyl trimellitic acid (4-MET) is used both as an adhesion promoter and demineralizing monomer [127,128]. 4-MET is known to improve wetting to metals, such as amalgam [129] or gold [130]. Its popularity is partially due to its easy synthesizing method and broad availability. 4-MET is available in anhydride form (4-META) which is a crystalline powder. After addition of water to 4-META powder, hydrolysis reaction occurs rapidly to form 4-MET. The two carboxylic groups bonded to the aromatic ring increase acidity thus demineralizing properties as well as wetting. The aromatic group, however, is hydrophobic and will moderate the acidity and the hydrophilicity of the carboxyl groups [77].

6.8.5 4-Acryloyloxyethyl Trimellitate Anhydride

4-Acryloyloxyethyl trimellitate anhydride (4-AETA) differs from the structure of 4-META slightly having an acrylate polymerizable group instead of a methacrylate group. The acrylate group is regarded as an advantage for polymerization because of higher reactivity [131]. Apart from facilitating resin penetration into dentin, the highly reactive acrylate group of 4-AETA is regarded as an advantage for better polymerization.

6.8.6 10-Methacryloyloxydecyl Dihydrogen Phosphate

10-Methacryloyloxydecyl dihydrogen phosphate (10-MDP) is a monomer that was originally synthesized by Kuraray (Osaka, Japan). Its main use is as an etching monomer, due to the dihydrogen phosphate group, which can dissociate in water to form two protons [112]. Structurally, the long carbonyl chain renders this monomer quite hydrophobic. Consequently, ethanol and acetone are most suitable solvents for this monomer. It is clear that 10-MDP is relatively hydrolysis stable. Yoshida et al. [105] demonstrated this monomer is capable of forming strong ionic bonds with calcium because of the low dissolution rate of its Ca-salt in its own solution.

6.8.7 Other Monomers

These monomers include 11-methacryloyloxy-1,10-undecanedicarboxylic acid (MAC-10). This monomer is hydrophobic, which may reflect in limited dissolution in water. Another compound is 2-(methacryloyloxyethyl) phenyl hydrogen phosphate (Phenyl-P) [132,133] which was used as one of the first acidic monomers in self-etching primers. It is seldom used in contemporary. Two other monomers are phosphates: di-2-hydroxyethyl methacryl hydrogen phosphate (Di-HEMA-phosphate) and 2-hydroxyethyl methacryl dihydrogen phosphate (HEMA-phosphate) [134]. Di-methacrylates are cross-linking agents and methacrylamides is an interesting matrix monomer because of its similarity to amino acids of which collagen consists [135] thus promoting the formation of hydrogen bonds between the carboxyl and amide groups of the monomer with the carboxyl groups of collagen.

References

[1] Troughton MJ. Handbook of plastics joining: a practical guide. 2nd ed. New York: William Andrew, Elsevier; 2009.

[2] Messler RW. Joining of materials and structures: from pragmatic process to enabling technology. Butterworth-Heinemann; 2004.

[3] Sastri VR. Plastics in medical devices properties, requirements and applications. New York: William Andrew, Elsevier; 2010.

[4] Perez R. Design of medical electronic devices. New York: Academic Press; 2002.

[5] Medical devices—use and safety, Churchill Livingstone. Oxford; 2006 and Ebnesajjad S, Landrock AH. Adhesives technology handbook. 2nd ed. William Andrew, Elsevier; 2008.

[6] Ebnesajjad S, Ebnesajjad CF. Surface treatment of materials for adhesion bonding. New York: William Andrew, Elsevier; 2006.

[7] New developments and trends in medical-grade adhesives, a report by Robert W Smith, Partner and Director, the Chemquest Group, Inc., on behalf of the Adhesive and Sealant Council, Inc., Business Briefing: Medical Devices Manufacturing & Technology; 2004.

[8] Bitton R, Josef E, Shimshelashvili I, Shapira K, Seliktar D, Bianco-Peled H. Int J Adhes Adhes 2012;33:89–97.

[9] Farndale RW, Sixma JJ, Barnes MJ, De Groot PG. The role of collagen in thrombosis and hemostasis. J Thromb Haemost 2004;2:561–73.

[10] Duarte AP, Coelho JF, Bordado JC, Cidadec MT, Gil MH. Prog Polym Sci 2012;37:1031–50.

[11] Society of Manufacturing Engineers (SME), Types of adhesives (Chapter 1). Adhesives in modern manufacturing. Bruno EJ, editors. SME; 1970.

[12] Henkel Corporation Student Center, History of adhesives, published at website, <www.stickwithhenkel.com/student/history.asp>; 2010.

[13] Petrie EM. Handbook of adhesives and sealants. 2nd ed. New York: McGraw Hill; 2006.

[14] Wake WC. Adhesion and the formation of adhesives. 2nd ed. London: Applied Science Publishers; 1982.

[15] Brumit TM. Cyanocrylate adhesives—when should you use them? Adhes Age 1975;18(2):17–22.

[16] Loctite 380 Technical Data Sheet, Henkel Loctite Corp. CT: Rocky Hill; 2004.

[17] Thermal cycling makes strong adhesive stronger. News Trends, Machine Design 1984;56(6): 10.

[18] Quinn JV, Drzewiecki AE, Li MM, et al. A randomized, controlled trial comparing a tissue adhesive with suturing in the repair of pediatric facial lacerations. Ann Emerg Med 1993;22:1130–5.

[19] Galil KA, Schofield I, Wright GZ. Effect of n-2butyl cyanoacrylate (Histoacryl blue) on the healing of skin wounds. J Can Dent Assoc 1984;50:565–9.

[20] Keng TM, Bucknall TE. A clinical trial of histoacryl in skin closure of groin wound. Med J Malaysia 1989;44:122–8.

[21] Mizrahi S, Bickel A, Ben-Layish E. Use of tissue adhesives in the repair of lacerations in children. J Pediatr Surg 1988;23:312–3.

[22] Applebaum JS, Zalut T, Applebaum D. The use of tissue adhesion for traumatic laceration repair in the emergency department. Ann Emerg Med 1993;22:1190–2.

[23] Kamer FM, Joseph JH. Histoacryl: its use in aesthetic facial plastic surgery. Arch Otolaryngol Head Neck Surg 1989;115:193–7.

[24] Halopuro S, Rintala A, Salo H, Ritsila V. Tissue adhesive versus sutures in closure of incision wounds. Ann Chir Gynaecol 1976;65:308–12.

[25] Osmond MH, Quinn JV, Sutcliffe T, et al. A randomized, clinical trial comparing butylcyanoacrylate with octylcyanoacrylate in the management of selected pediatric facial lacerations. Acad Emerg Med 1999;6(3):171–7.

[26] Gosain AK, Lyon VB. Plastic surgery educational foundation DATA committee. The current status of tissue glues: part II. For adhesion of soft tissues. Plast Reconstr Surg 2002;110(6):1581–4.

[27] <www.aesculapusa.com/default.aspx?pageid=423>; 2010.

[28] Eaglstein WH, Sullivan T. Cyanoacrylates for skin closure. Dermatol Clin 2005;23:193–8.

[29] The current status of tissue glues: part II. For adhesion of soft tissues. Plast Reconstr Surg 2002;110(6):1581–4.

[30] Singer AJ, Thode Jr. HC. A review of the literature on octylcyanoacrylate tissue adhesive. Am J Surg 2004;187:238–48.

[31] Ethicon, Inc, a Johnson & Johnson Company, <www.dermabond.com/applications/surgical-uses.html>; 2010.

[32] Blondeel PN, Murphy JW, Debrosse D, et al. Closure of long surgical incisions with a new formulation of 2-octylcyanoacrylate tissue adhesive versus commercially available methods. Am J Surg 2004;188:307–13.

[33] Maw JL, Quinn JV. Cyanoacrylate tissue adhesives. Amer J Cosmetic Surg 1997;14:413–6.

[34] Hall LT, Bailes JE. Using DERMABOND® for wound closure in lumbar and cervical neurosurgical procedures. Neurosurgery 2005;56(Suppl. 1):147–50.

[35] Toriumi DM, O'Grady K, Desai D, Bagal A. Use of octyl-2-cyanoacrylate for skin closure in facial plastic surgery. Plast Reconstr Surg 1998;102:2209–19.

[36] Branfield AS. Use of tissue adhesives in sport? A new application in international ice hockey. Br J Sports Med 2004;38:95–6.

[37] Am Fam Physician 2000;61:1383–8.

[38] Bruns TB, Mackworthington J. Using tissue adhesive for wound repair: a practical guide to Dermabond. Am Acad Family Phys 2000; March: <www.aafp.org/afp/20000301/1383.html>

[39] <www.dermabond.com>; 2010.

[40] Guidance for industry and FDA staff: class II special controls guidance document: tissue adhesive for the topical approximation of skin, issued May 30, 2008, Supersedes cyanoacrylate tissue adhesive for the topical approximation of skin—premarket approval applications (PMAs), dated Feb 13, 2004 (issued on: July 3, 2007), contact George J. Mattamal, Ph.D., at 240-276-3619 or by email at <george.mattamal@fda.hhs.gov>.

[41] Available from: www.adhesives.org/AdhesivesSealants/MarketsApplications/Medical.aspx.

[42] Available from: www.nature.com/ebd/journal/v4/n3/full/6400194a.html.

[43] Artzi N, Zeiger A, Boehning F, Ramos Ab, Vliet KV, Edelman ER. Tuning, adhesion failure strength for tissue-specific applications. Acta Biomater 2010;: doi: 10.1016/j.actbio., 2010.07.008

[44] Yoo J, Chandarana S, Cosby R. Clinical application of tissue adhesives in soft-tissue surgery of the head and neck. Curr Opin Otolaryngol Head Neck Surg 2008;16:312–7.

[45] Sze DY, Kao JS, Frisoli JK, McCallum SW, Kennedy II WA, Razavi MK. Persistent and recurrent postsurgical varicoceles: venographic anatomy and treatment with N-butyl cyanoacrylate embolization. J Vasc Interv Radiol 2008;19:539–45.

[46] Thouveny F, Aube C, Konate A, Lebigot J, Bouvier A, Oberti F. Direct percutaneous approach for endoluminal glue embolization of stomal varices. J Vasc Interv Radiol 2008;19:774–7.

[47] Rotondano G, Viola M, Orsini L, et al. Uncommon cause of early postoperative colonic fistula successfully treated with

endoscopic acrylate glue injection. Gastrointest Endosc 2008;67:183−6.
[48] Howell JM, Bresnahan KA, Stair TO, Dhindsa HS, Edwards BA. Comparison of effects of suture and cyanoacrylate tissue adhesive on bacterial counts in contaminated lacerations. Antimicrob Agents Chemother 1995;559−60.
[49] Eiferman RA, Snyder JW. Antibacterial effect of cyanoacrylate glue. Arch Ophthalmol 1983;101:958−60.
[50] Salasche SJ. Acute surgical complications: cause prevention and treatment. J Am Acad Dermatol 1986;15:1163−85.
[51] Olson ME, Ruseska I, Costerton JW. Colonization of n-butyl-2-cyanoacrylate by Staphylococcus epidermidis. J Biomed Mater Res 1988;22:485−95.
[52] Jorgensen JH, Cleeland R, Craig WA, et al. Methods for dilution antimicrobial susceptibility tests for bacteria that grow aerobically. 3rd ed. Approved standard, vol. 13. Villanova, Pa: National Committee for Clinical Laboratory Standards; 1993. p. 13−17.
[53] Madeo M, Lowry L, Cutler L. Cyanoacrylate dressings: are they microbiologically impermeable? J Hosp Inf 2010;75:136−47.
[54] Rocos B, Blom AW, Estela C, Bowker K, MacGowan A, Hardy JR. The passage of bacteria through surgical drapes. Ann R Coll Surg Engl 2000;82:405−7.
[55] Bady S, Wongworawat MD. Effectiveness of antimicrobial incise drapes versus cyanoacrylate barrier preparations for surgical sites. Clin Orthop Relat Res 2009;467:1674−7.
[56] Qu L, Jing Z, Wang Y. Sutureless anastomoses of small- and medium-sized vessels by medical adhesive. Eur J Vasc Endovasc Surg 2004;28:526−33.
[57] Ulusoy MG, Kankaya Y, Uysal A, Sungur N, Kocer U, Kankaya D, et al. "Lid technique": cyanoacrylate-assisted anastomosis of small-sized vessels. J Plastic Reconst Aesth Surg 2009;62:1205−9.
[58] Akhtar MS. Use of cyanoacrylate compounds in vascular anastomosis. J Plast Reconstruct Aesthet Surg 2010;63(6):1063−4.
[59] Barbalinardo RJ, Citrin P, Franco CD, et al. A comparison of isobutyl 2 ecyanoacrylate glue, fibrin adhesive and oxidized regenerated cellulose for control of needle hole bleeding from polytetrafluoroethylene vascular prostheses. J Vasc Surg 1986;4:220−3.
[60] Ellman P, Reece TB, Maxey T, et al. Evaluation of an absorbable cyanoacrylate adhesive as a suture line sealant. J Surg Res 2005;125:161−7.
[61] Rajimwale A, Golden BK, Oottomasathien S, Krishnamurthy M, Ullrich NO, Koyle MA. Octyl-2-cyanoacrylate as a routine dressing after open pediatric urological procedures. J Urol 2004;171:2407−8.
[62] Ryou M, Thompson CC. Tissue adhesives: a review. Tech Gastrointest Endosc 2006;8(1):33−7.
[63] Ryan BM, Stockbrugger RW, Ryan JM. A pathophysiologic, gastroenterologic and radiologic approach to the management of gastric varices. Gastroenterology 2004;126:1175−89.
[64] Lo GH, Lai KH, Cheng JS, et al. A prospective randomized trial of butyl cyanoacrylate injection versus band ligation in the management of bleeding gastric varices. Hepatology 2001;33:1060−4.
[65] Omar MM, Fakhry SM, Mostafa I. Immediate endoscopic injection therapy of bleeding oesaphageal varices: a prospective comparative evaluation of injecting materials in Egyptian patients with portal hypertension. J Egypt Soc Parasitol 1998;28:159−69.
[66] Sun JJ, Yeo W, Suen R, et al. Injection sclerotherapy for variceal bleeding in patients with hepatocellular carcinoma: cyanoacrylate versus sodium tetradecyl sulphate. Gastrointest Endosc 1998;47:235−9.
[67] Maluf-Filho F, Sakai P, Ishioka S, et al. Endoscopic sclerosis versus cyanoacrylate endoscopic injection for the first episode of variceal bleeding: a prospective, controlled, and randomized study in Child-Pugh class C patients. Endoscopy 2001;33:421−7.
[68] Lee KJ, Kim JH, Hahm KB, et al. Randomized trial of N-butyl-2-cyanoacrylate compared with injection of hypertonic saline-epinephrine in the endoscopic treatment of bleeding peptic ulcers. Endoscopy 2000;32:505−11.
[69] Yoshida T, Adachi K, Tanioka Y, et al. Dieulafoy's lesion of the esophagus correctly diagnosed and successfully treated by the endoscopic injection of N-butyl-2-cyanoacrylate. Endoscopy 2004;36:183−5.

[70] Rosa A, Sequeira C, Macas F, et al. Histoacryl® in the endoscopic treatment of severe arterial tumor bleeding. Endoscopy 2000;32:S69.

[71] Seewald S, Groth S, Sriram PV, et al. Endoscopic treatment of biliary leakage with n-butyl-2 cyanoacrylate. Gastrointest Endosc 2002;56:916–9.

[72] Lee YC, Na HG, Suh JH, et al. Three cases of fistulae arising from gastrointestinal tract treated with endoscopic injection of histoacryl. Endoscopy 2001;33:184–6.

[73] Seewald S, Brand B, Omar S, et al. Endoscopic sealing of pancreatic fistula by using N-butyl-2-cyanoacrylate. Gastrointest Endosc 2004;9:463–70.

[74] Ramond MJ, Valla D, Gotlib JP, et al. Endoscopic obturation of esophagogastric varices with bucrylate. I. Clinical study of 49 patients. Gastroenterol Clin Biol 1986;10:575–9.

[75] FrenchBattaglia G, Morbin T, Patarnello E, et al. Visceral fistula as a complication of endoscopic treatment of esophageal and gastric varices using isobutyl-2-cyanoacrylate: report of two cases. Gastrointest Endosc 2000;52:267–70.

[76] Cheah WK, So J, Chong SM, et al. Duodenal ulcer perforation following cyanoacrylate injection. Endoscopy 2000;32:S23.

[77] Vallieres E, Jamieson C, Haber GB, et al. Pancreatoduodenal necrosis after endoscopic injection of cyanoacrylate to treat a bleeding duodenal ulcer: a case report. Surgery 1989;106:901–3.

[78] Sato T, Yamazaki K, Toyota J, et al. Inflammatory tumor in pancreatic tail induced by endoscopic ablation with cyanoacrylate glue for gastric varices. J Gastroenterol 2004;39:475–8.

[79] Lee GH, Kim JH, Lee KJ, et al. Life-threatening intraabdominal arterial embolization after histoacryl injection for bleeding gastric ulcer. Endoscopy 2000;32:422–4.

[80] Tan YM, Goh KL, Kamarulzaman A, et al. Multiple systemic embolisms with septicemia after gastric variceal obliteration with cyanoacrylate. Gastrointest Endosc 2002;55: 276–8.

[80] Turler A, Wolff M, Dorlars D, et al. Embolic and septic complications after sclerotherapy of fundic varices with cyanoacrylate. Gastrointest Endosc 2001;53:228–30.

[82] Wahl P, Lammer F, Conen D, et al. Septic complications after injection of N-butyl-2-cyanoacrylate: report of two cases and review. Gastrointest Endosc 2004;59:911–6.

[83] Bhasin DK, Sharma BC, Prasad H, et al. Endoscopic removal of sclerotherapy needle from gastric varix after n-butyl-2-cyanoacrylate injection. Gastrointest Endosc 2000;51:497–8.

[84] Singer AJ, Quinn JV, Hollander JE. The cyanoacrylate topical skin adhesives. Am J Emergency Med 2008;26:490–6.

[85] Singer AJ, Thode Jr HC, Hollander JE. National trends in emergency department lacerations between 1992–2002. Am J Emerg Med 2006;24:183–8.

[86] US markets for current and emerging wound closure technologies, 2001–2011. Tuscan, CA: Medtech Insight; 2002.

[87] Singer AJ, Hollander JE, Quinn JV. Evaluation and management of traumatic lacerations. N Engl J Med 1997;337:1142–8.

[88] Osmond MH, Klassen TP, Quinn JV. Economic comparison of a tissue adhesive and suturing in the repair of pediatric facial lacerations. J Pediatr 1995;126 (6):892–5.

[89] Gordon CA. Reducing needle-stick injuries with the use of 2-octyl cyanoacrylates for laceration repair. J Am Acad Nurse Pract 2001;13:10–2.

[90] Singer AJ, Hollander JE, Valentine SM, Thode HC, Henry MC. Association of training level and short term cosmesis (appearance) of repaired lacerations. Acad Emerg Med 1996;3:378–83.

[91] Hollander JE, Singer AJ. Application of tissue adhesives: rapid attainment of proficiency. Acad Emerg Med 1998;5:1012–7.

[92] Laccourreye O, Cauchois R, Sharkawy EL, Menard M, De Mones E, Brasnu D, et al. Octylcyanoacrylate (Dermabond®) for skin closure at the time of head and neck surgery: a longitudinal prospective study. Ann Chir 2005;130:624–30 and Spauwen PH, de Laat WA, Hartman EH. Octyl-2-cyanoacrylate tissue glue (Dermabond®) versus Monocryl 6×0 sutures in lip closure. Cleft Palate Craniofac J 2006;43:625–7.

[93] Roberts AC. The tissue adhesive Indermil and its use in surgery. Acta Chir Plast 1998;40:22−5.
[94] Losi P, Burchielli S, Spiller. D, Finotti V, Kull S, Briganti E, et al. Cyanoacrylate surgical glue as an alternative to suture threads for mesh fixation in hernia repair. J Surg Res 2010;e1−6.
[95] Brown JK, Campbell BT, Drongowski RA, Alderman AK, Geiger JD, Teitelbaum DH, et al. Prospective, randomized comparison of skin adhesive and subcuticular suture for closure of pediatric hernia incisions: cost and cosmetic considerations. J Pediatric Surg 2009;44:1418−22.
[96] Nahas FX, Solia D, Ferreira LM, Novo NF. The use of tissue adhesive for skin closure in body contouring surgery. Aesth Plast Surg 2004;28:165−9.
[97] Farrar DF. Int J Adhes Adhes 2012;33:89−97.
[98] Van Landuyta KL, Snauwaertb J, De Muncka J, Peumansa M, Yoshidac Y, Poitevina A, et al. Systematic review of the chemical composition of contemporary dental adhesives. Biomaterials 2007;28:3757−85.
[99] Gaengler P, Hoyer I, Montag R, Gaebler P. Micromorphological evaluation of posterior composite restorations—a 10-year report. J Oral Rehab 2004;31(10):991−1000.
[100] Opdam NJ, Loomans BA, Roeters FJ, Bronkhorst EM. Five-year clinical performance of posterior resin composite restorations, placed by dental students. J Dent 2004;32(5):379−83.
[101] Van Meerbeek B, Vargas M, Inoue S, Yoshida Y, Peumans M, Lambrechts P, et al. Adhesives and cements to promote preservation dentistry. Oper Dent 2001;6:119−44.
[102] Asmussen E, Hansen EK, Peutzfeldt A. Influence of the solubility parameter of intermediary resin on the effectiveness of the gluma bonding system. J Dent Res 1991;70(9):1290−3.
[103] VanMeerbeek B, DeMunck J, Yoshida Y, Inoue S, Vargas M, Vijay P, et al. Buonocore memorial lecture. Adhesion to enamel and dentin: current status and future challenges. Oper Dent 2003;28(3):215−35.
[104] Nakabayashi N, Kojima K, Masuhara E. The promotion of adhesion by the infiltration of monomers into tooth substrates. J Biomed Mater Res 1982;16(3):265−73.
[105] Yoshida Y, Nagakane K, Fukuda R, Nakayama Y, Okazaki M, Shintani H, et al. Comparative study on adhesive performance of functional monomers. J Dent Res 2004;83(6):454−8.
[106] Peumans M, Kanumilli P, De Munck J, Van Landuyt K, Lambrechts P, Van Meerbeek B. Clinical effectiveness of contemporary adhesives: a systematic review of current clinical trials. Dent Mater 2001;21(9):864−81.
[107] Coessens V, Pintauer T, Matyjaszewski K. Functional polymers by atom transfer radical polymerization. Prog Polym Sci 2001;26(3):337−77.
[108] Sheldon RP. Composite polymeric materials. New York: Applied Science Publishers; 1982.
[109] Paul SJ, Leach M, Rueggeberg FA, Pashley DH. Effect of water content on the physical properties of model dentine primer and bonding resins. J Dent 1999;27(3):209−14.
[110] Asmussen E, Peutzfeldt A. Influence of selected components on crosslink density in polymer structures. Eur J Oral Sci 2001;109(4):282−5.
[111] Mabilleau G, Moreau MF, Filmon R, Basle MF, Chappard D. Biodegradability of poly(2-hydroxyethyl methacrylate) in the presence of the J774.2 macrophage cell line. Biomaterials 2004;25(21):5155−62.
[112] Hayakawa T, Kikutake K, Nemoto K. Influence of self-etching primer treatment on the adhesion of resin composite to polished dentin and enamel. Dent Mater 1998;14(2):99−105.
[113] Andreasson H, Boman A, Johnsson S, Karlsson S, Barregard L. On permeability of methyl methacrylate, 2-hydroxyethyl methacrylate and triethyleneglycol dimethacrylate through protective gloves in dentistry. Eur J Oral Sci 2003;111(6):529−35.
[114] Geurtsen W. Biocompatibility of resin-modified filling materials. Crit Rev Oral Biol Med 2000;11(3):333−55.
[115] Goossens A. Contact allergic reactions on the eyes and eyelids. Bull Soc Belge Ophtalmol 2004;292:11−7.
[116] Paranjpe A, Bordador LC, Wang MY, Hume WR, Jewett A. Resin monomer 2-

hydroxyethyl methacrylate (HEMA) is a potent inducer of apoptotic cell death in human and mouse cells. J Dent Res 2005;84 (2):172–7.
[117] Pashley EL, Zhang Y, Lockwood PE, Rueggeberg FA, Pashley DH. Effects of HEMA on water evaporation from water–HEMA mixtures. Dent Mater 1998;14(1):6–10.
[118] Nakabayashi N, Takarada K. Effect of HEMA on bonding to dentin. Dent Mater 1992;8(2):125–30.
[119] Nakabayashi N, Watanabe A, Gendusa NJ. Dentin adhesion of "modified" 4-META/MMA-TBB resin: function of HEMA. Dent Mater 1992;8(4):259–64.
[120] Burrow MF, Inokoshi S, Tagami J. Water sorption of several bonding resins. Am J Dent 1999;12(6):295–8.
[121] Hannig M, Reinhardt KJ, Bott B. Self-etching primer vs. phosphoric acid: an alternative concept for composite-to-enamel bonding. Oper Dent 1999;24(3):172–80.
[122] Hitmi L, Bouter D, Degrange M. Influence of drying and HEMA treatment on dentin wettability. Dent Mater 2002;18(7):503–11.
[123] Hasegawa T, Manabe A, Itoh K, Wakumoto S. Investigation of self etching dentin primers. Dent Mater 1989;5(6):408–10.
[124] Nakaoki Y, Nikaido T, Pereira PN, Inokoshi S, Tagami J. Dimensional changes of demineralized dentin treated with HEMA primers. Dent Mater 2000;16(6):441–6.
[125] Patel MP, Johnstone MB, Hughes FJ, Braden M. The effect of two hydrophilic monomers on the water uptake of a heterocyclic methacrylate system. Biomaterials 2001;22(1):81–6.
[126] Tay FR, King NM, Chan KM, Pashley DH. How can nanoleakage occur in self-etching adhesive systems that demineralize and infiltrate simultaneously? J Adhes Dent 2002;4(4):255–69.
[127] Nakabayashi N, Hiranuma K. Effect of etchant variation on wet and dry dentin bonding primed with 4-META/acetone. Dent Mater 2000;16(4):274–9.
[128] Chang JC, Hurst TL, Hart DA, Estey AW. 4-META use in dentistry: a literature review. J Prosthet Dent 2002;87 (2):216–24.
[129] Chang JC. Amalgam repair with a 4-META resin. J Prosthet Dent 2004;92(5):506–7.
[130] Ohno H, Endo K, Hashimoto M. New mechanical retention method for resin and gold alloy bonding. Dent Mater 2004;20 (4):330–7.
[131] Ikemura K, Endo T. Effects of a new 4-acryloxyethyltrimellitic acid in a visible light-cured dental adhesive on adhesion and polymerization reactivity. J Appl Polym Sci 1997;69:1057–69.
[132] Tani C, Itoh K, Hisamitsu H, Wakumoto S. Efficacy of dentin bonding agents combined with self-etching dentin primers containing phenyl-P. Dent Mater J 1993;12(2):219–24.
[133] Chigira H, Yukitani W, Hasegawa T, Manabe A, Itoh K, Hayakawa T, et al. Self-etching dentin primers containing phenyl-P. J Dent Res 1994;73(5):1088–95.
[134] Salz U, Zimmermann J, Zeuner F, Moszner N. Hydrolytic stability of self-etching adhesive systems. J Adhes Dent 2005;7 (2):107–16.
[135] Torii Y, Itou K, Nishitani Y, Yoshiyama M, Ishikawa K, Suzuki K. Effect of self-etching primer containing N-acryloyl aspartic acid on enamel adhesion. Dent Mater 2003;19 (4):253–8.

7 Silicones

Andrè Colas and Jim Curtis

OUTLINE

7.1 Chemical Structure and Nomenclature 131
   7.1.1 Historical Milestones in Silicone Chemistry 132
   7.1.2 Nomenclature 132
   7.1.3 Preparation 133
      7.1.3.1 Silicone Polymers 133
      7.1.3.2 Polymerization and Polycondensation 133
      7.1.3.3 Silicone Elastomers 136
      7.1.3.4 Silicone Gels 140

      7.1.3.5 Silicone Adhesives 140
      7.1.3.6 Silicone Film-in-Place, Fast-Cure Elastomers 141
   7.1.4 Physico-Chemical Properties 141

7.2 Conclusion 142

Acknowledgments 142

References 142

Silicone materials have been widely used in medicine for over 60 years. Available in a variety of material types, they have unique chemical and physical properties that manifest in excellent biocompatibility and biodurability for many applications. Silicone elastomers have remarkably low glass-transition temperatures and maintain their flexibility over a wide temperature range, enabling them to withstand conditions from cold storage to steam autoclaving. They have high permeability to gases and many drugs, advantageous respectively in wound care or in transdermal drug delivery. They have low surface tension and remarkable chemical stability, enabling biocompatibility and biodurability in many long-term implant applications.

However, versatile as they are, present-day silicone materials still have limitations. The mechanical properties of silicone elastomers, such as tensile strength or tear resistance, are somewhat lower than for other implantable elastomers such as polyurethanes (although generally speaking, polyurethanes are less biodurable). While resistant to a wide array of chemical environments, silicone elastomers are susceptible to degradation in very strongly basic or acidic conditions, such as those found in the stomach. Like all hydrophobic implant materials, silicones are quickly coated with proteins when placed in tissue contact; and a scar tissue capsule forms to surround an implant during wound healing, walling it off from the host. Additionally, silicone elastomers are thermosetting materials, requiring different processing from conventional thermoplastics, which can on occasion be seen as a drawback.

7.1 Chemical Structure and Nomenclature

Silicones are a general category of synthetic polymers whose backbone is made of repeating silicon-to-oxygen bonds. In addition to their links to oxygen to form the polymeric chain, the silicon atoms are also bonded to organic groups, typically methyl groups. This is the basis for the name "silicones," which was assigned by Kipping based on their similarity with ketones, because in most cases there is on average one silicone atom for one oxygen and two methyl groups [1]. Later, as these materials and their applications flourished, more specific nomenclature was developed. The basic repeating unit became known as "siloxane," and the most common silicone is polydimethylsiloxane, abbreviated as PDMS.

Table 7.1 Key Milestones in the Development of Silicone Chemistry

1824	Berzelius discovers silicon by the reduction of potassium fluorosilicate with potassium: $4K + K_2SiF_6 \rightarrow Si + 6KF$. Reacting silicon with chlorine gives a volatile compound later identified as tetrachlorosilane, $SiCl_4$: $Si + 2Cl_2 \rightarrow SiCl_4$.
1863	Friedel and Crafts synthesize the first silicon organic compound, tetraethylsilane: $2Zn(C_2H_5)_2 + SiCl_4 \rightarrow Si(C_2H_5)_4 + 2ZnCl_2$.
1871	Ladenburg observes that diethyldiethoxysilane $(C_2H_5)_2Si(OC_2H_5)_2$, in the presence of a diluted acid gives an oil that decomposes only at a "very high temperature."
1901–1930s	Kipping lays the foundation of organosilicon chemistry with the preparation of various silanes by means of Grignard reactions and the hydrolysis of chlorosilanes to yield "large molecules." The polymeric nature of the silicones is confirmed by the work of Stock.
1940s	In the 1940s, silicones become commercial materials after Hyde of Dow Corning demonstrates the thermal stability and high electrical resistance of silicone resins, and Rochow of General Electric finds a direct method to prepare silicones from silicon and methylchloride.

$$-\left(\begin{array}{c} R \\ | \\ Si-O- \\ | \\ R \end{array}\right) \text{ and if R is } CH_3, \quad -\left(\begin{array}{c} CH_3 \\ | \\ Si-O- \\ | \\ CH_3 \end{array}\right)_n$$

"siloxane"   "polydimethylsiloxane"

Many other groups (e.g., phenyl, vinyl, and trifluoropropyl) can be substituted for the methyl groups along the chain. The simultaneous presence of organic groups attached to an inorganic backbone give silicones a combination of distinctive properties, making their use possible as fluids, emulsions, compounds, resins, and elastomers in numerous applications and diverse fields. For example, silicones are common in the aerospace industry, due principally to their low and high temperature performance. In the electronics field, silicones are used as electrical insulation, potting compounds, and other applications specific to semiconductor manufacture. Their long-term durability has made silicone sealants, adhesives, and waterproof coatings commonplace in the construction industry. Excellent biocompatibility makes many silicones well suited for use in numerous personal care, pharmaceutical, and medical device applications.

7.1.1 Historical Milestones in Silicone Chemistry

Key milestones in the development of silicone chemistry, thoroughly described elsewhere by Lane and Burns [2], Rochow [3], and Noll [4], are summarized in Table 7.1.

7.1.2 Nomenclature

The most common silicones are the trimethylsilyloxy end-blocked polydimethylsiloxanes, with the following structure:

$$CH_3-\underset{\underset{CH_3}{|}}{\overset{\overset{CH_3}{|}}{Si}}-O-\left(\underset{\underset{CH_3}{|}}{\overset{\overset{CH_3}{|}}{Si}}-O\right)_n-\underset{\underset{CH_3}{|}}{\overset{\overset{CH_3}{|}}{Si}}-CH_3,$$

$$(n = 0,1,\ldots)$$

These are linear polymers and liquids, even for large values of n. The main chain unit, $-(Si(CH_3)_2O)-$, is often represented by the letter D for $(CH_3)_2SiO_{2/2}$, because with the silicon atom connected to two oxygen atoms this unit is capable of expanding within the polymer in two directions. M, T, and Q units are defined in a similar manner, as shown in Table 7.2.

Table 7.2 Shorthand Notation for Siloxane Polymer Units

M	D	T	Q
$(CH_3)_3SiO_{1/2}$	$(CH_3)_2SiO_{2/2}$	$CH_3SiO_{3/2}$	$SiO_{4/2}$

Table 7.3 Examples of Silicone Shorthand Notation

Structure	Notation
$H_3C-Si(CH_3)_2-O-[Si(CH_3)_2-O]_n-Si(CH_3)_3$ (MD$_n$M)	MD$_n$M
Cyclic tetramer [(CH$_3$)$_2$SiO]$_4$ (D$_4$)	D$_4$
Branched trisiloxane (TM$_3$)	TM$_3$
QM$_2$M^{H}M^{C_2H_5} structure	QM$_2$M^{H}M^{C2H5} or QM$_2$M^{H}M^{Et}

The system is sometimes modified by the use of superscript letters designating nonmethyl substituents, for example, D^H = H(CH$_3$)SiO$_{2/2}$ and M^ϕ or M^{Ph} = (CH$_3$)$_2$(C$_6$H$_5$)SiO$_{1/2}$ [5]. Further examples are shown in Table 7.3.

7.1.3 Preparation

7.1.3.1 Silicone Polymers

The modern synthesis of silicone polymers is multifaceted. It usually involves the four basic steps described in Table 7.4. Only step 4 in this table will be elaborated upon here.

7.1.3.2 Polymerization and Polycondensation

The linear [4] and cyclic [5] oligomers resulting from dimethyldichlorosilane [2] hydrolysis have chain lengths too short for most applications. The cyclics must be polymerized, and the linears condensed, to give macromolecules of sufficient length [4].

Catalyzed by acids or bases, cyclosiloxanes (R$_2$SiO)$_m$ are ring-opened and polymerized to form long linear chains. At equilibrium, the reaction results in a mixture of cyclic oligomers plus a distribution of linear polymers. The proportion of

Table 7.4 The Basic Steps in Silicone Polymer Synthesis

1. Silica reduction to silicon	$SiO_2 + 2C \rightarrow Si + 2CO$
2. Chlorosilanes synthesis	$Si + 2CH_3Cl \rightarrow (CH_3)_2SiCl_2$ [1] $+ CH_3SiCl_3$ [2] $+(CH_3)_3SiCl$ [3] $+ CH_3HSiCl_2 + \cdots$
3. Chlorosilanes hydrolysis	$Cl-Si(CH_3)_2-Cl + 2H_2O \rightarrow HO-(-Si(CH_3)_2-O-)_x-H + (-Si(CH_3)_2-O-)_{3,4,5} + HCl$ [1] linears [4], cyclics [5]
4. Polymerization and polycondensation	$(-Si(CH_3)_2-O-)_{3,4,5}$ cyclics [5] $\rightarrow (-Si(CH_3)_2-O-)_y$ polymer $HO-(-Si(CH_3)_2-O-)_x-H \rightarrow (-Si(CH_3)_2-O-)_z + zH_2O$ linears [4], polymer

cyclics depends on the substituents along the Si—O chain, the temperature, and the presence of a solvent. Polymer chain length depends on the presence and concentration of substances capable of giving chain ends. For example, in the KOH-catalyzed polymerization of the cyclic tetramer octamethylcyclotetrasiloxane $(Me_2SiO)_4$ ([5] or D_4 in shorthand notation), the average length of the polymer chains depends on the KOH concentration:

$x(Me_2SiO)_4 + KOH \rightarrow (Me_2SiO)_y + KO(Me_2SiO)_zH$

A stable hydroxy-terminated polymer, $HO(Me_2-SiO)_zH$, can be isolated after neutralization and removal of the remaining cyclics by stripping the mixture under vacuum at elevated temperature. A distribution of chains with different lengths is obtained. The reaction can also be made in the presence of $Me_3SiOSiMe_3$, which acts as a chain end-blocker:

∿∿ $Me_2SiOK + Me_3SiOSiMe_3$
$\rightarrow$ ∿∿ $Me_2SiOSiMe_3 + Me_3SiOK$

where ∿∿ represents the main chain.

The Me_3SiOK formed attacks another chain to reduce the average molecular weight of the linear polymer formed.

The copolymerization of $(Me_2SiO)_4$ in the presence of $Me_3SiOSiMe_3$ with Me_4NOH as catalyst displays a surprising viscosity change over time [4]. First a peak or viscosity maximum is observed at the beginning of the reaction. The presence of two oxygen atoms on each silicon in the cyclics makes them more susceptible to a nucleophilic attack by the base catalyst than the silicon of the end-blocker, which is substituted by only one oxygen atom. The cyclics are polymerized first into very long, viscous chains that are subsequently reduced in length by the addition of terminal groups provided by the end-blocker, which is slower to react. This reaction can be described as follows:

$Me_3SiOSiMe_3 + x(Me_2SiO)_4$
$\xrightarrow{cat} Me_3SiO(Me_2SiO)_nSiMe_3$

or, in shorthand notation:

$MM + xD_4 \xrightarrow{cat} MD_nM$

where $n = 4x$ (theoretically).

The ratio between D and M units defines the average molecular weight of the polymer formed.

Catalyst removal (or neutralization) is always an important step in silicone preparation. Most catalysts used to prepare silicones can also catalyze the depolymerization (attack along the chain), particularly at elevated temperatures in the presence of traces of water.

$$\sim\sim\sim(Me_2SiO)_n\sim\sim\sim + H_2O$$
$$\xrightarrow{cat} \sim\sim\sim(Me_2SiO)_y H + HO(Me_2SiO)_z\sim\sim\sim$$

It is therefore essential to remove all remaining traces of the catalyst, providing the silicone optimal thermal stability. Labile catalysts have been developed. These decompose or are volatilized above the optimum polymerization temperature, and consequently can be eliminated by a brief overheating. In this way, catalyst neutralization or filtration can be avoided [4].

The cyclic trimer $(Me_2SiO)_3$ has internal ring tension and can be polymerized without re-equilibration of the resulting polymers. With this cyclic, polymers with narrow molecular weight distribution can be prepared, as well as polymers only carrying one terminal reactive function (living polymerization). Starting from a mixture of cyclics with different internal ring tensions also allows preparation of block or sequential polymers [4].

Linears can combine when catalyzed by many acids or bases to give long chains by intermolecular condensation of silanol terminal groups [4,6].

$$\sim\sim\sim O-\underset{\underset{Me}{|}}{\overset{\overset{Me}{|}}{Si}}-OH + HO-\underset{\underset{Me}{|}}{\overset{\overset{Me}{|}}{Si}}-O\sim\sim\sim$$

$$\underset{+H_2O}{\overset{-H_2O}{\rightleftarrows}} \sim\sim\sim O-\underset{\underset{Me}{|}}{\overset{\overset{Me}{|}}{Si}}-O-\underset{\underset{Me}{|}}{\overset{\overset{Me}{|}}{Si}}-O\sim\sim\sim$$

A distribution of chain lengths is obtained. Longer chains are favored when working under vacuum or at elevated temperatures to reduce the residual water concentration. In addition to the polymers described above, reactive polymers can also be prepared. This result can be achieved when re-equilibrating oligomers or existing polymers to obtain a polydimethylmethylhydrogenosiloxane, $MD_zD^H_wM$.

$$Me_3SiOSiMe_3 + x(Me_2SiO)_4$$
$$+ Me_3SiO(MeHSiO)_ySiMe_3$$
$$\xrightarrow{cat} cyclics + Me_3SiO(Me_2SiO)_z(MeHSiO)_w$$
$$SiMe_3$$
[6]

Additional functional groups can be attached to this polymer using an addition reaction.

$$Me_3SiO(Me_2SiO)_z(MeHSiO)_wSiMe_3 + H_2C=CHR$$
[6]
$$\xrightarrow{Pt\ cat} Me_3SiO(Me_2SiO)_z(Me\underset{\underset{CH_2CH_2R}{|}}{Si}O)_wSiMe_3$$

All the polymers heretofore shown are linear or cyclic, comprising mainly difunctional units, D. In addition, branched polymers or resins can be prepared if, during hydrolysis of the chlorosilanes, a certain amount of T or Q units are included, which allow molecular expansion in three or four directions, as opposed to just two. For example, consider the hydrolysis of methyltrichlorosilane in the presence of trimethylchlorosilane, which leads to a branched polymer:

$$x\,Me-\underset{\underset{Me}{|}}{\overset{\overset{Me}{|}}{Si}}-Cl + y\,Me-\underset{\underset{Cl}{|}}{\overset{\overset{Cl}{|}}{Si}}-Cl \underset{-HCl}{\overset{+H_2O}{\longrightarrow}} z$$
$$\quad[3]\qquad\qquad[2]$$

$$Me-\underset{\underset{Me}{|}}{\overset{\overset{Me}{|}}{Si}}-O-\underset{\underset{O}{|}}{\overset{\overset{Me}{|}}{Si}}-O-\underset{\underset{OH}{|}}{\overset{\overset{Me}{|}}{Si}}-O\sim\sim\sim$$
$$Me-\underset{\underset{O}{|}}{Si}-O\sim\sim\sim$$
$$Me-\underset{\underset{Me}{|}}{Si}-Me$$

The resulting polymer can be described as $(Me_3SiO_{1/2})_x(MeSiO_{3/2})_y$ or M_xT_y, using shorthand notation. The formation of three silanols on the $MeSiCl_3$ by hydrolysis yields a three-dimensional structure or resin after condensation, rather than a linear polymer. The average molecular weight depends upon the number of M units that come from the trimethylchlorosilane, which limits the growth of the resin molecule. Most of these resins are prepared in a solvent and usually contain some residual hydroxyl groups. These groups could subsequently be used to cross-link the resin and form a continuous network.

7.1.3.3 Silicone Elastomers

Silicone polymers can easily be transformed into a three-dimensional network by way of a cross-linking reaction, which allows formation of chemical bonds between adjacent chains. The majority of silicone elastomers are cross-linked according to one of the following three reactions.

Cross-linking with radicals

Efficient cross-linking with radicals is achieved only when some vinyl groups are present on the polymer chains. The following mechanism has been proposed for the cross-linking reaction associated with radicals generated from an organic peroxide for the initiation, propagation, and termination steps [6]:

$$R^{\cdot} + CH_2=CH-Si\equiv \rightarrow R-CH_2-CH^{\cdot}-Si\equiv$$
$$RCH_2-CH^{\cdot}-Si\equiv + CH_3-Si\equiv$$
$$\rightarrow RCH_2-CH_2-Si\equiv + \equiv Si-CH_2^{\cdot}$$
$$\equiv Si-CH_2^{\cdot} + CH_2=CH-Si\equiv$$
$$\rightarrow \equiv Si-CH_2-CH_2-CH^{\cdot}-Si\equiv$$
$$\equiv Si-CH_2-CH_2-CH^{\cdot}-Si\equiv + \equiv Si-CH_3$$
$$\rightarrow \equiv Si-CH_2-CH_2-Si\equiv + \equiv Si-CH_2^{\cdot}$$
$$2\equiv Si-CH_2^{\cdot} \rightarrow \equiv Si-CH_2-CH_2-Si\equiv$$

where $\equiv$ represents two methyl groups and the rest of the polymer chain.

This reaction has been used for high-consistency silicone rubbers (HCRs), such as those used in extrusion or compression and injection molding, which are cross-linked at elevated temperatures. The peroxide is added before processing. During cure, some precautions are needed to avoid the formation of voids by the volatile residues of the peroxide. Post-cure may also be necessary to remove these volatiles, which can catalyze depolymerization at high temperatures.

Cross-linking by condensation

Although mostly used in construction sealants and caulks, condensation-cure silicone materials have also found utility in medical device manufacturing as silicone adhesives (facilitating the adherence to materials of silicone elastomers), encapsulants, and sealants.

One-part products are ready to apply and require no mixing. Cross-linking starts when the product is squeezed from the tube or cartridge and comes into contact with moisture, typically from humidity in the ambient air. These materials are formulated from a reactive polymer prepared from a hydroxy end-blocked polydimethylsiloxane and a large excess of methyltriacetoxysilane.

$$HO-(Me_2SiO)_x-H + excess\ MeSi(OAc)_3$$
$$\xrightarrow{-2AcOH} (AcO)_2MeSiO(Me_2SiO)_x OSiMe(OAc)_2$$
$$[7]$$

where
$$Ac = \begin{array}{c} CH_3 \\ | \\ -C=O \end{array}$$

Because of this excess, the probability of two different chains reacting with the same silane molecule is remote. Consequently, all the chains are end-blocked with two acetoxy functional groups. The resulting product is still liquid and can be packaged in sealed tubes and cartridges. Upon opening and exposing the sealant to room humidity, acetoxy groups are hydrolyzed to give silanols, which allow further condensation to occur.

$$\begin{array}{ccc}
\text{Me} & & \text{Me} \\
| & & | \\
\sim\sim O-Si-OAc & \xrightarrow[-AcOH]{+H_2O} & \sim\sim O-Si-OH \\
| & & | \\
\text{OAc} & & \text{OAc} \\
[7] & & [8]
\end{array}$$

$$\begin{array}{ccc}
\text{Me} & & \text{Me} \\
| & & | \\
\sim\sim O-Si-OH + AcO-Si-O\sim\sim \\
| & & | \\
\text{OAc} & & \text{OAc} \\
[8] & & [7]
\end{array}$$

$$\xrightarrow{-AcOH} \begin{array}{cc}
\text{Me} & \text{Me} \\
| & | \\
\sim\sim O-Si-O-Si-O\sim\sim \\
| & | \\
\text{OAc} & \text{OAc}
\end{array}$$

In this way, two chains have been linked, and the reaction continues from the remaining acetoxy groups. An organometallic tin catalyst is normally used, and the cross-linking reaction requires moisture to diffuse into the material. Accordingly, cure will proceed from the outside surface inward. These materials are called one-part RTV (room temperature vulcanization) sealants, but actually require moisture as a second component. Acetic acid is released as a by-product of the reaction. Problems resulting from the acid can be overcome by using other cure (cross-linking) reactions developed by replacing the methyltriacetoxysilane MeSi(OAc)$_3$ with oximosilane RSi(ON=CR′)$_3$ or alkoxysilane RSi(OR′)$_3$.

Condensation curing is also used in some two-part products where cross-linking starts upon mixing the two components (e.g., a hydroxy end-blocked polymer and an alkoxysilane such as tetra-n-propoxysilane, Si(OnPr)$_4$) [4]:

$$4 \; \sim\!\!\!\sim\!\!\!\sim \mathrm{Si(Me)_2-OH} + n\mathrm{PrO-Si(OnPr)_2-OnPr}$$

$$\xrightarrow[-4n\mathrm{PrOH}]{\mathrm{cat}} \text{cross-linked network}$$

Here, no atmospheric moisture is needed. Usually an organotin salt is used as a catalyst, but it also limits the stability of the resulting elastomer at high temperatures. Alcohol is released as a by-product of the reaction, leading to some shrinkage after cure at room temperature (0.5–2% linear shrinkage). Silicones with this cure system may not be suitable for the fabrication of parts with precise tolerances.

Cross-linking by addition

Use of an addition-cure reaction for cross-linking can eliminate the shrinkage problem mentioned above. In addition-cure, cross-linking is achieved by reacting vinyl end-blocked polymers with ≡Si–H groups carried by a functional oligomer such as described above [6]. A few polymers can be bonded to this functional oligomer [6] [6]:

$$\sim\!\!\!\sim\!\!\!\sim \mathrm{O-Si(Me)_2-CH=CH_2} + \mathrm{H-Si} \equiv$$

$$\xrightarrow{\mathrm{cat}} \sim\!\!\!\sim\!\!\!\sim \mathrm{O-Si(Me)_2-CH_2-CH_2-Si} \equiv \quad [5]$$

where ≡ represents the remaining valences of the Si in [6].

The addition occurs mainly on the terminal carbon and is catalyzed by Pt or Rh metal complexes, preferably as organometallic compounds to enhance their solubility. The following mechanism has been proposed (oxidative addition of the ≡Si–H to the Pt complex, H transfer to the double bond, and reductive elimination of the product):

$$\equiv\mathrm{Si-CH=CH_2} + \mathrm{H-Si} \equiv \xrightarrow{\mathrm{Pt}}$$
$$\equiv\mathrm{Si-CH=CH_2}$$
$$\qquad \mid$$
$$\qquad \mathrm{Pt}$$
$$\qquad /\,\backslash$$
$$\equiv\mathrm{Si} \quad \mathrm{H}$$
$$\rightleftarrows \equiv\mathrm{Si-CH_2-CH_2-Pt-Si}\equiv$$
$$\xrightarrow[-\mathrm{Pt}]{} \equiv\mathrm{Si-CH_2-CH_2-Si}\equiv$$

where, to simplify, other Pt ligands and other Si substituents are omitted.

There are no by-products with this reaction. Molded silicone elastomer components cured at room temperature by this addition-reaction mechanism are very accurate in terms of dimensional tolerance (i.e., there is no shrinkage). At elevated temperatures, some shrinkage occurs because of the thermal expansion during cure. However, handling these two-part products (i.e., Si–Vi polymer and Pt complex in one component, Si–Vi polymer and SiH oligomer in the other) requires some precautions. The Pt in the complex is easily bonded to electron-donating substances such as amine or organosulfur compounds to form stable complexes with these "poisons," rendering the catalyst complex inactive and inhibiting the cure.

The preferred cure system can vary by application. For example, silicone medical bonding adhesives use acetoxy cure (condensation cross-linking), while platinum cure (cross-linking by addition) is used for precise silicone parts with no by-products.

Elastomer filler

In addition to the silicone polymers described above, most silicone elastomers incorporate "filler." Besides acting as a material extender, as the name implies, filler acts to reinforce the cross-linked matrix. The strength of silicone polymers without filler is unsatisfactory for most applications [4]. Like most other noncrystallized synthetic elastomers, the addition of reinforcing fillers reduces the tackiness of the silicone, increases its hardness, and enhances its mechanical strength. Fillers might also be employed to affect other properties; for example, carbon black is added for electrical conductivity, or barium sulfate to increase radiopacity. These and other materials are used to pigment the otherwise colorless elastomer; however, care must be taken to select only pigments suitable for the processing temperatures and end-use application.

Generally, the most favorable reinforcement is obtained by using fumed silica, such as Cab—O—Sil®, Aerosil®, or Wacker HDK®. Fumed silica is produced by the vapor phase hydrolysis of silicon tetrachloride vapor in a hydrogen/oxygen flame:

$$SiCl_4 + 2H_2 + O_2 \xrightarrow{1800°C} SiO_2 + 4HCl$$

Unlike many naturally occurring forms of crystalline silica, fumed silica is amorphous. The very small spheroid silica particles (in the order of 10 nm in diameter) fuse irreversibly while still semi-molten, creating aggregates. When cool, these aggregates become physically entangled to form agglomerates. Silica produced in this way possesses remarkably high surface area (100–400 m^2/g), as measured by the BET method developed by Brunauer, Emmett, and Teller [4,7,8].

The incorporation of silica filler into silicone polymers is accomplished prior to cross-linking, by mixing the silica into the silicone polymers on a two-roll mill, in a twin-screw extruder, or in a Z-blade mixer capable of processing materials with this rheology.

Reinforcement occurs with polymer adsorption encouraged by the large surface area of the silica, and when hydroxyl groups on the filler surface lead to hydrogen bonds between the filler and the silicone polymer. In this way, reinforcing filler contributes to the high tensile strength and elongation

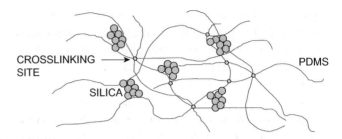

Figure 7.1 Silicone elastomer/silica network.

capability of silicone rubber [9]. The addition of filler increases the already high viscosity of the polymer. Uncured silicone elastomers can have viscosities from 10,000 to well over 100,000 mPa·s. Chemical treatment of the silica filler with silanes enhances its incorporation in, and reinforcement of, the silicone elastomer, resulting in increased material strength and tear resistance [2] (Figure 7.1).

> Silicone elastomers for medical applications normally use fumed silica as filler, and occasionally appropriate pigments or barium sulfate. Because of their low glass transition temperatures, these compounded and cured silicone materials are elastomeric at room and body temperatures without the use of plasticizers, unlike other medical materials such as PVC, which might contain phthalate additives.

Processing of silicone elastomers

In addition to the polymer blend with amorphous silica filler, other ingredients are needed: an initiator or cross-linker plus catalyst. To avoid premature cure during shipment and storage, these ingredients must be separated. Consequently, products for making silicone elastomers are generally supplied as two components or two-part kits, for example, a base and a peroxide paste, or a kit made of Part A containing polymer and catalyst, and Part B containing polymer and cross-linker. These two components are mixed at a fixed ratio at the point of use and formed into the desired shape before cure.

Silicone elastomers are thermosetting materials. They must be formed into the appropriate shape and configuration prior to cross-linking. Unlike a thermoplastic, which can be remelted and formed again, a cured silicone elastomer part cannot be reprocessed. Suitable processing methods for shaping silicone elastomers include casting, extrusion, and molding. The process selected depends on the viscosity of the feedstock elastomer material, and the shape and configuration of the desired cured elastomer product.

High Consistency Rubber (HCR). If very high molecular weight silicone polymers are used (silicone "gums" in the trade), the result is high consistency rubbers, which are desirable as they allow for high tear strengths and tensile elongations. Uncured HCRs are putty-like materials that require high shear equipment for processing. These are usually supplied in two parts to be mixed prior to use, either as a silicone base plus a peroxide initiator or as two-part kit using a Pt cure system. These parts are combined using high shear two-roll mills. The mixed material is then shaped into "preforms" before use in compression, transfer or injection molding at elevated temperature. *Compression molding* requires the simplest equipment: a preform is inserted in a mold and cured under high pressure at elevated temperature. The preform must be of an approximate shape that corresponds well to the mold cavity. This allows sufficient material to fill the cavity without producing excessive flash, the overflow material that remains attached to the parts from around the edge of the mold. Removal of flash requires post-processing. *Transfer molding* requires less preparation of the preform: a more precise but simply shaped preform is transferred from a receiving cavity to the mold cavity. *Injection molding* allows for more automation: an extruder system is used to inject a simple ribbon preform directly into the mold cavity. Typical considerations in this case are controlling the exact amount of material sent to the molding cavity to avoid flash, and maximizing speed but avoiding "scorching" (premature cure before the mold cavity is properly filled). HCRs are also used for *extrusion* to produce tubing, as they have enough "green strength" or mechanical integrity when leaving a cooled extruder and prior to enter a curing oven. When peroxides are used, post-cure in a well-ventilated oven is necessary to remove peroxide by-products, which could bloom at the surface and can reduce the stability of the cured elastomer. One part HCR materials, for which all ingredients have been premixed by the supplier, are also available, but have limited shelf-life depending on the cure system.

Liquid Silicone Rubber (LSR). If lower molecular weight silicone polymers are used, the silicone polymer/silica blend viscosities are lower, leading to liquid silicone rubber. These LSRs are provided as two-part materials that can be used in liquid injection molding—pumped, metered, mixed, and then directly injected in the molding cavity. Processing is eased by the shear-thinning effect that occurs during pumping and injection, reducing the viscosity of the LSR blend and the injection pressures compared to HCR processing. LSRs are particularly well-suited for long automated production runs. Mixing LSR Parts A and B from two 200-liter drums is typically automated using a static mixer prior to direct injection of the precise amount needed. In contrast with the handling of small quantities of HCR on a two-roll mill, preforming, and molding, LSR processing allows more automation. Yet liquid injection molding requires higher investment in the equipment to control the injected amount (to avoid under- or over-filling the mold) precisely. Precise mold cavity temperature control is needed, as cold material is quickly and repeatedly injected into a hot mold. With LSRs, complex molds are needed, preferably with cold runners to avoid premature cure in the feeding lines between injection cycles, with tight specifications still allowing venting (air escape from the mold cavity during injection). The molds may be equipped with complex ejectors to remove parts quickly at the end of the cure, enabling the processing of the next part without loosing thermal control of the mold. The acquisition cost of liquid injection molding machines and sophisticated molds is usually justified for large production runs, as they provide for more efficiency in terms of mold cycle time, overall processing time, and material usage. Cycle time is dependant on operator skills, equipment, and the part to be cured. Typical conditions for LSRs are 0.3–3.0 seconds injection time, 150–200°C cure temperature, and 3–5 sec/mm thickness cure time, depending on formulations [10].

> Fabricators of silicone elastomer parts should be aware that these LSRs and other addition-cure products contain an inhibitor, a substance that weakly bonds to the platinum catalyst to moderate its activity, permitting sufficient pot life by avoiding premature cure. If contamination occurs with substances capable of bonding more strongly to the platinum catalyst (e.g., amino or thio compounds), the catalyst (which is present in only minute quantities, typically about 10 ppm) may lose activity, resulting in inhibition of elastomer cure.

Room Temperature Vulcanizing (RTV) elastomers. In addition to HCRs and LSRs, which are designed to cure by exposure to heat, other silicone elastomers, known as RTVs, are intended to be cured at room temperature. Typically, RTV elastomers are provided in two-part systems and can be viewed as a variation of the LSRs, but with lower viscosity and less inhibitor. They can be mixed with a spatula and cast after de-airing, and are typically used for laboratory trials and commercially in medical applications for dental impression molding. RTVs are also available as one-part silicone elastomers provided ready to use, usually as adhesives. These materials rely on a condensation reaction and on moisture in the air as the second component to achieve cure.

7.1.3.4 Silicone Gels

Silicone gels are typically composed of a very lightly cross-linked silicone elastomer whose polymer network has been swollen with silicone fluids; however, these gels contain no silica or other fillers. Medical applications for silicone gels include breast, testicular, and other soft-tissue implants for tissue augmentation or to help restore one's appearance after cancer surgery. In addition, silicone gel external breast prostheses can be worn in or attached to garments, such as brassieres, for similar purposes. Silicone gel is often supplied in a two-part fluid system and cures via a platinum-catalyzed addition reaction. Parts A and B are mixed at a desired ratio and cured (usually by exposure to elevated temperature) to yield a sticky, cohesive mass of the desired consistency. The consistency of the material can be controlled by the degree of cross-linking, as well as quality and quantity of swelling fluid. After mixing but before curing, the mixture is still liquid and can be pushed through a large gauge needle, enabling the filling of a silicone elastomer implant shell or the thermoformed pouch of an external breast prosthesis made of a thin polyurethane film.

Beyond gel implants and external prostheses, silicone gels find application in skin-contacting sheet goods in wound and scar care.

In addition to gels composed entirely of silicone materials, the gel used in some gel pads for the prevention of pressure sores or for orthotic applications are comprised of a cross-linked silicone polymer network swollen with non-silicone fluids such as mineral oil.

7.1.3.5 Silicone Adhesives

Three basic types of silicone adhesives are used in medical applications: bonding, pressure-sensitive, and gel.

1. *Bonding adhesives.* Silicone bonding adhesives are used to attach components together and to seal seams and junctions. Electrical components can also be encapsulated and insulated using silicone bonding adhesive. Silicone bonding adhesives are most commonly formulated as one-part RTV elastomer systems that use a condensation cross-linking reaction, as described earlier in this chapter.

2. *Pressure-sensitive adhesives.* Silicone PSAs are typically formulated in solvent. A silanol end-blocked PDMS undergoes a polycondensation reaction with a silicate resin in the presence of ammonia as catalyst. The ammonia is stripped with heat, and usually the solvent is exchanged.

In some applications, a hot melt silicone PSA is used ostensibly without solvent.

Silicone PSAs have properties that make them well-suited for application in the medical area. Besides their biocompatibility, the materials are highly flexible and permeable to moisture vapor, CO_2, and oxygen. Silicone PSAs can provide strong adhesion to the skin, facilitating the attachment of hairpieces, prosthetics, and other devices to the body, and they are widely used in transdermal drug delivery. Due to compatibility concerns with amine-containing drugs, an additional class of silicone PSAs have been generated by the further reaction of the PSA with hexamethyldisilazane to convert the pendant $\equiv$ SiOH groups into $\equiv$ SiOSi(CH$_3$)$_3$.

3. *Gel adhesives.* Silicone gel adhesives, also known as soft skin adhesives, are used in wound care, and are found to be gentler and less traumatic on removal than the pressure-sensitive types. Unlike PSAs, which are typically formulated in solvent, silicone gel adhesives are supplied in solventless two-part systems. In addition to wound care applications, the materials are also used in the treatment of hypertrophic and keloid scars. Evidence suggests this therapy may reduce scar height and appearance [11].

7.1.3.6 Silicone Film-in-Place, Fast-Cure Elastomers

In addition to the cured silicone elastomers in skin contact applications, *in situ* cure materials have been developed. These materials form films when spread or sprayed on the skin, and then undergo RTV cure. Products such as spray-on wound dressings or drug-loaded lotions have been evaluated. The ability of silicone to spread and form films is related to its low surface tension as described in Section 7.1.4 below [12].

7.1.4 Physico-Chemical Properties

The position of silicon just under carbon in the periodic table led to a belief in the existence of analog compounds where silicon would replace carbon. Most of these analog compounds do not exist, or behave very differently from their carbon counterparts. There are few similarities between Si—X bonds in silicones and C—X bonds [2,6,13,14].

Between any given element and Si, bond lengths are longer than for the element and C. The lower electronegativity of silicon ($\chi_{Si} \approx 1.80$, $\chi_C \approx 2.55$) leads to a very polar Si—O bond compared to C—O. This bond polarity also contributes to strong silicon bonding; for example, the Si—O bond is highly ionic and has a high bond energy. To some extent, these values explain the stability of silicones. The Si—O bond is highly resistant to homolytic scission. On the other hand, heterolytic scissions are easy, as demonstrated by the re-equilibration reactions occurring during polymerizations catalyzed by acids or bases.

Silicones exhibit the unusual combination of an inorganic chain similar to silicates and often associated with high surface energy, but with side methyl groups that are very organic and often associated

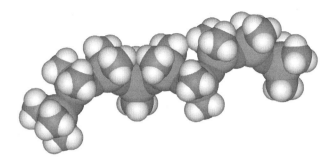

Figure 7.2 Three-dimensional representation of eicosamethylnonasiloxane, $Me_3SiO(SiMe_2O)_7SiMe_3$ or MD_7M. *(Courtesy T. Lane, Dow Corning.)*

with low surface energy [15]. The Si—O bonds are moderately polar, and without protection would lead to strong intermolecular interactions [6]. Yet, the methyl groups, only weakly interacting with each other, shield the main chain (see Figure 7.2).

The surface activity of silicones is evident in many ways [15]:

- Polydimethylsiloxanes have low surface tension (20.4 mN/m) and are capable of wetting most surfaces. With the methyl groups pointing to the outside, this configuration gives very hydrophobic films and a surface with good release properties, particularly if the film is cured after application. Silicone surface tension is also in the most promising range considered for biocompatible elastomers (20–30 mN/m) [16].

- Silicones have a critical surface tension of wetting (24 mN/m), higher than their own surface tension. This means silicones are capable of wetting themselves, which promotes good film formation and surface coverage.

- Silicone organic copolymers can be prepared with surfactant properties, with the silicone as the hydrophobic part (e.g., in silicone glycol copolymers).

The low intermolecular interactions in silicones have other consequences [15]:

- Glass transition temperatures are very low (e.g., 146°K for a polydimethylsiloxane compared to 200°K for poly-isobutylene, the analog hydrocarbon).

Continued

> —cont'd
> - The presence of a high free volume compared to hydrocarbons explains the high solubility and high diffusion coefficient of gas into silicones. Silicones have a high permeability to oxygen, nitrogen, or water vapor, even though liquid water is not capable of wetting a silicone surface. As expected, silicone compressibility is also high.
> - The viscous movement activation energy is very low for silicones, and their viscosity is less dependent on temperature compared to hydrocarbon polymers. Furthermore, chain entanglements are involved at higher temperature, and contribute to limit viscosity reduction [6].

This shielding is made easier by the high flexibility of the siloxane chain. Barriers to rotation are low, and the siloxane chain can adopt many configurations. Rotation energy around a H_2C-CH_2 bond in polyethylene is 13.8 kJ/mol, but is only 3.3 kJ/mol around a Me_2Si-O bond, corresponding to a nearly free rotation. In general, the siloxane chain adopts a configuration so that the chain exposes a maximum number of methyl groups to the outside, whereas in hydrocarbon polymers, the relative rigidity of the polymer backbone does not allow selective exposure of the most organic or hydrophobic methyl groups. Chain-to-chain interactions are low, and the distance between adjacent chains is also greater in silicones. Despite a very polar chain, silicones can be compared to paraffin, with a low critical surface tension of wetting [15].

7.2 Conclusion

Polydimethylsiloxanes are often referred to as silicones. They are used in many applications because of their stability, low surface tension, and lack of toxicity. Methyl group substitution or introduction of tri- or tetrafunctional siloxane units leads to a wide range of structures. Polymers are easily cross-linked at room or elevated temperature to form elastomers, without losing their advantageous properties.

Acknowledgments

Part of this chapter (here revised) was originally published in *Chimie Nouvelle*, the journal of the Société Royale de Chimie (Belgium), Vol. 8 (30), 847 (1990) by A. Colas and is reproduced here with the permission of the editor.

Bibliography

[1] Kipping FS. Organic derivative of silicon. Preparation of alkylsilicon chlorides. Proc Chem Soc 1904;20:15.

[2] Lane TH, Burns SA. Silica, silicon and silicones ... unraveling the mystery. Curr Top Microbiol Immunol 1996;210:3–12.

[3] Rochow EG. The direct synthesis of organosilicon compounds. J Am Chem Soc 1945;67:963–5.

[4] Noll W. Chemistry and technology of silicones. New York, NY: Academic Press; 1968.

[5] Smith AL. Introduction to silicones. The analytical chemistry of silicones. New York, NY: John Wiley & Sons; 1991. pp. 3–19

[6] Stark FO, Falender JR, Wright AP. Silicones. In: Wilkinson G, Sone FGA, Ebel EW, editors. Comprehensive organometallic chemistry, vol. 2. Oxford, UK: Pergamon Press; 1982. p. 288–97.

[7] Brunauer S, Emmett PH, Teller E. Adsorption of gases in multimolecular layers. J Am Chem Soc 1938;60:309.

[8] Cabot Corporation. CAB-O-SIL fumed silica properties and functions. Tuscola, IL: Cabot Corporation; 1990.

[9] Lynch W. Handbook of silicone rubber fabrication. New York, NY: Van Nostrand Reinhold; 1978. pp. 25–34

[10] Sommer JG. Elastomer molding technology: a comprehensive and unified approach to materials, methods, and mold design for elastomers. Hudson, OH: Elastech; 2003.

[11] O'Brien L, Pandit A. Silicon gel sheeting for preventing and treating hypertrophic and keloid scars. Cochrane Database Syst Rev 2006;(1):CD003826.

[12] Maxon BD, Starch MS, Raul VA. New silicone film-forming technologies for topical delivery and beyond. Proceedings of the 23rd International

Federation of the Society of Cosmetic Chemists (IFSCC) Congress. Orlando, FL; 2004

[13] Corey JY. Historical overview and comparison of silicon with carbon. In: Patai S, Rappoport Z, editors. The chemistry of organic silicon compounds. New York, NY: John Wiley & Sons; 1989. p. 1–56. part 1

[14] Hardman B. Silicones. Encyclopedia of Polymer Science and Engineering, vol. 15. New York, NY: John Wiley & Sons; 1989. p. 204

[15] Owen MJ. Why silicones behave funny. Chemtech 1981;11:288.

[16] Baier RE. Adhesion in the biologic environment. Biomater Med Devices Artif Organs 1985;12:133–59.

[17] Dow Corning Corporation. Fabricating with silastic high consistency silicone rubber. Midland, MI: Dow Corning Corporation; 2001 (accessible at dowcorning.com/content/rubber/rubberprocess).

8 Review of Research in Cardiovascular Devices

Zbigniew Nawrat

OUTLINE

8.1 Introduction 145
8.2 The Heart Diseases 150
8.3 The Cardiovascular Devices in Open-Heart Surgery 151
   8.3.1 Blood Pumps 151
   8.3.2 Valve Prostheses 162
   8.3.3 Heart Pacemaker 171
8.4 The Minimally Invasive Cardiology Tools 171
8.5 The Technology for Atrial Fibrillation 174
8.6 Minimally Invasive Surgery 175
   8.6.1 The Classical Thoracoscopic Tools 176
   8.6.2 The Surgical Robots 177
   8.6.3 Blood Pumps—MIS Application Study 182
      8.6.3.1 Minimally Invasive VAD Implantation 183
      8.6.3.2 The AORobAS Idea 184
      8.6.3.3 The Blood Pump Support in the Palliative (Pediatric) Surgery Study 185
8.7 The Minimally Invasive Valve Implantation 185
8.8 Support Technology for Surgery Planning 186
8.9 Conclusions 187
8.10 Acknowledgments 189
References 189

8.1 Introduction

Remarkable advances in biomedical engineering create new possibilities of help for people with heart diseases. This chapter provides an overview of research in cardiac surgery devices. An explosion in multidisciplinary research, combining mechanical, chemical, and electrical engineering with physiology and medicine, during the 1960s created huge advances in modern health care. This decade opened new possibilities in aerospace traveling and in human body organ replacement. *Homo sapiens* after World War II trauma became not only the hero of mind and progress but also the creator of the culture of freedom. Computed tomographic (CT) scanning was developed at EMI Research Laboratories (Hayes, Middlesex, England) funded in part by the success of EMI's Beatles records. Modern medical imaging techniques such as CT, nuclear magnetic resonance (NMR), and ultrasonic imaging enable the surgeon to have a very precise representation of internal anatomy as preoperative scans. It creates possibilities of realizing new intervention methods, for instance, the very popular bypass surgery. It was a revolution in disease diagnosis and generally in medicine. In cardiovascular therapy, lifesaving implantable defibrillators, ventricular assist devices (VADs), catheter-based ablation devices, vascular stent technology, and cell and tissue engineering technologies have been introduced.

Currently, the number of people on Earth is more than 6 billion: increasingly lesser number of living organisms and about million increasingly more "intelligent" robots accompany them.

Robotics, a technical discipline, deals with the synthesis of certain functions of the human using some mechanisms, sensors, actuators, and computers. Among many types of robotics is the medical and rehabilitation robotics—the latest but rapidly developing branch at present, which includes the manipulators and robots providing surgery, therapy, prosthetics, and rehabilitation. They help fight pareses in humans and can also fulfill the role of a patient's assistant. Rehabilitation manipulators can be steered using ergonomic user interfaces—e.g., the head, the chin, and eye movements. The "nurse" robots for patients and physically challenged persons' service are being developed very quickly. Partially or fully robotic devices help in almost all life actions, such as person moving or consuming meals, simple mechanical devices, science education, and entertainment activities. Help-Mate, an already existing robot-nurse, moving on the hospital corridors and rooms delivers meals, helps find the right way, etc.

On the one hand, robots are created that resemble the human body in appearance (humanoids), able to direct care; on the other hand, robotic devices are constructed—telemanipulators—controlled by the human tools allowing to improve the precision of human tasks. Robots such as ISAC (Highbrow Soft Arm Control) or HelpMate can replace several functions of the nurse, who will give information, help find the way, bring the medicines and the meal. In case of lack of qualified staff, to provide care for hospice patients at home, these robots will be of irreplaceable help.

Robotic surgery was born out of microsurgery and endoscopic experience. Minimally invasive interventions require a multitude of technical devices: cameras, light sources, special tools (offering the mechanical efficiency and tissue coagulation for preventing bleeding), and insufflations (thanks to advances in computer engineering, electronics, optics, materials, and miniaturization). The mobility of instruments is decreased [from seven, natural for human arm, to four degrees of freedom (DOFs)] due to the invariant point of insertion through the patient's body wall. Across the world, physicians and engineers are working together toward developing increasingly effective instruments to enable surgery using the latest technology. The leading technology presents robots intended to keep the surgeon in the most comfortable, dexterous, and ergonomic position during the entire procedure. The surgery is complex and requires precise control of position and force. The basic advantages of minimally invasive robot-aided surgery are safe, reliable, and repeatable operative results with less patient pain, trauma, and recovery time. Conventional open-heart surgery requires full median sternotomy, which means cracking of sternum, compromising pulmonary function, and considerable loss of blood.

	Milestones in the Evolution of Cardiac Devices
1628	William Harvey, St Bartholomew's Hospital, London, presented his theory of the circulatory system. He described the function of the heart, arteries, and veins. It is considered to be one of the greatest advances in medicine.
1812	Julien-Jean Cesar LeGallois, a French physician, proposed the idea of artificial circulation.
1882	German von Schröder introduced the first bubble oxygenator.
1929	Werner Forssmann, a German surgeon, developed the technique of cardiac catheterization, the first to document right heart catheterization in humans using radiographic techniques (won the Nobel Prize in 1956).
1934	Dr Michael DeBakey invented the DeBakey pump (peristaltic).
1937	Artificial heart designed by the Soviet scientist W.P. Demichow was first successfully applied on the dog for 5.5 h.
1949	IBM developed the Gibbon Model I heart—lung machine, delivered to Jefferson Medical College, Philadelphia, PA, USA. It consisted of DeBakey pumps and film oxygenator.
1952	Paul Zoll developed the first cardiac pacemaker.
1952	Charles Hufnagel sewed an artificial valve into a patient's aorta.
1953	Dr John H. Gibbon, Jr, Jefferson Medical College Hospital, Philadelphia, PA, USA, first successfully applied extracorporeal circulation in an 18-year-old female with an atrial septal defect.

(Continued)

—Cont'd

	Milestones in the Evolution of Cardiac Devices
1953	Dr Michael DeBakey, Baylor University, Houston, TX, USA, implanted a seamless, knit Dacron tube for surgical repairs and/or replacement of occluded vessels or vascular aneurysms.
1957	Wild et al. reported the use of ultrasound to visualize the heart noninvasively.
1957	Dr C. Walton Lillehei and Earl Bakken, an electronic engineer, developed the first portable pacemaker. Bakken later formed the Medtronics Corporation.
1957	Drs William Kolff and Tetsuzo Akutsu at the Cleveland Clinic implanted the first artificial heart in a dog. The animal survived for 90 min.
1958	Dr Mason Sones, a cardiologist at the Cleveland Clinic Foundation, developed coronary angiography.
1960s	Semm et al. developed laparoscopic instrumentation.
1960	Dr Albert Starr, an Oregon surgeon, developed the Starr–Edwards heart valve. One of the most successful heart valves produced until the late 1970s.
1967	René Favaloro, an Argentine surgeon in the United States, performed the first coronary bypass operation using the patient's native saphenous vein as an autograft.
1967	Christiaan Barnard performed the first heart transplantation.
1968	A. Kantrowitz et al. performed the first clinical trial in a man with intra-aortic balloon pumping.
1969	Dr Denton Cooley, Texas Heart Institute, Houston, TX, USA, implanted a total artificial heart (TAH) designed by Domingo Liotta. The device served as a "bridge" to heart transplantation until a donor heart was found, for 64 h. The heart transplant functioned for an additional 32 h until the patient died of pneumonia.
1971	White—ECMO on newborn babies using veno-venous bypass for up to 9 days.
1975	A. Gruentzing developed the first balloon catheter.
1975	Dr Willem Kolff, University of Utah, designed a nuclear-powered artificial heart (Westinghouse Corporation).
1975	BioMedicus BioPump (Centrifugal) introduced for clinical applications.
1975	Computerized axial tomography, the "CAT scanner," was introduced.
1977	Newer generations of mechanical prostheses included the mono-leaflet (Medtronic-Hall) and the bi-leaflet (St Jude Medical).
1979	The Jarvik TAH was designed using a flexible four-layer diaphragm and a structural design that fits in the human chest. This design was a larger 100 cc version of today's CardioWest TAH-t, which is 70 cc.
1981	Dr Denton Cooley implanted another pneumatically driven artificial heart designed by Dr Akutsu. This artificial heart was used for 27 h as a "bridge" to cardiac transplantation.
1982	Dr William DeVries implanted the Jarvik 7 into Barney Clark, DDS. Dr Clark lived for 112 days.
1984	Baby girl Faye's native heart, Loma Linda Medical Center, was explanted and replaced with a baboon heart. She survived for 3 weeks.
1984	First human implant and successful bridge-to-transplant—a Novacor® LVAS.
1985	The FDA gave approval for Hershey Medical Center to perform six PennState artificial heart implants as bridges to human heart transplantations. This heart is no longer used with human subjects.

(Continued)

—Cont'd

	Milestones in the Evolution of Cardiac Devices
1985	At the University of Arizona, Dr Jack Copeland implanted a prototype TAH in a patient who had rejected a recently transplanted heart.
1986	The first atherectomy devices that remove material from the vessel wall were introduced.
1987	Introduction of the first use of coronary stent (by 1997, more than 1 million angioplasties had been performed worldwide).
1990	First LVAS patient discharged home with a Novacor LVAS.
1990–1992	The FDA had withdrawn the Investigational Device Exemption (IDE) from Symbion for the clinical study of the Jarvik TAH. Symbion subsequently donated the TAH technology to University Medical Center (UMC), Tucson, AZ, USA, which reincorporated the company and renamed it CardioWest.
1994	First FDA-approved robot for assisting surgery [automated endoscopic system for optimal positioning (AESOP) produced by Computer Motion (CM; Goleta, CA, USA)].
1994	FDA approved the pneumatically driven HeartMate® LVAD (Thoratec Corporation, Burlington, MA, USA) for bridge to transplantation (the first pump with textured blood-contacting surfaces).
1994	HeartMate LVAS has been approved as a bridge to cardiac transplantation.
1996	REMATCH Trial (Randomized Evaluation of Mechanical Assistance for the Treatment of Congestive Heart failure, E. Rose principal investigator) initiated with HeartMate® VE (Thoratec Corp.). Results published in 2002 showed mortality reduction of 50% at 1 year as compared to patients receiving optimal medical therapy.
1998	Simultaneous FDA approval of HeartMate VE (Thoratec Corporation, Burlington, MA, USA) and Novacor LVAS (World Heart Corporation, Ontario, Canada), electrically powered, wearable assist systems for bridge to transplantation, utilized in more than 4000 procedures to 2002. Till now, we can estimate 4500 HeartMate XVE, more than 440 IVAD (Implantable Ventricular Assist Device) and more than 1700 Novacor in this kind of blood pump.
1998	First clinical application of next-generation continuous-flow assist devices. DeBakey (MicroMed Inc.) axial-flow pump implanted by R. Hetzer, G. Noon, and M. DeBakey.
1998	Carpentier and Loulmet performed first in the world endoscopic operation of single bypass graft between left internal thoracic artery and left anterior descending (LITA–LAD) and first operation inside the heart–mitral valve plastic and atrial septal defect closure was performed using surgical robot da Vinci (Intuitive Surgical, Sunnyvale, CA, USA).
1998	Mohr and Falk bypass surgery and mitral valve repairs in near endoscopic technique (da Vinci).
1999	First clinical application of a totally implantable circulatory support system. LionHeart LVAS implanted in a 67-year-old male recipient by R. Koerfer and W. Pae.
1999	D. Boyd first totally endoscopic coronary artery bypass graft (E-CABG) using Zeus robot (Computer Motion, CA, USA, currently intuitive surgical, not in the market).
2000	Physicians in Houston, USA, have realised the implantation and have got the first patient in the clinical investigation of the Jarvik 2000 Heart. Jarvik Heart, Inc. and the Texas Heart Institute began developing the Jarvik 2000 Heart in 1988.
2000	THI was granted permission by the Food and Drug Administration to evaluate the Jarvik 2000 Heart as a bridge to transplantation in five patients.
2000	The FDA gave permission to extend the study. Patients have been sustained for more than 400 days with this device. (http://www.texasheartinstitute.org/Research/Devices/j2000.cfm).

(Continued)

—Cont'd

	Milestones in the Evolution of Cardiac Devices
2001	The AbioCor was implanted in Robert Tools by cardiac surgeons Laman Gray and Robert Dowling on July 2, 2001, at Jewish Hospital in Louisville, Kentucky. L. Robert Tools aged 59 years with the artificial heart survived 5 months. He died because of the blood clot.
2001	Doctors Laman Gray and Robert Dowling in Louisville (KY, USA) implanted the first autonomic artificial heart—AbioCor (Abiomed, Inc., Danvers, MA, USA). The FDA approved the Abiocor for commercial approval under a Humanitarian Device Exemption in September, 2006. ABIOMED is also working on the next generation implantable replacement heart, the AbioCor II. Incorporating technology both from ABIOMED and Penn State, the AbioCor II is smaller and is being designed with a goal of 5-year reliability. The BVS 5000 was the first extracorporeal, or outside the body, ventricular assist device on the market and is still the most widely used bridge to recovery device with systems located in more than 700 institutions throughout the world. Abiomed also offers the Impella 2.5—a minimally invasive, percutaneous ventricular assist device that allows the heart to rest and recover (http://www.abiomed.com/products/faqs.cfm).
2001	Drs Laman Gray and Robert Dowling in Louisville (KY, USA) implanted the first autonomic artificial heart—AbioCor (Abiomed Inc., Danvers, MA, USA).
2001	The first transatlantic telesurgery—Lindbergh operation—surgeon from New York operated patients in Strasburg using Zeus system.
2001	The first full implantable TAH Lion Heart (the Texas Heart Institute in Houston, Abiomed in Danvers, US) was used. The first-ever human implant of the LionHeart™ left ventricular assist system took place October 26, 1999 at the Hearzzentrum NRW in Bad Oeynhausen, Germany. Eight patients have lived with the device for more than 1 year, and four patients have lived with the device for more than 2 years. The Food and Drug Administration approved the first series of US clinical trials for the Arrow LionHeart™ heart assist device in February 2001. Penn State Milton S. Hershey Medical Center implanted the device in the first US patient later that month (http://www.hmc.psu.edu/lionheart/clinical/index.htm).
2001	The first totally implantable TAH LionHeart (the Texas Heart Institute in Houston, TX, USA; Abiomed in Danvers, MA, USA) was used.
2002	FDA approved the HeartMate VE LVAD forpermanent use (Thoratec Corp.).
2002	Novacor LVAS became the first implanted heart assist device to support a single patient for longer than 5 years.
2002	The first percutaneous aortic valve replacement was performed by Alain Cribier in April of 2002.
2004	The CardioWest TAH-t becomes the world's first and only FDA-approved temporary total artificial heart (TAH-t). The indication for use is as a bridge to transplant in cardiac transplant patients at risk of imminent death from nonreversible biventricular failure. SynCardia Systems, Inc. (Tucson, AZ, USA) is the manufacturer of the CardioWest™ TAH-t. It is the only FDA- and CE-approved TAH-t in the world. It is designed for severely ill patients with end-stage biventricular failure. The TAH-t serves as a bridge to human heart transplant for transplant eligible patients who are within days or even hours of death. A New England Journal of Medicine paper published on August 26, 2004 (NEJM 2004; 351: 859–867), states that in the pivotal clinical study of the TAH-t, the 1-year survival rate for patients receiving the CardioWest TAH-t was 70% versus 31% for control patients who did not receive the device. One-year and 5-year survival rates after transplantation among patients who had received a TAH-t as a bridge to human heart transplant were 86% and 64%. The highest bridge to human heart transplant rate of any heart device is 79% (New England Journal of Medicine 2004; 351: 859–867). Over 715 implants account for more than 125 patient years on the TAH-t (http://www.syncardia.com).

(Continued)

—Cont'd

	Milestones in the Evolution of Cardiac Devices
2005	A total of about 3000 cardiac procedures were performed worldwide using the da Vinci system. This includes totally endoscopic coronary artery bypass grafting (TECAB), mitral valve repair (MVR) procedures, ASD closure, and cardiac tissue ablation for atrial fibrillation.
2006	The next-generation pulsatile VAD, the Novacor II, entered a key phase of animal testing with the first chronic animal implant.
2006	The FDA approved the first totally implantable TAH—developed by AbioCor—for people who are not eligible for heart transplantation and who are unlikely to live more than a month without intervention.
2006	Have experience with human implantation: Edwards Lifesciences (>100 patients) and Core Valve (>70 patients). (www.touchbriefings.com/pdf/ 2046/Babaliaros.pdf)
2006	US FDA approval to start pilot clinical trial for Impella 2.5 (Abiomed, Inc., Danvers, MA, USA). To date the Impella 2.5 has been used to support over 500 patients during high-risk PCI, post PCI, and with AMI with low cardiac output.
2007	More than 4,500 in 186 centers advanced heart failure patients worldwide have been implanted with the HeartMate XVE. Longest duration of support (ongoing patient on one device): 1,854 days, age range: 8–74 (average 51). The REMATCH (Randomized Evaluation of Mechanical Assistance for the Treatment of Congestive Heart Failure) clinical trial demonstrated an 81% improvement in two-year survival among patients receiving HeartMate XVE versus optimal medical management. A Destination Therapy study following the REMATCH trial demonstrated an additional 17% improvement (61% vs. 52%) in one-year survival of patients receiving the HeartMate XVE, with an implication for the appropriate selection of candidates and timing of VAD implantation.
2008	State of art in 2008, based on the experience almost 20–30 years shows among others: – future of long-term heart support methods will be connected with rotary pumps, the stop of activity in pulsating pump technology is observed (rotary pumps are smaller and comfortable in the implantation especially it is possible introduce mini invasive surgical methods) – the mono-leaflet disk valve are applied more and more seldom (they require during the implantation the definite orientation in the heart) in the comparison with bi-leaflet – the new kind of biological valve prostheses based on tissue engineering method get into the clinical experiment – the multiple companies have engineered percutaneous heart valves (PHV), primarily for aortic stenosis
2008	There have been 867 unit shipments worldwide—647 in the United States, 148 in Europe and 72 in the rest of the world (http://www.intuitivesurgical.com). Devices for "robotic surgery" are designed to perform entirely autonomous movements after being programmed by a surgeon. The *da Vinci* Surgical System is a computer-enhanced system that interposes a computer between the surgeon's hands and the tips of microinstruments. The system replicates the surgeon's movements in real time.

8.2 The Heart Diseases

The human biological heart has two sets of pumping chambers. The right atrium receives oxygen-depleted blood from the body, which is pumped into the lungs through the right ventricle. The left atrium receives aerated blood from the lungs, which is pumped out to the body through the left ventricle. With each heart beat, the ventricles contract together. The valves control the direction of blood flow through the heart.

Congestive heart failure, a condition in which the heart is unable to pump the blood effectively throughout the body, is one of the leading causes of death. This disease is caused by sudden damage from heart attacks, deterioration from viral infections, valve malfunctions, high blood pressure, and other problems. Although medication and surgical techniques can help control symptoms, the only cure for heart failure is heart transplantation. Artificial hearts and pump assist devices have thus been developed as potential alternatives.

Ischemic heart disease is caused by progressive atherosclerosis with increasing occlusion of coronary arteries resulting in a reduction in coronary blood flow. Blood flow can be further decreased by superimposed events such as vasospasm, thrombosis, or circulatory changes leading to hypoperfusion. Myocardial infarction (MI) is the rapid development of myocardial necrosis caused by a critical imbalance between the oxygen supply and the oxygen demand of the myocardium. Coronary artery bypass grafts (CABGs) are implanted in patients with stenosed coronary arteries to support myocardial blood flow.

Valvular heart disease is a life-threatening disease that affects millions of people worldwide and leads to valve repairs and/or replacements.

In the USA and Europe alone, with more than 600 million inhabitants and more than 6 million patients with heart failure, the prevalence of advanced heart failure, constituting 1–10% of the heart failure population, is estimated to total between 60,000 and 600,000 patients. More than 700,000 Americans die each year from heart failure, making it the number one cause of death in the USA, as well as worldwide. About half of these are sudden cardiac deaths, which occur so quickly that there is not enough time for intervention with a cardiac assist or replacement device. For the remaining half, heart transplantation is one of the few options available today. Though hundreds of thousands are in need, only about 2,000 people in the USA will be able to receive donor hearts every year. This consistent shortage in the supply of donor hearts in the USA demonstrates the need for an alternative to heart transplantation. The total potential market for the artificial heart is more than 100,000 people in the USA each year (http://www.abiomed.com).

8.3 The Cardiovascular Devices in Open-Heart Surgery

Cardiac surgery is surgery on the heart and/or great vessels. This surgery is a complex procedure requiring precise control of position and force. Conventional open-heart surgery requires full median sternotomy, which means cracking of sternum, compromising pulmonary function, and considerable loss of blood.

The repair of intracardiac defects requires a bloodless and motionless environment, which means that the heart should be stopped and drained of blood. Hence, the patient requires the function of the heart and lungs provided by an artificial method.

Modern heart–lung machines can perform a number of other tasks required for a safe open-heart operation. This system preserves the patient's own blood throughout the operation and the patient's body temperature can be controlled by selectively cooling or heating the blood as it flows through the heart–lung machine. Medications and anesthetic drugs can be administered via separate connections. The disadvantages include the formation of small blood clots, which increase the risk of stroke, pulmonary complications, and renal complications. The machine can also trigger an inflammatory process that can damage many of the body's systems and organs. Those risks push today's biomedical engineers to improve the heart–lung machine and oxygenator, while surgeons are developing advances that would eliminate the need for the machine altogether. One such advance is minimally invasive surgery (MIS).

The surgeons have begun to perform "off-pump bypass surgery"—coronary artery bypass surgery without the aforementioned cardiopulmonary bypass. The surgeons operate on the beating heart stabilized to provide an (almost) still work area. One of the greatest challenges in beating-heart surgery is the difficulty of suturing or sewing on a beating heart. A stabilization system makes it possible for the surgeon to work on the patient's beating heart carefully and, in the vast majority of cases, eliminates the need for the heart-lung machine.

8.3.1 Blood Pumps

The human heart is a pump that is made of muscle tissue. A special group of cells called the sinus node is located in the right atrium. The sinus node generates electrical stimuli that make the heart contract and pump out blood. The normal human heart beats about 75 times per minute (i.e., about 40 million times a year)—i.e., the heart pumps 5 l of blood per minute. The normal systemic blood pressure is 120/80 mmHg. The mechanical power (calculated by multiplying the pressure by the flow rate) of the human heart is about 1.3 W. However, to provide this mechanical power, the heart requires 10 times much higher rate of energy turnover, owing to its low mechanical efficiency (less than 10%).

However, the development in biotechnology can open the opportunity for tissue engineering (a branch of biotechnology)—a prospect of saving people with extremely complex or irreversible failure heart will still be realized using mechanical heart support devices.

During the last half-century, various blood pumps were introduced into clinical practice, which can partially support or replace the heart during open-heart surgery or considerably for a longer time period until heart recovers or until transplantation is performed. Several millions of people owe their health and lives to these devices. According to the American Heart Association, an estimated 5 million Americans are living with heart failure and more than 400,000 new cases are diagnosed every year. About 50% of all patients die within 5 years.

The first operation on a beating heart was performed by Gibbon in 1953 using a peristaltic pump. Since then, there has been rapid development in mechanical assist devices, leading to the realization of today's mechanical aid system for blood circulation, based on the requirements using the following:

- intra-aortic balloon pump (IABP)
- continuous blood flow devices—roll and centrifugal rotary pumps
- pulsating flow blood pumps—pneumatic or electro-control membrane pumps

The assumed time of blood pump using in the organism influences the construction and material used in its design. According to this criterion, the pumps can be divided into following categories:

- short-term (during the operation or in sudden rescue operations)
- medium-term—over several weeks or months (as a bridge to heart transplantation or treatment)
- long-term—several years (already at present) and permanently (in the intention) (as the target therapy)

The extracorporeal circulation (*perfusion*) and the controlled stopping of heart action make it possible to perform the open-heart operation. The peristaltic pumps are in common use, where the turning roll locally tightens the silicon drain to move a suitable volume of the blood. The disadvantages of this procedure, such as the damage to blood components, are eliminated or reduced by pump construction and material improvement. The patients with both heart and lung failure are assisted by the system consisting of pump and oxygenator. The method of time oxygenation (supply oxygen to the blood) for extracorporeal blood—extracorporeal membrane oxygenation (ECMO)—was applied the first time in 1972 by Hill. The blood pump, membrane oxygenator, heat exchanger, and a system of cannulas (tubes) for patient's vascular system connection are the elements of the system. Inner surface of all these parts are covered with heparin. The Extracorporeal Life Support Organization Registry has collected (since 1989) data on more than 30,000 patients, most of whom have been neonates with respiratory failure [7]. The currently available centrifugal pump VADs are BioMedicus BioPump (Medtronic, Minneapolis, MN, USA), CentriMag (Levitronix, Zürich, Switzerland), RotaFlow (Jostra, Hirrlingen, Germany), and Capiox (Terumo, Ann Arbor, MI, USA). These pumps have been available since 1989 to support neonates and older children with postoperative cardiac failure but competent lung function.

Centrifugal pumps benefit from the physical phenomena (centrifugal, inertia force) of blood acceleration during temporal rotational movement. These pumps consist of a driving unit and an acrylic head driven by a magnetic couple. Input and output blood flow channels are perpendicular to each other. The output velocity of the blood on the conical rotor depends on the input rotary speed, preload, and afterload. Based on vortex technology, these pumps use turbine spins of 10,000–20,000 rpm to create a flow of 5–6 l/min and have generally been applied for temporary assistance of stunned myocardium of the left ventricle. The construction of working pump and its environment conditions influence the blood hemolysis during its use. According to the results of in vitro experiment, with the pump working as VAD and extracorporeal circulation (CPB and ECMO), the use of the pump as VAD caused the least degree of hemolysis, and the hemolysis of pumps in the time to ECMO strongly depends on the kind of oxygenator used. Pumps with the conical rotor caused a greater degree of hemolysis working with small flows and large pressures (ECMO). On the contrary, a lesser degree of hemolysis was observed for pumps with the flat rotor, regardless of its purpose.

The *intra-aortic balloon* was introduced as a tool for coronary circulation assistance in works of Maulopulos, Topaz, and Kolff in 1960. In 1968, Kantrowitz was the first to prove the clinical effectiveness of intra-aortic counterpulsation. It became the classic method in the 1970s, thanks to Datascope Company for its first device (System 80) for their clinical applications. The balloon (30—40 ml) placed in the aorta, synchronically with the heart, is filled up and emptied by raising the diastolic pressure and the perfusion of coronary arteries. As a result, the myocardial contractility is improved, and hence, the cardiac output is bigger. This is one of the basic devices in cardiosurgery units. The balloon, rolled up on a catheter, is introduced through the artery. Kantrowitz introduced to cardiosurgery also another type of pump called the *aortic patch*, which has been in clinical use for many years, and uses the natural localization of heart valve. The balloon, which is sewn to cut the descending aorta, is connected through the skin with the pneumatic driver unit. The aortic blood flow is improved by the pulsate balloon filling and the aortic valve blocked the backflow to the ventricle.

New constructions of TAHs and VADs offer new hope for millions of heart patients whose life expectancy is greatly reduced because the number of patients waiting for a transplant far exceeds the donated hearts available. An artificial heart or VAD is made of metal (typically titanium—aluminum—vanadium alloy), plastic, ceramic, and animal parts (valve bioprostheses). A blood-contacting diaphragm within the pump is made from a special type of polyurethane that may also be textured to provide blood cell adherence.

The VAD (Figure 8.1) is an extracorporeal pneumatic blood pump, invented to assist a failure left or right ventricle, or the whole heart until it

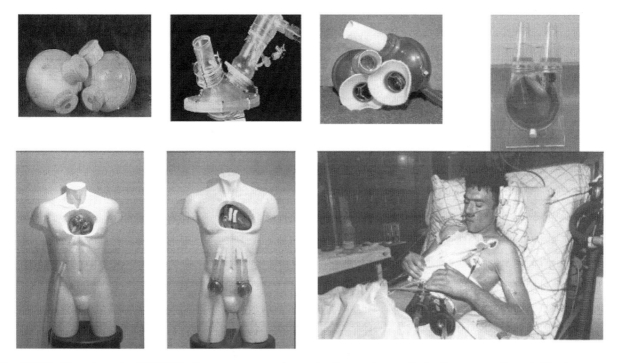

Figure 8.1 The steps in POLTAH design process (model after cadaver study, transparent model for laser visualization investigation, first polyurethane model for starting animal experiments). Nonsymmetrical shape of POLVAD proposed and designed creates a very good internal flow condition. The first successful POLVAD implantation was performed in 1993 in T. Gruszczyński. Until now, more than 200 POLVAD clinical implantations have been performed, the longest time successful application being over 200 days. Pneumatically driven artificial heart (POLTAH) and ventricular assist device (POLVAD).

recovers or until a replacement by transplantation is performed. A mechanical heart assist is used to support the heart during failure caused by the ischemia of the heart muscle, the small cardiac output, cardiomyopathy, or heart valve diseases. The role of these aid pumps is to support the life function of the brain and other organs and heart treatment (thanks to the devices that partly take over its role) by improving hemodynamic conditions. It is fitted with inflow and outflow cannulas for connecting the VAD with heart and vascular system in parallel with the biological heart ventricle being assisted. The VAD consist one or two ventricles placed outside the body (failing heart is left in place) connected to the control unit.

The TAH (Figure 8.2) is designed for emergency replacement of irreversible damaged natural heart. Because the natural heart is completely removed, the TAH must ensure the hemodynamic, regulatory, and control functions of the circulatory system.

If the total replacement artificial heart is to mimic the function of the natural human heart, it meet the following requirements [1]:

1. Two separate pumps duplicating the left and the right heart
2. Output range of 5–10 l/min from each side
3. Aortic arterial pressure range of 120–180 mmHg
4. Pulmonary arterial pressure range of 20–80 mmHg
5. Physical dimensions permitting easy surgical insertion within the pericardium
6. Low weight to minimize restraints
7. A minimum of noise and vibration
8. A heat output of less than 25 W
9. A low degree of hemolysis
10. Inert to body chemicals

The artificial heart, designed by the Soviet scientist W.P. Demichow, was first successfully applied on a dog for 5.5 h in 1937. Several study groups in the United States in the 1950s performed the first clinical experiments. In 1957 T. Akutsu and W. Kolff (Figure 8.3) made the pneumatically driven artificial heart. The artificial heart constructed by D. Liotta with the same drive type successfully replaced the patient heart for 64 h, before heart transplantation in 1969. On 4 April 1969, Dr Denton A. Cooley performed the first human implantation of a TAH when he used a device developed by Dr Domingo Liotta to sustain the life

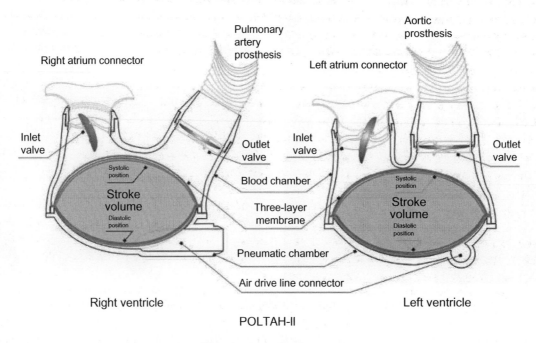

Figure 8.2 Schematic diagram of an artificial heart.

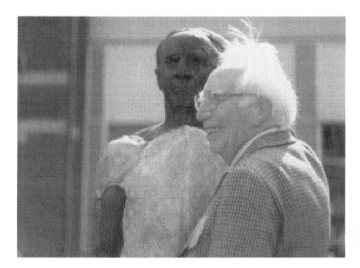
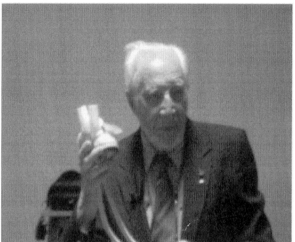

Figure 8.3 William Kolff in Kampen and in Gent (*photo taken by the author*).

of Mr Haskell Karp. After having undergone resection of a left ventricular aneurysm, the 47-year-old patient developed cardiac failure. The Liotta heart supported him for nearly 3 days until a suitable donor heart was available and successfully transplanted. This case demonstrated the feasibility of bridging to transplantation with a mechanical circulatory support system.

In 1982 William DeVries (UT, USA) implanted the artificial heart designed by R. Jarvik, cooperating in that time with W. Kolff, *called Jarvik* 7 in a patient for 112 days. The Jarvik heart was pneumatically driven (driver unit called COMDU) through a drain carried out by the skin. Four disk valves from Medtronic-Hall were fixed in the polyurethane body. The inner surface of ventricle was covered with a smooth layer of polyurethane (Biomer, Ethicon Inc.) and a four-layer membrane made from Biomer that separated the pneumatically driven part from the part having contact with the blood. There were two types of these VADs: Jarvik 7–70 and Jarvik 7–100 with 70 and 100 ml of stroke volume, respectively. Since 1993, these types of the artificial heart after a little modification have been clinically used [now under the name CardioWest (the technology transferred from the firm Symbion to CardioWest Technologies Inc., Tuscon, AZ, USA currently Syncardia Systems, Inc. Tucson, AZ, USA) and is marked C-70 and C-100, respectively]. The pump can operate at 30–199 bpm and also has variable systolic duration, delay, and stroke volume. By 1989, such devices had largely become a bridge to human heart transplantations. In a pivotal clinical study [2], these patients were successfully transplanted 79% of the time. The 1-year and 5-year survival rates after heart transplantation among these patients were 86 and 64%, respectively.

In Europe, the hospital La Pitié in Paris has the biggest experiences in implanting the artificial heart in patients. From April 1986 to June 2000, there had been 120 implantations of pneumatically driven Jarvik VADs (with the trade name TAH *Symbion* and at present TAH CardioWest). The total time of the implantation was more 3000 days (with the longest being 607 days implantation). Another type of pneumatically driven TAH named *PennState* was made at the Pennsylvania State University, where ventricles were also made from Biomer, but sacks were used instead of membrane-type construction. PennState VAD with the Björk–Shiley (B–S) disk valves was considerably not as often applied as the Jarvik heart.

As a next stage, the electrically powered PennState artificial heart was constructed. In this device, a DC brushless motor turns over the helical (screw) drive, which causes compression and expansion of segment polyurethane sack resulting in an 8 l/min volume flow with 16–22 W of consumed power. The total animal experimentation time is about 5 years at present, the longest trial being more than 5 months. Searching for the biocompatible and durable biomaterials in 1969, Y. Nose made the steel heart covered with Teflon (so-called *Green Heart*), which he implanted in the ram for 50 h. There were also trials to use properly prepared heart pericardium for the internal structure of the ventricle. Electrohydraulic artificial heart (Japan) *EHTAH* is equipped with ellipsoidal ventricle membranes made from nonthrombogenic, segmented polyurethane, 21 and 23 mm B−S valves and vascular Dacron grafts (Medox Medical, USA). *Baylor* TAH (Baylor College of Medicine, USA) is the electromechanical pump (the rotation of the screw causes the movement of membrane). The membrane is made from polyolefin rubber, the ventricle body from epoxy Hysol (Dexter Electronic Materials, USA) or at present from coal fibers, which is lighter and stronger. In the laboratory of Kolff, small ventricles with semielastic shell were worked out. They were made from Pellethane 80AE/2363 (Dow Chemical, Japan) by the vacuum forming and glued by dielectric welding. Valves are made from Isoplast, covered with Pellethane, and glued. W. Kolff sent the sets of ventricles to many centers in the world, for realization experiments, to Poland as well. In Zabrze comparative in vitro investigations were carried out with these ventricles to detect the extent of artificially induced thrombogenesis.

AbioCor implantable replacement heart (Abiomed, Inc., Danvers, MA, USA) is a fully implantable, electrically driven artificial heart. The rotary pump forces the movement of liquid, which by means of a second motor is directed to the left or right ventricle causing cramp of polyurethane sacks with two polyurethane valves. It does not require a compliance chamber (the internal hydraulic platform was rather applied). The normal flow is 4−8 l/min up to a maximum of 10 l/min. Internal implanted batteries enable 30−60 min of work. The pump regulates automatically its work frequency in the range 60−140 bpm. As a pump biomaterial tested for the last 20 years, the elastomer Angioflex was applied. After successful laboratory investigations on implantation in animals, the clinical experiment begun. On 3 July 2001, Drs Laman Gray and Robert Dowling in Louisville (KY, USA) implanted the first autonomic artificial heart (AbioCor). It consists of two ventricles separated by the pumping mechanism. Four original polyurethane valves are used to direct the flow (identical valves like these had been applied for many years in the Abiomed BVS pump). Energy from the external battery is wirelessly transferred through the skin port. The final goal of AbioCor applications is to reach the 5-year, statistical survival of patients with the replaced natural heart. Unlike the Jarvik 7, the AbioCor is powered by electrical energy that is transmitted from a battery across the skin to an internal coil and a backup battery. Because an opening in the skin is not needed to allow passage for tubes or wires, the risk of infection is greatly reduced. In addition, the external battery pack is designed to be worn on a belt or suspenders, enabling the patient to be mobile. From 2001 to 2004, the patients who had received the heart and survived the operation lived for 5 months, on average, the longest being not more than 17 months. In 2006, the AbioCor was approved for use in patients who do not qualify for a heart transplantation if their life expectancy as a result of heart failure is less than a month; the device is also approved as a temporary measure for patients awaiting a transplant.

The Abiomed Company designed AbioCor based on experience with application blood assist pumps. *Abiomed BVS 500* (Abiomed, Inc., Danvers, MA, USA) is pneumatically driven, two-chamber pump one atrium without any power support and the other pneumatically driven ventricle for pumping freely (means not pneumatically driven, under the natural blood pressure) filled atrium with the freely filled atrium, vertically fixed to the patient's bed. Relatively long cannulas are used for establishing the patient's circulatory system connection. It is relatively easy to adjust, with the full ejection mode (80 ml). As a first, the company introduced the polyurethane valves to the pump (had been in clinical use for more than 10 years). Cannulas are made from Angioflex, which is a nontoxic and durable material (can withstand 100,000 beats/day). Endings of the cannulas sewn to the atrium have a special armature and the shape preserving collapsing the atrium walls or the blocking of the cannula inlet. From the output side, the arterial cannulas have special Dacron collars facilitating their sewing.

In Europe, the most developed construction of implantable artificial heart is located in Aachen and in Berlin. In Poland, apart from pneumatically driven artificial heart POLTAH, in the Artificial Heart Laboratory of Foundation for Cardiac Surgery Development in Zabrze, promising construction of implantable electrohydraulic pump project is being led. According to plan, this project will give as a result a totally implantable VAD with all driven and control units inside the patient's body.

In 1966, the pump designed by M. DeBakey, who was also the constructor of the first roll pump applied to the perfusion of the heart during surgery, was a first successfully implanted membrane VAD for left heart ventricle support. The future of implantable pumps is based on the electric drive. The first VAD of this type was *Novacor* (Novacor Division, World Heart Corporation, Ontario, Canada) with electromagnetic driving system. The blood flows in the rhythmically compressed sack, made from Biomer (polyurethane) having two biological valves (made from pericardium 25 mm or porcine 21 mm from the Edwards Laboratories, Baxter Inc.) working as the one-way flow valves. The controller provides electrical energy, via the percutaneous lead, to actuate the driver during the ejection cycle. The driver's balanced, symmetrical solenoid (electromagnet) converts this electrical energy into mechanical energy, stored in a pair of springs. The spring forces act directly on the blood pump's dual symmetrically opposed pusher plates, pressurizing the blood within the pump, and propelling it into the aorta to support systemic circulation. The ventricle body was made from polyester resin, strengthened by glass fibers. It is located in the left upper square of the stomach. The blood flows into the ventricle from Dacron cannula placed in the apex of the left ventricle and is ejected to the system through the Dacron cannula as well to the side wall of the ascending aorta. It works synchronically with the heart. The pump/drive unit can eject from all-fill volumes (from 25 ml to its maximum capacity of 70 ml), to match the stroke volume received from the left ventricle. A small residual blood volume, proportional to afterload (systemic pressure), remains in the blood pump at the end of ejection. The system can thereby adapt to the natural heart's function without depending on an ECG signal or other physiological measurement. Currently, WorldHeart's Novacor LVAS has been implanted in nearly 100 medical centers worldwide in more than 1700 patients, and is the first mechanical circulatory support device to support a single patient for more than 6 years. Also, 172 primarily bridge-to-transplant patients have been supported by Novacor LVAS for more than 1 year, 45 have been supported for more than 2 years, 24 for more than 3 years, 11 for more than 4 years, and 1 for more than 6 years. Only 1.4% of the pumps have needed replacement. No patient deaths have been attributed to Novacor LVAS failure.

Another type of the implantable VAD used for several years as a pneumatically and electrically driven pump is *HeartMate VAD* (HE HAS; Thermo Corporation, Burlington, MA, USA (http://www.thoratec.com/vad-trials-outcomes)). *HeartMate* is the family of ventricles. First FDA on the mechanical VAD (Pneumatic HeartMate® I) in the United States was designed as the platform to the transplantation. Electrically driven HeartMate received FDA in 1998. All ventricles were made from the especially rough surface facilitating the formation of natural endothelium. This VAD is implanted in abdominal space between the heart apex and the ascending aorta and the power supply is transferred by the wire through the skin. The second pipe (through the same skin port) is used to deaerate the chamber or in emergency states allows an external person to manually drive the pump. The volume flow is up to 11 l/min. Closed in titan body motor through the cam system causes the pulsator to move up and down the synthetic sack filled with the blood, closed at two sides by biological pig valves (25 mm, Medtronic). This company also introduced different solution, assuring biocompatibility of membrane. Instead of focusing on achieving the maximal smoothest of polyurethane bag, they worked out material with built-in network of the fibers that facilitates the creation of natural endothelium. Currently, similarly to R. Jarvik, this company works out the artificial heart with turbine axial pump.

PennState LionHeart, *LionHeart LVD LVAS* (Arrow International, Inc., Reading, PA, USA), is an implantable pulsating pump that has developed since 1994. The stroke volume is automatically controlled, resulting in the 3–7 l/min of flow. A set of external batteries (3.5 kg weight) is adequate for 6 h of work. It was first clinically used in Germany in October 1999.

Thoratec® VAD (Thoratec Laboratories, Inc., Pleasanton, CA, USA) is an external pump, applied to the short and long support comparatively often. The new implantable version has streamlined shapes, body made of polished titanium, and rest made from polyurethane and the sack through which the blood will flow from Tharalon. It is supplied pneumatically from the mobile, handy driver, connected through the skin by 9 mm drain. This relatively small VAD is also suitable for the biventricular assistance, weighs 339 g, and has an external volume of 252 ml.

The Thoratec PVAD (Paracorporeal Ventricular Assist Device) provides short-to-intermediate, uni- or biventricular support with the option and benefit of home discharge. With more than 20 years of clinical use, the PVAD has been well established as a Bridge-to-Transplantation or Post-Cardiotomy Recovery option for advanced heart failure patients of any age or size. Around 69% of PVAD patients were successfully supported to cardiac transplantation or device removal for myocardial recovery. More than 4,000 patients implanted at over 240 medical centers in 26 countries, the longest duration of support: 1,204 days (858 days discharged to home), smallest patient: 17 kg (BSA 0.73 m^2).

The IVAD (Implantable Ventricular Assist Device) provides intermediate-to-chronic support and is the only biventricular, implantable, and home-dischargeable VAD. It is indicated for Post-Cardiotomy Recovery and Bridge-to-Transplantation. Patients implanted: More than 440 patients at 95 medical centers in 9 countries, longest duration of support: 735 days, smallest patient: BSA 1.31 m^2.

As Thoratec's first-line intermediate-to-chronic left ventricular assist device, the HeartMate II has been extensively studied as Bridge-to-Transplantation for advanced heart failure. Over 1,200 worldwide patients implanted, longest duration of support (ongoing patient on one device): 3.6 years, transplanted, recovered, or supported to 180 days: 80%. World Heart registry (http://www.worldheart.com).

In the nearly 100 medical centers worldwide that use Novacor LVAS, it is renowned for its reliability, durability and predictability of wear. Of the more than 1,700 Novacor LVAS recipients to date, 172 primarily Bridge-to-Transplant patients have been supported by Novacor LVAS for more than one year. Among these recipients, 45 have been supported for more than two years, 24 for more than three years, 11 for more than four years and 1 for more than six years. Only 1.4% of the pumps have needed replacement. No patient deaths have been attributed to Novacor LVAS failure. In Germany, the 1,500th patient was implanted with Novacor® LVAS in 2004.

Medos-HIA VAD from Aachen is made from biocompatible polyurethane (project led by Helmut Reul). It is similar to natural trileaflet valves also made from polyurethane, but with the valve cusp optimization resulting in a conical shape (natural are spherical). Ventricles are made in the full row of sizes, from 60 to 9 ml (pediatric ventricle). Medos was clinically used in more than 100 cases. The investigations carried out in 1994 allowed to guarantee the minimum time of valve functioning of half-year (18 million of cycles). Since 1990, in Aachen, the HIA TAH has been developed, which is based on electromechanical driving unit. The inclination of the plate on which the membrane is fixed about 2 cm allows to reach the 65 ml stroke volume. Brushless motor rotates in only one direction (similar to the case of HeartMate, but the construction of the cam unit is different). The pump allows to reach above 10 l/min (with the frequency of 140 bpm under physiological conditions).

HeartSaver VAD (WorldHeart Corporation, Ottawa, ON, Canada) is the pulsate pump with hydraulic drive (project led by Tofy Mussivand). In 2000, it was almost ready for the starting of clinical experiments. Different types were prepared: the axial pumps for continuous flow and VADs and TAHs for pulsating pumps. All models are driven electrohydraulically (rotor). The external volume of the VAD is approximately 530 ml, the membrane is made from smooth polyurethane, and Medtronic-Hall mechanical valves are used, which according to plan will be replaced with the less thrombogenic biological Carpentier–Edwards valves. The working liquid in this pump is the silicon oil, which is currently not in use.

Berlin Heart is a series of external, pneumatically driven, ventricle assist devices, with the 50, 60, or 80 ml ejection, equipped with B−S mechanical valves or the polyurethane valves. Berlin Heart VADs have comfortable silicone cannulas with the wire armature, which renders cannulas a suitable shape. This type of VADs had been successfully in vitro tested for 5 years (more than 210 million cycles), mainly in Berlin. Berlin Heart VAD was used in Poland by Z. Religa's team in first successful mechanical support of heart as a bridge to transplantation.

The pneumatically driven membrane-type Polish ventricle assist devices *POLVAD* (U-shaped) and artificial heart *POLTAH* (spherical) were developed in Zabrze, Poland. Until now, more than 200 VAD implantations have been performed. First successful bridge to transplantation was constructed by Z. Religa's team. The implantation of BVAD produced by Berlin Heart LVAD was performed in May 1991. The patient T. Gruszczyński was awaiting heart transplantation. After 11 days of support, the heart transplantation was performed and patient returned home. Unfortunately, rejection occurred and the patient needed a second, new heart. In the meantime, author (physicist) designed and B. Stolarzewicz (chemist) performed a new Polish ventricular assist pump named POLVAD. After tests, POLVAD was ready for clinical applications. It happened that the first patient to use POLVAD was the same patient T. Gruszczyński (the heart was rejected after 2 years). Fortunately, the POLVAD worked very well, and after 21 days, the heart transplantation was performed. Unfortunately, the patient died during surgery (second heart transplantation).

In pulsate blood pumps, the part producing mechanical energy is separated from the blood by a biocompatible and durable membrane. Membrane-type VADs have it fixed to the hard or half-elastic body. They divide the artificial chamber in two almost even parts. However, in the ventricle with sack, the membrane is shaped into this bag hung in stiff chamber. The artificial ventricles can be driven pneumatically, hydraulically, or electromechanically. The trials of the nuclear power source introduction failed. The VADs are used for supporting patient's life as a bridge to transplantation or to natural heart recovery. At the end of this procedure, the cannulas connecting VAD to the patient's circulatory system are operationally removed. The TAHs are used in these cases, when heart transplantation is the only rescue for the patient or as a target therapy.

Distinct from above described pulsate pumps, the Jarvik 2000 and MicroMed–DeBakey are the currently used implantable axial pumps with continuous flow. The first axial flow pump to be introduced into clinical practice for intermediate to long-term treatment of end-stage heart failure in adults was the DeBakey VAD®. *MicroMed–DeBakey VAD* is the rotor, axial pump (flow up to 5 l/min), connected by the cable through the skin to the driver unit held on the patient's belt. It is implanted between the heart apex and aorta (ascending or descending). The DeBakey VAD is 30 mm × 76 mm, weighs 93 g, and is approximately 1/10th the size of pulsatile products on the market. In 2000, the first successful usage was performed in Vienna.

Jarvik 2000 is a small (2.5/5.5 cm) rotor pump (the electromagnetic rotor covered by titanium layer). It fits directly into the left ventricle, which may eliminate problems with clotting. The outflow graft connects to the descending aorta. The device itself is nonpulsatile, but the natural heart continues to beat and provides a pulse. The rotor has ceramic bearings, which are washed by the blood (smearing and the receipt of warmth). The angular velocity of 9000–16,000 rpm ensures 3–6 l/min of output flow with the aortic pressure of 80 mmHg and power consumption of 4–10 W. The system is powered by external batteries remotely through skin using electromagnetic field created by a set of coupled coins or using the wire carried out through the "port" in the skull safety plugged with the pyrolytic carbon. On 25 April 2000, physicians in Houston, TX, USA, have realized the implantation and introduced the first patient in the clinical investigation of the Jarvik 2000. For lifetime use, the Jarvik 2000 has also had proven successful in treating a target population of patients suffering from chronic heart failure due to a prior heart attack or cardiomyopathy. Many have been rehabilitated to a dramatically improved life at home, and in some cases patients have even returned to work. So far, the Jarvik 2000 FlowMaker has been used to treat more than 200 patients in the United States, Europe, and Asia. Of those, roughly 79% received the Jarvik 2000 as a bridge to transplantation and 21% as a permanent implant, with a number of patients in each group being terminally ill, near-death cases. Nearly 70% of those patients were supported successfully. Several surgeons reports have described placement of continuous flow devices without cardiopulmonary bypass. Frazier described a patient in whom he placed this pump while briefly fibrillating the heart and placement of the Jarvik 2000 with an anterior, intraperitoneal approach without bypass. This technique is attractive in reoperative situations.

The University of Pittsburgh–Thermo Cardiosystems *HeartMate® II* is an axial rotary pump with the stone bearing with a volume of 89 ml, weighs 350 g, and the estimated time of use is 5–7 years. As intermediate-to-chronic left ventricular assist device, the HeartMate II (now Thoratec's) has been extensively studied as Bridge-to-Transplantation for advanced heart failure. Over 1,200 worldwide patients implanted, longest duration of support (ongoing patient on one device): 3.6 years, transplanted, recovered, or supported to 180 days: 80%. The third-generation, HeartMate III, will be the centrifugal pump with the rotor levitating in the magnetic field (without mechanical bearings).

There have been several scientific groups working in the field of artificial heart in Japan, Australia, Austria, Argentina, France, Germany, Poland, Czech Republic, Russia, and so on. But from the market point of view, there is not easy business. Currently, the strongest company offering the wide range of products in the area of blood pumps is Thoratec. Thoratec Corporation is engaged in the research, development, manufacturing, and marketing of medical devices for circulatory support, vascular graft, blood coagulation, and skin incision applications. The Thoratec VAD system is the device that is approved for left, right, or total heart support and that can be used both as a bridge to transplantation and for recovery from open-heart surgery. More than 4300 of these devices have been used in the treatment of over 2800 patients worldwide. With the introduction of the Implantable Ventricular Assist Device (IVAD™), Thoratec delivers the first and only implantable VADs for left, right, and biventricular support for bridge to transplantation and for postcardiotomy recovery. The HeartMate® XVE Left Ventricular Assist System (LVAS) is now FDA approved as a long-term permanent implant, called destination therapy. In addition, the accompanying Thoratec TLC-II® Portable VAD Driver provides hospitals with the first mobile system that allows these univentricular or biventricular VAD patients to be discharged home to await cardiac transplantation or myocardial recovery. The company is also a leader in implantable LVADs. Its air-driven and electric HeartMate LVAD, which has been implanted in more than 4100 patients worldwide, are implanted alongside the natural heart and take over the pumping function of the left ventricle for patients whose hearts are too damaged or diseased to produce adequate blood flow.

WorldHeart is a developer of mechanical circulatory support systems (e.g., Novacor) with leading next-generation technologies. The Levacor is a next-generation rotary VAD. It is the only bearingless, fully magnetically levitated implantable centrifugal rotary pump with clinical experience. An advanced, continuous-flow pump, the Levacor uses magnetic levitation to fully suspend the spinning rotor, its only moving part, inside a compact housing.

WorldHeart's Novacor II LVAS is a next-generation, pulsatile VAD. It can be fully implanted without a volume displacement chamber, thereby reducing the risk of complications by eliminating the need to perforate the skin. The operation of the pump drive unit is very interesting. When the pusher plate is driven to the right (pumping stroke), the prechamber expands, filling from the left ventricle. Simultaneously, the pumping chamber is compressed, ejecting blood into the body. When the pusher plate returns to the left (transfer stroke), the prechamber is compressed while the pumping chamber expands; blood transfers from the prechamber to the pumping chamber, with no inflow or outflow. Because the total volume of the two chambers remains constant as one fills and the other empties, the system can operate without a volume compensator or venting through the skin. WorldHeart's Novacor II LVAS is not currently available. In 2005, WorldHeart conducted the first animal implant of the Novacor II LVAS—ahead of schedule. WorldHeart Company currently focuses on new products—especially for pediatric patients. The PediaFlow VAD is an implantable, magnetically levitated blood pump based on WorldHeart's proprietary rotary VAD MagLev™ technology. In its pediatric configuration, the device is designed to provide a flow rate from 0.3 to 1.5 l/min. The PediaFlow VAD is being developed to provide medium-term (less than 1 year) implantable circulatory support to patients from birth to 2 years of age with congenital or acquired heart disease.

Pneumatic pulsatile VADs have been available in pediatric sizes since 1992. At Herzzentrum Berlin, VADs are used lasting from several days to 14 months in 70 infants and children with myocarditis and cardiomyopathy, leading to a notable rise in survival in the past 5 years. It is possible to discharge 78% of the infants under 1 year old [3].

Several types of VADs have been used in children and adolescents whose body surface area is greater than $1.2\ m^2$—that is, generally in children older than 5 years. The Thoratec VADs (Thoratec Laboratories, Inc.) have been available since the early 1980s for adult use, but they can also be implanted in older children and adolescents. Several other adult-size VADs, such as the Novacor (Baxter Healthcare Corporation, Irvine, CA, USA), have been applied in adolescents, and a version of the axial flow DeBakey VAD

(MicroMed Technology Inc., The Woodlands, TX, USA) has been developed that is suitable for use in children and has been implanted in several patients. Two miniaturized extracorporeal, pneumatically driven VADs designed specifically for smaller children and infants have been introduced in Europe so far: the Berlin Heart Excor (Berlin Heart AG, Berlin, Germany) in 1992 and the Medos HIA device (Medos Medizintechnik AG, Stolberg, Germany) in 1994. The first reported implantation of a Medos VAD as a bridge to transplantation in a child took place in 1994. Only the extracorporeal, pneumatically driven Berlin Heart Excor and the Medos HIA pulsatile systems have so far proven successful in children of all ages. The pediatric version of the Berlin Heart Excor VAD is mounted with trileaflet polyurethane valves and is available with pump sizes of 10, 25, 30, 50, 60, and 80 ml. The 10-ml pumps are suitable for neonates and infants with body weight of up to 9 kg (body surface area 0.43 m), and the 25 and 30 ml pumps can be used in children up to the age of 7 years (weight 30 kg and body surface area of about $0.95\ m^2$); adult-sized pumps can be implanted in older children. The adult pump has a stroke volume of 80 ml and tilting disk valves. Pediatric-sized pumps are suitable for children with a body weight of 3–9 kg. This pump has a stroke volume of 10 ml and polyurethane trileaflet valves [3].

Several other pulsatile devices developed for the adult population are used in school-aged children: the HeartMate I (Thoratec Laboratories, Inc.), Toyobo (National Cardiovascular Center Tokyo, Japan), Abiomed BVS 5000 (Abiomed Inc., Delaware, MA, USA), and Novacor (World Heart Corporation, Ontario, Canada). Two continuous flow rotary VADs that use axial flow or centrifugal flow—the Incor VAD (Berlin Heart) and the DeBakey VAD—have been introduced into routine clinical care. Some further devices are still being subjected to clinical trials: Jarvik 2000 (Jarvik, New York, NY, USA), HeartMate II, Duraheart® (Terumo Kabushiki Kaisha Corporation, Shibuya-ku, Japan), VentrAssist (Ventracor, Chatswood, NSW, Australia), and CorAid® (Cleveland Clinic, Cleveland, OH, USA) [3].

The Incor device (Berlin Heart AG) is 146 mm long and 30 mm wide and weighs 200 g. MicroMed modified the adult pump to fit children and in 2004 received FDA humanitarian device exemption status, enabling implantation of the DeBakey VAD Child pump for persons, aged 5–16, awaiting heart transplantation.

Berlin Heart AG products are Incor, Excor cannulas, and driving units. In June 2002, the worldwide first implantation of the Incor device took place in the German Heart Center DHZB. By July 2005, no less than 300 Incor devices had been implanted (two patients have been living with the device for 3 years). Excor is an extracorporeal, pulsatile VAD. Various types and sizes of blood pumps and a wide range of cannulas allow us to meet all clinical needs and treat all patients, regardless of their age.

The VentrAssist, which is made by the Australian company Ventracor, has a moving part—a hydrodynamically suspended impeller. It has been designed to have no wearing parts or cause blood damage. It weighs just 298 g and measures 60 mm in diameter, making it suitable for both children and adults. VentrAssist also has an advantage over its one competitor, Incor made by the German company Berlin Heart. The VentrAssist is less likely to damage red blood cells because it moves the blood more slowly with a bigger impeller.

The term VAD has been applied to a wide variety of mechanical circulatory support systems designed to unload the heart and provide adequate perfusion of the organs.

Short-term circulatory support with an LVAD may be indicated for patients with end-stage heart failure (of any etiology) who are awaiting a donor heart for transplantation, and for patients with a severe acute heart failure syndrome from which myocardial recovery is anticipated (such as acute myocarditis). An LVAD is sometimes used if weaning from cardiopulmonary bypass after cardiac surgery fails. In the active arm of a nonrandomized controlled study, 78% (32/41) of patients survived for a mean of 215 days with LVAD support. In another comparative study, 81% (13/16) of patients survived to transplantation (duration of support not stated). One case series showed that at 30 days of bridging to transplantation with an LVAD, survival was 83%, falling to 19% after 24 months' support.

In a nonrandomized controlled trial, posttransplant survival of patients bridged on LVAD support was 66% (21/32) at 41 months, compared with 67% (98/146) of patients at 36 months who had a transplant without circulatory support, although patients in the latter group were significantly older. One case series of 243 patients in whom LVADs were used to bridge to transplantation reported actuarial post-transplant survival of 91% at 1 year, 70% at 5 years, and 40% at 10 years. Results from case series included in a systematic review showed that between 60% (12/20) and 83% (5/6) of patients survived to transplantation or were still alive awaiting transplantation on LVAD support. Of the total cases of bridge to recovery reported, 58% (7/12) of patients survived to final follow-up; successful explantation of the device or weaning from support was achieved in all these patients [4].

The randomized controlled study showed a reduction of 48% in the risk of death from any cause in the group that received left VADs as compared with the medical therapy group [relative risk 0.52; 95% confidence interval (CI) 0.34–0.78; $P = 0.001$]. Randomly assigned 129 patients with end-stage heart failure were ineligible for cardiac transplantation to receive a left VAD (68 patients) or optimal medical management (class IV heart failure). The rates of survival at 1 year were 52% in the device group and 25% in the medical therapy group ($P = 0.002$), and the rates at 2 years were 23% and 8% ($P = 0.09$), respectively. The frequency of serious adverse events in the device group was 2.35 (95% CI 1.86–2.95) times that in the medical therapy group, with a predominance of infection, bleeding, and malfunctioning of the device. The quality of life was significantly improved at 1 year in the device group. The use of a left VAD in patients with advanced heart failure resulted in a clinically meaningful survival benefit and an improved quality of life. A left VAD is an acceptable alternative therapy in selected patients who are not candidates for cardiac transplantation [5].

All mechanical circulatory support systems are associated with a wide range of possible complications: bleeding, infection, device malfunction, hemolysis, peripheral ischemia, and perforation of a ventricle or the aorta, of which bleeding and thromboembolic complications are the most frequent and most serious. Infections, hemolysis, pulmonary edema, and multiorgan failure have also been reported. It was also noted that implantation of an LVAD could unmask previously subclinical right ventricular dysfunction. Damage to the blood pump equipment rarely causes harm to the patient. As examples, one Jarvik 2000 patient broke a cable connector when he slammed it in a car door; another accidentally cut his cable with scissors while changing his bandage; yet another patient lost connection to his battery and controller when a purse snatcher grabbed his shoulder bag and ran off with it. Fortunately, in all these cases, the patient suffered no harm. Their own natural hearts were able to sustain them until they could connect to their backup equipment. But it can be noticed that the longest-running Jarvik 2000 FlowMaker patient has been supported by the device longer than any patient in the world with any other type of mechanical heart, either TAH or VAD—i.e., more than 4 years.

In September 2006, the FDA approved the first totally implantable TAH (AbioCor) for people who are not eligible for a heart transplant and who are unlikely to live more than a month without intervention. It is a big success, but it also means that many problems are awaiting to be solved in laboratories (Figure 8.4) in the near future.

8.3.2 Valve Prostheses

Valvular heart disease is a life-threatening disease that affects millions of people worldwide and leads to approximately 250,000 valve repairs and/or replacements every year. Almost 90,000 Americans a year need surgery for valve disease. Malfunctioning of a native valve impairs its efficient fluid mechanical/hemodynamic performance. Human heart valves act as check valves, controlling the direction of blood flow through the heart. The aortic valve is between the left ventricle and the aorta and the mitral valve is between the left atrium and the left ventricle. It opens and closes to control the blood flow into the left side of the heart. The normal aortic valve area is 3.0–4.0 cm^2. In general, severe aortic stenosis has been defined as a valve whose area was reduced to 0.75–1.0 cm^2. In general, mean transvalvular pressure gradients greater than 50 mmHg represent severe aortic stenosis, while mean gradients less than 25 mmHg suggest mild aortic stenosis. Mitral stenosis causes leaflet/chordal thickening and calcification, commissural fusion or shortening, chordal fusion, or a combination of these processes. The normal mitral valve area (MVA) is 4.0–5.0 cm^2. Accordingly, mild mitral stenosis is defined as a condition with an MVA of 1.5–2.5 cm and a mean gradient at rest less than 5 mmHg. Moderate and severe mitral stenoses are defined as conditions with an MVA 1.0–1.5 and less than 1.0 cm^2, respectively, with mean gradients greater than 5 mmHg [6].

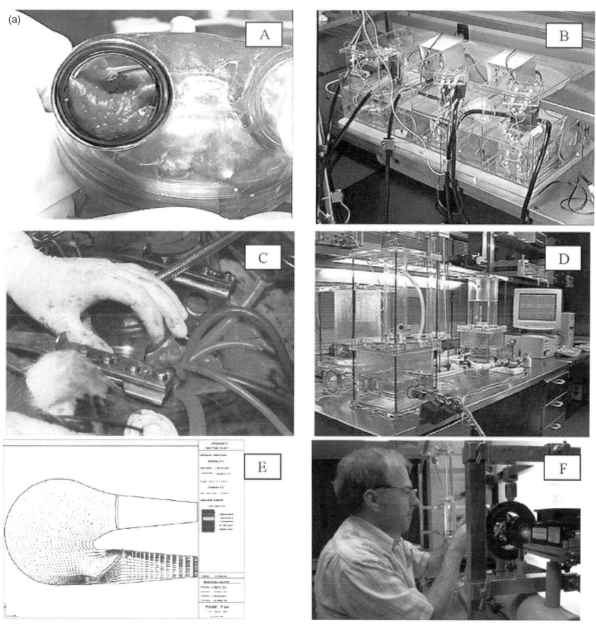

Figure 8.4 (a) The in vitro cloth formation and hemolysis test [A,B]. The artificial heart POLTAH in vivo (calf) implantation [C] and in vitro blood circulation test stand [D]. Computer flow simulation method (Fidap software) [E] and laser anemometry, flow visualization stand (constructor Z. Małota) [F]. (b) One of the problems that are not satisfactorily solved was the interpretation of laser flow visualization pictures. Proposed by the author in the 1990s, functional analyzing method (FAM) method involves monitoring the quality of a flow system. The artificial heart is a pump that should cause fluid flow from the inlet (atrial) to the outlet channel and provide blood with a determined amount of energy to overcome the load, in order to create clinically desired pressure-flow state in the circulatory system. Both goals must be achieved, while conserving the safe transportation of morphotic blood elements, which is essential for long-term blood pumps. Therefore, it must minimize the undesired phenomena occurring at the blood–artificial surface interface. (c) The chamber was divided into areas where, for a given section, and for every local flow velocity, vectors are assigned with its components in the direction of an outlet V_o and inlet V_i channel as well as the component V_r tangent to the chamber's wall. The results depend on the phase of work cycle. The analysis of time changes of the first two components

(Continued)

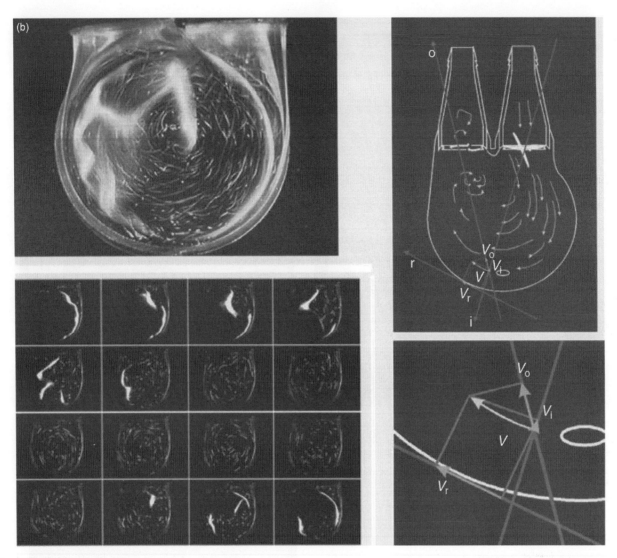

Figure 8.4 (*Continued*)

Valve repair is now the method of choice for surgical treatment of valve disease, thanks to improvements in techniques over the past 40 years. Starr and associates first reported a technique for aortic repair in 1960. In the early 1980s, surgeons who performed percutaneous balloon valvotomy became more involved in aortic valve repair after annular disruptions, and other balloon-induced injuries caused acute insufficiency in young patients requiring immediate repair. Balloon valvotomy may be appropriate for children and adolescents with congenital aortic stenosis, but not for adults with calcific aortic stenosis.

The application of mitral and tricuspid valve repair method allows to maintain the natural anatomy of the heart valve. The surgeon repairs the tissue of the damaged valve and usually implants an *annuloplasty ring* to provide extra support to the valve.

◀ allows to track down the dynamics of flow structure organization during an entire cycle, to detect inertial effects and passage time, while the tangent component is responsible for a good washing of wall vicinity areas. The full analysis makes possible the classification of obtained pictures (since digital picture recording is suitable for computer analysis and gives results that are easy to interpret), so that the conclusions regarding the causes of phenomena and their regulation may be drawn easily.

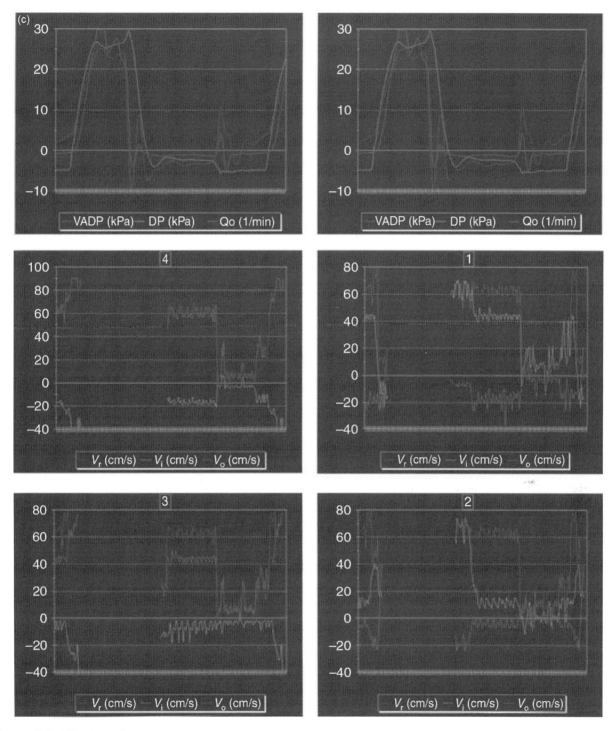

Figure 8.4 (*Continued*)

Natural valve leaflets are constructed from layers of connective tissue lined with endothelium. The zones of stress concentration are reinforced with bands of collagen fibers. Artificial heart valves should be designed to mimic the natural function and flow dynamics that are optimized in the course of million years of evolution.

The prosthetic valve must be durable and biocompatible, should quickly change phase (close to open, or vice versa), and must allow adequate blood flow with a minimum pressure gradient (energy dissipation), turbulence, and stagnation zones (Figure 8.5). Optimum leaflet valve design creates minimal stress concentration in leaflets, and

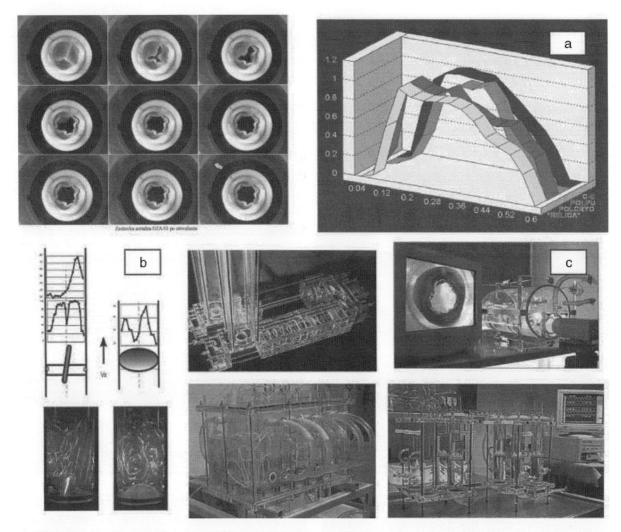

Figure 8.5 Results of valve test tester designed and introduced in Institute Heart Prostheses, FCSD. The opening area valve test and comparison in one cycle of working biological Religa, Polcryo, and synthetic Polpu prototypes with Carpentier–Edwards bioprotheses (a). The laser visualization and laser anemometer test results of Polish disk valve prototype (b). Several testing apparatus used in our laboratories (c).

optimal cusp shape effects smooth washout, minimal pressure gradient, and adequate longevity. The geometry and the construction of the valve should be surgically convenient to insert in the heart. Most number of valves, including natural ones, are constructed from three leaflets. The simplest configuration (Figure 8.6) shows that it is due to the Π number whose value is about 3.

There are two main types of prosthetic valves: mechanical and biological. Mechanical valves can cause various complications, including thrombosis, ischemia, and turbulent flow. Advantages of bioprosthetic valves (porcine and bovine xenografts) include their durability and low incidence of

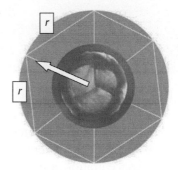

Figure 8.6 The simplest configuration of a valve:. An open valve ideally constructed using three leaflets lies on the perimeter of the wheel created by the aorta's cross section ($2\pi r$ is equal to about $2r + 2r + 2r$).

thromboembolism. Complications associated with bioprosthetic heart valves include hemorrhage and stiffening of the leaflets.

For over 50 years, materials and construction of cardiovascular prosthesis have been under investigation. Hufnagel was the first to implant a valvular prosthesis in the descending aorta for the treatment of aortic insufficiency (in 1952).

The first artificial heart valve prosthesis for routine prosthetic valve replacement clinical use was the Starr–Edwards mechanical valve, which was introduced in the 1960s. The problem of lifelong anticoagulation therapy in mechanical heart valves was solved with the introduction of biological valves in the 1970s: porcine or pericardial. The most popular tissue valves, the Hancock and the Carpentier–Edwards prostheses, are porcine xenografts. However, their durability was limited and age dependent with faster degeneration at younger age.

In 1977 the new generations of mechanical prostheses were introduced: the mono-leaflet Medtronic-Hall and the bi-leaflet St Jude Medical valves and next CarboMedics valves. Currently, mechanical heart valve prostheses account for 60–70% of the prosthetic heart valves implanted worldwide, with bi-leaflet tilting disk prostheses accounting for the majority.

The development of flexible polymeric heart valves started as early as in 1958 (Roe implanted valves made of silicone rubber). Between 1961 and 1963, 23 patients underwent aortic valve replacement with a tricuspid polytetrafluoroethylene (PTFE) prosthesis by Braunwald et al. Again, mortality was high, and the explanted valves showed severe thickening and rupture of the leaflets. Next aortic prosthesis made of Dacron and silicone was implanted by Roe in 1966, but only four patients survived the operation and lived for 33–61 months. In 1977, Hufnagel implanted a single leaflet aortic prosthesis made of Dacron into the aortic position. Most valves failed, but some patients survived up to 15 years. Embolic complications and fatigue failure were observed frequently in silastic, collagen, and PTFE valves; the latter also exhibited shrinkage. Calcification was also observed frequently, hinting at a destruction of the chemical integrity of the polymer. Polyurethanes have demonstrated the best biocompatibility, durability, and resistance to thromboembolism among all polymers and are, therefore, also used for a variety of medical devices [7].

Currently, some polymeric valves have proven efficacious in assist devices (Abiomed, Medos, and Berlin Heart). However, so far no flexible polymeric heart valve has proven durability for long-term implantation.

All mechanical valves are made up of an orifice ring and occluders, either one or two leaflets through which blood flows through the heart in a forward direction. Because of susceptibility to thromboembolic events, mechanical devices are used in a lifelong anticoagulation therapy (using agents such as Heparin, Warfarin, or Coumadin that delay the clotting of blood, which can cause a heart attack or stroke). The abovementioned drawbacks are minimized or eliminated when bioprostheses are implanted.

Tissue valves (bioprosthetic valves) are made of human or animal tissue. There are three types of tissue valves: pig tissue (porcine), cow tissue (bovine), and human tissue (e.g., aortic or pulmonary valves obtained from human cadavers), or autografts (e.g., the patient's own pulmonary valve, pericardium, or fascia lata). Homograft aortic or pulmonary valves (and associated portions of aortic or pulmonary root) obtained from human cadavers are cryopreserved and implanted directly in place without a synthetic frame.

Heterograft tissue valves for aortic or mitral valve replacement (MVR) are made from natural, animal tissue (porcine aortic valve or bovine pericardium) fixed, usually in dilute glutaraldehyde (GA) and mounted on a synthetic stent—a semi-rigid frame comprising a base ring and struts.

The technically more difficult to implant, similar to the homograft valve, porcine stentless valve is used only for aortic valve replacement.

The mechanical valves are made from Stellite 21, Haynes 25, Titanium (the housing/strut), Delrin, pyrolytic carbon, carbon/Delrin composite, and an ultra-high-molecular polyethylene (UHMPE) (the leaflet).

In bioprostheses, leaflets are made from porcine aortic valve or porcine pericardial tissue fixed by stabilized GA mounted on stents (polypropylene stent covered with Dacron and Elgiloy wire and nylon support band covered with polyester and Teflon cloth).

The sewing ring is made from Dacron and soft silicone rubber insert covered with porous, seamless Teflon cloth or PTFE fabric over silicone rubber filter.

The physical properties of material, valve geometry, stress—strain distribution in leaflets, and the local pressure and flow values near the valve influence the risk of valve failure and can cause damage to the blood components. Dangerous for blood local space are associated with shear velocities and shear stress reaching critical values for morphotic blood elements. For soft (biological) valve durability, the stress on leaflets is the most important factor, which lead to calcifications and, as a result, valve damage.

The global geometry of valve is enforced by the fit criteria and is characteristic of physical nature of work. The biological valve design made from donors (humans or animals) is limited by anatomical valve tissue and heart geometry.

The use of xenograft and allograft biomaterials has typically required chemical or physical pretreatment aimed at preserving and sterilizing the materials and reducing the immunogenicity of the tissue. Multiple chemical and physical cross-linking techniques have been explored to stabilize the collagen-based structure of the tissue, maintaining its mechanical integrity and natural compliance. Bioprotheses are mainly prepared from animal structures, e.g., valves or pericardium, composed primarily of collagen. The main advantage of xenogenic bioprotheses is their structural similarity to human tissues. However, in order to improve prosthesis durability reflected by the enhanced resistance to enzymatic degradation and reduced immunogenicity, animal tissues must be chemically or physically pretreated (fixed). Fixation procedures are connected with crosslinking of tissue proteins. Among chemical methods of crosslinking, the most commonly accepted is treatment with GA. This five-carbon bifunctional aldehyde reacts with free amino groups of proteins—mainly ε-amino groups of collagen lysyl residues—forming inter- or intrachain crosslinks. Prostheses obtained after tissue treatment with GA reveal remarkable reduction in immunogenicity and sensitivity to in vivo degradation.

Patients with mechanical valves require long-term anticoagulant therapy owing to the risk of thromboembolic complications. Reports of strut failure, material erosion, and leaflet escapes as well as pitting (cavitations) and erosion of valve leaflet and housing have resulted in numerous investigations on the closing dynamics of mechanical valves and the pressure distribution on the leaflets and impact forces between the leaflets and guiding struts. This requires the flow through the clearance between the leaflet and the housing in closing position influencing the hemolysis and thrombus initiation.

The valve-related problems are as follows:

- *Mechanical valves:* thromboembolism, structural failure, red blood cell and platelet destruction, tissue overgrowth, damage to endothelial lining, para/perivalvular leakage, tearing of sutures, infection
- *Bioprosthetic valves:* tissue calcification, leaflet rupture, para/perivalvular leakage, infection

The cause of valve failure can be related to the valve components (Figure 8.7).

The probability of survival 5 and 10 years following heart valve replacement is approximately 70 and 50%, respectively. Prosthesis-associated complications often lead to reoperation such that replacements currently account for 15—25% of all valve operations. Thrombotic deposits may form on heart valve prostheses, which is more likely to occur in mechanical heart valves which are more thrombogenic than tissue valves. Hemorrhage rates are higher in patients with mechanical valves in the aortic site than in patients with aortic tissue valves. However, these rates are similar for mechanical and tissue valves in the mitral location. Rates of infection (1—6%) do not differ significantly between tissue and mechanical prostheses. In tissue valves, infection may be localized in the vicinity of the sewing ring. However, the cusps may also be a focus of infection [6].

From the early generation of heart valves, only the Starr—Edwards ball valve design remains in clinical use today. Currently available mechanical valves have been designed with a lower profile and a more effective orifice area, to improve hemodynamics.

The initial design of tilting disk valve consisting of Delrin disk exhibited good wear resistance and mechanical strength. But due to the swelling phenomenon, it was replaced by pyrolytic carbon. Structural dysfunction of the B—S (Shiley Inc., USA) 60° and 70° convexo-concave mechanical heart valve prosthesis occurred at a relatively high frequency (2.2—8.3%). The B—S tilting disk design has been withdrawn from the market, while the Duromedics bi-leaflet prosthesis was reintroduced as the Edwards—Tekna (Edwards Lifesciences,

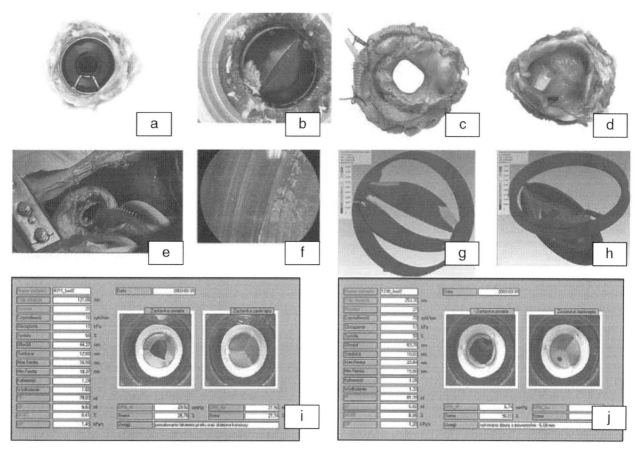

Figure 8.7 The samples of explanted valves collected in the Institute of Heart Prostheses, FCSD (COST Action 537 project). One-disk (a) and two-disk mechanical valve (b) and two bioprostheses (c,d). The in vivo valve test on ship (e). The microscopic evaluation of valve's disk (f) and modeling of mechanical valves— equivalent elastic strain values (g,h). The effect of biological heart valve prosthesis damage on hemodynamic efficiency has been investigated and analyzed: improper functioning due to leaflet calcification—the opening area of "calcified" (leaflets partially glued (i)) valve decreased by 44%, while the pressure gradient grew up to 22 mmHg. Perforation of a leaflet (j)—significant perforation (hole area 6.68 mm^2) of leaflet caused increase in back-leakage of 147% to 8.38 (6.8 ml).

USA) valve following design modifications. The failure mode of the B−S prosthesis is due to failure of the welded outlet strut with resultant embolization of the disk. Fracture of the carbon component in a small number of mechanical valves, including the Edwards−Duromedics (Edwards Lifesciences, USA) and St Jude Medical (St Jude Medical Inc., USA) bi-leaflet tilting disk valves, has also been reported [6].

The most common cause of failure during implantation is leaflet fracture. The most common causes of mechanical valve failure are pannus formation and thrombosis. Structural dysfunction occurs more commonly with tissue valves than with contemporary mechanical valves [6].

The rate of bioprosthetic valve failure increases over time, particularly after the initial 4−5 years after implantation. At 10 years after implantation, 20−40% of porcine aortic valves implanted in either aortic or mitral sites require replacement for primary tissue failure. Up to 50% of such valves fail after 10−15 years. Calcification, cuspal tears, or both are the most common manifestations of tissue failure in bioprosthetic porcine aortic valves.

Stentless bioprosthetic porcine aortic valves have shown minimal cuspal calcification or tissue degeneration for periods up to 8 years following implantation. As with bioprosthetic porcine valves, bioprosthetic heart valves made from bovine pericardium develop both calcific and noncalcific tissue failure. The second generation of bovine pericardial prostheses, such as the Carpentier–Edwards pericardial valve, have increased durability compared with first-generation pericardial valves [Ionescu–Shiley (Shiley Inc., USA), Mitroflow (CarboMedics, Canada), and Hancock] and excellent hemodynamics. Cryopreserved human homograft (or allograft) aortic valves have equivalent or slightly better durability than contemporary bioprosthetic porcine valves with valve survival rates of approximately 50–90% at 10–15 years [6].

Technology continues to improve the durability of bioprostheses and to reduce the thrombogenic effects of mechanical prostheses.

The most significant changes in mechanical heart valves over the last decade have focused on the sewing ring and the ability to rotate the valve after implantation. The St Jude Medical Regent prosthesis and CarboMedics Top Hat improve valve hemodynamics by introducing modification that allows for the placement of the device in a supra-annular position. The St Jude Medical Silzone (silver nitrate incorporated in the sewing cuff) was withdrawn from the clinical trials due to increased incidence of paravalvular leak in the silzone cohort. The newer generation mechanical prostheses, e.g., the Edwards–MIRA (Edwards Lifesciences, USA) (Sorin Bicarbon mechanical prosthesis with a modified sewing ring), ATS (Advancing the Standard) (ATS Inc., USA), and On-X (Medical Carbon Research Institute, USA), have just completed regulatory clinical trials [6].

The most significant changes in biological heart valves over the last decade have focused on the stent construction and tissue treatment method (changing fixation pressure and chemicals). Stent mounting produces higher transvalvular gradients and also causes premature valve failure. In the brief period in which homografts were stented, the average life expectancy of the valve was less than 10 years (about 90% homografts have a 10-year freedom from valve degeneration). Furthermore, to date, in two large international trials, no Medtronic Freestyle (Medtronic Inc.) and Toronto SPV (St Jude Medical Inc.) stentless valves have been explanted because of primary structural failure [6].

The valves fixed at zero pressure retain a collagen architecture virtually identical to that of native unfixed porcine aortic valve cusps. The 10-year experience with the Medtronic Intact (Medtronic Inc.) (zero pressure fixed) valve reported no cases of primary structural degeneration in patients over 60 years of age and only one case of valve failure in individuals over 40 years of age. The exposed amine residues of the GA molecule promote tissue calcification. Surfactants, particularly sodium dodecyl sulfate (T6) (Hancock II, Medtronic Inc., USA), polysorbate 80 (Carpentier-Edwards standard and supra-annular porcine bioprostheses; Edwards Lifesciences, USA), and toluidine blue (Medtronic Intact, Medtronic Inc.), have been incorporated in the preservation process. No-React detoxification process has been proposed as a method of preventing calcification of GA fixed tissue. Detoxification with homocysteic acid is used in Sorin products (Sorin Group Inc.) [6].

The Carpentier–Edwards PERIMOUNT Pericardial Bioprosthesis, made of bovine pericardial tissue that has been preserved in a buffered GA solution and mounted on fully extensible stents and distensible struts, decreases shearing stresses on valve leaflets and maintains physiologic aortic ring movements to reduce flow turbulence and vibrations. Both the frame and the sewing ring are covered with a knitted PTFE cloth. This material helps facilitate the healing and ingrowth of tissue around the implanted valve.

The Medtronic Company is currently manufacturing two new bioprostheses. One valve is stentless (Freestyle aortic root bioprosthesis) and the other incorporates a stent design (Mosaic bioprosthesis). Both represent new concepts in the manufacture of bioprostheses, specifically, zero-pressure fixation and α-amino oleic acid antimineralization treatment. CarboMedics is investigating a Photofix bioprosthetic valve: a patented trileaflet, central-flow prosthesis, with each leaflet mounted on a flexible support frame. The leaflets are prepared from bovine pericardium treated with a unique patented dye-mediated photo-oxidation process. This new fixation process results in collagen crosslinking without the use of GA, a suspected contributor to the calcification failures of other clinically available tissue valves.

The *choice* of prosthesis is again a decision to be made by the surgeon and the patient, with full knowledge of the advantages and disadvantages of the different types available.

From a clinical point of view, the use of bioprosthetic valves is recommended for older patients (over 65–70 years) because of the increased risk of bleeding in the elderly and the low probability of structural failure of the bioprosthesis in the remaining expected life of these patients. Mechanical prostheses are indicated for patients 70 years of age or younger, even though there is significant valve-related morbidity. The outcomes 15 years after valve replacement with a mechanical versus a bioprosthetic valve have been reported by the Veterans Affairs randomized trial. All-cause mortality was not different after MVR with mechanical prostheses versus bioprostheses. Structural valve deterioration was greater with bioprostheses for MVR in all age groups but occurred at a much higher rate in those less than 65 years of age. Thromboembolism rates were similar in the two valve prostheses, but bleeding was more common with the mechanical prostheses. In 2003, the Edinburgh randomized trial extrapolated results to 20 years. The prosthesis type did not influence survival, thromboembolism, or endocarditis. Major bleeding was more common with mechanical prosthesis [6].

Thanks to EU grant COST Action 537—"Core Laboratories for the improvement of medical devices in clinical practice from the failure of the explanted prostheses analysis (FEPA)"—organized in Europe. The goal is to improve medical devices in clinical practice from the FEPA—systematic studies of medical evaluation of cardiovascular implants requiring an explantation and assessment of generalized (immunological, inflammatory) and/or remote biological effects in patients with cardiovascular implants and with complications.

Living tissue valve replacements would solve many of the existing problems. In the future, natural biomaterials repopulated with autologous or genetically engineered cells will be used as ideal templates for the design of living tissue grafts. To date, the knowledge about these new materials is not very wide.

Further developments toward the alternative biological valve prostheses based on biological cell-free matrices as ideal valve substitutes using tissue engineering would potentially eliminate the known disadvantages of current valve prostheses. The endothelial cells harvested from the patient may be cultured in laboratory and incorporated into the synthetic scaffolds (polyglycolic acid, polyhydroxyalkanoate, and poly-4-hydroxybutrate) or both heterograft and allograft valvular decellularized tissues.

An ideal heart valve substitute should possess the following characteristics: absolute biocompatibility, long-term durability, nature-like biomechanical properties, no thrombogenic or teratogenic effects, sufficient availability in all common sizes, and moreover, particularly for pediatric patients the growth potential is crucial. Regions of stress concentration on the leaflets during the complex motion of the leaflets have been implicated in the structural failure of the leaflets with bioprosthetic valves. Computational fluid dynamics (CFD) has emerged as a promising tool, which, alongside experimentation, can yield insights of unprecedented detail into the hemodynamics of prosthetic heart valves.

8.3.3 Heart Pacemaker

The pacemaker was the first electronic device ever surgically implanted inside a human. In 1950, John Hopps, an electrical engineer, built the first pacemaker. The first successful attempts at designing a totally implantable pacemaker were reported by W. Chardack, A. Gage, and W. Greatbatch (New York). The group's work was recognized by Medtronic, which in 1960 signed a contract with Chardack and Greatbatch to produce an implantable pulse generator. These pacemakers and batteries have improved and saved the lives of millions of people worldwide. The pacemaker was applied for the first time in 1952 (P. Zoll) to stimulate the heart muscle through electrodes placed on the patient's chest. On the next stage, endocavitary electrodes were introduced into the right ventricle through the vein and a new, more effective way of controlling the system was carried out. The size and the weight of pacemakers and their durability had improved after replacing mercury batteries with lithium batteries, which have to be replaced every 10 years. Currently, the average weight of the device is about 15–30 g and 2.5 mm in diameter. In order to reduce the risk of system distortion, the bipolar electrodes should be fixed to endocardium using special methods. The electrode tips are made of special metal alloys and have a porous surface.

8.4 The Minimally Invasive Cardiology Tools

Minimally invasive cardiology requires a separate set of tools allowing the surgeon to operate through vessels. For surgical interventions, the following devices can be used: the guideline (diameter 2–3 mm), catheters (the balloon catheter has a diameter of 0.8 mm), balloons (the balloon has to hold out an inflation up to 20 atm), and broadening vascular stents and devices (about 2 mm in diameter covered with diamond particles) for drilling out and excising the atherosclerotic plaques in coronary vessels, all under X-ray control.

The human circulatory system consists of the heart and the network of vessels transporting blood throughout the body. A pathological state of the aorta, which in more advanced stage blocks the blood flow, can be treated by vascular prosthesis implantation, replacing the damaged fragment of the vessel. Tissue implants (autogenic, allogenic, xenogenic) and synthetic vessels can be used as vascular prostheses in the surgery of vessels and cardiosurgery. If the main aim is to preserve the life of the cells, then depending on the time of tissue treatment, they are stored in antibiotic bath, nutritious liquids, or in hypothermia; or deep-freezed in liquid nitrogen. The blood cannot be used as a preservation solution, because at room temperature, unoxygenated blood becomes toxic. In some cases, vascular stents can also be used, which are constructions for vessel wall supporting to preserve its physiological diameter. They are pipes with diameter up to several centimeters, made of biocompatible materials (Dacron) fixed on a steel frame, assembled in the vessel during operation.

The narrowing or blockage in one or more coronary arteries (those supplying the blood to the heart muscle) can be a direct cause of the coronary artery disease. Currently, several treatment methods are available: e.g., using bypass techniques, vessel stents and minimally invasive, mechanical cloth, or by calcification removing. Pharmacological therapy and tissue engineering are very promising tools for contemporary and future treatment.

The catheter can be brought to the desired location via navigation, propulsion, and steering to perform several functions:

— actuation (ablation of material, balloon angioplasty, deployment of stent)
— sensing (pressure)
— transportation of material or energy (contrast fluid, embolization material, or signal from sensors for diagnostic purposes)

and that it can be retrieved again from the body [8]. The physical contact of the interventionist with the patient's tissue is established by using catheter, and the visual observation is mediated by the X-ray imaging.

Since the origin of the field of interventional cardiology in 1966 with balloon atrial septostomy, a procedure directed at treating congenital heart diseases, pediatric interventional cardiologists have developed percutaneous techniques for treating congenital valvular and great vessel stenoses and transcatheter closure of aberrant vascular channels. Balloon angioplasty [percutaneous transluminal coronary angioplasty (PTCA)] is widely used for treatment of the blockages of coronary artery. Percutaneous coronary intervention (PCI) encompasses a variety of procedures used to treat patients with diseased arteries of the heart. The catheter with balloon is inserted into the vessel (most often the femoral artery) through a small prick in artery. After transferring the balloon to the destination place, it is filled with a physiological saline mixture up to several atmospheric pressure. Due to this pressure, the balloon will expand, thus compressing the plaque, and hence, the narrowed vessel will also expand. The effectiveness of coronary angioplasty can be improved by using vessel prosthesis—a stent that is placed in vessel supports it and prevents it from closing. Typically, PCI is performed by threading a slender balloon-tipped tube—a catheter—from an artery in the groin to a trouble spot in an artery of the heart (this is referred to as the PTCA, coronary artery balloon dilation, or balloon angioplasty). The balloon is then inflated, compressing the plaque and dilating (widening) the narrowed coronary artery so that blood can flow more easily. This is often accompanied by inserting an expandable metal stent. Stents are wire mesh tubes used to prop open arteries after PTCA. The stent is collapsed to a small diameter and put over a balloon catheter. It is then moved into the area of the blockage. When the balloon is inflated, the stent expands, locks in place, and forms a scaffold. This holds the artery open. The stent remains in the artery permanently, holds it open, improves blood flow to the heart muscle, and relieves symptoms (usually chest pain). Within a few weeks of the time the stent was placed, the inner lining of the artery (the endothelium) grows over the metal surface of the stent. More than 70% of coronary angioplasty procedures also include stenting. Some blockages in the arteries are hard, calcified deposits that do not respond to balloon angioplasty or stent implantation. In this case, the rotablator technique may be introduced. This is a small device used inside of the coronary arteries to "drill" through the calcified blockage. It breaks the calcium into microscopic pieces and disintegrates the blockage.

Percutaneous balloon dilation of isolated congenital semilunar valvular stenoses has proven to be highly effective in providing long-term hemodynamic and symptomatic benefit in neonatal, pediatric, and adult patient populations. Kan and associates described the first clinical application of balloon valvuloplasty in 1982, in which drastic improvement in transvalvular gradient was achieved in five children with pulmonary valve stenosis.

Percutaneous balloon valvuloplasty has thus been proposed as a less invasive means of treating mitral stenosis (Figure 8.8). The valve is usually approached in an anterograde direction via an interatrial septal puncture, although a retrograde technique has been reported. One or two tubular balloons or a specialized nylon-rubber (Inoue) balloon is advanced to position across the mitral valve and repetitive inflations are performed until the balloons have fully expanded.

Hemodynamic improvement following mitral valvuloplasty occurs immediately, with valve area increasing on average by $1.0\,cm^2$, with a prompt drop in pulmonary pressures.

A randomized trial comparing mitral balloon valvuloplasty to open surgical commissurotomy among patients with favorable valvular anatomy demonstrated comparable initial hemodynamic results and clinical outcomes among patients treated with either technique, although hemodynamic findings at 3 years were more favorable in the balloon valvuloplasty group.

Pulmonary artery stenosis or hypoplasia may be effectively treated using catheter-based technologies. Success rates following balloon dilation of these vessels have ranged from 50 to 60%, with failures due primarily to elastic recoil. There has also been a limited experience with balloon angioplasty or stent placement for management of aortic coarctation, venous obstruction, or stenoses of Fontan shunts.

Advances in the technology for percutaneous coronary revascularization have been accompanied by a dramatic increase in the number of procedures carried out in the world.

Intravascular stenting of arteries is one of the most frequent operations in cardiovascular surgery. Stents are inserted into a vessel with injured inner wall to avoid its destruction, thrombus formation, or vasoconstriction. Vascular stents should have a shape rendering it relatively elastic and durable with respect to the vessel (Figure 8.9). There have to be (e.g., gold) marker lines, allowing stent observation during procedure (RTG monitoring). Stents are made from metal alloys using various techniques. They can be formed from the wire or through excising from tubes using laser. More recent research uses shape memory alloys (Nitinol). Such stents in cooled stage are transported to the target place, where after warming up to physiological temperature, they reach the final shape. One of the first stents clinically applied (Wiktor-GX stent, Medtronic Interventional Vascular, Holland) is an

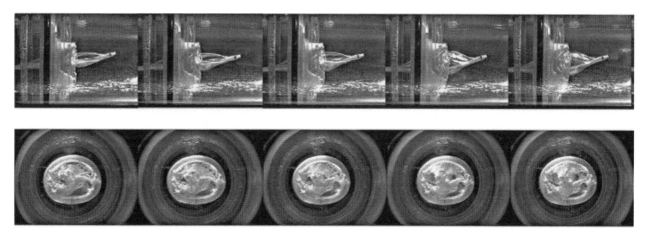

Figure 8.8 The physical percutaneous balloon valvuloplasty simulation on polyurethane and mitral valve.

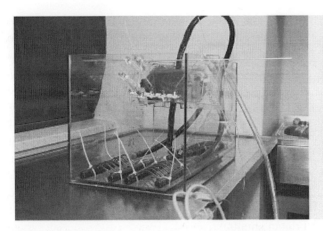 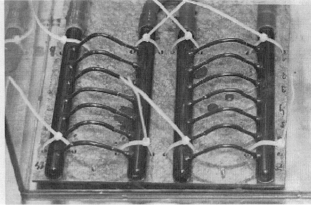

Figure 8.9 Fatigue tests on the nanocrystalline diamond and steel coronary stents were carried out: Tyrode's physiologic solution; frequency 180 cpm; 3 months. Coronary arteries were simulated using a tube of inner diameter 3 mm and wall thickness 1 mm. After investigations, the corrosion resistance tests of the implants have been additionally performed.

original project of Pole, Dominick Wiktor, in the United States. This stent was created from wire with sinusoidal shape wounded on the cylinder. It is made from tantalum, instead of steel, because of its better contrast in RTG visualization and the electronegative surface improving thromboresistance of the stent. The first clinical implantation of stent was performed in 1989. The materials used for the construction of these stents have changed dramatically over the past 10 years. Unfortunately, metal stents induce thrombus formation. Stent biocompatibility can be enhanced by either modifying the metal surface of the implant or applying biocompatible coatings. To improve its biocompatibility and to prevent the closing of renewed vessel, the surface of stents is covered with heparin. Stenting procedures can also be connected with genetic therapy by covering its surface by a layer of polymer, which when placed into the vessel wall releases the genetic material, which blocks the cell growth. In Poland, the multidisciplinary team works on original vascular stents covered with a layer of nanocrystalline diamond.

Currently, multiple research projects are focused on the design of a stent with better radiopacity, reduced stent-vessel wall contact area, and improved elasticity, and thrombogenic effects are lowered when the stent is coated with the proper antithrombotic substances. The problem that plagues about one-third of patients who receive angioplasty with or without stents is "restenosis"—the recurrence of the narrowing of the blood vessel.

The new drug-coated stents release a medication that blocks this scarring process.

Novel technologies will be introduced and developed, directed at the efficient removal or modification of arterial plaques with minimal arterial trauma or at site-specific drug delivery to inhibit thrombosis and restenosis. Concurrently, intravascular ultrasound and angioscopy will be further refined and integrated into revascularization devices, allowing precise guidance and optimization of plaque ablation or remodeling while limiting associated coronary injury. Finally, understanding of the vascular biology of percutaneous revascularization, thrombosis, and restenosis will be improved, leading to pharmacological therapies designed to ameliorate adverse thrombotic, proliferative, and remodeling responses.

8.5 The Technology for Atrial Fibrillation

The evolving technologies for ablation of atrial fibrillation include radio frequency, cryotherapy, microwave, laser, and ultrasound. The efforts directed at isolating and ablating percutaneous catheter pulmonary vein have essentially been abandoned because of the extensive length of procedures and the high incidence of pulmonary vein stenosis. The newer technologies have been developed to create transmural lesions during cardiac surgery [6].

Radiofrequency used in ablation: Radio frequency corresponds to the frequency of unmodulated alternating current delivered in the range of 0.5–1.0 MHz between two electrodes, one located on the endocardial surface and the other on the skin. Its heating effect produces homogeneous lesions that measure a few millimeters in diameter and depth. It has been demonstrated that reliable and effective ablation is performed at 70°C for 60 s. The goal temperature should never be set at more than 95°C to avoid potential tissue disruption.

Cryoablation: Cryoablation has an excellent clinical safety record, although its use in atrial fibrillation surgery has been limited to creating spot lesions over the tricuspid and mitral valve annuli. The salient features of the procedure are rapid freezing, and slow thawing with repeated freeze–thaw cycles. The coldest temperature (the prime determinant of cell death) may range from −50°C to −150°C and the application time can vary between 0.5 and 5 min, depending on the area of application.

Laser ablation: The laser lesion formation is thermal through photon absorption at the surface, with deeper myocardial sites heated through passive conduction. The wavelength chosen for good penetration is 980 nm (using a 980-nm diode laser). This wavelength ablates tissue with absorption of actual laser energy as deep as 4 mm into the tissue and further ablation by conductive heating mechanisms. The lesion times are for 36 s utilizing 5 W/cm, but ablation cannot be longer than 5 cm.

Microwave ablation: The electromagnetic microwaves occur at 2.45 GHz to generate frictional heating by induction of dielectric ionic movements. The microwave device can provide a range of 40–45 W of power for 20–30 s, generating a consistent 3–6 mm lesion depth sufficient to produce transmural ablation.

Ultrasound ablation: This technology uses an ultrasound transducer to deliver mechanical pressure waves at high frequency. The tissue destruction is thermal and lesion depth corresponds to vibrational frequency. The ultrasound wave emitted from the transducer travels through tissue causing compression, refraction, and particle movement, resulting in kinetic energy and heat [6].

8.6 Minimally Invasive Surgery

Minimally invasive surgery, a keyhole surgery, is an operation technique in which access to the inside of the patient's body is achieved via small incisions. The long rigid instruments inserted via trocars can be used to move, retract, and cut tissue in abdomen (laparoscopy), chest (thoracoscopy), blood vessels (angioscopy), gastrointestinal tract (colonoscopy), uterus (hysteroscopy), and joints (artheroscopy). Insufflation of the body cavity may be carded out and maintained by seals on the trocar port, which allow tool manipulation without excessive loss of insufflation gas [8]. The trocars may be sized to provide ports of differing sizes, typically of about 5–11 mm diameter. Currently, tools such as retractors, forceps, graspers, suture needles, scissors, different types of knives, laser incision instruments, and specimen bags are available. A video camera is generally operated through a trocar port for visualization and control of the procedures in the cavity. High-definition video cameras and monitors are then attached to the camera and a surgical team can obtain a clear picture of the affected internal area without resorting to radical, disfiguring surgical incisions to physically open the patient. Another benefit of laparoscopic surgery is the significantly reduced recovery time, when compared to standard surgical procedures, due to the minuscule size of the scalpel incisions and avoidance of the massive internal traumatization known in standard surgical procedures.

Due to fixed entry points of the instruments in the abdominal wall, the DOF is reduced, and the movements are mirrored and scaled. The coupling between observation and manipulation, the hand-eye coordination is disturbed, tactile information about tissue properties partially, due to friction and the poor ergonomic design of instruments, lost. The future is open for semiautomatic tools for MIS. As an example, Medtronic, Inc., has introduced the world's first minimally invasive epicardial lead placement tool. The Medtronic Model 10626 Epicardial Lead Implant Tool allows for perpendicular alignment to the heart from different angle approaches. The tool furthers the trend moving away from invasive sternotomy procedures. Laparoscopy reduces patient trauma, but eliminates the surgeon's ability to directly view and touch the surgical environment. This is reason that the surgeon introduced the small-incision surgery when they have a direct view of the tissue.

The rapid development and growing interest in MIS methods impelled creation of modern, complicated tools: cardiosurgical robots.

8.6.1 The Classical Thoracoscopic Tools

Laparoscopic or thoracoscopic surgery requires that surgeons perform complex procedures using a standardized set of tools. For laparoscopic procedures, special sewing devices, ligating instruments, knot pushers, clips, and clip appliers have been developed. The clamp is an essential tool for stopping or controlling blood flow to an organ during surgery. There is a need for a secure and easy method of suturing in laparoscopic surgery. Laparoscopic suturing can be performed with a suture, using automatic sewing devices or clips. When a surgeon wants to suture laparoscopically in the traditional way by using a Roeder knot for instance, the tying of the knot requires some expertise and makes the procedure more complicated and time-consuming. The vascular clips provide a very easy (and secure) method of stopping blood flow while performing procedures on vessels. The locking forceps allows easy, precise, and secure grasping of the surgical clips. The risky point of a clip is the open end of its U-shaped design, which makes it possible for the clip to slip off. Sutures avoid this risk by totally enclosing the structure to be occluded. Knotting instruments require a two-forcep technique, whereas sewing devices require only one working channel.

There has been a tremendous interest in the development of *anastomotic devices* for coronary surgery. Coronary artery disease is a major health problem worldwide, with approximately 850,000 bypass procedures being performed every year. The current methods of coronary bypass surgery can be time-consuming and technically difficult especially when minimally invasive instruments for suturing the blood vessels (the connection is called anastomosis) are used. Alexis Carrel, who many consider the father of anastamoses, received a Nobel Prize for the suturing of blood vessels about 100 years ago. More than 5 million vascular anastomoses are performed annually in the world and more than 70% often are on the CABG market [9].

The requirements of anastomotic devices include reproducibility, ease of use, and a short anastomotic time (less than 1 min). The anastomotic device ideally would work with either vein or artery and so the proximal or distal order of anastomoses should be interchangeable. The device should facilitate a wide range of surgical access points and should have patency comparable to that of hand-sewn techniques [9].

There are manual and automatic anastomotic devices. The manual proximal anastomotic devices Heartstring *Aortic Occluder*™ from Guidant (that acts as an umbrella inside an aortotomy) and the Enclose™ device from Novare Medical (require a separate insertion through the aorta) create a dry area for conventional suturing in aortotomies.

The Symmetry™ Bypass System Aortic Connector is the first in a line of sutureless anastomoses devices for CABG developed by St Jude Medical, Inc., Cardiac Surgery Division—Anastomotic Technology Group (ATG), formerly Vascular Science, Inc. (VSI). There have been more than 50,000 implants performed.

CardioVations™ has released the *Corlink*™ proximal device in Europe. This is a Nitinol-based stent device. The major difference in comparison with Symmetry is that the Corlink device sits outside of the vein graft wall and the Symmetry device lies inside the vein graft wall.

The *Passport*™ automatic proximal device consists of an integrated system that performs the aortotomy, delivers the graft to the aorta, and deploys a stainless-steel connector end-to-side the graft using a delivery device. The stainless-steel stent (more rigid than Nitinol) creates a widely patented anastomosis.

Another proximal anastomotic device is the *Magnaport* from Ventrica. This is also a one-step anastomotic device using rare earth magnets.

Coalescent Surgical™ has developed an automatic proximal anastomotic device, called the *Spyder*® based on their proprietary Nitinol (nickel–titanium) clip technology.

The first distal device to market (launched in 2000) was the manual *Coalescent U-CLIP*™. This is a self-closing, penetrating device with bailout. The U-CLIP device is designed to provide an alternative to conventional suture and surgical clips in a variety of applications including anastomosis creation and tissue approximation. The device consists of a self-closing surgical clip attached to a conventional surgical needle by a flexible member. U-CLIP device placement is easy and requires only standard surgical instrumentation. The self-closing clip eliminates the requirement for knot-tying and suture management. A fresh, sharp needle is provided with each clip. The clip is easily removed. The U-CLIP anastomotic device technology consistently facilitates the interrupted technique in both on-pump (or surgery performed with a cardiopulmonary bypass machine) and off-pump (also known as beating-heart, CABG procedures). Independent core laboratory analysis demonstrated that the left internal mammary artery to the left anterior descending coronary artery (LIMA to LADA) anastomoses created with the U-CLIP anastomotic device were 100% perfectly patented at 6 months [9].

The Spyder device provides fast, automated proximal anastomotic connection by simultaneous delivery of six U-CLIP devices without the use of a side-biting clamp or second manipulation of the aorta. The *JoMed Solem* connector consists of a stented "T"-shaped PTFE graft connected to the internal mammary artery. The *St Jude* distal connector consists of a stent that is deployed with a balloon using a side-to-side technique to create a distal coronary anastomosis. The *Converge Medical* device consists of outer and inner Nitinol couplers that are placed on the vein graft. This device allows for an angled anastomosis and creates elliptical interface. Magnetic Vascular Positioner (MVP), developed by Ventrica (received CE Mark approval in February 2002), uses magnetic attraction to form an instantaneous self-aligning, self-sealing connection between two blood vessels. The elliptical magnets are placed inside the conduit and native vessel. The MVP device connects the "bypass graft" to the coronary artery in seconds, and is designed to be used in the distal, or smallest, portion of the coronary arteries.

Anastomotic devices in OPCAB may play their most important role in the proximal anastomosis. The major meta-analyses reveal the significant benefits of performing OPCAB (off-pump coronary artery bypass) over CCABG (conventional coronary artery bypass) for certain patient populations requiring myocardial revascularization procedures. The technology has potential benefits as a replacement for sutures due to shorter procedure times, uniform and repeatable connections, and the potential to allow for significantly smaller incisions. This would allow proximal anastomoses to be performed with minimal aortic manipulation, which may result in a lower rate of intra- and postoperative embolism. An automated distal device could facilitate lateral wall grafting in OPCAB. In total endoscopic coronary artery bypass (TECAB), a distal automatic device could be critical in evolving the endoscopic procedure. Currently, the Ventrica device is being modified for deployment in a robotic environment. Finally, in multivessel TECAB procedures, distal anastomotic devices are predicted to make a major contribution. Most minimally invasive procedures in the future will be facilitated by an automated anastomotic device. The automated anastomotic device will level the playing field and allow for more surgeons to perform more perfect anastomoses. Wolf concluded that with continued evolution of these devices, it is easy to anticipate that in the near future the majority of anastomoses may be performed with a manual or automatic device as opposed to the current conventional suture technique [9]. The leaders of clinical trials of these new methods are Randall K. Wolf and Volkmar Falk, MD.

Since 1997, Medtronic has been a pioneer in minimally invasive, beating-heart surgery with the introduction of the Octopus tissue stabilizer system and its family of products, and most recently with the release of the Starfish2 heart positioner.

In traditional open-heart surgery, the heart is stopped and an artificial pump is used to maintain blood circulation. This is highly traumatic as the blood flow is rerouted through a machine. Many patients with coronary heart disease undergo open-heart operations, especially bypass surgery. These are traditionally performed with a heart–lung machine. The machine serves as a substitute for the patient's own beating heart and lungs, allowing the organs to function while surgeons operate on a "still" heart.

Endoscopic surgery in a major cavity in the body requires space for manipulation and local cardiac wall immobilization for coronary artery grafting on the working heart. One of the revolutionary instrument used in beating-heart surgery is Octopus. The name comes from its suction device of two arms and a series of "suckers," which allow to position the heart in various places with the chest open.

8.6.2 The Surgical Robots

About 4 million MISs are performed in the world every year. The aim is to limit the operative field and spare surrounding tissue, which would be damaged if a traditional surgical technique was used. The number of endoscopic procedures, less invasive than traditional surgery, performed through natural orifices in the patient's body, or through special openings called ports, is on the rise.

The success of the procedures largely depends on the instruments used. Unfortunately, typical endoscopic (laparoscopic) instruments reduce precision and make the surgery more difficult because they add to hand tremor and almost completely eliminate the natural sense of touch. Additionally, the surgeon does not have a direct view of the operative field—a camera inserted into the body through a third opening transmitting the image to a display. So the surgeon's task is not easy. An ideal noninvasive surgery can be compared to renovating a house through a keyhole without disturbing the household members. Across the world, physicians and engineers are working together toward developing increasingly effective instruments to enable surgery using the latest technology. But how can one enhance instrument precision and maneuverability, which are so important in the case of surgery on the beating heart, for instance? Surgical robots provide such capabilities.

Surgical robots improving precision and facilitating minimally invasive access to the area of the operation make up a great potential instrument for the surgery. Currently, these are mainly telemanipulators, where on the "master" side is the surgeon giving the instructions (movements, tasks), on the "slave" side is the end-effector as a surgery tool tip executing tasks in the definite working space, and in the middle of these "actors" is a control system, which reads, processes the input data, enriches them, and computes the output commands.

Currently, two types of medical robotic systems are used in the surgery:

Robots replacing the assistant during the operation: By using systems such as AESOP (Computer Motion – production stopped at present) or EndoAssist (Armstrong Healthcare Ltd, High Wycombe, UK), the surgeon can unaidedly control the position of endoscopic camera, serving as their "eyes" in the closed area of the operation field.

Surgical robots: Robots invented for less minimally invasive cardiac surgery are computer-controlled devices, located between surgeon's hands and the tip of a surgical instrument (Figure 8.10). Currently used cardiac surgery robots fulfill the role of telemanipulators, the main task of which is to detect and scale up or down the surgeon's hand movements and precisely translate them to the movements of robot's arm equipped with tools. A cardio-robot was invented in the United States in the 1990s. Two companies, currently merged, Computer Motion (Computer Motion) and Intuitive Surgical (Intuitive Surgical, Mountain View, CA, USA),

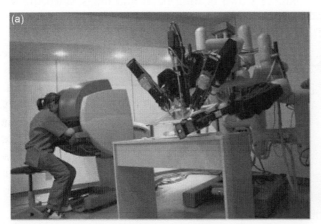 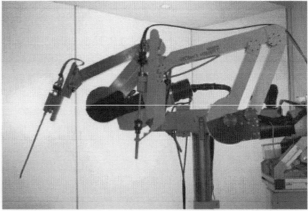

Figure 8.10 (a) Robot daVinci (*left*) and Robin Heart cardiosurgery robot (*right*). (b) Comparison of different tools: Robin Heart 0,1 and laparoscopic tools; test of Robin Expert advisory system (presented by the author); and the test using animal tissue. (c) Evaluation of Robin Heart robot is carried out using the following measurements: vibration (new accelerometer sensors) [A]; linear movement (using digital micrometer) [B]; system of external trajectory recording (several digital cameras, markers, and image analysis methods) [C]; and physical [D] and computer surgery simulation (*bottom:* general range of robot mobility and workspace equipped with [E] standard laparoscopic tool and [F] Robin Heart I instrument).

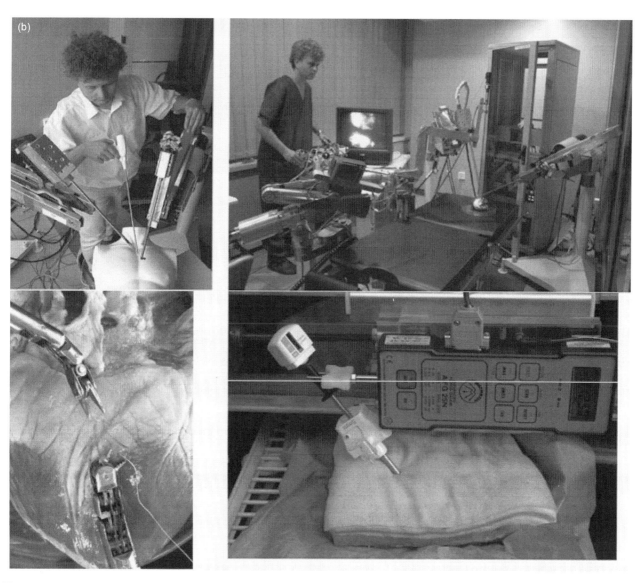

Figure 8.10 (*Continued*)

were set up based on Star Wars project technologies developed by NASA and Pentagon. In Europe, Poland, the Robin Heart family robots are developed (Figure 8.10). The Foundation of Cardiac Surgery Development (FCSD) in Zabrze in 2000 started issuing the grant for realizing the prototype of a robot useful for cardiac surgery. The multidisciplinary team including specialists in medicine and techniques prepared until now four robot prototypes named Robin Heart [10].

An application of teleoperation allows to remove the tremor and to introduce the scaling of hand movement range via interface of manipulator on exact movements of tool inside the body, thus improving the ergonomics and precision. Supervision is held using visual observation via voice- or manually controlled endocamera (2D or 3D). American cardiosurgical robots have been produced by two, currently merged, companies, Computer Motion and Intuitive Surgical, which was firstly clinically used in Europe.

The first mechanical assistant of surgeon—voice-controlled endoscope positioner AESOP 1000 (automated endoscopic system for optimal positioning)—was introduced by firm CM in 1994. In January–May 1998, a French team in Paris and a German group from Leipzig performed using da Vinci (Figure 8.10a) (IS) telemanipulator the first endoscopic operation of single coronary bypass and

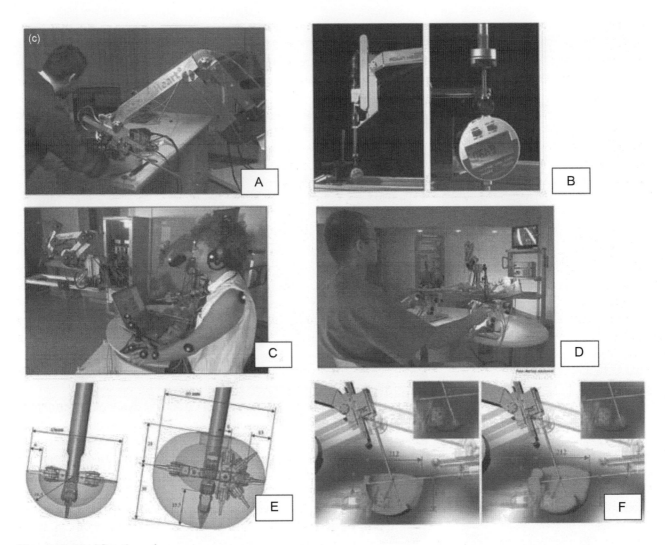

Figure 8.10 (*Continued*)

mitral valvuloplasty. About 1000 surgical and endocamera robots were installed in clinics; to date, more than 130,000 minimally invasive procedures, across a wide range of surgical applications such as general surgery, gynecology, spinal, urology, and cardiothoracic surgery, have been performed in several counters (also in Poland, Katowice) [11].

In 1999, the Zeus surgical system made history in the world's first robot-assisted beating-heart bypass surgery, by Douglas Boyd, MD. In 2001, the first transatlantic telesurgical procedure was performed using the Zeus system. The doctors in New York removed a gallbladder of a 68-year-old patient in Strasbourg, France, and the procedure was successful with no complications.

In traditional laparoscopic surgery, the operating surgeon does not have direct visual control of the operative field due to manual camera control by an assistant. Ideally, the surgeon should have full control of operative instruments and the operative field. Camera holders should return camera control to the surgeon and stabilize the visual field during minimally invasive procedures. The active and passive camera holders offer the surgeon an alternative and better tool to control the operating surgeon's direct visual field. One of the first, active teleoperated robots introduced into clinical practice was produced by Computer Motion (US) Company. Currently, more than 1500 of Computer Motion's robotic systems (AESOP, Zeus) are in use worldwide in 900 hospitals by more than 3000 surgeons in 32 countries. The Zeus system consists of three robotic arms mounted onto an operating table. Two arms hold surgical instruments, and the third arm holds and positions the endoscope via voice control. All three arms are connected to a master console where the surgeon telemanipulates the arms. The handles used to control the movement of the surgical instruments are similar to the instruments used in conventional surgery. The surgeon's manual movements are filtered and scaled for the slave instruments to perform precise microsurgery. The Zeus system can be used in combination with an independent 3D visualization system (AESOP). More than 300,000 surgical procedures have been performed with Computer Motion's robotic systems assistance. The AESOP system is both CE marked and FDA approved and has been used in more than 100,000 laparoscopic and endoscopic procedures. The duration of several types of endoscopic surgery was reportedly faster using the AESOP; voice control was considered to be more efficient and faster than either the foot or hand control.

The disadvantages for the AESOP include the constant voice commands, which may be distracting. In addition, the voice control is slower compared to the rapid camera movements achieved by an experienced assistant. The AESOP is intended to facilitate solo-surgeon laparoscopic procedures; however, the surgeon may still need an assistant to control the fourth laparoscopic port. The Intuitive Surgical Inc. (US) da Vinci telemanipulator consists of three or four robotic arms in one set fixed on one common column, placed near the operating table.

In contrast to the AESOP system, da Vinci arm for camera holding is integrated with all robotic arms. Today approximately 400 da Vinci systems have been installed worldwide, and its applications have been described in thousands of scientific publications and presentations. It is CE marked and FDA approved and used in more than 300 hospitals in America and Europe. The da Vinci was used in at least 16,000 procedures in 2004 and sells for about $1.3 million.

In Europe, the Armstrong Healthcare Ltd (UK) produced telemanipulator EndoAssist. A robot system EndoAssist holds a conventional laparoscopic telescope and camera, coordinated by the surgeon's head movements. EndoAssist (CE marked and approved by FDA) has also been used in telesurgical applications with control via a joystick communicating with the robot over a telephone line. About 30 systems installed worldwide now has been used in several thousand clinical procedures.

The future of robotic surgery has significant potential that has been proven in many clinical applications. The procedure completed without the need for an additional assistant is called a "solo surgery." Robotic assistance has enabled a solo surgery approach. The basic principle of manipulator construction is that of a serial architecture of joints and links with a fixed remote center in the corporeal wall. For instance, the da Vinci robot have seven DOFs: three (yaw, pitch, and insertion) have surgical manipulators provide motion coupling to the end-effector, an exchangeable instrument that adds four DOFs (roll, pitch, yaw, and grip) by means of a cable-driven mechanical wrist. The surgeon controls the movements of tools via a human machine. The slave is capable of detecting force feedback (tissue contact, collision of manipulator) greater than 2.2 N. Scaling is useful in the range from 1:1 to 10:1, in combination with tremor filtering greater than 6 Hz [12].

The computer and laboratory tests are required to design a new, smart surgery robot and expanding its applications to the field of medicine. The 3D computer simulation and physical modeling will continue to be supported on Polish grants.

The use of conventional endoscopic instruments allows a limited range of motion by the trocars through which the instruments are introduced and by reduction to only four DOFs for tools. Long and rigid instruments are harder to control and amplify tremor.

Six DOFs are required to perform a free motion. For instance, suturing perpendicular to the four-DOF tool's shape becomes impossible. The study shows that using four-DOF robot (Zeus system, Computer Motion) the 1.5 mm tube anastomosis was performed in 46 min compared to only 12 min performed by six-DOF robots (da Vinci). Endoscopic tissue manipulation and suturing using four-DOF instrumentation requires skill and training.

Cardiac surgery is carried out on soft tissues. Results obtained from surgical action analysis allowed to determine the maximum values of forces needed for typical procedures performed in heart area, using different types of tools. This can be the basis for cardiac surgery robot design assumption, in the field connected with controlling of robot tool movements. The penetration of soft tissue involves actions such as cutting, slicing, inserting a needle, and knotting. The difficulty with soft tissue is that it deforms and changes shape. The map of force resistance during pricking for left and right heart chamber was obtained (i.e., the basic mechanical properties of typical surgical actions; from the FCSD). For example, the maximal force value for surgical needle Prolene 3/0 during pricking through papillary muscle reached the 150 G, the measured load value equaled 200 G (2 cm depth) during scalpel cutting procedure for the left ventricle (the mitral valve ring), and up to 200 G with 0.1 mm/s test speed for sewing tests—the knot-tying using Prolene needle.

One of the limitations of current surgical robots used in surgery is the lack of haptic feedback. Although current surgical robots improve surgeon dexterity, decrease tremor, and improve visualization, they lack the necessary fidelity to help a surgeon characterize tissue properties for improving diagnostic capabilities. Many research groups focus on the development of tools and software that will allow haptic feedback to be integrated in a robot-assisted surgical procedure.

The surgeon needs assistants of next robot arm during operation mainly for stabilization of the heart (beating-heart bypass grafting) or another tissue. Several trials using two da Vinci consoles delivered good results. In response, the IS prepared the da Vinci S model with four arms.

The devices providing an "inside equipment store" for the surgeon are also needed. A self-sufficient Cargo Module was developed as a transportation and depot device by Dresden group. With the Assist Module, the surgical equipment, tissue, and vessels can be positioned on a desired place in the operating field. This module provides the surgeon an "assistant" inside the closed chest.

Potential applications of robotics in cardiac surgery includes aortic valve replacement (standard or percutaneous technology); tricuspid valve repair; descending thoracic aortic surgery; transmyocardial laser revascularization; ventricular septal defect, patent ductus arteriosus, coarctation; and intramyocardial delivery platform for biological agents such as stem cells, molecular therapeutics, genetic vectors, and AORobAS (Artificial Organs Robotically Assisted Surgery).

In the Institute of Heart Prostheses, FCSD, surgeries related to artificial organ (AO) implantation are performed. Our future plans, AORobAS, include carrying out a robotically assisted less invasive procedures to implant pumps and valves.

The da Vinci system is therefore the only surgical telemanipulator that is currently clinically being used. Due to the actual range of the system acceptance, the number of endoscopic cardiac procedures performed in 2005 worldwide (reported in a company-based registry) was 2984 and it increased steadily. This includes TECAB procedures or small access single- or multivessel coronary artery bypass procedures with endoscopic uni- or bilateral ITA harvest (1784 procedures). The number of MVR increased to about 450 cases in 2004, to more than 600 in 2005, to 850 in the first 10 months of 2006 (reported in a company-based registry) [13].

The number of procedures performed may increase due to development of and improvement in facilitating anastomotic devices (MVP magnetic coupling device) and augmented reality with preoperative planning and intraoperative navigation. Based on the preoperation cardiac surgery simulation results, the optimization of cardiac surgery procedures can be achieved.

The *effectiveness* and *expansion* of robot's application fields requires searching the most effective cardiac robots in the wide application range, building the strategy of its usage, simulating the operation results, and creating the knowledge base supporting the robot's arm navigation and cardiac surgeon decision making, and studying image processing methods for optimal robot's arm navigation [13].

8.6.3 Blood Pumps—MIS Application Study

The use of the mechanical circulatory support systems (TAHs and VADs) has evolved significantly over the last 30 years, with more than 10,000 patients being supported by these devices (TAH 2%). The devices have evolved from extracor-poreal devices (such as Jarvik 7, Thoratec, Abiomed systems), driven by large pneumatic consoles, to electrically driven partially implantable devices with portable controllers carried by the patient (such as Novacor, HeartMate).

The future prospects of the mechanical circulatory support clearly lie in three major areas:

1. active left ventricular pump system, which supports and stabilizes the heart in extremely critical situations (e.g., acute heart attack), and can be implanted for a period of up to 5 days (e.g., Impella® Acute)

2. devices as a bridge to recovery (e.g., pulsatile pumps: Novacor, HeartMate; rotary pumps: MicroMed, Jarvik-Heart, Nimbus-HeartMate II)

3. devices as an alternative to the cardiac transplantation and conventional therapy (e.g., destination therapy: LionHeart, AbioCor TAH)

8.6.3.1 Minimally Invasive VAD Implantation

Dr J. Donald Hill of the California Pacific Medical Center (San Francisco, CA, USA) has successfully performed the less invasive Thoratec LVAD surgery on several patients.

The patient is placed on the cardiopulmonary bypass using the right or left femoral artery or vein. The VAD cannulation system is placed in the left ventricular apex (VAD inflow) and the ascending aorta (VAD outflow), using two separate incisions. The procedure offers the following advantages: no sternotomy, easier reoperation, less blood use, reduced risk of sensitization, and it is psychologically more acceptable (according to Dr Hill, the Thoratec Laboratories).

General steps in VAD implantation are as follows: anesthesia is administered to the patient; preparing the operating area—cardiopulmonary bypass (if required) and lung deflation; choosing the exit site for LVAD—depending on the need of LVAD alone or of BiVAD, one or two outflow and inflow grafts will be necessary; aortic and pulmonary artery anastomoses performed; left and right ventricular apical or atrial cannulation performed; connecting the VAD to the cannulas, deaerating the VAD; gradually discontinue cardiopulmonary bypass and allow the VAD to run in "fill-to-empty" mode; completing surgery.

Our plans include carrying out robotically assisted less invasive procedures to implant VADs (Figure 8.11), TAHs, valves, and vessel prostheses. The rapid evolution of MIS techniques for heart prostheses will have implications for designing and construction of heart prostheses. Our team works on the designing of heart pumps and valves particularly for robot and MIS applications and special tools of robot are being constructed. I am sure that

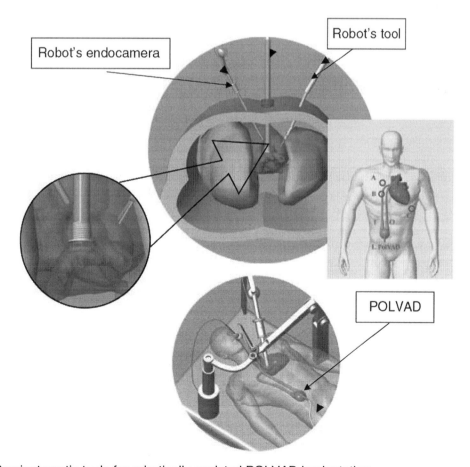

Figure 8.11 Semiautomatic tools for robotically assisted POLVAD implantation.

this is the future of this domain of biomedical engineering.

8.6.3.2 The AORobAS Idea

Currently used VADs, pumps, valves, and pacemakers require to be replaced and repaired throughout the patient's life. A better solution seems to be application of MIS at once by designing AOs with construction ready to easy assembly and disassembly as well as to ensure an access to replace the used parts. For external pumps, an MIS technique of cannula implantation should be performed.

In 2000, a new type of blood pump was introduced into clinical practice. In robot-assisted surgery, the use of the small, axial heart assist pump is very promising. The Jarvik 2000 VAD and the DeBakey VAD, which have been approved for evaluation as a bridge to transplantation, are valveless devices that are electrically powered miniature axial flow pumps. These fit directly into the left ventricle, which may eliminate problems with clotting. The outflow graft connects to the descending aorta. The DeBakey VAD is 30 mm × 76 mm, weighs 93 g, and is approximately 1/10th the size of pulsatile products on the market. The development of this idea causes changes in requirements for blood pump. It should be folding device, with dimension not exceeding the port hole incision diameter. It means that this part must be a cylinder with about 1 cm diameter and the technology for quick mounting of this part on the whole pump inside the chest must be developed. Robots also require special constructions of semiautomatic tools. The surgical procedure requires faster and efficient connection to pulmonary bypass apparatus, because the surgery is performed on a stopped heart. Of course, there are many problems to solve, but this type of surgery has wide perspectives. In our laboratory, the design and simulation study has been conducted. I work on the realization of the following procedure:

- *Stages of AO implantation and assembly:* Parts of the AO, put into capsule through mechanically or pneumatically controlled channel, run into pumped balloon, where they are assembled. The balloon has valves that allows for insertion of additional tools into the workplace. The balloon is supported mechanically or by compressed CO_2. In the next stage, the balloon is removed and the AO is implanted. Pumps that fulfill the role of a vessel bypass seem to be most suited to this procedure because their implantation does not require stopping (and hence external circulation) of the heart.

- *Stages of repairing of replacing of the AO:* Laparoscopic tool inserts a tight balloon around the AO, which is removed after repairing. The parts for replace are inserted in special capsules.

Great progress in MIS technique will influence the design and construction of implantable AOs. The goal of this work expresses the evolution of telemanipulator and AOs dedicated to the MIS. The system is named AORobAS (Figure 8.12). The future plans regarding development of Polish robot Robin Heart include carrying out of a robotically assisted MIS to implant AOs, VADs, TAHs, valves, and vessel prostheses. Currently used blood pumps, valves, and pacemakers require to be replaced and repaired throughout the patient's life. This is only a temporary solution. Probably, in the near future, the progress in the subject of biocompatible, long-term durable materials and mechanical construction will not solve this problems. The best for patient will be realization of conception minimally invasive service of AO. Robots may be ideal for this task. The solution seems to be application of robotically assisted MIS at once by designing AOs with

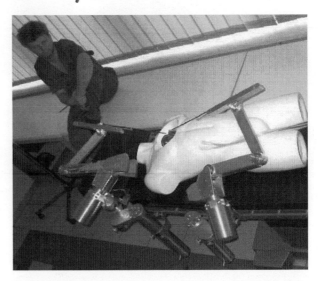

Figure 8.12 Artificial Organs Robotically Assisted Surgery (AORobAS) system.

construction ready to easy assembly and disassembly and to ensure an access to replace used parts. The development of this idea causes changes in requirements for blood pump. It should be folding device, with dimension not exceeding the port hole incision diameter. It means that this part must be a cylinder about 1 cm diameter and the technology for quick mounting of this part on the whole pump inside the chest must be developed. Robots also require special constructions of semiautomatic tools.

8.6.3.3 The Blood Pump Support in the Palliative (Pediatric) Surgery Study

The aim of the palliative procedure is to increase pulmonary blood flow in children with a congenital heart defect. As a result of a shunt operation [Blalock−Taussig (B−T) shunt or Glenn procedure], the oxygen level in the child's blood is improved. The main problem of such surgery is the small shunt effectiveness and lack of possibility of flow regulation. Our idea is to apply advanced computer simulation methods to give the information to the cardiac surgeon—which procedure will be optimal before realization of the operation. A small axial blood pump can be introduced into B−T shunt or Glenn in order to control the blood flow and prevent the growth of graft stenosis. Based on the results obtained using physical and computer 3D simulation based on finite element method (FEM) (Figure 8.13), it can be concluded that the module graft with axial pump makes possible the exact regulation of blood flow and blood pressures in the pulmonary artery. Its use allowed to decrease the afterload of left heart ventricle. Palliative procedures are only a temporary solution. As a child grows, the graft does not grow, and the size of graft (flow through graft) may be not sufficient. The use of axial pump across regulation blood flow allows to extend the time between necessary operations.

8.7 The Minimally Invasive Valve Implantation

Percutaneous (pulmonary and aortic) valve replacement has recently opened new perspectives on transcatheter replacement of cardiac valves. Typically, a bioprosthetic valve is dissected and sutured into an autoexpandable Nitinol stent (which has an initial aortic diameter, for instance, 25 mm) or mounted within a balloon-expandable stent. It has been used in patients who are at high risk for valve replacement surgery. Percutaneous valve repair is also being developed for mitral regurgitation. Direct leaflet repair and percutaneous annuloplasty are being employed in clinical trials. All the percutaneous approaches are based on existing surgical techniques and offer less invasive alternatives. This marked the beginning of the era of percutaneous valve therapy, and ongoing trials will define the clinical role for these new therapeutic modalities. Percutaneous catheter-based systems for the treatment of valvular heart disease have been designed and studied in animal models for several

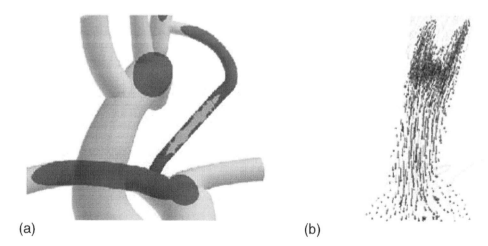

Figure 8.13 Pulmonary artery axial blood pump used to control blood flow in Blalock−Taussig (B−T): (a) the axial pump in B−T graft and (b) velocity vectors on inlet from pump in B−T graft. The simulations have been performed by Z. Małota.

years. Bonhoeffer et al. were the first to perform percutaneous implantations of artificial valves, using a bovine jugular vein valve mounted within a stent, in children with right ventricle to pulmonary prosthetic conduits. The first human case report of percutaneous transcatheter implantation of an aortic valve prosthesis for calcific aortic stenosis appeared in 2002 [14].

A percutaneously implanted heart valve (PHV) composed of three bovine pericardial leaflets mounted within a balloon-expandable stent was developed (Percutaneous Valve Technologies, Inc.). Using an antegrade transseptal approach, the PHV was successfully implanted within the diseased native aortic valve, with accurate and stable PHV positioning, without impairing the coronary artery blood flow or the mitral valve function, and a with no mild paravalvular aortic regurgitation. Immediately and at 48 h after implantation, valve functioning was excellent, resulting in a marked hemodynamic improvement. Nonsurgical implantation of a prosthetic heart valve can be successfully achieved with immediate and midterm hemodynamic and clinical improvement.

8.8 Support Technology for Surgery Planning

Modern medical imaging techniques such as CT, NMR, and ultrasonic imaging enable the surgeon to have a very precise representation of internal anatomy as preoperative scans.

For surgery robots (telemanipulators), the following distinct phases can be realized:

- *Preoperative planning:* The optimal strategy is defined using the 3D computer model.
- *Robot-assisted intervention:* A calibration routine brings robot, patient, and image system to a common frame of reference, for example, using anatomical (or artificial) landmarks.
- *Feedback and replanning:* The robot starts to operate under the supervision of surgeon. Sensor information ensures that the anatomy is as expected and stored by a model in computer. If deviations occur, the surgeon asks for a revised strategy, or for permission to continue.

Computer flow simulation method is important for diagnosing the heart disease development, for optimizing the surgery for a particular patient, and for long-term functioning of graft prognosis. During simulation, the input data (biochemical data, diagnostic data, geometrical data, biophysical data) are transformed into test output data (the hemodynamic pressure and flows or another characterization of biological object modified by surgery).

Remote-control manipulators are proposed for cardiac surgery using a computer-based advisory system. Information in a prepared database (an online expert system) may be of help to a surgeon in decision making. The first step is to simulate the robot-assisted surgery using both computer and physical models of a particular operation type. Based on the preoperation cardiac surgery simulation results, the optimization of the procedures can be achieved.

The main issues of computer simulation support to surgery robots are as follows:

1. *The operation planning:* Based on diagnostic data (images, pressure and flow signals, etc.), computer and physical models can be created. In vitro simulations performed on them may be used to find the optimal way of operation (the joint point localization, the graft selection). A prepared report can be presented to the surgeon as a hint for robot choreography planning. This stage should also include input port localization on patient skin, the type of tools, and the way of removing and preparing the graft branch.

2. *Advisory and control system:* During the operation, diagnostic images or simulation results from various sources can be called by surgeon and superimposed on the real operating image.

The introduction of robots to cardiac surgery created the possibility of direct and practical use of simulation results of surgical procedures in the robot information system.

Surgical planning and augmented reality are likely to enhance robotic surgery in the future. The interesting case of applying preoperatively in robotically assisted cardiac surgery planning, intraoperative registration, and augmented reality was performed by Falk et al. [15]. The regions of interest (i.e., the heart, ribs, coronaries, ITA) were segmented semiautomatically to create a virtual model of the animal. In this model, the target regions of the total endoscopic bypass procedure along with the ITA and anastomotic area were defined. Algorithms for assessing visibility, dexterity, and *collision avoidance* were developed after defining nonadmissible areas using the virtual model of the manipulator. Intraoperatively, registration of the animal and the telemanipulator was performed using encoder data of the telemanipulator by pointing to the fiducial points. After pericardiotomy, the reconstructed coronary tree was projected onto the videoscopic image using a semiautomatic alignment procedure. In dogs, the total endoscopic bypass procedure was successful on the beating heart.

For medical applications, matching procedures between diagnostic images and off-line intervention planning and real execution are very important. Many problems still remain for soft tissue surgery where deformations may occur. The navigation and guidance of the instruments highly depends on the surgeon's skill who has to combine their intraoperative views with the information extracted from the preoperative images.

Several scientific groups work on *computer method for preparing quasi-stationary view*. The da Vinci robot uses a two-camera endoscope that feeds images to the surgeon's viewer. Images from the left and right cameras are fed to each of the surgeon's eyes separately, providing a 3D view of the tissue being operated on. The Mylonas system exploits this principle by fitting an infrared eye tracker to the viewer. This ensures that each eye detects precisely where the surgeon is looking, and then calculates the distance to the point their gaze is fixed upon using triangulation. The software first constructs a 3D model of the heart by tracking the surgeon's eyes as they move over the organ. Then it creates a real-time moving image by recording the changes in the surgeon's focal point as the heart beats. The endoscope is calibrated to move forward and backward in time with this image, thus making the heart to appear stationary to the surgeon viewing it through the two cameras. The surgical instruments are also calibrated to move in synchrony with the beating heart, removing the need to constantly move them back and forward, and allowing the surgeon to concentrate on performing the operation. The software has so far been tested only on an artificial silicone heart using a robotic arm.

According to surgeons and device executives, surgeon training is the key to the future success of the robotics industry. Because modern surgery is very challenging, the surgeon training will become comparable to fighter pilot training while the robotic systems are having a huge impact on surgical education, and, without doubt, will be integrated into surgeons' future education process. Currently for clinical use of the da Vinci surgical system, the FDA requires a 2-day training course to understand the setup, maintenance, and applications of the surgical system, in addition to animated laboratory training. The device manufacturers have training programs in place to advance the skill sets of both new and experienced surgeons.

Both the *virtual* (Figure 8.14) and the *real* station are used for MIS education. As examples, commercial products include LapTrainer z SimuVision (Simulab Inc., Seattle, WA, USA; www.simulab.com), ProMIS (Haptica Inc., Boston, MA, USA; www.haptica.com), Laparoscopic Surgical Workstation and Virtual Laparoscopic Interface (Immersion Inc., Gaithersburg, MD, USA; www.immersion.com), Phantom devices (SensAble Technologies Inc., Woburn, MA, USA; www.sensable.com), Xitact LS500 Laparoscopy Simulator (Xitact S.A., Lausanne, Switzerland; www.entice.com), Lapmentor (Simbionix Inc., Cleveland, OH, USA; www.simbionix.com); Surgical Education Platform (SEP) (SimSurgery, Oslo, Norway; www.simsurgery.no; www.meti.com), LapSim (Surgical Science Ltd, Gothenburg, Sweden; www.surgical-science.com), Procedus MIST (Mentice AB, Gothenburg, Sweden; www.mentice.com), EndoTower (Verefi Technologies Inc., Elizabethtown, PA, USA; www.verefi.com), Reachi Laparoscopic Trainer (Reachin Technologies AB, Stockholm, Sweden; www.reachin.se), Vest System (Virtual Endoscopic Surgical Trainer; Select-IT VEST Systems AG, Bremen, Germany; www.select-it.de), and Simendo (Simulator for endoscopy; DeltaTech, Delft, Netherlands; www.simendo.nl).

8.9 Conclusions

Notable achievements in cardiovascular research and devices that are currently under investigation and expected in the near future are listed below:

1. New pediatric devices, such as the axial-flow pumps and small-diameter valve prostheses, have been introduced, and some are under

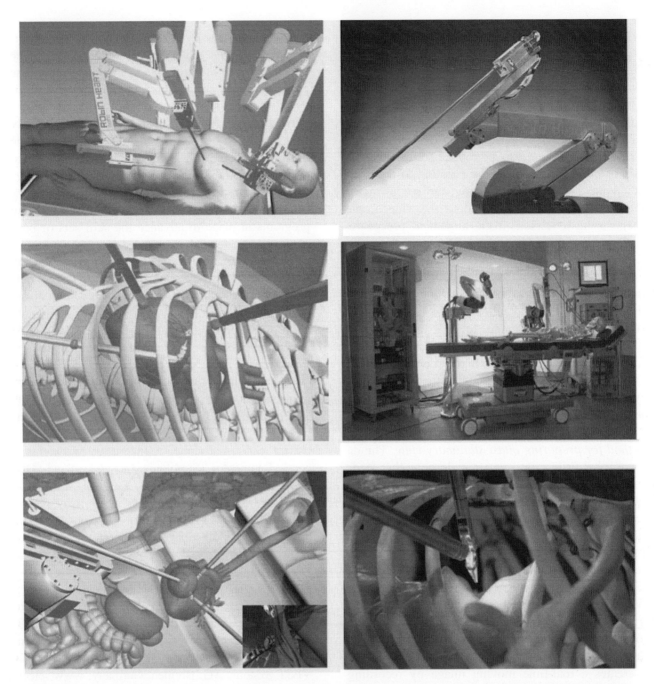

Figure 8.14 The virtual and the real condition for testing the Robin Heart robot. Using avirtual reality (VR) technology, an interactive model of surgery room equipped with a Robin Heart system was created using EON Professional software. This computer modeling method allows for an advanced procedure training and will be used as a low-cost training station for surgeons in the future. The model allows for a better understanding process of less invasive surgery treatment and a robot behavior. This type of modeling and a computer-aided design (CAD) technique use an accurate CAD robot model in a VR software together with a precise reflection of workspace geometry. This approach gives a surgeon easy and intuitive way to understand the technical details and use it to optimize and plan medical process. The next step in FCSD research work will be establishing the surgery workshops based on the newest technology, and some new projects using affordable semiautomatic robotic tools. Presented model of operating room in VR environment has been successfully used during Surgery Workshop in FCSD (May 2006). This system is intuitive for a user and gives them a very realistic 3D visualization.

construction. As the devices become more and more reliable, mechanical circulatory support will play an increasingly important role, not only for rescue therapy but also for safe treatment of the most complex congenital heart diseases, not only with the aim of bridging to cardiac recovery or transplantation but, eventually, as a permanent solution.

2. The effective miniature blood pumps have been commonly used in minimally invasive cardiology. Transported to the destination place through the arteries, the smart pump mainly for short-term heart support can play an important role in an emergency.

3. New types of devices create possibilities of pump and blood oxygenation introduction into clinical practice. The idea is not new, but thanks to new materials (durable, semiconductive silicon membranes) that are being rapidly developed.

4. New "biomechanical" valves and vessels completely synthetic/artificial, but flexible and durable, will be introduced. The development of small-caliber vascular grafts is very important for bypass and graft surgery.

5. A significant improvement in technical support for preplanning and control surgical interventions, including telemedicine technology, will be observed.

6. Bioartificial myocardial grafts will be introduced in which perfusion by a macroscopic core vessel will be applicable.

7. Improved cell-culture techniques may render human aortic myofibroblasts a native tissue-like structure.

8. Tissue-engineered bioprosthethic valves will be commonly used in clinics.

As the field of surgery robots controlled by surgeons expands, the economical cost is expected to reduce, which will allow surgeons to more commonly use teleoperation in situations that warrants professional staff assistance such as wars, epidemics, and space trips. The situation of "no contact" between the medical personnel and the patient will reduce the risk of loss of health because of the infection(s) from the side of the operating staff.

It is most probable that contemporary telemanipulators will be replaced by adaptive robots in the near future. Currently, the trials of shifting from passive to active systems can be seen. To be clear, let's define the basic concepts: Teleoperators are remotely controlled by operator robot transferring on distance motoric and sensoric functions, whereas adaptive robots have more advanced control system with sensoric and learning abilities. However, creating the next-generation "intelligent" robots is a true challenge. These robots must be able to work unaidedly in various environments, gathering information from their senses. Optimization of their behavior and the effectiveness of given task realization will depend on "self-learning control algorithm," which will more resemble systems based on "instincts" in relation to living creatures and contact with surroundings by means of "senses," zoom, touch sensors (inductive, supersonic, optical, pneumatic, and microwave). I am convinced that they will not be similar to contemporary cardiosurgical robots, but they will be able to replace them considerably. Probably, they will be microrobots that are able to reach, e.g., a given human internal diseased organ (e.g., the heart).

8.10 Acknowledgments

This chapter has been illustrated with the experimental data obtained in the Institute of Heart Prostheses, FCSD, Zabrze. The research was supported by the Polish State Committee for Scientific Research and Foundation. The author thanks his numerous collaborators, including R. Kustosz, M. Koźlak, P. Kostka, Z. Małota, L. Podsędkowski, Z. Religa, and M. Jakubowski (special thanks for excellent photography), who prepared the artwork of this chapter.

References

[1] Morris D, Couves C. Experiences with a sac-type artificial heart. Can Med Assoc J 1971;105:483–7.

[2] Copeland JG, Smith RG, Arabia FA, et al. For the cardiowest total artifical heart investigators. Cardiac replacement with a total artificial heart as a bridge to transplantation. N Engl J Med 2004;351:859–67.

[3] Hetzer R, Stiller B. Technology insight: use of ventricular assist devices in children. Nat Clin Pract Cardiovasc Med 2006;3:377–86.

[4] Short-term circulatory support with left ventricular assist devices as a bridge to cardiac transplantation or recovery. National Institute for Health and Clinical Excellence June 2006; ISBN 1-84629-233-6. Available from: <www.nice.org.uk/ip059overview>.

[5] Rose E, Gelijns A, Moskowitz A, et al. from the randomized evaluation of mechanical assistance for the treatment of congestive heart failure (REMATCH) study group. Long-term use of a left ventricular assist device for end-stage heart failure. N Engl J Med 2001;345(20):1435–43.

[6] Jamieson E, Cartier P, Allard M, et al. Primary panel members. Surgical management of valvular heart disease 2004. Can J Cardiol 2004;20(Suppl. E):7E–120E.

[7] Daebritz S, Sachweh J, Hermanns B, et al. Introduction of a flexible polymeric heart valve prosthesis with special design for mitral position. Circulation 2003;108:II-134.

[8] Dankleman J, Grimbergen CA, Stassen HG. Engineering for patient safety. Issues in minimally invasive procedures. London: Lawrence Erlbaum Associates; 2005.

[9] Wolf R. Anastomotic devices for coronary surgery. CTSNet 2005; January(14):. Available from: <www.ctsnet.org/sections/innovation/minimallyinvasive/articles/article-9.html>

[10] Nawrat Z. Perspectives of computer and robot assisted surgery for heart assist pump implantation. Planning for robotically assisted surgery. Darowski M, Ferrari G, editors. Lecture notes of the ICB Seminars. Assessment and mechanical support of heart and lungs. Warsaw; 2001. p. 130–50.

[11] Nawrat Z, Kostka P. The Robin Heart vision, telemanipulator for camera holding preliminary test results. J Autom Mobile Rob Intell Syst 2007;1(1):48–53.

[12] Falk V, McLoughin J, Guthart G, Salisbury JK, Walther T, Mohr FW. Dexterity enhancement in endoscopic surgery by a computer-controlled mechanical wrist. Minim Invasive Ther Allied Tech 1999;8:235–42.

[13] Jacobs S, Falk V, Holzhey D, Mohr FW. Perspectives in endoscopic cardiac surgery. Comp Biol Med 2007;37(10):1374–6 (Epub 20 December 2006; doi: 10.1016/ j.compbiomed.2006.11.007)

[14] Bauer F, Derumeaux G, Anselme F, et al. Percutaneous transcatheter implantation of an aortic valve prosthesis for calcific aortic stenosis: first human case description. Circulation 2002;106:3006–8.

[15] Falk VD, Mourgues F, Adhami L, et al. Cardio navigation: planning, simulation, and augmented reality in robotic assisted endoscopic bypass grafting. Ann Thorac Surg 2005;79:2040–7.

9 Endotracheal Tube and Respiratory Care

Thomas C. Mort and Jeffrey P. Keck Jr.

OUTLINE

9.1 Introduction — 192
9.2 Properties of the Endotracheal Tube — 192
   9.2.1 Anatomy of the Endotracheal Tube — 192
   9.2.2 Development and Properties of the Endotracheal Tube — 194
   9.2.3 Physiologic Effects of Endotracheal Tube Placement — 194
   9.2.4 Complications of Endotracheal Tube Placement — 195
9.3 Endotracheal Tubes and Other Airway Adjuncts — 195
   9.3.1 Choice of Endotracheal Tube Size — 195
      9.3.1.1 Small Tubes and Airway Resistance — 195
      9.3.1.2 Large Tubes and Trauma — 196
   9.3.2 Potentially Beneficial Alternatives to the Standard Endotracheal Tube — 196
      9.3.2.1 Preformed and Reinforced Tubes — 196
      9.3.2.2 Laser Tubes — 197
      9.3.2.3 Subglottic Suctioning Evac Endotracheal Tubes — 198
      9.3.2.4 Double-Lumen Endotracheal Tubes — 199
      9.3.2.5 Supraglottic Airways — 200
9.4 Proper Safeguarding of the Airway — 200
   9.4.1 Airway Evaluation: Predicting the Difficult Airway — 200
   9.4.2 Identifying Proper Position of the Endotracheal Tube — 201
      9.4.2.1 Detection of Esophageal Intubation — 201
      9.4.2.2 Confirmation of Appropriate Depth of Insertion — 203
      9.4.2.3 Cuff Pressure Monitoring — 204
      9.4.2.4 Evaluation of an Audible Cuff Leak — 204
      9.4.2.5 Documentation of Placement — 205
   9.4.3 Stabilization of the Endotracheal Tube — 206
      9.4.3.1 Taping — 206
      9.4.3.2 Commercially Available Devices — 209
      9.4.3.3 Stapling for Facial Burns — 209
   9.4.4 Rapid Response Cart for Airway Emergencies — 209
9.5 Maintenance of the Endotracheal Tube — 210
   9.5.1 Heat and Humidity of Inspired Gas — 210
   9.5.2 Suctioning — 212
   9.5.3 Subglottic Care — 213
   9.5.4 Bronchoscopy — 213
   9.5.5 Biofilm Management — 214
9.6 Respiratory Therapies for the Intubated Patient — 215
   9.6.1 Secretion Clearance and Control Therapies — 215
      9.6.1.1 Mucolytic Agents — 215
      9.6.1.2 Chest Physiotherapy — 215
   9.6.2 Overcoming Work of Breathing Imposed by Endotracheal Tubes, Tracheostomy Tubes, and Ventilator Circuits — 217
      9.6.2.1 Pressure Support — 217
      9.6.2.2 Continuous Positive Airway Pressure — 217
      9.6.2.3 Automatic Tube Compensation — 217
   9.6.3 Pharmacologic Treatments — 218
      9.6.3.1 Inhalation Drug Delivery — 218
      9.6.3.2 Inhaled Bronchodilators — 219
      9.6.3.3 Anticholinergics — 219
      9.6.3.4 Corticosteroids — 220
      9.6.3.5 Inhaled Antibiotics — 220
   9.6.4 Positioning of the Patient — 220
9.7 Conclusions — 221
9.8 Clinical Pearls — 221
References — 222

9.1 Introduction

The earliest recorded use of airway manipulation with an artificial device dates back to early Roman civilization when Asclepiades performed a tracheostomy for laryngeal edema. Today it is clear that the role of the endotracheal tube (ETT) in medicine is as invaluable as that of any other medical device created to date. The establishment of a definitive airway via the ETT in both elective and emergency situations has allowed for the delivery of immediate life-sustaining therapies during resuscitation, the maintenance of oxygenation and ventilation in prolonged illness, and the (temporary) delivery of inhaled anesthesia [1]. This chapter begins with a brief history of the development of the ETT. It describes the various ETTs available along with their indications for use and respective limitations. It reviews basic airway anatomy with regard to ETT placement, proper positioning and stabilization of the ETT, and complications attributed to its use. Finally, it addresses respiratory care of the intubated and mechanically ventilated patient.

9.2 Properties of the Endotracheal Tube

9.2.1 Anatomy of the Endotracheal Tube

Between the time of Asclepiades and the present, ETTs have been constructed of a variety of materials, including reed, brass, and steel. Eventually, in 1917, Magill and Rowbotham manufactured them from rubber for the purpose of administering anesthesia [2]. In 1928, when Guedel and Waters added a protective cuff to prevent aspiration, the modern ETT was born. Rubber, however, had limitations in this application, such as increased stiffness with rising temperature and limited adhesive properties with different polymers, which required the cuffs to be manufactured from the same polymer as the tube [3]. These shortcomings led to the search for alternative materials. In 1967, polyvinyl chloride (PVC) was popularized by Dr. S. A. Leader, and it has since been the material most commonly used. One property that makes PVC attractive is that it provides stiffness to an ETT at room temperature to assist with intubation yet becomes more malleable with the increased temperature in situ. Other properties include the ability to embed radiopaque lines in the material to assist with positioning and recognition on a radiograph. Because it accepts many materials, the addition of an exteriorized inflation line to connect the pilot balloon to the cuff can allow for varied cuff materials. Finally, it simply is much lower in cost than other available materials [3].

The 15-mm adapter allows for universality between ventilating devices such as a bag-mask ventilation system, anesthesia circuit, or ventilator circuit. The adapter fits ETTs as large as 12 mm internal diameter and as small as 3 mm, thereby providing further commonality among multiple ETTs and ventilating devices. Having one standard size also allows for interchange between devices made for tracheostomies or ETTs. The adapter is removable to allow for passage of intraluminal devices (e.g., bronchoscope, suction catheter) or to allow passage of the ETT via a supraglottic airway device such as a laryngeal mask airway (LMA, LMA North America, San Diego, CA). Adapter removal may facilitate the extraction of extensive biofilm accumulation or mucus plugs. Additionally, some clinicians choose to resize (shorten) the ETT [4].

The Murphy eye, so named for Peter Murphy, an English anesthetist, is designed to provide an extra (secondary) portal for ventilation should the most distal lumen become opacified by bodily fluids, foreign bodies, or soft tissue prolapse. The most typical manifestation of this phenomenon occurs when the distal lumen abuts soft tissue of the tracheal tree, thereby occluding distal flow, or when secretion build-up occludes the distal opening. However, both native and foreign materials are also capable of creating such a dilemma, including mucus, blood, and foreign bodies. Management of such an obstruction is discussed later in this chapter.

The cuffs on the early ETTs were, like the tubes themselves, composed of rubber. The rubber ETT cuffs had limitations such as the need for elevated inflation pressures (high pressure, low volume [HPLV]) to fill the cuff and occlude the airway surrounding the ETT. These high inflation pressures result in the transmission of high lateral pressures to the tracheal wall, albeit in a very minimal contact area, to maintain a seal. The trachea is not circular but rather D-shaped. HPLV cuffs inflate in a circular manner, thereby altering the structure of the trachea; the high pressure exerted on the

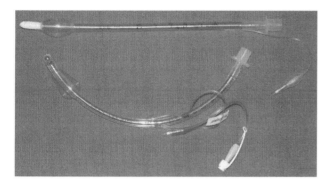

Figure 9.1 Structural comparison of the intubating laryngeal mask airway (ILMA) high-pressure, low-volume (HPLV) cuff (*top*) and a high-volume, low-pressure (HVLP) cuff (*bottom*). *(Courtesy of LMA North America, San Diego, CA.)*

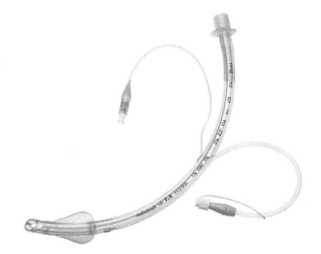

Figure 9.2 Taperguard endotracheal tube cuff. *(Courtesy Covidien, Boulder, CO.)*

tracheal wall impairs capillary pressure and possibly results in greater mucosal ischemia [5]. The most commonly used HPLV cuffs in today's practice are the reusable silicone ETTs found with intubating LMAs (ILMAs) (Figure 9.1). Caution should be exercised when using these ETTs for prolonged periods, given their inherent risk of tracheal mucosal damage. The introduction of PVC-based cuffs reduced this problem because the cuff wall was more supple and thinner, allowing the cuff to accommodate high volume and low pressure (HVLP) and thus providing an adequate seal with lower lateral wall pressures [3,5,6]. The main value of the HVLP cuff is its ability to conform to the irregular borders of the trachea [7–9]. Polyurethane is even thinner and more pliable, with increased tensile strength, allowing for higher volumes, larger contact areas, and minimal mucosal pressures [10]. Foam-based cuffs exist and provide maximal conformation to the tracheal walls, but they do little for the prevention of microaspiration [9].

Remodeling of the cuff has been particularly driven by the desire to improve prevention of ventilator-associated pneumonia (VAP), and the shape of the cuff has also been altered. The Mallinckrodt TaperGuard Evac ETT (Covidien, Boulder, CO) is a new option that has been demonstrated in randomized, controlled trials to reduce microaspiration by as much as 83%, compared with traditional HVLP barrel shaped cuffs (Figure 9.2) [8]. It is postulated that a barrel-shaped tube tends to wrinkle and fold in an attempt to conform to the tracheal wall, allowing small channels for potential microaspiration, whereas the bulbous, conical shape of the TaperGuard ETT may reduce wrinkling and thus decrease the incidence of microaspiration. Continued work in this area may lead to improved tracheal wall sealing capabilities at safe levels of pressure while minimizing potential pathways for the translocation of oronasal and gastric secretions, which is thought to be the prime etiologic pathway for VAP [11].

The pilot balloon of an ETT functions as an indirect volume gauge for the ETT cuff, relative to the amount of air located in the cuff (inflated or deflated). The pilot balloon does not provide information about the absolute volume insufflated or the pressure exerted on the tracheal mucosa. When a pilot balloon fails or is an impediment to an intubation, options are generally limited to a tracheal tube exchange [12–14]. Pilot balloon failures have multiple causes. Shearing along the ETT connection (usually due to contact with dentition), cracked inflation valves (from syringe manipulation or trauma), material aging, and pilot tubing laceration due to biting all cause the ETT cuff to lose air over time [15–18]. Simple techniques have been described to replace a pilot balloon in a variety of clinical situations using equipment readily available in the operating room. Needles or intravenous catheters with stopcocks or claves, epidural clamp connectors, and commercially available repair kits (Figure 9.3) provide reliable substitutions for incompetent pilot balloons when they are connected

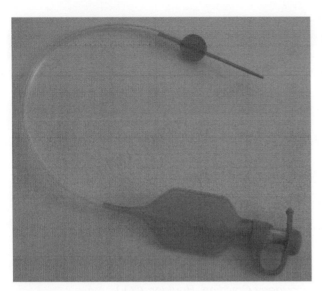

Figure 9.3 Pilot balloon repair device. *(Courtesy Instrumentation Industries, Bethel Park, PA.)*

to the pilot-cuff inflation line [19,20]. The procedure for replacing an incompetent valve is as follows: cut the inflation tube distal to the pilot balloon; insert a needle or intravenous catheter into the cut end (or affix the hub of an epidural catheter to the cut end); and use a stopcock or clave (an item capable of stemming the entrance of air) on the needle or catheter after insufflation, paying careful attention not to overinflate.

9.2.2 Development and Properties of the Endotracheal Tube

The purpose of the ETT has always been the same, and it has always had the same inherent problems. Technology continues to advance the standard ETT for improved function and decreased physiologic insult. Rather than compensate for the resistance produced by a rubber or PVC ETT, a newly designed ETT has been produced of ultrathin polyurethane that is reinforced with wire to resist collapsing and kinking. This wire is unique in that it has an elastic shape memory to prevent deformation. The internal diameter is increased without compromising the rigid shape of the ETT. The result is a tube with a resistance similar to that of the upper airway that is lighter, offers less airflow resistance, and, when compressed, forms an egg shape rather than an oval [21]. Experimentally, this new design has been shown to decrease inspiratory and expiratory resistance by 60% each and the inspiratory, expiratory, and total work of breathing (WOB) by 70%, 47%, and 45%, respectively [22,23].

The use of the ETT continues to expand. No longer is it expected to be simply a conduit for ventilation. As the technology has advanced, the original ETT has steadily been outfitted with a host of successful innovations to improve patient care, whether for convenience or necessity. For example, modifications to the cuff to improve occlusion of the trachea in an effort to prevent microaspiration, coupled with an extra subglottic suctioning port (and other patient care maneuvers), have served to vastly reduce the incidence of VAP [7–9]. Another example is the modification of the surfaces of the ETT to minimize bacterial adhesion and thereby minimize biofilm accumulation [24]. As for bells and whistles, there are ETTs with fiberoptic cameras distally, allowing for ease of placement and the possibility of continued intratracheal surveillance. Another example is the addition of multiple sensors, for so-called bioimpedance cardiography, that are capable of monitoring stroke volume variation, cardiac output, systemic vascular resistance, and arterial pressures (due to the close proximity of the ETT and the aorta) and thereby, at least theoretically, preventing the need for further invasive technologies. Continued study of these modifications may provide justification to adapt these technologies to patient care.

9.2.3 Physiologic Effects of Endotracheal Tube Placement

The placement of an ETT, whether oral, nasal, or translaryngeal, is unnatural. Certain physiologic changes occur that must be addressed, including those created by the ETT itself and those modified by its presence. The properties inherent to the ETT are relatively obvious: it causes a partial obstruction, resulting in a decrease in the normal airway circumference and the possibility of turbulent air flow patterns. Additionally, the narrowed conduit leads to higher pressure relationships with lower flows, possibly leading to damaged mucosa distally. The presence of the ETT is a nidus for the inflammatory cascade. Despite its relatively hypoallergenic profile, it is still a recognizable foreign body and as such triggers well-defined host responses. Placement of the device, regardless of the care used in placing it, still results in mechanical trauma to all of the periglottic mucosalized regions and therefore decreases the ability of the respiratory mucosa to protect itself. Finally, the ETT may cause airway alteration secondary to pressure injury.

The body's response to the ETT is also multifaceted, affecting mechanics, structure, and physiologic function. Loss of humidity and heat is the most obvious effect of replacing the regular mucosa with a foreign conduit. The gas that is delivered is already dry and cool, but bypassing the patient's natural ability to heat and humidify leads to problems more distally, including reduced ciliary function, inspissated secretions, and increased mucus plugging. The normally motile respiratory cilia are essentially paralyzed, leading to impaired secretion management. The body lacks its normal ability to move debris in a proximal direction, and collection sites develop within the tracheobronchial tree, leading to multiple potential areas for infection. Additionally, these partially or completely occluded areas may result in lobar collapse and, consequently, a ventilation-perfusion mismatch. This obstruction can also create an inability to completely exhale, leading to breath stacking and auto-PEEP (positive end-expiratory pressure) and possibly resultant barotrauma.

9.2.4 Complications of Endotracheal Tube Placement

Complications associated with ETT placement should be grouped into three major subcategories: those that occur at intubation, those that occur with the ETT in situ, and postextubation sequelae [25]. The problems associated with placement are numerous and can be worsened in emergencies, with multiple attempts, use of a variety of devices, or inexperience of the operator [26]. Problems at placement include dental and oral problems, maxillofacial damage, displacement of the arytenoid cartilages, vocal cord ulceration or dysfunction, airway perforation, autonomic hyperactivity, and, of course, failed intubation. Structural damage is unlikely to be repaired until the patient no longer requires intubation, unless the damage interferes with ventilation and oxygenation. Problems that occur as a result of an in situ ETT include those related to the ETT, such as aspiration, vocal cord paralysis, or transient nerve palsy; ulceration and granuloma formation in the trachea and on the cords; tracheal synechiae; subglottic stenosis; laryngeal webbing; tracheomalacia; tracheoesophageal, tracheoinnominate, or tracheocarotid fistula; and recurrent and superior laryngeal nerve damage [27]. Other complications are related to mechanical ventilation facilitated by the ETT and include aspiration, barotrauma (pneumothorax, pneumomediastinum), VAP, and dislodgement [28]. Finally, postextubation complications can lead to long-term morbidity or the urgent need for reintubation. Many of the postextubation culprits have already been encountered as complications of ETT placement or presence, particularly subglottic stenosis, vocal cord injury, and hoarseness [28,29].

9.3 Endotracheal Tubes and Other Airway Adjuncts

9.3.1 Choice of Endotracheal Tube Size

In selecting an ETT, consideration must be given to the functional reason for placement as well as patient-specific factors such as body height, gender, airway integrity, airway pathology, and previous airway manipulation or instrumentation. Theoretically, short-term placement for anesthesia should be different than placement for prolonged support with mechanical ventilation or for fiberoptic bronchoscopy to aid therapy. Generally, the trachea of an adult female accepts a tube of 7.5 to 8.0 mm and that of a male accepts one of 8.5 to 9.0 mm, but typically a 7.0-mm ETT is used for females and an 8.0-mm tube for males, at least in the United States. It is also generally accepted that an ETT of at least 8.0 mm is needed for competent use of an adult-based bronchoscopic investigation [30].

9.3.1.1 Small Tubes and Airway Resistance

The physics of laminar gas flow through a conduit are described by the Hagen-Poiseuille equation, which reflects the relationship of resistance varying inversely with the fourth power of tube radius. Despite the fact that gas flow through ETTs is often turbulent rather than laminar, the effect on resistance to gas flow represented by each millimeter decrease in tube size is considerable, ranging from 25% to 100% [31]. Airway resistance is affected by more than tube diameter: the presence of secretion within the tube, ETT kinking, and positioning of the head and neck can also increase the tendency for turbulent flow [32,33]. The fundamental principle of which to be mindful is that airway resistance induced by an ETT is inversely proportional to the tube size—hence, the mantra that the largest tube is usually the best size [34].

Airway resistance increases with decreasing ETT diameter, whether due to internal occlusion, smaller size, or external compression. As airway resistance increases, WOB also increases [31]. The increase in WOB associated with a 1-mm reduction in ETT diameter varies in accordance with tidal volume and respiratory rate at a given minute ventilation and can range from 34% to 154% [31]. When ventilation is controlled, the increase in WOB related to ETT resistance is seldom of any consequence, because it is overcome by ventilator adjustments. However, small-diameter tubes create greater difficulty for patients in weaning from ventilatory support due to the higher levels of resistance encountered when attempting to breathe spontaneously [35,36]. It has been suggested that an inability to spontaneously ventilate due to the increased WOB imposed by a 7-mm ETT might indicate that extubation will fail regardless of tube size [37,38].

Increased airway resistance associated with a smaller-diameter ETT may also be associated with inadvertent PEEP. Patients with high oxygen consumption, increased carbon dioxide production, or ventilation-perfusion relationships that produce high dead space ventilation often require higher minute ventilations to achieve appropriate ventilation and oxygenation. The gas flows necessary to maintain such a minute ventilation are also quite high, and the resistance imposed by a smaller-diameter ETT further prohibits the completion of expiratory flow before initiation of the subsequent inspiration. This breath stacking results in air trapping and unwanted PEEP, magnifying the risk of mechanical ventilation because barotrauma and subsequent intrathoracic overpressure could result in circulatory compromise [39].

The restriction to gas flow through any ETT increases dramatically when devices such as a suction catheter or bronchoscope are placed in the lumen. The cross-sectional area of the tube is effectively reduced by an amount equal to the cross-sectional area of the device inserted into the tube. The limitation of gas flow has consequences for both the inspiratory and expiratory phases: inspiratory flow may be inadequate to maintain oxygenation and ventilation during the procedure, and retarded expiratory flow may lead to overdistention resulting in barotrauma or circulatory compromise [40].

9.3.1.2 Large Tubes and Trauma

Whereas smaller-diameter ETTs have disadvantages related to gas flow and airway resistance, larger tubes are more frequently associated with traumatic placements and damage to both the laryngeal structures and the tracheal mucosa [37,38,41]. Larger ETTs are associated with a higher incidence of sore throat after general anesthesia, compared with smaller-diameter tubes, but this difference is relatively negligible with long-term intubation [42]. With prolonged intubation, laryngeal trauma is more likely. Women, because of the inherently smaller size of their airway, are more susceptible to injury than men [43,44].

Laryngeal structures at particular risk for trauma are the arytenoid cartilages and the cricoid cartilage. Trauma results not only from the shape discrepancy between the round ETT and the angular, wedge-shaped glottic opening but also from direct contact and pressure on these structures and from repetitive tube movement, which leads to ulceration or erosion of the protective mucosa [44–46]. Tracheal mucosal injury can also occur because of the irregular surfaces created by wrinkling and folding of the ETT cuff or the externalized pilot tube used to fill the ETT cuff. If the tracheal lumen is "overcrowded," airway injury is more likely to occur when large tubes are used and little cuff volume is required to seal the airway [47].

9.3.2 Potentially Beneficial Alternatives to the Standard Endotracheal Tube

9.3.2.1 Preformed and Reinforced Tubes

Modifications to the ETT that are made in the operating room setting to accomplish specific surgeries are often developed in response to interference and access issues. The ability to work without disturbing the ETT has led to several variations of the ETT that can be placed safely and remove the risk of inadvertent advancement, dislodgement, kinking, or obstruction. ETTs used in remote locations also have airway access issues associated with tube kinking and partial occlusion, which typically are related to positioning problems and associated comorbidities. In part because of less stringent vigilance, unintended consequences of ETT use outside the operating room may result in more drastic outcomes. In response to these dilemmas, a variety of tubes have been developed to maintain their shape and patency in locations where distortion might cause kinking and occlusion.

Rigid, preformed tubes such as those developed for long-term use in tracheostomy were known to maintain their patency despite the need for angulation. Preformed tubes have been developed for specific application in anesthesia practice as well. The Ring-Adair-Elwyn (RAE) tubes (Mallinckrodt Inc., Pleasanton, CA), both oral and nasal (Figure 9.4), maintain a fixed contour similar to the average facial profile, allowing for head and neck surgery while minimizing surgical field interference. Their contour also reduces the risk of pressure injury to the posterior pharynx when repositioning is desired. The intra-airway length is tied to the size of the ETT, with a relatively appropriate depth based on the average size of a patient for whom the tube might be selected [48,49].

An anode or armored tube with an embedded wire coil is designed to minimize kinking even with quite severe position-induced angulation. Armored tubes are popular for use in head and neck surgery where remote airway access and the potential for kinking of the ETT are concerns. Placement of an armored tube through a tracheostomy for procedures such as laryngectomy is a common practice; it allows placement during surgical procedures such that the tube can be mobilized or the circuit draped away from the field without a high risk of tube kinking. The other common use of a wire-reinforced tube is with the ILMA. These tubes are designed to facilitate placement through the device and to be used for short periods of time. The HPLV cuff and the theoretical possibility of kinking and resultant airway obstruction make the long-term use of ILMAs risky.

The embedded wire concept of the armored ETT has also been developed for long-term tracheostomy use. Although the armored tracheostomy tube is not free of risks, one advantage is that its flexibility allows its length and intratracheal depth to be adjusted, which may be beneficial if tracheomalacia at the level of the cuff develops [50]. These

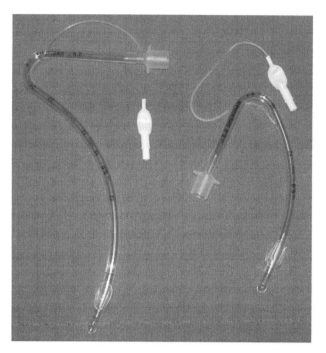

Figure 9.4 Nasal (*left*) and oral (*right*) Ring-Adair-Elwyn (RAE) preformed endotracheal tubes. *(Courtesy Covidien, Mansfield, MA.)*

tracheostomy tubes are also popular for use in morbidly obese patients, in whom, because of the depth of tissue, preformed tracheostomy tubes may not have the shape required to fit an individual patient. One major consequence of this type of reinforced ETT may occur when external pressure is applied to the wire-reinforced component (i.e., by patient biting). Once a compression threshold is reached, the luminal support provided by the wire may be compromised, and a permanent, irreparable dent remains that can significantly endanger ventilation and suctioning capabilities.

9.3.2.2 Laser Tubes

Progress in laser technology has advanced surgical capabilities, particularly for airway surgery. To protect patients and health care providers from laser-induced injury to eyes and airways, special precautions are required. Fire is the most serious danger associated with the use of lasers in the operating room, especially when a laser is used in airway surgery [30,51–53]. A major complication related to the use of lasers for laryngeal surgery is ignition of the ETT [54]. The laser beam may ignite the tube by direct penetration or indirectly if burning tissue is

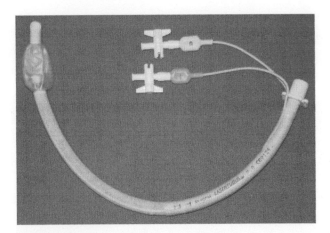

Figure 9.5 Rusch Lasertubus laser-safe endotracheal tube. *(Courtesy Teleflex Medical, Durham, NC.)*

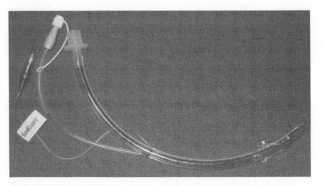

Figure 9.6 Mallinckrodt Sealguard Evac Endotracheal Tube. *(Courtesy Covidien, Mansfield, MA.)*

inhaled into the tube [30,51,52,55]. The ease of ignition is related to the ETT material, the concentration of oxygen in use, and any other adjunctive materials or gases that could support combustion [30,52,55]. Most ETTs are constructed of PVC, which is highly flammable. Ideally, PVC tubes should not be used for airways when a laser is employed [51,55,56].

ETTs can be laser-proofed or protected from the laser beam by wrapping them with either reflective metal tape or muslin. Ideally, they should be constructed from noncombustible materials. In particular, the ETT cuff is vulnerable to puncture by the laser beam and should be filled with saline or water, which allows more energy to be absorbed before disruption [30,52,55]. One trick to enhance appreciation of a penetrated, defective cuff, is to place a dye indicator, such as methylene blue, into the solution that is instilled into the cuff. Any leakage will clearly mark the airway and alert the provider to the potential dangers [57]. Protecting the tube from the laser beam by wrapping it with a foil tape has proved effective (commercial devices are available) (Figure 9.5) [58]. Tubes made of materials such as metal and silicone and those with special double cuffs also reduce the risk of airway fires and injury during laser airway surgery [51,58].

9.3.2.3 Subglottic Suctioning Evac Endotracheal Tubes

Hospitalized patients who require mechanical ventilation are susceptible to the development of aspiration pneumonia. VAP is known to increase hospital length of stay, health care costs, and mortality [59]. Organisms that grow in pooled subglottic secretions above the inflated cuff of the ETT, but beneath the glottis, have previously been unmeasurable with any reliability and are now demonstrated to be a major impetus for VAP. Several nursing care measures may be taken to reduce the incidence of VAP caused by this route, including improved oral care, patient positioning by elevating the head of the bed past 30 degrees, frequent suctioning, and ensuring postpyloric tube feedings, but none of these measures completely stops the production [60].

The presence of these pooled collections has led to the development of specific ETTs that possess a dedicated suction system capable of emptying this area of debris. Drainage of subglottic secretions has been shown to prevent VAP [61–64]. The currently available subglottic drainage ETTs have a suction lumen that opens on the external (posterolateral) surface of the ETT immediately above the cuff (Figure 9.6). The lumen is attached to constant or intermittent suction for active drainage of the space. Although these ETTs are beneficial, their efficacy is not 100%, and therefore all of the aforementioned nursing care actions remain vital to good hygiene and prevention of VAP. The subglottic drainage tubes have been further developed to include variations in cuff construction (materials, shapes, volumes, locations) that help to prevent aspiration of the subglottic debris.

Subglottic secretions are not the only recognized cause for VAP. Biofilm is an accumulation of debris adhered to the internal circumference of the

ETT that is composed of tissue, secretions, mucus, and undetermined bacteria load. Biofilm can be aspirated, leading to a nidus for infection or causing an area of obstruction to airflow. Biofilm removal and reduction by hygiene care are currently better researched than prevention. However, there is a growing interest in the reduction of biofilm through construction of ETTs impregnated with antimicrobial agents [65–67]. The ability of such developments to affect the incidence of VAP has not yet been proved.

9.3.2.4 Double-Lumen Endotracheal Tubes

The uses of a double-lumen endotracheal tube (DLT) (Figure 9.7) can be separated into relative and absolute indications. The absolute indications are isolation, to avoid soilage or contamination of the contralateral lung tissue when dealing with infections or frank hemoptysis from a unilateral location, bronchoalveolar lavage, and one-lung ventilation (OLV). The most common reason for placement is OLV for surgical exposure, but OLV can also be important in cases of bronchopleural or bronchocutaneous fistula, unilateral pulmonary hemorrhage, giant unilateral bulla or cyst, and severe unilateral ventilation-perfusion mismatch. The relative indications all deal with surgical exposure. Complementing the DLT as another option for lung isolation, particularly if a DLT cannot be placed, are bronchial blocking devices. However, the DLT has an advantage because of the ability to pass suctioning catheters or fiberoptic devices into the area on collapse without drastically jeopardizing OLV or contaminating the contralateral side.

Relative contraindications to the placement of a DLT are fairly minimal. They include patient refusal (likely due to risk of trauma secondary to the large size), a known difficult airway, and the speed with which an isolated airway must be established. In patients with difficult airways, specially designed airway exchange catheters (Cook Medical, Bloomington, IN) (Figure 9.8) can be used after placement of a conventional ETT to facilitate DLT placement. Additionally, some makers of video laryngoscopic technologies have developed specific DLT devices. The time required for placement is usually the biggest detractor to their use. Situations such as frank hemoptysis may be better served by a rapid-sequence induction and placement of a contralateral, main stem, single-lumen ETT for stabilization.

This technique is not ideal for long-term management. The long-term use of the DLT in the

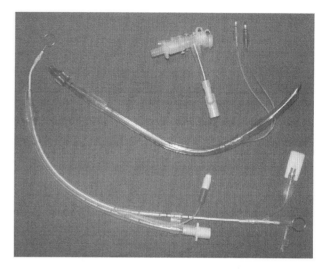

Figure 9.7 Endobronchial blocking devices for lung isolation. Mallinckrodt Endobronchial Tube (*top*). (Covidien, Mansfield, MA); Fuji TCB Univent Tube (*bottom*). (Phycon Products, Tokyo, Japan).

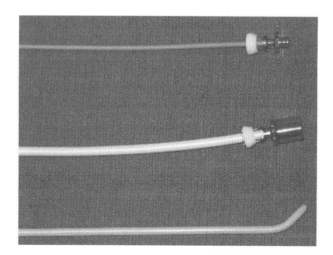

Figure 9.8 A selection of airway exchange catheters. Double-lumen airway exchange catheter (*top*), Aintree Intubation Catheter (*center*) and Portex Single-Use Bougie (*bottom*). *(Aintree courtesy Cook Medical, Bloomington, IN; Portex courtesy Smiths Medical, Carlsbad, CA.)*

intensive care unit (ICU) setting (>24 to 48 hours) must be approached with caution, because the two smaller-diameter lumens are at significantly increased risk for partial or complete occlusion. Consideration should be given to close monitoring of luminal patency with fiberoptic evaluation on a regular basis and optimization of luminal hygiene to reduce mucus or biofilm accumulation.

9.3.2.5 Supraglottic Airways

Supraglottic devices are continually coming onto the market. Largely designed for shorter surgical procedures to deliver general anesthesia, their use seems to be growing past their original intent. Supraglottic airways (Figure 9.9) such as the LMA, the esophageal-tracheal Combitube (ETC, Tyco Healthcare, Mansfield, MA), the King LT (King Systems, Noblesville, IN), and other variants have provided valuable means of establishing an (unsecured) airway in an emergency. Equally important is their ability to function as a conduit for endotracheal intubation. For example, the ILMA is a blind passage device that is designed to place an ETT through the LMA. Recently, use of the LMA as a conduit for fiberoptic bronchoscopy and subsequent ETT placement has also been demonstrated in emergency situations [68]. Although these devices do not provide classically definitive airways, their utility is unsurpassed in helping to manage the difficult airway.

9.4 Proper Safeguarding of the Airway

9.4.1 Airway Evaluation: Predicting the Difficult Airway

The decision to intubate, whether for airway protection, ventilatory failure, inadequate oxygenation, or medication delivery, is often difficult, but equally difficult can be the decision of how to intubate. Each patient and airway is unique, as is the clinical setting and the judgment, skill, and equipment of the airway team that responds. Outside the operating room, time often does not allow a comprehensive evaluation and establishment of a plan complete with contingencies before the decision to intubate must be made. Performance of a proper airway evaluation before intubation is attempted can dramatically improve outcomes.

However, a difficult airway should be assumed when one approaches the patient outside the controlled setting of the operating room. An airway physical examination is paramount to predicting a successful attempt. Criteria such as dental status, mouth opening, thyromental distance, cervical range of motion, Mallampati score, and neck circumference are all standard examination points. However, the emergent intubation presents a host of new, potentially detrimental issues not seen in operating room intubations. For example, hemodynamics may not allow for the controlled process typically seen in the operating room. Trauma patients may have actively unstable facial fractures or cervical vertebral injuries that merit inline stabilization and modified techniques for tube placement. Neurosurgical patients may have external fixators to stabilize injuries or intracranial monitoring devices that make it difficult to position the head. The type of bed a patient is in can also create access issues with intubation. A bariatric bed with an inflatable mattress can be very difficult to properly ramp, thereby making positioning suboptimal. Last, but not least, is the patient with failed extubation who must be reintubated. Issues with anxiety, hypoxemia, decreased functional residual and closing capacities, copious

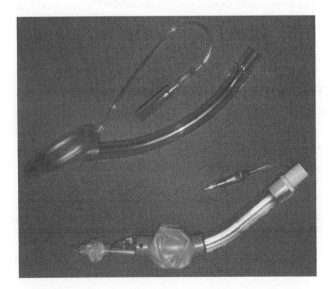

Figure 9.9 Supraglottic devices. LMA Unique (*top*), (Courtesy USA) King LT Supraglottic Device (*bottom*). *(LMA Unique courtesy LMA North America Inc., San Diego, CA; King LT courtesy King Systems, Noblesville, IN.)*

secretions, residual airway edema, and subglottic stenosis all make a repeat attempt more difficult than the first pass [28].

9.4.2 Identifying Proper Position of the Endotracheal Tube

9.4.2.1 Detection of Esophageal Intubation

Once the clinician has deemed intubation necessary and has performed the intervention, confirmation of proper ET placement must be provided expeditiously. An incorrectly positioned ETT can produce adverse effects, especially in an already apneic patient. Unrecognized esophageal intubation can have disastrous consequences with a reported incidence as high as 8% in critical patients [69]. Therefore, a brief discussion of verification of ETT placement is warranted.

Once intubation has been accomplished, confirmation of proper placement of the ETT in the trachea needs to be achieved, ideally by the detection of end-tidal carbon dioxide ($Etco_2$) in expired gases using capnography or other capnometric (colorimetric) methods [70]. The detection of $Etco_2$ is not fail-safe and does not guarantee that the ETT is positioned within the tracheal lumen (e.g., the tip may lie above the vocal cords). After three to five breaths, the absence of $Etco_2$ suggests a nontracheal placement. Blockage or soilage of the $Etco_2$ detection device can hamper efforts. $Etco_2$ detection should be complemented with indirect maneuvers such as auscultation, ETT misting or fogging, bag compliance, chest wall excursions, lack of phonation, and improved oxygen saturation. The dependence of any $Etco_2$ detection device on adequate cardiac output has spurred utilization of an esophageal detector device (Figure 9.10). It is essentially an air-filled bulb placed on the end of an in situ ETT. After a vacuum has been created by squeezing the bulb, immediate re-expansion should occur when the bulb is placed on an ETT in the trachea (any column of air). If the ETT is esophageal, the suction created by the bulb will draw the pliable esophageal tissue into the distal lumen of the ETT, preventing full expansion of the bulb on top of the ETT (column of soft tissue) [71–73].

If intubation is to occur in a patient with cardiac arrest, capnometry may be fallible given the amount of down time and the lack of any life-sustaining cardiac output. If cardiopulmonary resuscitation (CPR)

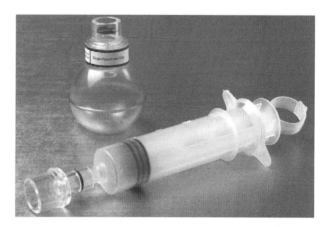

Figure 9.10 Esophageal bulb detector and a homemade syringe device. *(Courtesy Wolfe-Tory Medical, Inc.)*

is adequate, this technicality is likely to be moot. However, esophageal bulb detectors can be helpful in this situation, although false-positives and false-negatives do occur and confound ETT verification. Still other methods that are independent of carbon dioxide and cardiac output exist, such as a tracheal whistle to verify correct placement (Box 9.1), but not one is without limitations [72–77]. Ideally, two methods are to be considered fail-safe: direct or indirect visualization of the ETT traversing the vocal cords and fiberoptic verification via the ETT lumen. The limitation of direct laryngoscopy is the operator's line of sight to the glottic opening. The key is to identify the ETT positioned in the glottis, not simply to see it go in. An indirect method such as video laryngoscopy does improve the validity of ETT passage. Fiberoptic verification is hampered by equipment availability at the bedside, any airway or ETT soilage, time constraints, and operator skill. Chest rise and condensation from expired gas found in the ETT have also been used, but these signs may occur in esophageal intubations as well [77]. Therefore, the gold standard used today is the presence of $Etco_2$ in expired gases as demonstrated by capnography or other colorimetric techniques [70].

Capnography yields quantifiable measurements of inspired and expired gases in addition to a waveform generated with each tidal volume. Although not without limitations (e.g., lack of portability, need for a power source), capnography reliably identifies initial proper placement of the ETT (non-esophageal) and provides a continuous verification

> **Box 9.1** Methods used to Verify Endotracheal Tube Placement
> Sustainable, exhaled CO_2 by capnography or colorimetric methods
> Fiberoptic visualization of carina
> Videolaryngoscopic visualization of translaryngeal endotracheal tube position
> Direct laryngoscopic visualization of translaryngeal position
> Positive response with esophageal bulb detector device or syringe method
> Auscultation of breath sounds in bilateral lung fields and absence of same in epigastric area
> Visualization of chest wall movement with spontaneous patient efforts
> Reservoir bag synchrony with spontaneous patient efforts
> Palpable ballottement of cuff in suprasternal notch
> Acoustic reflectometry
> Transtracheal illumination
> Chest roentgenogram
> Condensation in endotracheal tube
> Lack of phonation in the nonparalyzed, semiconscious patient
> Bougie passage to distinguish between tracheobronchial tree and esophagus

of ETT security. If esophageal intubation has occurred, a gradual reduction in height of the capnograph waveforms is observed with successive breaths. False-positive results during esophageal intubations may occur in situations of ingested CO_2-containing or -liberating substances (e.g., carbonated beverages) before intubation, bag-mask ventilation with inflation of expired air into the stomach, or intubation of the supralaryngeal hypopharynx [78]. Inappropriate extubations may occur due to misinterpretation of a false-negative situation because an $Etco_2$ waveform is lacking despite proper placement. This error may occur with unrecognized circuit disconnections, an obstructed or kinked ETT, a disconnected or contaminated gas sampling line (water, secretions, entrainment of room air), equipment failure, severe bronchospasm, or inadequate cardiac output. Unquestionably, capnography is dependent on pulmonary blood flow. In the absence of perfusion (e.g., cardiac arrest), the utility of capnography can be limited; however, even in very low-flow states (e.g., CPR, separation from cardiopulmonary bypass), it has been shown to provide effective detection. Ornato and colleagues used an animal model to evaluate the relationship between cardiac output (CO) and $Etco_2$. Through manipulation of CO, with inotropes or controlled hemorrhage, a logarithmic relationship between CO and $Etco_2$ was demonstrated [50]. This finding shows that capnography is useful in cardiac resuscitation to assist with evaluation of low-flow states and adequacy of perfusion.

To alleviate the logistic concerns with capnography in emergency situations—mainly the lack of portability and the need for a power source—a portable and reliable means of detecting $Etco_2$ was developed. Colorimetric $Etco_2$ uses a detector impregnated with metacresol purple (Figure 9.11). This indicator is pH sensitive and changes color, from purple to yellow, in the presence of CO_2. The devices are disposable, attach between the ETT and the circuit or bag, and provide a rapid and reliable indication of CO_2 concentration on a graded scale: A (purple) corresponds to an $Etco_2$ level of 0.5%, B (tan) to a level of 0.5% to 2%, and C (yellow) to a level greater than 2% [70,77]. Limitations of this method are that it is ineffective with exposure to humidified gases, vomitus, or secretions and in cases of prolonged cardiac arrest or low-perfusion states. False-positive results can occur as well, just as in capnography. Delays in recognition of esophageal intubation with colorimetric capnometry have been reported far more often than with capnography, particularly in patients with prolonged bag-mask ventilation or ingestion of $Etco_2$-containing substances before intubation. Therefore, capnography simply is

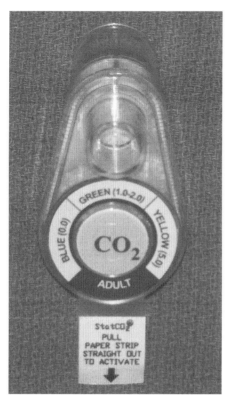

Figure 9.11 Example of a colorimetric capnometric device. *(Courtesy Mercury Medical, Clearwater, FL.)*

the best method for detection of esophageal intubation [79].

As mentioned previously, the esophageal bulb detector capitalizes on the physical characteristics of the esophagus, which, unlike the trachea, collapses when negative pressure is applied. Commercial devices exist, but a homemade version can be improvised using a syringe that attaches to the end of the ETT. When the plunger is withdrawn, resistance is appreciated if an esophageal intubation has occurred, because the walls of the esophagus collapse around the ETT. Unencumbered aspiration of the plunger occurs with proper tracheal placement [71]. Bulb detector devices are reported to be reliable and effective, with one study demonstrating a sensitivity of 100% and a specificity of 99% [72]. However, other studies have reported limitations and false-negative results in patients with copious or aspirated secretions, gastric distention, vomitus in the airway, morbid obesity, or reduced functional residual capacity [71,80–83].

A little used but highly effective method of detecting proper ETT location is the passage of a catheter (e.g., bougie) via the ETT to decipher a straight smooth muscle pathway (esophagus without pathology) or a more rigid, angulated tube with reduction in the luminal diameter (tracheobronchial tree). A bougie can be used in this fashion, particularly at the time it is being used as an adjunct to intubation, or later if necessary. Gentle advancement to 28 to 34 cm (in adults) typically results in contact with the carina or a main stem bronchus. Further advancement down a main stem bronchus should be limited by the secondary lobar carina. Gentle unopposed advancement of the bougie beyond 35 cm suggests esophageal placement (assuming no esophageal pathology).

9.4.2.2 Confirmation of Appropriate Depth of Insertion

After correct tracheal placement of the ETT has been verified, it is imperative to identify the correct depth of the ETT to ensure adequate ventilation of each lung [49]. Before addressing the various methods that assist in confirmation of appropriate ETT depth, a brief discussion of what is considered to be the correct depth is warranted. Malpositioning of ETTs occurs frequently, with unrecognized right main stem intubation occurring in approximately 4% of chest radiographs [49,69,84]. The generally accepted depth of insertion of the ETT is between 2 and 7 cm above the carina, optimally between 4 and 7 cm above the carina with the head and neck in a neutral position [49,77,85–87]. It is important to realize this, because flexion-extension movements of the neck can displace the ETT upward or downward with resultant extubation or main stem intubation, respectively. Typically the right main stem bronchus is entered, given its straighter trajectory in relation to the trachea. If endobronchial intubation remains undetected, an inadvertent hyperinflation of the ipsilateral lung can occur with subsequent pneumothorax and concomitant atelectasis of the hypoventilated contralateral lung. Indeed, it has been reported that up to 15% of chest radiographs reveal malpositioned ETTs in intubated patients [84,88,89]. This is more frequently seen after difficult airway management.

In the operating room, chest radiographs are not used to confirm proper position; rather, indirect clinical assessment methods are used (i.e., auscultation of bilateral breath sounds, visualization of equal chest expansion, and direct visualization of the ETT tip placed just below the vocal cords). The

ETT is also manufactured with distance measurements to aid with the depth of insertion. In orally intubated patients, a depth of 23 cm at the teeth or corner of the mouth has been advocated for men and 21 to 22 cm for women [90,91]. In nasotracheal intubations, a depth of 26 cm at the nares in women and 28 cm in men should be sufficient for proper tracheal position [92]. Other methods used include direct visualization of the ETT tip in reference to the carina with a fiberoptic scope or catheter [69], transtracheal illumination, and ballottement of the ETT cuff in the suprasternal notch [93–96].

9.4.2.3 Cuff Pressure Monitoring

Probably the most often overlooked parameter in daily airway care is cuff pressure [97,98]. Almost universally, this measurement is neglected in operating room intubations. However, it is well documented that excessive forces applied to the tracheal mucosa can cause necrosis and ulceration [9,99,100]. Cuff pressures of 30 cm H_2O for 4 hours have been shown to damage ciliary motility for at least 3 days [100–102]. In addition, animal studies have revealed diminished circulation in the tracheal mucosa with a pressure of just 20 cm H_2O, exaggerated greatly in the presence of hypotension [103].

Normal occlusive pressures should be between 20 and 30 cm H_2O to avoid complications while maintaining an adequate seal in the tracheal lumen circumferentially around the cuff to prevent microaspiration and ultimately VAP [100]. Depending on the type of cuff used, the same pressure range seems to be effective at accomplishing this task both in vitro and during in vivo animal studies. For example, standardized HVLP cuffs have been demonstrated to be ineffective at preventing microaspiration with pressures as high as 60 cm H_2O [7], whereas polyurethane tubes seem to be effective down to 15 cm H_2O [7,10,104].

As was previously discussed, ETTs are not without risks. However, it appears that most of the morbidity is related to either inappropriate inflation of an ETT cuff or a defective ETT cuff [98–100]. An often dreaded scenario that leads to increased morbidity is frequent ETT exchanges for suspected cuff leaks. Trended values for cuff pressure could help to alleviate some of these unnecessary procedures. Most importantly, it has been demonstrated that manual palpation of the cuff or instillation of a

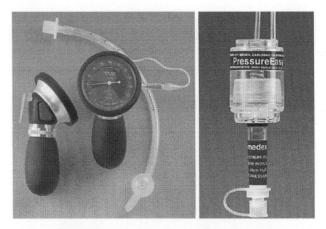

Figure 9.12 Posey Cufflator aneroid manometer (*left*) and the PressureEasy Pressure Controller Device (*right*) for monitoring endotracheal tube cuff pressure. *(Cufflator courtesy Posey Company, Arcadia, CA; PressureEasy courtesy Smiths Medical, Dublin, OH.)*

standard volume of air often underestimates the actual occlusive pressure delivered, leading to unrecognized complications [97,98,100]. Therefore, it is recommended that frequent examination of the cuff pressure be documented and trended using manometry.

Reusable aneroid manometers can be onerous to calibrate and are often difficult to locate; in addition, they pose a recurring risk of cross-contamination for each patient. The manometers currently in use in most ICUs provide only a single data point at the time of collection. A commercially available disposable, precalibrated device that constantly measures airway cuff pressures is available. The PressureEasy device (Smiths Medical, St. Paul, MN), among others, attaches to the pilot balloon and exhibits a mark in a fixed window when the measured cuff pressure is in the optimal range of 20 and 30 cm H_2O (Figure 9.12) [97–100].

9.4.2.4 Evaluation of an Audible Cuff Leak

Although ETT cuff leaks pertain most often to the ICU or postanesthesia care unit (PACU) setting and longer-duration intubations, short-term tracheal intubation in the operating room may also fall prey to an apparent leak. The most relevant question is, When is a cuff leak really a cuff leak? The audible leak implies that air is escaping from the presumably

Table 9.1 Causes and Solutions for Apparent ETT Cuff Leaks

Problem	Solution	Risk Level
Cuff perforation (pilot balloon deflation)	Exchange ETT (only feasible choice)	High
Incompetent pilot valve	Exchange ETT	High
	Clamp line (Kelly, hemostat)—short term solution	Low
	Place stopcock or cap on valve	Low
	Replace pilot balloon–line assembly	Low
Broken pilot line	Exchange ETT	High
	Clamp line (Kelly, hemostat)—short-term solution	Low
	Replace pilot balloon line assembly (homemade vs. commercial)	Low
Displaced ETT (intact pilot balloon)	Perform fiberoptic evaluation—diagnostic	Low-moderate
	Blindly advance ETT	Very high
	Videolaryngoscopy evaluation	Low-moderate
	Blindly pass airway exchange catheter	High
	Perform direct laryngoscopy (suboptimal line of sight)	Low-moderate

ETT, *Endotracheal tube.*

closed ETT system. The leak may be caused by a defective ETT cuff that has failed, ripped, or is microperforated (in which case the pilot balloon deflates spontaneously). Equally possible is a defective pilot balloon–line assembly. The valve on the pilot balloon may be faulty and incompetent, the balloon may have a perforation, the line may be cracked or broken or may become disjointed at the tube end or the valve end. Moreover, the intermittent or continuous audible leak may represent an ETT cuff that fails to seal the airway due to malpositioning, deranged shape, or laxity and deformation of the tracheal wall (e.g., tracheomalacia, tracheitis, tracheal erosion). The ETT cuff (intact pilot balloon) may be subglottic, between the vocal cords, or supraglottic, having been displaced during patient movement, transport, repositioning, "tonguing" (dislodging the ETT by moving it with the tongue) of the ETT, excessive coughing, excessive tension on the ETT by the ventilator circuit, or, commonly, positioning for radiography. Once the ETT is partially displaced upward, an audible leak may prompt further ETT cuff insufflation, leading to further displacement. Head and neck movement by the patient may be all that is required to further displace the ETT into the hypopharyngeal region. This must be diagnosed before disaster strikes.

The various sources of a suspected cuff leak require investigation because each necessitates a different solution. Any one solution, incorrectly applied, may lead to morbidity or mortality. For example, a cuff leak resulting from a herniated cuff above the vocal cords may prompt the team to order a chest radiograph. Further displacement may take place during lifting and repositioning of the patient for the examination. Conversely, if an ETT is malpositioned in the hypopharynx (intact pilot balloon) but is assumed to be a properly positioned ETT with a cuff perforation, an exchange catheter passed via the ETT (presumably into the trachea) may exit the supraglottic ETT and enter the esophagus, leading to airway compromise. Table 9.1 highlights the possible causes and potential solutions, with relevant risk assessments for an apparent cuff leak evaluation.

9.4.2.5 Documentation of Placement

Clinicians who care for patients who are intubated for long periods in the ICU may find it onerous to obtain pertinent airway management details.

This can be especially detrimental to future care providers who are faced with a patient with a known or suspected difficult airway. This situation could result for a number of reasons: lack of relevance (routine intubation before the patient's surgery), lack of continuity (the intubator is no longer involved in the patient's care), or an incomplete or total lack of documentation.

As an ICU course progresses, the details surrounding the original ETT placement may prove less relevant because the patient's clinical status and airway are dynamic, not static. A previously easy airway may remain so, but difficulty often increases as edema, trauma, secretion management, and patient status decline to confound an airway intervention. Anatomic abnormalities may be hidden or exaggerated by excessive fluid administration or a capillary leakage phenomenon in the critically ill patient, and examination of the airway may become impossible. Appreciation of the airway adjuncts that have been attempted is imperative for the incoming airway team. Immediate availability of pertinent historical airway management details may prove helpful in delivering better care. Documentation of airway interventions and procedures on a specific sheet (Figure 9.13) may provide the incoming airway team perspective on what to expect in a single concise location.

9.4.3 Stabilization of the Endotracheal Tube

After verification and confirmation of proper tracheal placement and position have been achieved, care should be focused on securing the ETT in its proper position, and frequent assessments should be made to recognize malpositioning [105,106].

At the most basic level, recording and confirming the depth of the ETT at the patient's teeth or lips in centimeters should be routine. This measurement should be documented on the respiratory care flow sheet. In patients requiring prolonged mechanical ventilation, the depth should be assessed and documented frequently (e.g., every shift, every 4 hours), along with clinical assessments of ETT patency and hygiene, appropriate chest expansion, and auscultation findings.

Securing and surveillance of the ETT are important not only to ensure proper depth and positioning but also to reduce the incidence of inadvertent extubation [105]. Unplanned extubation is primarily a problem in the ICU. It has a reported incidence of approximately 2% to 16%, with 80% of those extubated requiring reintubation, and contributes to a higher rate of airway-related complications, hemodynamic alterations, patient morbidity, and mortality [48,107–109]. The most frequently identified cause is inadequate sedation of a mechanically ventilated patient, and only a few studies have specifically addressed techniques used to secure ETTs. In a study comparing four such techniques, Levy and Griego concluded that the use of simple adhesive tape split at both ends and secured to both the ETT and patient's face was more effective than proprietary methods and allowed more effective nursing care, improved oral hygiene, and greater comfort for the patient [106]. However, Barnason and colleagues found no statistical difference between two methods studied in preventing unplanned extubation, allowing oral hygiene, or maintaining facial skin integrity [110].

Attention to proper ETT stabilization primarily focuses on the reduction of unplanned extubation, improved comfort for the patient with prolonged ventilatory requirements, minimization of iatrogenic complications related to the method of fixture, and ease of nursing and respiratory care. One study addressed massive air leaks and contributing factors. The authors defined a massive air leak as one that requires extubation. Over a 2-year period, 18 ETTs were removed for massive air leaks, of which 61% were found to be free of mechanical defects (intact cuff). Fourteen of the 18 patients required reintubation; 2 of them aspirated gastric contents on replacement, and 1 suffered severe epistaxis from a blind nasal reintubation, resulting in a 21% complication rate [111]. The authors concluded that malpositioning was the most plausible explanation for the apparent air leaks. This study reinforces the importance of securing the ETT and daily vigilance to ensure that proper depth and positioning are confirmed and maintained.

Despite these studies, no consensus exists concerning the best method of securing the ETT.

9.4.3.1 Taping

The classically described methods are a "barber's pole" technique for operating room intubations, a simple split tape technique (Figure 9.14), and a more secure "four-point" technique for intubations anticipated to last for 24 hours or longer. In each of

Department of Anesthesiology Airway Management Note

Airway Management Procedure:
[ ] Elective [ ] Urgent [ ] Emergent
[ ] Cardiac or Respiratory Arrest
[ ] Intubation [ ] ETT Exchange [ ] Extubation [ ] Other: _____

Date: _____ Call Time: _____ Arrival Time: _____
Location: _____ Staff: _____

Height: _____ Weight: _____ NPO Status: _____
BP: _____ HR: _____ Oxy Sat: _____ on... _____ %
[ ] Room Air [ ] Nasal [ ] Facemask [ ] NRB [ ] NIPPV

Isolation Precautions: [ ] Contact [ ] Droplet [ ] Airborne
  [ ] Vector [ ] Common Vehicle

Condition Upon Arrival (check all that apply):
[ ] Awake   [ ] Hypoxemic   [ ] Dyspnea   [ ] Secretions
[ ] Sedated…   [ ] Hypercarbic   [ ] Tachypnea   [ ] Vomitus
[ ] Agitated   [ ] Stridorous   [ ] Bradypnea   [ ] Blood
[ ] Unconscious   [ ] Wheezing   [ ] Apnea   [ ] Foreign Matter…
[ ] Other/Comments: _____

Underlying Pathologies/Co-Morbidities (if known, mark all that apply):
Neurologic: [ ] CVA   [ ] Increased ICP   [ ] ICH/SDH   [ ] Seizure
             [ ] SCI   [ ] Δ Mental Status [ ] Drug Overdose
Pulmonary: [ ] Asthma   [ ] COPD   [ ] ARDS   [ ] OSA   [ ] PE
             [ ] PNA…   [ ] CAP   [ ] VAP   [ ] Pulm. Contusion
             [ ] Pneumo/Hemothorax   [ ] Upper Airway Issue…
             [ ] Post-operative Respiratory Failure   [ ] NPPE
Cardiac: [ ] AMI   [ ] CHF   [ ] Dysrhythmia…   [ ] Tamponade
Metabolic: [ ] Acidosis…   [ ] Electrolyte…   [ ] Alcohol Withdrawal
             [ ] UGIB or LGIB   [ ] SBO   [ ] Mesenteric Ischemia
Infectious: [ ] Immune compromised   [ ] Sepsis   [ ] PTA
             [ ] Tonsil/Epiglottitis   [ ] Tracheitis/Bronchitis
Trauma: [ ] Cranial/Spinal…   [ ] Thoracic…   [ ] Abdominal…
             [ ] Orthopedic…
Other/Comments: _____

Airway Management Procedural Documentation:
Preoxygenation: [ ] Room Air   [ ] Facemask/NRB   [ ] 100%, Bag-Mask
Ventilation: [ ] Assisted   [ ] Controlled   [ ] Easy [ ] Difficult
                 [ ] Oral Airway   [ ] Nasal Airway   [ ] Two-person
Positioning: [ ] Supine   [ ] Ramped   [ ] Elevated HOB
                 [ ] Sitting   [ ] Other: _____
Induction: [ ] Awake [ ] Sedated   [ ] General Anesthesia   [ ] None
                 [ ] Topical Anesthesia   [ ] Airway Block…   [ ] Paralysis…
                 [ ] Rapid Sequence Induction   [ ] Cricoid Pressure
                 [ ] Other: _____
Medications: [ ] Etomidate _____ mg   [ ] Propofol _____ mg
                 [ ] Ketamine _____ mg   [ ] Other: _____
                 [ ] Succinylcholine _____ mg [ ] Rocuronium _____ mg
1st Attempt: [ ] DL: MAC _____ MILLER _____   [ ] Glidescope/VL   [ ] FOB
                 Other: _____
                 C-L View: [ ] 1   [ ] 2a   [ ] 2b   [ ] 3a   [ ] 3b   [ ] 4
                             [ ] Secretions   [ ] Blood   [ ] Edema
                 AirwayAdjuncts: [ ] Bougie   [ ] ILMA   [ ] LMA
                 Other/Comments: _____

Figure 9.13 Example of a detailed airway record for emergency intubations.

2nd Attempt: [ ] DL: MAC _____ MILLER _____ [ ] Glidescope/VL [ ] FOB
Other: _____
C-L View: [ ] 1   [ ] 2a   [ ] 2b   [ ] 3a   [ ] 3b   [ ] 4
           [ ] Secretions   [ ] Blood   [ ] Edema
AirwayAdjuncts: [ ] Bougie   [ ] ILMA   [ ] LMA
Other/Comments: _____

3rd Attempt: [ ] DL: MAC _____ MILLER _____ [ ] Glidescope/VL [ ] FOB
Other: _____
C-L View: [ ] 1   [ ] 2a   [ ] 2b   [ ] 3a   [ ] 3b   [ ] 4
           [ ] Secretions   [ ] Blood   [ ] Edema
AirwayAdjuncts: [ ] Bougie   [ ] ILMA   [ ] LMA
Other/Comments: _____

Airway Device Ultimately Placed: [ ] ETT...   [ ] LMA...   [ ] Combitube
   Size: _____ Type: [ ] Standard   [ ] ORAE   [ ] NRAE
                        [ ] Subglottic EVAC   [ ] ECOM
   Placement Location: _____ cm @ lip
Confirmation: [ ] Esophageal bulb device   [ ] ETCO$_2$ [ ] Direct Visual
                    [ ] Bilateral BS   [ ] Bronchoscopy   [ ] Chest X-ray

Post-Procedure Vital Signs:
BP: _____ HR: _____ Oxy Sat: _____ on... _____ %

Other/Comments: _____

Signature: _____ Date/Time: _____

Figure 9.13 (*Continued*)

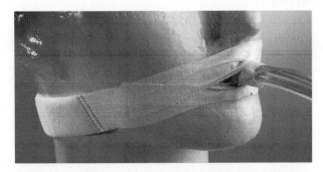

Figure 9.14 The split-tape method of taping the endotracheal tube.

these methods, tape is used to anchor the ETT to the face. Moisture, in the form of sweat, secretions, or vomitus, can jeopardize the integrity of the bond between adhesive and skin, putting the security of the ETT at risk [105]. Additionally, patient comfort is an issue when tape is used for this purpose. Skin breakdown due to allergic reactions, pressure necrosis, or repetitive trauma has been documented as a potential problem from the use of this method. The four-point method is more secure than the barber's pole technique because the tape encircles the patient's head and is not as susceptible to moisture because it is anchored to itself as well as to the patient's skin.

9.4.3.2 Commercially Available Devices

Although several options are available, a proprietary device has been developed to help secure the ETT and provide increased patient comfort while facilitating airway care. This device, the AnchorFast (Hollister Inc., Libertyville, IL) (Figure 9.15), incorporates an ergonomically designed frame to minimize well-known pressure points, a latex-free adhesive on a pad, and a padded Velcro-style retaining strap that encircles the head. Preliminary studies comparing this device against classic adhesive tapes showed reduced skin breakdown, fewer lip ulcers, and improved patient comfort [106,112].

Another commercial device used to secure the ETT has been postulated; it mimics the nasal bridling technique used for nasogastric tubes. This product is still in development.

9.4.3.3 Stapling for Facial Burns

The overall incidence of burn patients in most practices is very small, and this creates an unfamiliarity with their care, particularly as it relates to airway management. The focus of this section is to discuss the unique situation presented by the facial burn. Aside from the obvious difficulties of tube placement initially, replacement of an ETT after a burn resuscitation is far more challenging due to a multitude of unique injuries. The two major problems with securing an ETT for the patient with a facial burn are the increased (and increasing) edema due to ongoing inflammatory processes and continued resuscitation, which makes the face ever expanding, and the actual burned skin, which is constantly weeping and often débrided or sloughing. It should be obvious that adhesive devices, both simple tape and proprietary devices, are ineffective in this situation. A well-documented and accepted method in these patients is to secure the ETT with tape and anchor it to the skin by stapling the tape to the burned areas. This is surprisingly well tolerated, but more importantly it is very reliable to maintain the airway and is easy to care for.

One important airway management caveat should be understood regarding proper ETT position at the gum line or lips in all intubated patients: the ETT marking at these locations only assures the location

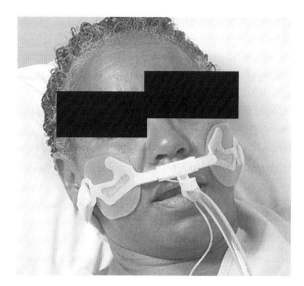

Figure 9.15 The AnchorFast system for endotracheal tube stabilization. *(Courtesy of Hollister Inc., Libertyville, IL.)*

of the proximal end; it does not guarantee the depth and location of the distal ETT tip. Although this problem pertains most often to the ventilated PACU or ICU patient, an ETT located at 25 cm at the gum line and seemingly secured by tape or a commercial device does not guarantee tracheal intubation (with or without a cuff leak). Typically, a continuous or intermittent apparent cuff leak leads to further insufflation of the pilot balloon to fix the leak. An intact (inflated) pilot balloon, in this clinical situation, should arouse suspicion that the distal tip is abnormally located outside the glottis. The potential for an airway catastrophe is extreme, especially in the patient with a difficult airway, compounded by significant mechanical ventilatory requirements. Proper assessment of the ETT position, preferably with flexible bronchoscopy for diagnostic and therapeutic maneuvers, is indicated.

9.4.4 Rapid Response Cart for Airway Emergencies

Areas in which care for intubated patients is provided need to have a dedicated set of supplies to establish emergency airways in the event of primary respiratory failure or cardiac arrest to reestablish lost, previously secured airways. The responding airway team must be knowledgeable and competent in advanced management techniques and provided with immediate access to such equipment. Infrequent or casual airway managers should ask for assistance early in the management process or even immediately, before starting. The American Society of Anesthesiologists difficult airway algorithm (Figure 9.16) should be close at hand to guide less experienced individuals who encounter problems [113]. Supplies on the cart may differ based on personal preference and facility purchase, but there are some items that must be present to help save a life.

Laryngoscopy, ETT exchange, pulmonary toilet, and a "cannot intubate, cannot ventilate" (CICV) scenario must all be covered in the equipment selection. Laryngoscopy includes both conventional (direct) and video laryngoscopy; it is used to assist the team with replacing the ETT after an inadvertent extubation, augmenting the exchange of a damaged ETT over an airway exchange catheter, improving the ability to assess ETT location within the airway, and interrogating the physiologic integrity of an airway slated for extubation [114].

An airway exchange catheter, coupled with video laryngoscopy, greatly reduces the complication rates for necessary airway exchanges in ICU patients, thereby earning its place in an airway response cart within the ICU [114]. A fiberoptic bronchoscope should be available for confirmation purposes, for awake intubation procedures, and for deeper pulmonary toilet needs to improve ventilation and oxygenation [115]. Supraglottic airway devices should be available for situations in which mask ventilation is difficult or as a conduit to facilitate the placement of an endotracheal airway [116]. Lastly, equipment for the placement of a surgical airway must be provided. Despite all of the options available, a scalpel may be the only device capable of establishing the airway. In cases of a known or suspected difficult airway, it is helpful to immediately contact someone with the ability to place a surgical airway should other conventional or advanced noninvasive means fail.

Box 9.2 delineates the contents of a proposed difficult airway cart, which should be readily available in case of any airway catastrophe.

9.5 Maintenance of the Endotracheal Tube

There is currently no alternative to the placement of an oral, nasal, or transtracheal ETT, whether to maintain airway patency, perform ventilation, improve oxygenation, remove secretions, or deliver necessary therapies. However, the ETT is only as good as its most pristine state. Despite the unavoidable decision, some still look on the placement of an ETT as a necessary evil. The conundrum arises in preserving or remastering the physiologic function of the host tissues while combating their inherent defenses aimed at reacting to the new artificial airway and protecting the new foreign device to maintain its optimized function as in its original condition.

The presence of the ETT bypasses the host defenses of the upper airway, eliminates the humidification of inspired gases, increases the WOB, limits the administration of medications, and prevents prophylactic oral hygiene. All of these changes promote bacterial colonization, inflammation, and sputum production. Inability to actively clear secretions because of a poor cough or increased difficulty of passive removal by health care personnel can lead to plugging of proximal and distal airways as well as the ETT. These retained secretions may result in the formation of atelectasis, ventilation-perfusion mismatching in the form of a shunt or dead space, hypoxemia, and increased respiratory load, thereby prolonging the duration of mechanical ventilation [117,118]. Therefore, aggressive respiratory care must be provided for the intubated patient to avoid these complications and further morbidity.

9.5.1 Heat and Humidity of Inspired Gas

During normal breathing, the air is delivered to the carina at a temperature of 32°C and an absolute humidity of 30.4 mg H_2O/L [119]. The insertion of an ETT via the nose, mouth, or trachea bypasses the upper airway and causes the natural ability to heat and humidify inspired gas to be lost. The American Association for Respiratory Care states that devices should provide a minimum of 30 mg of H_2O/L of delivered gas at 30°C [120]. If inspired air is not warmed and humidified, the result is a dry, cool gas that is damaging to the respiratory tract and impedes mucociliary function. Secretions may become dry and inspissated, possibly leading to partial or complete occlusion of the ETT lumen. If left unrecognized, this occlusion may lead to barotrauma and death [93]. The most common method to protect against this situation is the use of

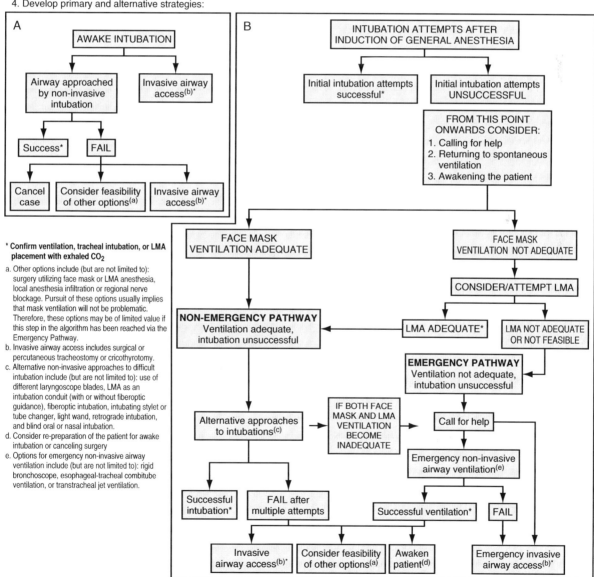

Figure 9.16 American Society of Anesthesiologists difficult airway algorithm. *LMA*, Laryngeal mask airway. *(Courtesy of American Society of Anesthesiologists, Park Ridge, IL.)*

> **Box 9.2 Contents of a Difficult Airway Cart**
> Fiberoptic bronchoscope and video monitoring system (optional), adult and pediatric sizes
> Magill and Krause forceps
> Solution atomizer
> Ovassapian and Williams airways
> Video laryngoscopy (various products available) blades, sizes for neonate to large adult
> Direct laryngoscopy Miller and Macintosh blades, sizes 1–4
> Intubating laryngeal mask airways, sizes 3–5 (or equivalent)
> Standard laryngeal mask airways, sizes 3–5 (or equivalent)
> Esophageal-tracheal Combitube (or King LT or EasyTube by Rüsch)
> Gum elastic bougies (various manufacturers)
> Airway exchange catheters, multiple sizes
> Endotracheal tubes, sizes 6–9, standard and Evac types (pediatric sizes if appropriate)
> Capnometric devices
> Cricothyroidotomy kit (purchased or hospital standardized)
> Retrograde intubation kit (Cook Critical Care)
> Percutaneous tracheostomy kit
> Medications kit (etomidate, propofol, ketamine, succinylcholine, rocuronium, intravenous and viscous lidocaine, atropine)

an active heated humidifier or a passive heat and moisture exchanger (HME) (Figure 9.17) [121].

HMEs are typically cylindrical devices that are fitted to the ventilator circuit, usually just proximal to the ETT connector and the Y-piece, with limited changes on airway mechanics [122,123]. This is the most effective HME placement for maximizing humidity and temperature retention in the patient circuit [121,124]. The materials provide heat, humidification, and filtering properties, earning the device the nickname, "artificial nose" [125]. They are lightweight and inexpensive, require no power source, and reduce circuit condensation, making them attractive alternatives to the more expensive heated humidifiers.

Use of heated humidifiers is associated with the production of almost 100% humidity in the inspiratory gas and is thus more effective than use of HMEs. These units require an external power source and additional circuitry, increasing cost. Accidental overheating can occur and may create additional damage to the airway if temperatures are not frequently monitored. There is no consensus about the proper duration of use of these implements. Multiple studies have failed to show a correlation of increased incidence of pneumonia with heated humidifiers versus HMEs or with frequent changes of HMEs or heated humidifiers. Therefore, frequent changes (i.e., more often than every 7 days) of ventilator circuits, unless they are visually soiled, is neither cost-effective nor medically efficacious [73,126–129].

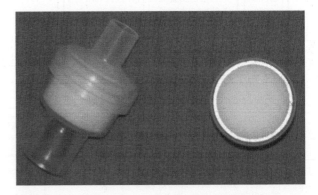

Figure 9.17 A heat and moisture exchanger.

9.5.2 Suctioning

Perhaps the simplest and most logical means of assisting with secretion clearance is direct suctioning. This modality is safe, but when it is performed carelessly, complications may occur, including soft tissue or airway trauma, aspiration, laryngospasm, increased intracranial pressure, bronchospasm, hypoxemia, and cardiac dysrhythmias [130]. Hypoxemia can be minimized with preoxygenation using a fraction of inspired oxygen (F_{IO_2}) of 100%. In patients with intracranial hypertension, mild hyperventilation or blunting of the cough reflex with instilled intravenous lidocaine just before suctioning may reduce the risks of additional increases in intracranial pressure. The evacuation procedure should be brief and intermittent. The vacuum should be applied only after the suction catheter has been advanced to its distal position. After each pass of the catheter, lung re-expansion with a few gentle manual breaths should be administered. Suctioning can be applied by a single-use open system in which the catheter is unprotected and open to the environment or by a closed system (Figure 9.18) that sheathes the catheter in a sterile protective covering.

Closed systems are usually incorporated into the ventilator breathing circuit at the junction of the Y-piece and the ETT or tracheostomy tube, allowing continued ventilation during suctioning with no need to disconnect the circuit. The advantage of not having to disconnect is important for patients who require aggressive ventilator management (e.g., high PEEP therapy), making them less susceptible to alveolar derecruitment compared with open suctioning. The retractable catheter does not add any additional restriction to airflow (when not deployed). There are concerns that colonization of these devices with aspiration of bacterial particles and cross-contamination may predispose to VAP [131]. Such concerns have led to differing opinions on the appropriate timing of any system changes. Kollef and coworkers randomly assigned patients to scheduled changes every 24 hours or to no change except when there was a malfunction or visible soiling [132]. In both groups, 15% of patients developed VAP. The only difference was in total cost: US$11,016 in the group with scheduled changes and US$837 in the group with no scheduled changes [132,133].

9.5.3 Subglottic Care

Secretion management has, by necessity, moved beyond the ETT lumen. Suctioning of secretions that are pooled above the ETT cuff, in the

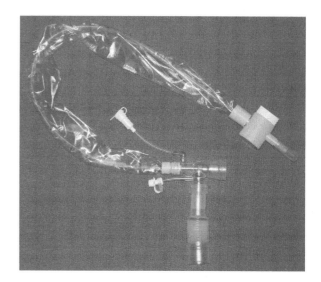

Figure 9.18 The Ballard closed endotracheal tube suctioning system.

subglottic space, is an important step in good tracheal care and is paramount in the prevention of VAP [111,132–137]. Subglottic suctioning has been shown to decrease the incidence of VAP in the ICU from 16% to 4% [135]. Specialized ETTs with dedicated subglottic suctioning ports are more expensive ($15 compared with $1 for a standard ETT) [138]. An interesting cost analysis done in 2003 demonstrated that despite this increased cost, the estimated cost benefit of an ETT with a subglottic suction port was $4,992 per case of VAP saved [138]. The U.S. Centers for Disease Control and Prevention (CDC) universally recommends the use of subglottic suctioning tubes in the ICU to help reduce the rate of VAP [139].

Subglottic suctioning can be done with small suction catheters that are advanced down the trachea until resistance is met from the ETT cuff. Another option is using ETTs with a subglottic port positioned just above the cuff. These specialized ETTs are certainly not infallible and do not replace vigilant airway care. It has been demonstrated that dysfunction of the suction lumen can occur almost 50% of the time [140]. In 43% of cases, the cause of the suction loss was determined to be prolapse of the tracheal mucosa into the subglottic suction port [140].

9.5.4 Bronchoscopy

The use of fiberoptic bronchoscopy for routine secretion management is not advocated. It is expensive, requires proficient training, and may produce

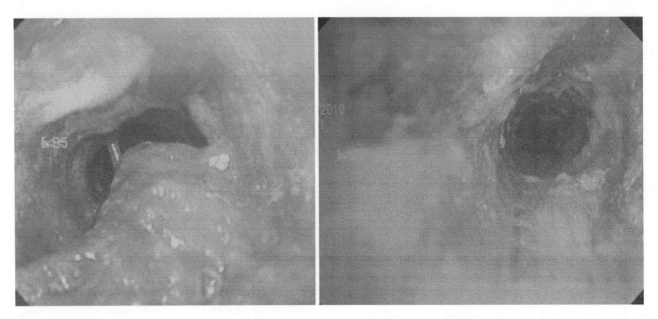

Figure 9.19 Examples of biofilm accumulation inside the lumen of an endotracheal tube.

complications such as barotrauma secondary to a marked reduction or cessation in expiratory airflow (depending on the relative airway caliber) in intubated patients [4]. It should be reserved for assisting with lobar collapse caused by mucus plugging or inspissated secretions not amenable to conventional mucolysis, to perform so-called pulmonary toilet bronchoscopy that may be needed after an inhalation injury to evaluate for tracheobronchial injury, to aid in the diagnosis of significant hemoptysis, or to assist with specimen procurement when clinical suspicion merits sampling.

9.5.5 Biofilm Management

Biofilm and adherence of secretions (Figure 9.19) within the ETT have been implicated in the development of VAP, increased WOB, delays in extubation, and other complications [141–144]. Biofilm can easily be identified by bronchoscopy on insertion of the scope into the ETT. Newer technologies using acoustic reflectometry have also been developed to help with monitoring the accumulation of biofilm and evaluating the integrity of the intubated airway. The SonarMed airway monitoring device (SonarMed, Indianapolis, IN) employs this technology to assess ETT positioning and movement as well as ETT patency hampered by either internal or external agents.

Traditional methods used to manage biofilm include catheter suctioning, bronchoscopic lavage, and ETT exchange. Catheter suctioning is often ineffective for biofilm removal, because its presence frequently evades detection as the suction catheter navigates the patent channel formed by the biofilm concretions, thereby leaving the impression that the lumen is patent. Bronchoscopic lavage and ETT exchange are hampered by significant costs and hazards for both practitioners and patients. Another option is a device that essentially scrapes the biofilm from the luminal surface of the ETT. The Complete Airway Management (CAM) Rescue Cath by Omneotech (Tavernier, FL) (Figure 9.20) resembles a Fogarty catheter used to remove a thrombus. This product has an inflatable balloon at the distal end of a catheter that is encased in a latticed netting to provide "traction" and atraumatic "abrasion" of the lumen. It is introduced into the ETT and advanced to the distal end (based on ETT and CAM depth markings); the balloon is then inflated, and the catheter is fully withdrawn back out through the proximal end of the catheter, along with any luminal biofilm. This device and procedure may prove to be a useful option in already hypoxic or PEEP-dependent patients in whom time-consuming bronchoscopies could be hazardous. The CAM Rescue Cath is also a good option for patients with a potentially difficult airway, in whom ETT exchange can pose a considerable risk [145].

Information on the prevention of biofilm formation is rife with conflicting data. One study showed no difference in rate of *Pseudomonas aeruginosa*

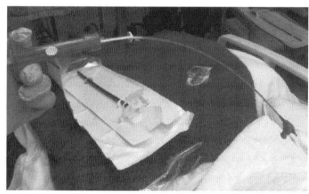
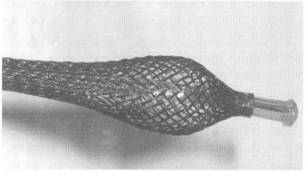

Figure 9.20 The Omneotech Complete Airway Management (CAM) Rescue Cath catheter. *(Courtesy of Omneotech, Tavernier, FL.)*

and *Staphylococcus epidermidis* biofilm formation among different ETT materials including PVC, silicone, stainless steel, and sterling silver [146]. More recently, however, ETTs coated in silver and chlorhexidine showed significantly reduced rates of biofilm colonization in a nonclinical setting [23,147]. The preventive management of biofilm may not be far in the future, but chlorhexidine-coated ETTs are currently not available. For now, the best strategy to manage biofilm is increased vigilance, fastidious respiratory care, and new technologies aimed at minimization and safe clearance.

9.6 Respiratory Therapies for the Intubated Patient

9.6.1 Secretion Clearance and Control Therapies

9.6.1.1 Mucolytic Agents

Agents used to decrease the viscosity of tracheobronchial secretions and assist with their reduction and clearance have been used for decades. The primary agent in use is *N*-acetylcysteine (NAC, Mucomyst). NAC is a sulfhydryl-containing compound; therefore, it is classified as a thiol. It has extensive first-pass metabolism in the gastrointestinal tract and liver when administered orally and is almost completely absorbed; only minimal amounts are excreted in the feces. The plasma half-life is approximately 2 hours, with virtually no detectable NAC at approximately 12 hours [148].

Most of NAC's biochemical effects appear to be related to its sulfhydryl group, which reduces the production hydroxyl radicals [148,149]. This effect has provided many uses for NAC beyond that of a mucolytic agent, including hepatic protection in acetaminophen overdose and renal protection against contrast-induced nephropathy [52,150]. NAC's effects on mucus viscosity result from its ability to disrupt the disulfide bridges and render them more liquid [133,148]. NAC is usually delivered by nebulizer in combination with a β_2-adrenergic agonist because it can induce bronchospasm [151]. Clinically, its effects have been variable in patients with chronic bronchitis, for whom oral NAC is used to assist with exacerbations and symptomatic relief [152–154]. Direct instillation of NAC during bronchoscopy may assist in secretion removal.

Another important factor in mucus viscosity is DNA content. DNA contributes to secretion viscosity because it accumulates from the degradation of bacteria and neutrophils. An agent that is considered mostly a mucokinetic agent, recombinant deoxyribonuclease (DNase, Pulmozyme), has been used in nebulized form in patients with bronchiectasis caused by cystic fibrosis with good results; however, it is expensive, and its use beyond this population of patients is not indicated [117,155,156].

One interesting therapy used in the population of burn patients who have an associated inhalation injury is nebulized heparin. Heparin assists with decreasing and removing bronchial casts that form with inhalation injury. Heparin's anticoagulant effects assist with removal of casts, and it may act as a free radical scavenger with anti-inflammatory effects. Although studies have not consistently shown a significant change in pulmonary function, cast formation and removal are favorably altered [157,158].

9.6.1.2 Chest Physiotherapy

Chest physiotherapy encompasses a variety of techniques that include position changes, percussion and vibration of the chest wall, and stimulation of a cough response. These are relatively dogmatic approaches that have historically provided poor results. They also tend to be burdensome to both the respiratory therapist and the patient. Newer, alternative techniques show promising results.

Percussion and Postural Drainage

Used extensively in patients with cystic fibrosis, the technique of percussion with postural drainage utilizes external percussion of the chest wall overlying the affected lung region. Percussion can be applied manually with a cupped hand or by an automated, usually pneumatic, device. The application of percussion or vibration, or both, to the chest wall functions to loosen the secretions in the bronchi and facilitate their mobilization [94,159]. A steep Trendelenburg position of 25 degrees or more is employed—less if the patient cannot tolerate that angle—to facilitate the gravitational effects on mucus clearance [77,160].

Relative contraindications to the postural component of this therapy are the presence of increased intracranial pressure; the possibility of an unprotected airway and the potential for aspiration; recent esophageal, ophthalmic, or intracranial surgery; congestive heart failure; and uncontrolled hypertension [120]. As for the application of percussion or vibration, placement of the technique over recent surgical sites (e.g., split-thickness skin grafts, rib fractures or chest trauma, pulmonary contusions, burns, unstable spine fractures) or in the presence of coagulopathies, subcutaneous emphysema, or bronchospasm are all relative contraindications [160]. Hazards include hypoxemia and accidental extubation.

Clinically and experimentally, the use of percussion with postural drainage in cystic fibrosis patients is well supported [161–163]. However, patients' compliance remains a concern, because the technique is burdensome for patients and caregivers.

Positive End-Expiratory Pressure Therapy

PEEP therapy, as a secretion clearance technique, creates a restriction to expiratory flow by means of a face mask or mouthpiece. The resistance is adjusted to 10 to 20 cm H_2O of back pressure during expiration, which allows airflow to move into distal airways and associated lung units, forcing past secretions and causing them to move toward the larger airways, where suctioning is more feasible. The maneuver is used with gentle and forceful coughs lasting up to 20 minutes and aerosolized medications that can be administered concurrently. Patients with an increased WOB or severe dyspnea may have difficulty performing this technique due to temporary lapses in ventilation. PEEP therapy is at least as effective for secretion clearance as percussion with postural drainage, if not more effective, and patient satisfaction is markedly more favorable [125,164,165].

Intrapulmonary Percussive Ventilation

Intrapulmonary percussive ventilation (IPV) can be delivered through a mouthpiece or to the end of the ETT. Its high-frequency percussive oscillations function to loosen retained secretions, expand airways and lungs, and reduce atelectasis. Conceptualized and designed by Dr. Forrest Bird, IPV uses a "phasetron"—a sliding venturi device capable of providing 5 to 35 cm H_2O pressure during oscillations of 2 to 5 Hz [166]. Aerosolized medications may also be delivered during IPV treatments. Favorable results have been reported for secretion clearance and lung expansion in patients with cystic fibrosis, as well as in other disorders with an increased incidence of thickened secretions [167,168]. IPV offers an advantage to patients who lack the ability to perform percussion with postural drainage or high PEEP therapies.

High-Frequency Chest Wall Compression

Therapy with high-frequency chest wall compression entails the wearing of an inflatable vest around the chest. Air is instilled into the vest bladder and then rapidly withdrawn in a cyclic manner, essentially creating an artificial cough. The high-frequency oscillations that are produced range from 5 to 25 Hz and can generate pressures as high as 50 cm H_2O. These oscillations create a gentle "squeezing" of the patient's chest that mimics small coughs. The frequency of the oscillations can be adjusted, and sensors in the vest can reduce the pressure delivered when the patient's chest expands (as with a sigh breath or a deep cough) [141]. Secretion clearance and improvement in mucus rheology have also been reported [169,170]. Perhaps the biggest drawback of this method is its cost, estimated at US$15,900 for each unit.

9.6.2 Overcoming Work of Breathing Imposed by Endotracheal Tubes, Tracheostomy Tubes, and Ventilator Circuits

With any translaryngeal intubation, the upper airway is bypassed and the resistance it imparts is thereby removed; however, there is still a substantial amount of work performed by the patient in an effort to ventilate. WOB is minimal during normal, quiet breathing, accounting for about 5% of the total oxygen consumption at rest. With increases in WOB, oxygen consumption can be markedly increased to as much as 30% or more [155]. This newly acquired increased demand may not be well tolerated by the critically ill patient. The additional WOB (WOB_{add}) imposed by the artificial airway and ventilator apparatus not only hinders weaning and liberation from mechanical ventilation but also impairs tissue oxygenation and alters critical blood flow, which may lead to worsened organ dysfunction [86]. To initiate a "breath" from the ventilator, a pressure differential across the ETT and circuit must be produced. The patient must overcome this resistance to initiate the demand flow needed for ventilation to occur. It has been shown experimentally that the ETT, the ventilator circuit, and the ventilator itself all add varying degrees of additional work for the patient to overcome, on top of the problems that initially necessitated intubation and mechanical ventilation [32,171].

9.6.2.1 Pressure Support

Various modalities have been designed to overcome WOB_{add} imposed by the artificial airway and ventilator [155]. One is pressure support (PS), which is used as either an adjunct or as a mode of ventilation to help the spontaneously breathing patient overcome the WOB_{add} imposed by an artificial airway [21,168,172]. A preset, flow-triggered inspiratory pressure chosen by the clinician is added to the airway opening pressure when inspiration is triggered by the patient. Because it is flow cycled, the patient can control the duration and depth of inspiration, and the PS ceases when some preset gas flow has diminished, usually about 25% of the maximal peak flow achieved [173]. PS has been shown to decrease WOB_{add} even with normal lungs [173,174]. However, in patients with obstructive pulmonary disease and expiratory flow limitation, breath stacking, or auto-PEEP, flow may not decelerate quickly enough, and active exhalation may be necessary to terminate the PS, thereby creating additional WOB [175]. The amount of inspiratory pressure added is usually 4 to 15 cm H_2O. Currently, it is recommended that PS be applied for all spontaneously breathing, intubated patients to assist with overcoming the resistance of the ETT or tracheostomy tube [176]. Additional PS may be necessary if tidal volumes or respiratory rates, or both, are inadequate to support oxygenation. Most patients tolerate PS well, but decreased tolerance in patients susceptible to expiratory flow limitation must be appreciated and accounted for in any management strategy.

9.6.2.2 Continuous Positive Airway Pressure

Continuous positive airway pressure (CPAP) is applied at end-exhalation in spontaneously breathing patients. Much like PEEP, CPAP is designed to offset the degree of atelectasis that occurs inherently in the intubated, supine patient. CPAP ranging from 4 to 10 cm H_2O should be provided for all spontaneously breathing patients in an effort to compensate for the loss of expiratory lung volumes and further promote oxygenation. So-called physiologic PEEP, an amount thought to rectify the aforementioned atelectasis, is theoretical but is estimated to be equivalent to 4 cm H_2O in the normal lung. The reduction in WOB seen with CPAP has been appreciated primarily in the setting of expiratory airflow reductions; in such cases, CPAP offsets the auto-PEEP, thereby reducing the work required to generate the next inspiratory effort [177]. The type of flow-triggered mechanism and the location at which the flow differential is measured (typically at the tracheal end of the ETT) have been shown experimentally to decrease the inspiratory WOB as well [178]. CPAP is usually applied in combination with added PS.

9.6.2.3 Automatic Tube Compensation

As stated previously, the ETT imposes a substantial degree of resistance to inspiration. The modalities described thus far assist with decreasing some of the work needed to overcome this burden. Added PS and PS ventilation help compensate for the resistance primarily encountered during inhalation but not during exhalation, and they are not consistently provided because of the varying flow across the ETT during normal breathing [179]. Much resistance to exhalation is also produced by the presence of an ETT. Indeed, the internal diameter of the ETT greatly affects this phenomenon, as do other factors such as gas flow rates, gas density and viscosity, and luminal secretions adherent to the ETT wall. Automatic tube compensation (ATC) is a feature on some newer ventilators. It is designed to assist with the resistance imposed by the ETT or tracheostomy tube during both the inspiratory and expiratory phases of the respiratory cycle. By altering the PS delivered—raising it during inspiration and lowering it during expiration according to the pressure-flow characteristics of the ETT—ATC adjusts for the resistance and the pressure drop across the ETT during spontaneous breathing. A computer assists by calculating the pressure difference across the ETT (ΔP^{ETT}) based on ETT size, measuring gas flow and airway pressure, and selecting the resistive properties of the ETT [179]. Unlike PS, ATC cannot be used as a ventilatory mode; it is merely an adjunct component to mechanical ventilation.

One drawback to ATC is the inability to correct for the reductions in airway diameter that can occur with secretions or kinking. This limitation results in an inaccurate measurement of ΔP^{ETT} such that ATC undercompensates for the pressure difference across the airway. A high index of suspicion is necessary to monitor for this possibility. Clinically, ATC has been shown to decrease the WOB_{add} encountered with ETTs and tracheostomy tubes [28]. When these modalities were used to assist with weaning and extubation of patients in a T-piece trial, there was no difference in the workload encountered with ATC and T-piece alone, whereas adding PS to the T-piece trial at 7 cm H_2O unloaded this additional work [180].

9.6.3 Pharmacologic Treatments
9.6.3.1 Inhalation Drug Delivery

The presence of an ETT does not limit drug delivery to the lungs and may actually enhance it. Many clinicians take advantage of this route of administration. The two predominant methods used to deliver agents are metered-dose inhalers (MDIs) and nebulizers. The drugs delivered by these devices are most commonly bronchodilators, mucolytics, corticosteroids, and antibiotics. For pulmonary ailments, inhaled drugs achieve efficacy comparable to or exceeding that of systemically delivered drugs with a smaller dose [181–183]. Tracheal administration of some traditionally systemic drugs often requires much higher doses to ensure absorption.

Inhalation drug delivery has other advantages over systemic administration. Systemic side effects can be reduced, because systemic absorption is markedly decreased. Variable reports regarding penetration and distribution of an aerosol to the lower respiratory tract range from 0% to 42% with nebulizers and 0.3% to 98% with MDIs. However, when the delivery method was standardized, the amount delivered in either method was similar, about 15% [184–186].

Particle size also plays an important role in delivery. The larger the particle, the less likely it is to be delivered distally to the alveoli. Aerosol particles ranging between 1 and 5 μm are optimal for proper deposition [181,182,185,187]. The density of the gas carrying the aerosol also influences the delivery in an inverse relationship. Improvement in delivery has been reported when a mixture of helium and oxygen was used in the ventilator circuits of both MDIs and nebulizers [183,188].

Nebulizers

The performance of a nebulizer depends on multiple factors including the model, operating pressure, flow rate, and volume of diluent utilized. Nebulizers are capable of generating aerosols with particle sizes of 1 to 3 μm, and the size produced is inversely influenced by the flow rate or pressure used: the greater the flow rate, the smaller the particle [181,182]. Nebulizers may be used continuously or intermittently. Intermittent use appears to be more efficient than continuous delivery, with less waste of aerosol demonstrated [189]. Placing a nebulizer upstream from the Y-piece and ETT also increases drug delivery [187,189,190]. Interestingly, the use of continuous drug nebulization may impair the ability of the patient to initiate a negative-pressure inspiratory effort in the PS mode of ventilation, thereby leading to hypoventilation [168,191].

Metered-Dose Inhalers

An MDI delivers medication in combination with a mixture of pressurized propellants, preservatives, flavoring agents, and surfactants. The final concentration of active drug constitutes about 1% of the total volume in the canister [181]. When the stem on the MDI canister is depressed, a finite amount of drug is released at a certain velocity, and a spray cloud develops. Various adapters are available that fit in line with the ventilator circuit or on the end of the ETT as so-called elbow adapters to aid in the administration of inhalational therapies. Chambers or spacers appear to provide better delivery of aerosol compared with the more commonly used elbow adapters [192]. MDIs typically cause more aerosol deposition on the ETT than nebulizers do, decreasing the amount of drug delivered. These particles, in turn, adhere to the ETT. This problem can be reduced by using a spacer and performing the administration with meticulous attention to timing of the ventilatory cycle: it is most effective during inspiration and when synchronized with the patient's spontaneous effort. Dhand and Tobin reported excellent results with their technique of MDI delivery [189].

When comparing the overall efficacy of nebulizers versus that of MDIs, several factors favor the use of MDIs in mechanically ventilated patients. Nebulizers may become colonized with bacteria and help to deliver an aerosolized inoculum. Bowton and colleagues reported a potential saving of US$300,000 annually with the use of MDIs compared with nebulizers [193].

9.6.3.2 Inhaled Bronchodilators

Airway reactivity is a ubiquitous consequence of airway manipulation that hinders respiratory function and prolongs the duration of mechanical ventilation. Additional pathophysiologic processes attributed to persistent bronchospastic disease that serve to prolong mechanical ventilation include mucosal inflammation that persists and promotes further mucus production, airway hyperemia and resultant edema, and the consequent narrowing of small airways leading to an increase in closing volume. These processes adversely affect oxygenation as functional residual capacity is decreased and CO_2 elimination, as expiratory flow, is limited. At extremes of expiratory flow limitation, generous amounts of intrinsic PEEP (auto-PEEP) are generated; this can impede cardiac filling by reducing preload, and hypotension and cardiac arrest may result. The physical effects of auto-PEEP are not limited to the cardiovascular system. The obvious effects of alveolar overdistention include an increased physiologic dead space and the potential for barotrauma, especially when controlled positive-pressure mechanical ventilation is instituted. Pneumothorax, pneumomediastinum, and pneumoperitoneum may all occur as a result, as may patient-ventilator dysynchrony.

Many maneuvers are available to reduce the effects of bronchospasm (and higher airway pressures), including decreasing the respiratory rate, prolonging the expiratory time, decreasing the tidal volume, and increasing the inspiratory flow rate. Pharmacologically, the use of β-adrenergic agonists, specifically $β_2$-agonists such as albuterol, is the mainstay therapy. $β_2$-receptors on bronchial smooth muscle promote relaxation and dilation of the airway diameter when stimulated. Systemic methylxanthines such as theophylline do not add much benefit in the acute stage of treating bronchospasm or reactive airways. Their narrow therapeutic window and vast side effect profile increase potential toxicity.

$β_2$-agonists also have a beneficial effect on respiratory cilia in that they cause an increase in ciliary beat frequency [194]. This phenomenon is mediated by β-adrenergic receptors and can be attenuated with nonselective beta-blocking agents. An increase in the frequency of ciliary beating promotes mucus clearance over the respiratory epithelium. Other effects include increased water secretion onto the airway surface, which facilitates mucus clearance [195]. Indeed, the beneficial effects of β-agonists on bronchial reactivity and mucociliary clearance are evident. However, there are data suggesting a more robust effect in healthier airways than in chronically diseased airways such as those seen in patients with chronic bronchitis, possibly due to downregulation and chronic attenuation [196]. Newer formulations of inhaled β-agonists such as levalbuterol may have reduced side effect profiles and possibly improved outcomes.

9.6.3.3 Anticholinergics

Although inhaled β-agonists are pivotal in the reduction of airway reactivity, the use of inhaled anticholinergics such as ipratropium bromide or the newer tiotropium bromide needs to be emphasized, given their obvious synergistic effect with β-agonists. It is well appreciated that many of the mechanisms of airway reactivity and inflammation associated with bronchospastic disease are cholinergically mediated. In patients with chronic obstructive pulmonary disease, the use of these agents alone or in combination with β-agonists is the foundation for rescue therapy and a mainstay in chronic management [183].

9.6.3.4 Corticosteroids

Inhaled glucocorticoid therapy has become a mainstay of treatment in various obstructive respiratory ailments, including chronic obstructive pulmonary disease and asthma. This class of medicines unquestionably has disease-specific effects at the target organ. Equally interesting is the fact that administration in an aerosol preparation magnifies their effects while markedly reducing their side effect profile, leading to a lower risk-benefit value. Targeted efficacy with minimal adverse effects helps to quantify an appropriate risk-benefit value [197,198]. High lung deposition or targeting, high receptor binding, longer pulmonary retention, and high lipid conjugation are among the pharmacokinetic parameters that lead to improved efficacy of these compounds and should be considered. A low or negligible oral bioavailability, smaller particle size leading to a relatively inactive drug at the oropharynx, higher plasma protein binding, increased metabolism rates, higher clearances, and lower systemic concentrations are associated with lower risks for adverse effects [197–199].

For individuals who require long-term care with inhaled glucocorticoids during ventilator dependency, therapy should be continued to minimize the underlying disease process and thereby decrease the number of new variables, including adrenal insufficiency, in the treatment equation with inhaled or intravenous formulations [200]. Despite all of these perceived benefits, inhaled glucocorticoids do not seem to reduce mortality [201]. Acute exacerbations tend to be treated with intravenous or oral preparations due to the higher doses required.

9.6.3.5 Inhaled Antibiotics

Inhaled antibiotics have been used for decades, falling in and out of favor over the years. They are used primarily for treatment and suppression of chronic airway bacterial colonization. Their theoretical advantages are improved drug delivery and higher concentrations at the site of infection, leading to improved efficacy and better bacterial eradication compared with systemic administration [90,202–204]. The primary concern with this therapy is development of bacterial resistance.

Results differ on efficacy. Inhaled antibiotics, mainly aminoglycosides, have been used extensively in cystic fibrosis patients with good results [90,202–205]. Palmer and colleagues reported a marked reduction in the volume of airway secretions and a decrease in the laboratory markers of inflammation in a prospective study of mechanically ventilated patients with chronic respiratory failure [90,205]. However, their study lacked power and was not randomized.

Other studies have failed to show similar benefits but rather have demonstrated poor, unpredictable drug delivery [206]. Unequal ventilation, atelectasis, lobar collapse, and consolidation impair even drug distribution. Bronchospasm with chest tightness has also been reported [134]. Use of inhaled antibiotics should be limited to selected patients, such as those with cystic fibrosis. Routine use to assist with secretion reduction and clearance in the mechanically ventilated patient is not recommended.

9.6.4 Positioning of the Patient

The appropriate position in which to maintain the patient requiring mechanical ventilation has been debated. Current recommendations from the CDC state that elevating the head 30 to 40 degrees reduces the risk of VAP. A study examining head elevation and the rate of VAP concluded early after interim analysis showed an incidence of microbiologically confirmed pneumonia of 5% in semirecumbent patients versus 23% in supine patients [207]. The semirecumbent position has also been supported with regard to facilitating nursing care and decreasing gastric reflux and resultant aspiration. It has not been shown to have an effect on the hemodynamic status of the patient, although this remains a common theoretical concern [208].

Special beds that provide continuous lateral rotation have been used for patients who cannot be repositioned easily, such as those with severe head or traumatic brain injury, bariatric patients, and those who are pharmacologically paralyzed (e.g., patients with acute respiratory distress syndrome [ARDS]). These beds are advertised to enhance skin care, reduce thrombotic events, and improve pulmonary function. Their use is proposed to reduce atelectasis and, hence, pneumonia formation; however, studies' results have remained conflicting [209,210].

Occasionally, in severe cases of ARDS, alternative positioning (prone) may be necessary to facilitate ventilation and oxygenation. This method attempts to combat the physiologic shunt that is responsible for the observed hypoxemia. The prone position improves oxygenation by increasing lung volume, recruiting posterior lung fields, and redistributing perfusion [211]. No statistical difference was shown in a meta-analysis of the data for prone positioning of patients, although a small subset of patients with severe ARDS has been shown to benefit [212,213]. However, prone positioning is not without risks, particularly an increased risk for bed sores and ETT complications such as dislodgement [212]. Recently, a bed has become commercially available that possesses the ability to fully prone the patient, making use of this potentially beneficial intervention more dependent on necessity than caregiver feasibility. (Rotoprone, KCI Therapeutic Support Systems, San Antonio, TX.)

9.7 Conclusions

The establishment and maintenance of a secure and dependable airway is paramount in the care of the critically ill patient. From the very onset of admission to the ICU, care of the airway should begin with surveillance and a determination of which airways will be difficult to secure or difficult to maintain. The proper choice of an artificial airway not only facilitates ventilatory requirements for improved oxygenation but protects the patient from untoward iatrogenic problems encountered with instrumentation. Regardless of the intervention, an unfettered vigilance is the key to improved outcomes. Proper ETT care, early performance of a tracheostomy (when indicated), frequent pulmonary hygiene, and the use of established protocols and proven preventive measures should help to ensure safe and successful outcomes in critically ill patients.

9.8 Clinical Pearls

- Polyurethane endotracheal tube (ETT) cuffs that have high-volume, low-pressure (HVLP) cuffs are capable of conforming to the irregular borders of the tracheal lumen and therefore are more effective at preventing microaspiration.
- ETT placement has mechanical and physiologic consequences. Vigilant surveillance of skin hygiene, airway patency, cuff integrity, and ventilatory support must be realized to minimize injury and maximize support.
- Confirmation of ETT placement is necessary to aid in proper resuscitation efforts. Verification by the presence of end-tidal carbon dioxide, whether by capnography or capnometry or by direct or indirect visualization, is mandatory to ensure appropriate placement.
- Cuff leak evaluation is a multifaceted endeavor requiring vigilance, diligence, and skill. An appropriate analysis of the potential cause, scrutinized against the risks and benefits of ETT exchange, must occur with limited interference to homeostasis.
- ETT exchange, whether for biofilm accumulation and luminal obstruction, ETT cuff damage (cuff leak), or other ETT mechanical failure (e.g., kinking) is a high-risk ordeal. The decision to exchange an ETT should be assessed against newer, currently available technologies, such as biofilm extraction, that are designed to salvage damaged ETTs. Should the decision to perform an exchange arise, airway adjuncts such as an airway exchange catheter and video laryngoscopy have proved invaluable for achieving higher success rates.
- Once an ETT is in place, efforts must be aggressive and perpetual to decrease the risk of ventilator-associated pneumonia (VAP); these efforts range from acid-suppression therapies to use of specially designed ETTs to advanced nursing care regimens. VAP appears to be more multifaceted than previously believed. Subglottic suctioning and biofilm management are just the beginning steps.
- Any area of a facility that deals with intubated patients should have a readily accessible difficult airway cart. The cart should be well outfitted but tailored to the types of airways managed and familiar as well as specific for the providers who respond to such emergencies.

- As with pulmonary artery catheters, it is not the difficult airway cart that manages the airway but the personnel who utilize it.
- It is better to investigate any perceived ETT problem electively than to deal with its consequences after it becomes an acute emergency.
- The landscape of ETT design, construction, and maintenance has changed and will continue to change over the next decade. Not all variations will prove effective, but improved patient care will take place.

References

[1] Macewan W. Rep Br Med J 1880;2:122.
[2] Condon HA, Gilchrist E. Stanley rowbotham: twentieth century pioneer anaesthetist. Anaesthesia 1986;41:46−52.
[3] Wong J, Keens T, Wannamaker E, et al. Effects of gravity in tracheal transport rates in normal subjects and in patients with cystic fibrosis. Pediatrics 1977;60:146−52.
[4] Matsushima Y, Jones R, King E, et al. Alterations in pulmonary mechanics and gas exchange during routine fiberoptic bronchoscopy. Chest 1984;86:184.
[5] Lotano R, Gerber D, Aseron C, et al. Utility of postintubation radiographs in the intensive care unit. Crit Care 2000;4:50−3.
[6] Sim WS, Chung IS, Chin JU, et al. Risk factors for epistaxis during nasotracheal intubation. Anaesth Intens Care 2002;30:449−52.
[7] Dullenkopf A, Gerber A, Weiss M. Fluid leakage past tracheal tube cuffs: evaluation of the microcuff endotracheal tube. Intens Care Med 2003;29:1849−53.
[8] Mulier J, Van den Brande F, Dilleman B, et al. Tracheal cuff leak in morbidly obese patients intubated with a Taperguard™, Hi-Lo™ Cuffed and Hi-Lo™ Cuffed and lubricated tracheal tube. Abstract P-9108. Presented at the 63rd PostGraduate assembly. New York; December 12, 2009.
[9] Spiegel JE. Endotracheal tube cuffs: design and function. Anesthesiology news guide to airway management. New York: McMahon Publishing; 2010; pp 51−58.
[10] Poelart J, Depuydt P, De Wolf A, et al. Polyurethane cuffed endotracheal tubes to prevent early postoperative pneumonia after cardiac surgery: a pilot study. J Thorac Cardiovasc Surg 2008;135:771−6.
[11] TaperGuard Evac endotracheal tube FDA 510 (k) application K090352. U.S. Food and Drug Administration 2009.
[12] Ho AM, Contardi LH. What to do when an endotracheal tube cuff leaks. J Trauma 1996; 40:486−7.
[13] Short JA. An unusual cause of tracheal tube cuff damage. Anaesthesia 1997;52:93−4.
[14] Verborgh C, Camu F. Management of cuff incompetence in an endotracheal tube. Anesthesiology 1987;66:441.
[15] Chua WL, Ng AS. A defective endotracheal tube. Singapore Med J 2002;43:476−8.
[16] Gettelman TA, Morris GN. Endotracheal tube failure: undetected by routine testing. Anesth Analg 1995;81:1313.
[17] Heusner JE, Viscomi CM. Endotracheal tube cuff failure due to valve damage. Anesth Analg 1991;72:270.
[18] Mesa A, Miguel R. Hidden damage to a reinforced LMA-Fastrach endotracheal tube. Anesth Analg 2000;90:1250−1.
[19] Kovatsis PG, Fiadjoe JE, Stricker PA. Simple, reliable replacement of pilot balloons for a variety of clinical situations. Pediatr Anesth 2010;20:490−4.
[20] Sprung J, Bourke DL, Thomas P, et al. Clever cure for an endotracheal tube cuff leak. Anesthesiology 1994;81:790−1.
[21] Kuhlen R, Max M, Dembinski R, et al. Breathing pattern and workload during automatic tube compensation, pressure support and T-piece trials in weaning patients. Eur J Anaesthesiol 2003;20:10−6.
[22] Adair CG, Gorman SP, O'Neill FB, et al. Selective decontamination of the digestive tract (SDD) does not prevent the formation of microbial biofilms on the endotracheal tubes. J Antimicrob Chemother 1993;31:689−97.
[23] Chastre J, Fagon JY. Ventilator-associated pneumonia. Am J Respir Crit Care Med 2002;165:867−903.
[24] Balazs DJ, Triandafillu K, Wood P, et al. Surface modification of PVC endotracheal tube surfaces to reduce *Pseudomonas aeruginosa* adhesion: plasma processing and chemical methods. Eur Cells Mater 2003;6 (Suppl. 1):86.

[25] Divatia JV, Bhowmick K. Complications of endotracheal intubation and other airway management procedures. Indian J Anaesth 2005;49:308–18.

[26] Mort TC. Emergency tracheal intubation: complications associated with repeated laryngoscopic attempts. Anesth Analg 2004;99:607–13.

[27] Gelman JJ, Aro M, Weiss SM. Tracheo-innominate artery fistula. J Am Coll Surg 1994;179:626–34.

[28] Hawkins DB. Glottic and subglottic stenosis from endotracheal intubation. Laryngoscope 1977;87:339.

[29] Weber S. Traumatic complications of airway management. Anesth Clin North Am 2002;20:503–12.

[30] Sois M, Dillon F. What is the safest foil tape for endotracheal tube protection during Nd-YAG laser surgery? A comparative study. Anesthesiology 1990;72:553.

[31] Bolder PM, Healy TE, Bolder AR, et al. The extra work of breathing through adult endotracheal tubes. Anesth Analg 1986;65:853–9.

[32] Bersten AD, Rutten AJ, Vedig AE, et al. Additional work of breathing imposed by endotracheal tubes, breathing circuits, and intensive care ventilators. Crit Care Med 1989;17:671–7.

[33] Gal TJ, Suratt PM. Resistance to breathing in healthy subjects following endotracheal intubation under topical anesthesia. Anesth Analg 1980;59:270–4.

[34] Demers RR, Sullivan MJ, Paliotta J. Airflow resistance of endotracheal tubes. JAMA 1977;237:1362.

[35] Schwartz DE, Lieberman JA, Cohen NH. Women are at a greater risk than men for malpositioning of the endotracheal tube after emergent intubation. Crit Care Med 1994;22:1127–31.

[36] Tanigawa K, Takeda T, Goto E, et al. The efficacy of esophageal detector devices in verifying tracheal tube placement: a randomized cross-over study of out-of-hospital cardiac arrest patients. Anesth Analg 2001;92:375–8.

[37] Sahn SA, Lakshminarayan S, Petty TL. Weaning from mechanical ventilation. JAMA 1976;235:2208–12.

[38] Stout DM, Bishop MJH, Dwersteg JF, et al. Correlation of endotracheal tube size with sore throat and hoarseness following general anesthesia. Anesthesiology 1987;67:419–21.

[39] Shapiro BA. Chest physical therapy administered by respiratory therapists. Respir Care 1981;26:655–6.

[40] Miller AB, Pavia D, Agnew JE, et al. Effect of oral N-acetylcysteine on mucus clearance. Br J Dis Chest 1985;79:262–6.

[41] Bryce DP, Briant TD, Pearson FG. Laryngeal and tracheal complications of intubation. Ann Otol Rhinol Laryngol 1968;77:442–61.

[42] Sullivan M, Paliotta J, Saklad M. Endotracheal tube as a factor in measurement of respiratory mechanics. J Appl Physiol 1976;41:590–2.

[43] Henschke CI, Yankelevitz DF, Wand A, et al. Accuracy and efficacy of chest radiography in the intensive care unit. Radiol Clin North Am 1996;34:21–31.

[44] Hilding AC. Laryngotracheal damage during intratracheal anesthesia. Ann Otol Rhinol Laryngol 1971;80:565–81.

[45] Bishop MJ, Weymuller EA, Fink BR. Laryngeal effects of prolonged intubation. Anesth Analg 1984;63:335–42.

[46] Stone DJ, Bogdonoff DL. Airway considerations in the management of patients requiring long-term endotracheal intubation. Anesth Analg 1992;74:276–87.

[47] Stenqvist O, Sonander H, Nilsson K. Small endotracheal tubes: ventilator and intratracheal pressures during controlled ventilation. Br J Anaesth 1979;51:375–81.

[48] Carrion MI, Ayuso D, Marcos M, et al. Accidental removal of endotracheal and nasogastric tubes and intravascular catheters. Crit Care Med 2000;28:63–6.

[49] Roberts JR, Spadafora M, Cone DC. Proper depth placement of oral endotracheal tubes in adults prior to radiographic confirmation. Acad Emerg Med 1995;2:20–4.

[50] Ornato JP, Garnett AR, Glauser FL. Relationship between cardiac output and the end-tidal carbon dioxide tension. Ann Emerg Med 1990;19:1104–6.

[51] Hermens JM, Bennett MJ, Hirschman CA. Anesthesia for laser surgery. Anesth Analg 1983;62:218–29.

[52] Sosis MB, Dillon FX. Saline-filled cuffs help prevent laser-induced polyvinylchloride

endotracheal tube fires. Anesth Analg 1991; 72:187—9.
[53] Stamm AM. Ventilator-associated pneumonia and frequency of circuit changes. Am J Infect Control 1998;26:71—3.
[54] Cozine K, Rosenbaum LM, Askanazi J, et al. Laser-induced endotracheal tube fire. Anesthesiology 1981;55:553—83.
[55] Sosis MB. Hazards of laser surgery. Semin Anesth 1990;9:90.
[56] Smilkstein MJ, Knapp GL, Kulig KW, et al. Efficacy of oral N-acetylcysteine in the treatment of acetaminophen overdose: analysis of the national multicenter study (1976—1985). N Engl J Med 1988;319:1557—62.
[57] Barash PG, Cullen BF, Stoelting RK, editors. Clinical anesthesia. 6th ed. Philadelphia: Lippincott-Raven; 2009.
[58] Sole ML, Poalillo FE, Byers JF, et al. Bacterial growth in secretions and on suctioning equipment of orally intubated patients: a pilot study. Am J Crit Care 2002;11:141—9.
[59] Baughman RP. Diagnosis of ventilator-associated pneumonia. Microbes Infect 2005; 7:262—7.
[60] Grap MJ, Cantley M, Munro CL, et al. Use of backrest elevation in critical care: a pilot study. Am J Crit Care 1999;8:475—80.
[61] Berra L, De Marchi L, Panigada M, et al. Evaluation of continuous aspiration of subglottic secretion in an in vivo study. Crit Care Med 2004;32:2071—8.
[62] Dezfulian C, Shojania K, Collard HR, et al. Subglottic secretion drainage for preventing ventilator-associated pneumonia: a meta-analysis. Am J Med 2005;118:11—8.
[63] Kollef MH, Shapiro SD, Boyd V, et al. A randomized clinical trial comparing an extended-use hygroscopic condenser humidifier with heated-water humidification in mechanically ventilated patients. Chest 1998; 113:759—67.
[64] Manthous CA, Chatila W, Schmidt GA, et al. Treatment of bronchospasm by a metered-dose inhaler albuterol in mechanically ventilated patients. Chest 1995;107:210—3.
[65] Berra L, De Marchi L, Yu ZX, et al. Endotracheal tubes coated with antiseptics decrease bacterial colonization of the ventilator circuits, lungs, and endotracheal tube. Anesthesiology 2004;100:1446—56.
[66] Pacheco-Fowler V, Gaonkar T, Wyer PC, et al. Antiseptic impregnated endotracheal tubes for the prevention of bacterial colonization. J Hosp Infect 2004;57:170—4.
[67] Pai VB, Nahata MC. Efficacy and safety of aerosolized tobramycin in cystic fibrosis. Pediatr Pulmonol 2001;32:314—27.
[68] Keck JP, Mort TC. Supraglottic airway devices for rescue during emergency airway management in the remote location. Abstract 476. Presented at the 40th annual congress of the society for critical care medicine. San Diego, CA; January 2011.
[69] Seegobin RD, van Hasselt GL. Endotracheal cuff pressure and tracheal mucosal blood flow: endoscopic study of effects of four large volume cuffs. Br Med J 1984;288:965—8.
[70] Goldberg JS, Rawle PR, Zehnder JL, et al. Colorimetric end-tidal carbon dioxide monitoring for tracheal intubation. Anesth Analg 1990;70:191—4.
[71] Kasper CL, Deem S. The self-inflating bulb to detect esophageal intubation during emergency airway management. Anesthesiology 1998;88:898—902.
[72] Lang DJ, Wafai Y, Salem MR, et al. Efficacy of the self-inflating bulb in confirming tracheal intubation in the morbidly obese. Anesthesiology 1996;85:246—53.
[73] Tanigawa K, Takeda T, Goto E, et al. Accuracy and reliability of the self-inflating bulb to verify tracheal intubation in out-of-hospital cardiac arrest patients. Anesthesiology 2000;93:1432—6.
[74] Cook RT, Moglia BB, Consevage NW, et al. The use of the beck airway airflow monitor for verifying intratracheal endotracheal tube placement in patients in the pediatric emergency department and intensive care unit. Pediatr Emerg Care 1996;12:331—2.
[75] Cook RT, Stene JK, Marcolina B. Use of a beck airway airflow monitor and controllable-tip endotracheal tube in two cases on nonlaryngoscopic oral intubation. Am J Emerg Med 1995;13:180—3.
[76] Cook RT, Stene JK. The BAAM and endotrol endotracheal tube for blind oral intubation. Beck airway air flow monitor. J Clin Anesth 1993;5:431—2.

[77] Schwartz DE, Matthay MA, Cohen NH. Death and other complications of emergency airway management in critically ill adults: a prospective investigation of 297 tracheal intubations. Anesthesiology 1995;82:367–76.

[78] Andersen KH, Hald A. Assessing the position of the tracheal tube: the reliability of different methods. Anaesthesia 1989;44:984–5.

[79] Rao S, Wilson DW, Brooks RA. Acute effects of nebulization of N-acetylcysteine on pulmonary mechanics and gas exchange. Am Rev Respir Dis 1970;102:17–22.

[80] Andres AH, Langenstein H. The esophageal detector device is unreliable when the stomach has been ventilated. Anesthesiology 1999;91:566–8.

[81] Leigh JM, Maynard JP. Pressure on the tracheal mucosa from cuffed tubes. Br Med J 1979;1(6172):1173–4.

[82] Tasaki O, Mozingo DW, Dubick MA, et al. Effects of heparin and lisofylline on pulmonary function after smoke inhalation injury in an ovine model. Crit Care Med 2002;30:637–43.

[83] Tepel M, Van Der Giet M, Schwarzfeld C, et al. Prevention of radiographic-contrast-agent-induced reductions in renal function by acetylcysteine. N Engl J Med 2000;343:180–4.

[84] Goodman LR, Conrardy PA, Laing F, et al. Radiographic evaluation of endotracheal tube position. AJR Am J Roentgenol 1976;127:433–4.

[85] Grenvik A, Ayres SM, Holbrook PR, editors. Textbook of critical care. 4th ed. Philadelphia: WB Saunders; 2000.

[86] Haberthur C, Fabry B, Stocker R, et al. Additional inspiratory work of breathing imposed by tracheostomy tubes and non-ideal ventilator properties in critically ill patients. Intens Care Med 1999;25:514–9.

[87] Reed DB, Clinton JE. Proper depth of placement of nasotracheal tubes in adults prior to radiographic confirmation. Acad Emerg Med 1997;4:1111–4.

[88] Hill BB, Zweng TN, Maley RH, et al. Percutaneous dilational tracheostomy. J Trauma 1996;41:238–44.

[89] Scott LR, Benson MS, Bishop MJ. Relationship of endotracheal tube size to auto-PEEP at high minute ventilation. Respir Care 1986;31:1080–2.

[90] Palmer LB, Smaldone GC, Simon SR, et al. Aerosolized antibiotics in mechanically ventilated patients: delivery and response. Crit Care Med 1998;26:31–9.

[91] Salem MR. Verification of endotracheal tube position. Anesthesiol Clin North Am 2001;19:813–39.

[92] Ricard JD, Le Miere E, Markowicz P, et al. Efficiency and safety of mechanical ventilation with a heat and moisture exchanger changed only once a week. Am J Respir Crit Care Med 2000;16:1104–9.

[93] Mehta S. Transtracheal illumination for optimal tracheal tube placement: a clinical study. Anaesthesia 1989;44:970–2.

[94] Mortensen J, Falk M, Groth S, et al. Effects of postural drainage and positive expiratory pressure physiotherapy on tracheobronchial clearance in cystic fibrosis. Chest 1991;100:1350–7.

[95] Pattnaik SK, Bodra R. Ballottability of cuff to confirm the correct intratracheal position of the endotracheal tube in the intensive care unit. Eur J Anaesthesiol 2000;17:587–90.

[96] Puntervoll SA, Søreide E, Jacewicz W, et al. Rapid detection of oesophageal intubation: take care when using colorimetric capnometry. Acta Anaesthesiol Scand 2002;46:455–7.

[97] Curiel-Garcia JA, Guerrero-Romero F, Rodriguez-Moran M. Cuff pressure in endotracheal intubation: should it be routinely measured. Gac Mex Med 2001;137:179–82.

[98] Stewart S, Secrest JA, Norwood BR, et al. A comparison of endotracheal tube cuff pressures using estimation techniques and direct intracuff measurement. AANA J 2003;71:443–7.

[99] Hoffman RJ, Parwani V, Hahn IH. Experienced emergency medicine physicians cannot inflate or estimate endotracheal tube cuff pressure using standard techniques. Am J Emerg Med 2006;24:139–43.

[100] Sengupta P, Sessler DI, Maglinger P, et al. Endotracheal tube cuff pressure in three hospitals and the volume required to produce appropriate cuff pressure. BMC Anesthesiol 2004;4(1):8.

[101] Habib MP. Physiologic implications of artificial airways. Chest 1989;96:180–4.

[102] Levine SA, Niederman MS. The impact of tracheal intubations on host defenses and risks for nosocomial pneumonia. Clin Chest Med 1991;12:523–43.

[103] Dobrin P, Canfield T. Cuffed endotracheal tubes: mucosal pressures and tracheal wall blood flow. Am J Surg 1977;133:562–8.

[104] Lorente L, Lecuona M, Jiménez A, et al. Influence of an endotracheal tube with polyurethane cuff and subglottic secretion drainage on pneumonia. Am J Respir Crit Care Med 2007;176:1079–183.

[105] Clarke T, Evans S, Way P, et al. A comparison of two methods of securing an endotracheal tube. Aust Crit Care 1998;11:45–50.

[106] Levy H, Griego L. A comparative study of oral endotracheal tube securing methods. Chest 1993;104:1537–40.

[107] Chevron V, Menard JF, Richard JC, et al. Unplanned extubation: risk factors of development and predictive criteria for reintubation. Crit Care Med 1998;26:1049–53.

[108] Coppolo DP, May JJ. Self-extubations: a 12-month experience. Chest 1990;98:165–9.

[109] Tomkiewicz RP, App EM, De Sanctis GT, et al. A comparison of a new mucolytic N-acetylcysteine L-lysinate with N-acetylcysteine: airway epithelial changes and mucus changes in dog. Pulm Pharmacol 1995;8:259–65.

[110] Barnason S, Graham J, Wild MC, et al. Comparison of two endotracheal tube securement techniques on unplanned extubation, oral mucosa, and facial skin integrity. Heart Lung 1998;27:409–17.

[111] Kollef MH, Prentice D, Shapiro SD, et al. Mechanical ventilation with or without daily changes of in-line suction catheters. Am J Respir Crit Care Med 1997;156:466–72.

[112] Kaplow R, Bookbinder M. A comparison of four endotracheal tube holders. Heart Lung 1994;23:59–66.

[113] American Society of Anesthesiologists Task Force on Difficult Airway Management: practice guideline for management of the difficult airway. Anesthesiology 2003;98:1269–77.

[114] Keck JP, Mort TC. Video laryngoscopy vs. direct laryngoscopy for airway evaluation prior to extubation. Abstract A906. Presented at the American Society of Anesthesiologists annual meeting. New Orleans, LA; October 2009.

[115] Peruzzi WT, Smith B. Bronchial hygiene therapy. Crit Care Clin 1995;11:79–96.

[116] Pollack Jr CV. The laryngeal mask airway: a comprehensive review for the emergency medicine physician. J Emerg Med 2001;20:53–66.

[117] Barker AF, Bronchiectasis N. Engl J Med 2002;346:1383–93.

[118] Bartlett RH. Postoperative pulmonary prophylaxis: breathe deeply and read carefully. Chest 1982;81:1–3.

[119] McFadden ER, Pichurko BM, Bowman HF, et al. Thermal mapping of the airways in humans. J Appl Physiol 1985;58:564–70.

[120] American Association for Respiratory Care: AARC clinical practice guideline: postural drainage therapy. Respir Care 1991;36:1418–25.

[121] Chiaranda M, Verona L, Pinamonti O, et al. Use of heat and moisture exchangers filters in mechanically ventilated ICU patients: influence on airway flow resistance. Intens Care Med 1993;19:462–6.

[122] Emergency Care Research Institute: heat and moisture exchangers. Health Devices 1983;12:155–66.

[123] Villafane MC, Cinnella G, Lofaso F, et al. Gradual reduction of endotracheal tube diameter during mechanical ventilation via different humidification devices. Anesthesiology 1996;85:1341–9.

[124] Inui D, Oto J, Nishimura M. Effect of heat and moisture exchanger (HME) positioning on inspiratory gas humidification. BMC Pulm Med 2006;6:19.

[125] Martin C, Papazian L, Perrin G, et al. Performance evaluation of three vaporizing humidifiers and two heat and moisture exchangers in patients with minute ventilation 10 L/min. Chest 1992;102:1347–50.

[126] Dreyfuss D, Djedaini K, Gros I, et al. Mechanical ventilation with heated humidifiers or heat and moisture exchanges: effects on patient colonization and incidence of nosocomial pneumonia. Am J Respir Crit Care Med 1995;151:986–92.

[127] Kolobow T, Tsuno K, Rossi N, et al. Design and development of ultra-thin walled, nonkinking endotracheal tubes of a new

"no-pressure" laryngeal seal design: a preliminary report. Anesthesiology 1994;81: 1061–7.
[128] Constant M, Stern R, Doershuk C. Efficacy of the Flutter device for airway mucus clearance in patients with cystic fibrosis. J Pediatr 1994;124:689–93.
[129] Ring WH, Adair JC, Elwyn RA. A new pediatric endotracheal tube. Anesth Analg 1975;54:273–4.
[130] Demers RR. Complications of endotracheal suctioning procedures. Respir Care 1982;27: 453–7.
[131] Steen JA. Impact of tube design and materials on complications of tracheal intubation. In: Bishop MJ, editor. Problems in anesthesia. Vol. 2: *physiology and consequences of tracheal intubation*. Philadelphia: JB Lippincott; 1988. p. 211–23.
[132] Kollef MH, Skubas NJ, Sundt TM. A randomized clinical trial of continuous aspiration of subglottic secretions in cardiac surgery patients. Chest 1999;116:1339–46.
[133] Kollef MH, Shapiro SD, Fraser VJ, et al. Mechanical ventilation with or without 7-day circuit changes. Ann Intern Med 1995;123: 168–74.
[134] Mahul P, Auboyer C, Jospe R, et al. Prevention of nosocomial pneumonia in intubated patients: respective role of mechanical subglottic secretions drainage and stress ulcer prophylaxis. Intens Care Med 1992; 18:20–5.
[135] Smulders K, van der Hoeven H, Weers-Pothoff I, et al. A randomized clinical trial of intermittent subglottic secretion drainage in patients receiving mechanical ventilation. Chest 2002;121:858–62.
[136] Valles J, Artigas A, Rello J, et al. Continuous aspiration of subglottic secretions in preventing ventilator-associated pneumonia. Ann Intern Med 1995;122: 179–86.
[137] Coffin SE, Klompas M, Classen D, et al. Strategies to prevent ventilator associated pneumonia in acute care hospitals. Supplement article SHEA/ISDA practice recommendation. Infect Control Hosp Epidemiol 2008;29(Suppl. 1):S31–40.
[138] Shorr AF, O'Malley PG. Continuous subglottic suctioning for the prevention of ventilator-associated pneumonia: potential economic implications. Chest 2001;119:228–35.
[139] Tablan OC, Anderson LJ, Besser R, et al. Guidelines for preventing health-care associated pneumonia, 2003. Recommendations of CDC and the healthcare infection control practices advisory committee. MMWR Recomm Rep 2004;53(RR-3):1–36.
[140] Dragoumanis CK, Vretzakis GI, Papaloannou VE, et al. Investigating the failure to aspirate subglottic secretions with the Evac endotracheal tube. Anesth Analg 2007;105:1083–5.
[141] Kapadia FN. Factors associated with blocked tracheal tubes. Intens Care Med 2001;27: 1679–81.
[142] Kapadia FN, Bajan KB, Raje KV. Airway accidents in intubated ICU patients: an epidemiological study. Crit Care Med 2000; 28:659–64.
[143] Kirton OC, DeHaven CB, Morgan JP, et al. Elevated imposed work of breathing, masquerading as ventilator weaning intolerance. Chest 1995;108:1021–5.
[144] Puntervoll SA, Soreide E, Jacewicz W, et al. Rapid detection of oesophageal intubation: take care when using colorimetric capnometry. Acta Anaesthesiol Scand 2002;46: 455–7.
[145] Mort T, Aldo F, Kopp GW. Managing the unusual airway—Case studies in complexity: clearing luminal occlusions. Anesthesiol News 2010;36(8):64–5.
[146] Jarrett WA, Ribes J, Manaligod JM. Biofilm formation on tracheostomy tubes. Ear Nose Throat J 2002;81:659–61.
[147] Mohamed JA, Reitzel R, Hachem R, et al., Activity of antimicrobial-coated endotracheal tubes (ETT) in preventing the biofilm colonization of resistant bacteria in a biofilm model with neutralizing broth. Abstracts 66, Presentation 467: healthcare- and community-acquired infections and infection control. Presented at the 48th annual meeting of the Infectious Diseases Society of America. Vancouver, Canada; October 22, 2010.
[148] Kelly GS. Clinical applications of N-acetylcysteine. Altern Med Rev 1998;3: 114–27.
[149] DeVries N, DeFlora S, N-Acetyl-1-cysteine J. Cell Biochem 1993;17F:S270–7.

[150] Tomkiewicz RP, App EM, Coffiner M, et al. Mucolytic treatment with N-acetylcysteine L-lysinate metered dose inhaler in dogs: airway epithelial changes. Eur Respir J 1994; 7:81–7.

[151] Rasmussen JB, Glennow C. Reduction in days of illness after long-term treatment with N-acetylcysteine controlled-release tablets in patients with chronic bronchitis. Eur Respir J 1988;1:351–5.

[152] British Thoracic Society Research Committee: oral N-acetylcysteine and exacerbation rates in patients with chronic bronchitis and severe airway obstruction. Thorax 1985;40:832–5.

[153] Mukhopadhyay S, Staddon GE, Eastman C, et al. The quantitative distribution of nebulized antibiotic in the lung in cystic fibrosis. Respir Med 1994;88:203–11.

[154] Reisman J, Rivington-Law B, Corey M, et al. Role of conventional therapy in cystic fibrosis. J Pediatr 1988;113:632–6.

[155] Fabry B, Hapeerthur C, Zappe D, et al. Breathing pattern and additional work of breathing in spontaneously breathing patients with different ventilatory demands during inspiratory pressure support and automatic tube compensation. Intens Care Med 1997; 23:545–52.

[156] Warwick W, Hansen L. Long-term effect of high-frequency chest compression therapy on pulmonary complications of cystic fibrosis. Pediatr Pulmonol 1991;11:265–71.

[157] Cox CS, Zwischenberger JB, Traber DL, et al. Heparin improves oxygenation and minimizes barotraumas after severe smoke inhalation in an ovine model. Surg Gynecol Obstet 1993;176:339–49.

[158] Tindol GA, DiBenedetto RJ, Kosciuk L. Unplanned extubation. Chest 1994;105: 1804–7.

[159] Gondor M, Nixon PA, Mutich R, et al. Comparison of Flutter device and chest physical therapy in the treatment of cystic fibrosis pulmonary exacerbation. Pediatr Pulmonol 1999;28:255–60.

[160] Ranieri VM, Grasso S, Fiore T, et al. Auto-positive end-expiratory pressure and dynamic hyperinflation. Clin Chest Med 1996;17: 379–95.

[161] Desmond K, Schwenk F, Thomas E, et al. Immediate and long term effects of chest physiotherapy in cystic fibrosis. J Pediatr 1983;103:538–42.

[162] Homnick D, Shite F, deCatro C. Comparison of effects of an intrapulmonary percussive ventilator to standard aerosol and chest physiotherapy in treatment of cystic fibrosis. Pediatr Pulmonol 1995;20:50–5.

[163] Ricard JD, Markowicz P, Djedaini K, et al. Bedside evaluation of efficient airway humidification during mechanical ventilation of the critically ill. Chest 1999;115: 1646–52.

[164] Shah C, Kollef MH. Endotracheal tube intraluminal volume loss among mechanically ventilated patients. Crit Care Med 2004;32: 120–5.

[165] Owens RL, Cheney F. Endobronchial intubation: a preventable complication. Anesthesiology 1987;67:255–7.

[166] Wright PE, Marini JJ, Bernard GR. In vitro versus in vivo comparison of endotracheal airflow resistance. Am Rev Respir Dis 1989;140:10–6.

[167] Birnkrant D, Pope J, Lewarski J, et al. Persistent pulmonary consolidation treated with intrapulmonary percussive ventilation: a preliminary report. Pediatr Pulmonol 1996; 21:246–9.

[168] Jubran A, Van de Graaff WB, Tobin MJ. Variability of patient-ventilator interaction with pressure support ventilation in patients with chronic obstructive pulmonary disease. Am J Respir Crit Care Med 1995;152: 129–36.

[169] Wanner A, Salathe M, O'Riordan TG. Mucociliary clearance in the airways. Am J Respir Crit Care Med 1996;154: 1868–902.

[170] White G. Equipment theory for respiratory care. Albany, NY: Delmar; 1996.

[171] Skinner MW, Waldron RJ, Anderson MB. Normal laryngoscopy and intubation. In: Hanowell LH, Waldron RJ, editors. Airway management. Philadelphia: Lippincott-Raven; 1996. p. 81–96.

[172] MacIntyre NR. Respiratory function during pressure support ventilation. Chest 1986; 89:677–83.

[173] Mahlmeister M, Fink J, Hoffman G, et al. Positive-expiratory-pressure mask therapy: theoretical and practical considerations and a

[174] Tomkiewicz RP, Biviji A, King M. Rheologic studies regarding high-frequency chest compressions (HFCC) and improvement of mucus clearance in cystic fibrosis [abstract]. Am J Respir Crit Care Med 1994; 149:A669.

[175] Kearl RA, Hooper RG. Massive airway leaks: an analysis of the role of endotracheal tubes. Crit Care Med 1993;21:518–21.

[176] Brochard L, Rua F, Lorino H, et al. Inspiratory pressure support compensates for the additional work of breathing caused by the endotracheal tube. Anesthesiology 1991; 75:739–45.

[177] Raphael DT. Acoustic reflectometry profiles of endotracheal and esophageal intubation. Anesthesiology 2000;92:1293–9.

[178] Banner MJ, Blanch PB, Kerby RR. Imposed work of breathing and methods of triggering a demand-flow, continuous positive airway pressure system. Crit Care Med 1993;21: 183–90.

[179] Harrison GA, Tonkin JP. Prolonged (therapeutic) endotracheal intubation. Br J Anaesth 1968;40:241–9.

[180] Langenderfer B. Alternatives to percussion and postural drainage. J Cardiopulm Rehabil 1998;18:283–9.

[181] Duarte AG, Dhand R, Reid R, et al. Serum albuterol levels in mechanically ventilated patients and healthy subjects after metered-dose inhaler administration. Am J Respir Crit Care Med 1996;154:1658–63.

[182] Duarte AG, Fink JB, Dhand R. Inhalation therapy during mechanical ventilation. Respir Care Clin North Am 2001;7:233–60.

[183] Fink JB, Dhand R, Duarte AG, et al. Deposition of aerosol from metered-dose inhaler during mechanical ventilation: an in vitro model. Am J Respir Crit Care Med 1996;154:382–7.

[184] Diot P, Morra L, Smaldone GC. Albuterol delivery in a model of mechanical ventilation: comparison of metered-dose inhaler and nebulizer efficiency. Am J Respir Crit Care Med 1995;152:1391–4.

[185] Fernandez A, Lazaro A, Garcia A, et al. Bronchodilators in patients with chronic obstructive pulmonary disease on mechanical ventilation: utilization of metered-dose inhalers. Am Rev Respir Dis 1990;141:164–8.

[186] Frederiksen B, Koch C, Hoiby N. Antibiotic treatment of initial colonization with *Pseudomonas aeruginosa* postpones chronic infection and prevents deterioration of pulmonary function in cystic fibrosis patients. Pediatr Pulmonol 1997;23:330–5.

[187] Dhand R, Tobin MJ. Inhaled bronchodilator therapy in mechanically ventilated patients. Am J Respir Crit Care Med 1997;156: 3–10.

[188] Goode ML, Fink JB, Dhand R, et al. Improvement in aerosol delivery with helium-oxygen mixtures in mechanical ventilation. Am J Respir Crit Care Med 2001; 163:109–14.

[189] Dhand R, Tobin MJ. Bronchodilator delivery with metered-dose inhalers in mechanically-ventilated patients. Eur Respir J 1996;9: 585–95.

[190] Dhand R. Special problems in aerosol delivery: artificial airways. Respir Care 2000;45: 636–45.

[191] Beaty CD, Ritz RH, Benson MS. Continuous in-line nebulizers complicate pressure support ventilation. Chest 1989;96:1360–3.

[192] Martin C, Perrin G, Gevaudan M, et al. Heat and moisture exchangers in the intensive care unit. Chest 1990;97:144–9.

[193] Bowton DL, Goldsmith WM, Haponik EF. Substitution of metered-dose inhalers for hand-held nebulizers: success and cost savings in a large, acute-care hospital. Chest 1992;101:305–8.

[194] Watson WF. Development of the PVC endotracheal tube. Biomaterials 1980;1:41–6.

[195] Davis B, Marin MG, Yee JW, et al. Effect of terbutaline on movement of Cl− and Na+ across the trachea of the dog. Am Rev Respir Dis 1979;120:547–52.

[196] Bennett WD. Effect of beta-adrenergic agonists on mucociliary clearance. J Allergy Clin Immunol 2002;110:S291–7.

[197] Rohatagi S, Derendorf H, Zech K. Risk-benefit value of inhaled corticosteroids: a pharmacokinetic/pharmacodynamic perspective. Chest 2003;123:430s–1s.

[198] Rohatagi S, Appajosyula S, Derendorf H, et al. Risk-benefit value of inhaled glucocorticoids: a pharmacokinetic/pharmacodynamic

perspective. J Clin Pharmacol 2004;44: 37–47.
[199] Hubner M, Hochhaus G, Derendorf H. Comparative pharmacology, bioavailability, pharmacokinetics, and pharmacodynamics of inhaled glucocorticosteroids. Immunol Allergy Clin North Am 2005;25(3):469–88.
[200] Todd GRG, Acerini CL, Ross-Russell R, et al. Survey of adrenal crisis associated with inhaled corticosteroids in the United Kingdom. Arch Dis Child 2002;87:457–61.
[201] Barnes PJ. Inhaled corticosteroids are not beneficial in chronic obstructive pulmonary disease. Am J Respir Crit Care Med 2000; 161:342–4.
[202] Fuller HD, Dolovich MB, Posmituck G, et al. Pressurized aerosol versus jet aerosol delivery to mechanically ventilated patients: comparison of dose to the lungs. Am Rev Respir Dis 1990;141:440–4.
[203] Maddison J, Dodd M, Webb AK. Nebulized colistin causes chest tightness in adults with cystic fibrosis. Respir Med 1994;88:145–7.
[204] Pappas JN, Goodman PC. Predicting proper endotracheal tube placement in underexposed radiographs: tangent line of the aortic arch. AJR Am J Roentgenol 1999;173:1357–9.
[205] Itokazu GS, Weinstein RA. Aerosolized antibiotics: another look. Crit Care Med 1998; 26:5–6.
[206] Oberwalder B, Evans JC, Zach MS. Forced expiration against a variable resistance: a new chest physiotherapy method in cystic fibrosis. Pediatr Pulmonol 1986;2:358–67.
[207] Drakulovic MB, Torres A, Bauer TT, et al. Supine position as a risk factor for nosocomial pneumonia in mechanically ventilated patients: a randomized trial. Lancet 1999; 354:1851–8.
[208] Guttmann J, Haberthur C, Mols G. Automatic tube compensation. Respir Care Clin North Am 2001;7:475–501.
[209] Anzueto A, Peters JI, Seidner SR, et al. Effects of continuous bed rotation and prolonged mechanical ventilation on healthy, adult baboons. Crit Care Med 1997;25:1560–4.
[210] Clemmer RP, Green S, Ziegler B. Effectiveness of the kinetic treatment table for preventing and treating pulmonary complications in severely head-injured patients. Crit Care Med 1990;18:614–7.
[211] Pelosi P, Brazzi L, Gattinoni L. Prone position in acute respiratory distress syndrome. Eur Respir J 2002;20:1017–28.
[212] Kopterides P. Siempos II, Armaganidis A: prone positioning in hypoxemic respiratory failure: meta-analysis of randomized controlled trials. J Crit Care 2009;24:89–100.
[213] Sud S, Friedrich JO, Taccone P, et al. Prone ventilation reduces mortality in patients with acute respiratory failure and severe hypoxemia: systematic review and meta-analysis. Intens Care Med 2010;36:585–99.

10 Applications of Polyaryletheretherketone in Spinal Implants: Fusion and Motion Preservation

Steven M. Kurtz, PhD

OUTLINE

10.1 Introduction	231
10.2 Origins of Interbody Fusion and the "Cage Rage" of the Late 1990s	233
10.3 CFR-PEEK Lumbar Cages: The Brantigan Cage	233
10.4 Threaded PEEK Lumbar Fusion Cages	237
10.5 Clinical Diagnostic Imaging of PEEK Spinal Cages and Transpedicular Screws	239
10.6 Subsidence and Wear of PAEK Cages	240
10.7 Posterior Dynamic Stabilization Devices	240
10.7.1 Interspinous Process Spacers	241
10.7.2 Pedicle-Based Posterior Stabilization (PEEK Rods)	242
10.7.2.1 Early Pedicle-Based Systems: Graf Ligaments and Dynesys	242
10.7.2.2 PEEK Rods	243
10.8 Cervical and Lumbar Artificial Discs	244
10.9 Summary	246
Acknowledgments	246
References	247

10.1 Introduction

The orthopedic and biomaterials literature of the 1990s reflects an early academic curiosity in implant applications of polyaryletherketone (PAEK) biomaterials [1,2]. However, widespread commercial applications for PAEK biomaterials in the human body were first realized with cage implants intended to promote intervertebral body (interbody) fusion of the lumbar spine. Success of PAEK with interbody implants would later inspire applications in a broad variety of spinal implant applications, including posterior fusion, dynamic stabilization, and disc arthroplasty.

Fusion is now considered a standard of care for intractable low back pain arising from degenerative disc disease and/or spinal instability. In the cervical spine, anterior decompression and fusion is the standard treatment for degenerative disc disease, myelopathy, and radiculopathy. Whether in the lumbar or cervical spine, fusion consists of first immobilizing the painful spine segments by encouraging bone growth across the immobilized level. Spine fusion was first performed without instrumentation using bone grafts, often obtained from the patient's own body, such as iliac crest. Harvesting bone from the patient was undesirable, because it is a second procedure and has associations with complications, including donor site pain. Also, the operated level was unstable until fusion occurred, and required local immobilization. Posterior instrumented fusion, using rods, plates, and screws, was developed to provide immediate rigid stability to the spine while the bone fused across the treated level [3].

Since the 1990s, the incidence of spinal fusion has grown substantially in the United States [4], reflecting both an increased prevalence of the degenerative disc disease and growing acceptance of the procedure (Figure 10.1). In 2008, an estimated 286,000 thoracolumbar fusions and 180,000 cervical fusions were performed in the United States based on the data from the Nationwide Inpatient Sample (NIS), and that the number is projected to increase to millions of procedures a year within the next two decades [5].

Polyaryletheretherketone (PEEK) interbody cages represent a considerable commercial, as well

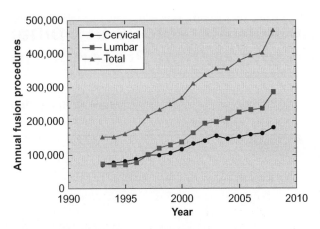

Figure 10.1 Incidence of spinal fusions in the United States based on NIS data from 1993 to 2008. (*Source: http://hcupnet.ahrq.gov.*)

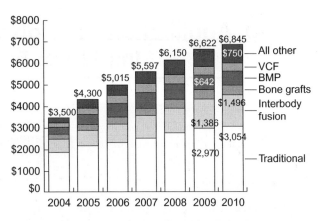

Figure 10.2 2004–2010 spinal implant US sales ($ millions) by segment. (*Reproduced with permission from the* Orthopedic Network News *[6].*)

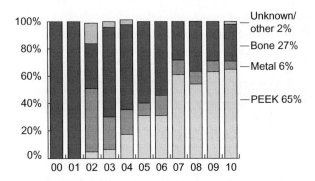

Figure 10.3 Trends in materials used in interbody fusion devices, 2000–2010. (*Reproduced with permission from the* Orthopedic Network News *[6].*)

as clinical, success. The US market for interbody fusion products has increased from 0.6 billion US$ in 2004 to 1.5 billion US$ in 2010 (Figure 10.2) [6]. The positioning of PEEK cages within the interbody market has likewise expanded since Food and Drug Administration (FDA) approval in 2001. By 2010, PEEK cages accounted for 65% of interbody devices, representing a market of approximately 1 billion US$ in the United States alone (Figure 10.3) [6]. PEEK cages have also contributed to the growth of the $613 m recombinant human bone morphogenetic protein-2 (BMP) market (Figure 10.2). The use of BMP for facilitating interbody fusion was approved by the FDA in 2002 for the threaded titanium LT-Cage [7], but it has been increasingly used "off label" with other spinal fusion devices [8]. Metal cages, such as the LT-Cage fabricated from titanium, are estimated to constitute 10% of the interbody market (Figure 10.3) [6]. Thus, the vast majority of BMP use for interbody fusion is accomplished using PEEK rather than metal cages. Compared with other synthetic biomaterial solutions, PEEK biomaterials now dominate the design space for interbody cages and are the principal implant delivery system for BMP.

In recent years, there has been great interest in finding ways to halt the degenerative cascade following fusion surgery [9,10]. Because fusion results in unnatural motion at adjacent levels, researchers have proposed that preserving normal motion in the spine will help alleviate, and perhaps even prevent, adjacent segment degeneration. Consequently, a variety of new implant technologies have developed to preserve, limit, or enhance motion of the spine. Although previous fusion technologies have been referred to as "static" or rigid fusion, new fusion technologies that employ a more flexible instrumentation systems are gaining clinical acceptance. Interspinous implants, such as the X-STOP (Kyphon, Sunnyvale, CA), have been developed with PEEK-OPTIMA components to treat back pain caused by spinal stenosis [11]. Artificial discs, developed with PEEK components, represent another novel implant technology that is intended to preserve motion of the treated spine [12].

Motion preservation spine technology, while perhaps no longer in its infancy, still remains in the very early years of development and clinical acceptance. In 2008, an estimated 5000 interspinous process implants, 800 posterior pedicle-based stabilization devices, and 4900 total disc replacements (TDRs, including both cervical and lumbar) were performed in the United States based on data from the NIS. Reimbursement for surgeons and hospitals for performing motion preserving spinal surgery continues to be extremely challenging in the United States. Thus, motion preservation should be viewed through the lens of an early development in the spine field; fusion procedures currently dominate the clinical practice of spine surgery.

This chapter focuses on the variety of spinal implant applications of PEEK. We begin with an overview of interbody fusion and historical development of the first carbon fiber-reinforced (CFR)-PEEK spinal implant, the Brantigan I/F lumbar fusion cage. More recent applications of PEEK in the spine, including dynamic stabilization devices and artificial discs, are also reviewed.

10.2 Origins of Interbody Fusion and the "Cage Rage" of the Late 1990s

Although lumbar and cervical fusions are today considered common procedures, the surgical techniques have evolved considerably since 1911 when fusion was first suggested as a treatment for Pott's disease [13]. During the first half of the 20th century, posterior fusion techniques for treatment of back pain included resection of the posterior elements and implantation of bone fragments harvested from the patient's pelvis [14]. Dissatisfaction with the stability and outcomes of these early posterior surgical techniques led to the development of interbody fusion between adjacent lumbar and cervical vertebral bodies during the 1930s and 1950s [15–17]. Early interbody fusions were accomplished by removal of the disc and implantation of bone graft, either from the patient or from newly created bone banks of cadaver bone [16]. However, the success of early interbody fusion surgery also proved to be variable [18]. A key limitation for interbody fusion remained the strength and stability afforded by the bone graft. Along with the development of posterior instrumentation, the invention of interbody implants, known as cages, would help expand the acceptance of both cervical and lumbar fusion surgery starting in the 1990s.

The first interbody implants were used in horses, not humans. George Bagby M.D. [19] developed a cylindrical stainless steel implant in 1982 known as the "Bagby Basket" to fuse unstable spine segments in race horses that had become paralyzed or otherwise neurologically impaired. The concept of an interbody implant for humans was developed in the 1980s and 1990s as the "Bagby and Kuslich" (BAK) technique. The BAK cage of the 1990s was a threaded, fenestrated titanium cylinder that could be filled with bone graft. The BAK cage was manufactured by Spine-Tech, Inc., Minneapolis, MN. The stand-alone threaded cage was approved by the FDA in 1996 after a rigorous multicenter clinical trial for implantation by a direct anterior approach, a posterior lumbar interbody fusion (PLIF), and a laproscopic approach [20]. In the FDA investigational device exemption (IDE) clinical trial, Kuslich et al. [20] reported that 91.7% of patients were fused at 2 years and 95.1% of patients were successfully fused at 4 years.

For a short time, the stand-alone BAK cage was widely used. However, the clinical results of the threaded cage after FDA approval did not match high expectations raised by the prospective clinical trial [21–23]. The poor results of the BAK cage that were reported following FDA approval are now thought to be largely due to poor patient selection by surgeons, technical difficulties with implantation, and its stand-alone indication [24]. Consequently, the period of the late 1990s is sometimes referred to as the "Cage Rage" by some members of the spine community. Regardless, Bagby and Kuslich are credited for developing the first FDA-approved interbody fusion cage as a stand-alone device in combination with bone graft. The second-generation threaded cage, the LT-Cage (Medtronic Spinal and Biologics, Memphis, TN), was approved in 2002 in combination with BMP. In retrospect, the Cage Rage of the late 1990s set the stage for the introduction of PEEK into this dynamic and growing field of spine surgery.

10.3 CFR-PEEK Lumbar Cages: The Brantigan Cage

In parallel with the development of threaded titanium cages, PAEK biomaterials for interbody spinal cages were also developed for posterior lumbar interbody fusion (PLIF) in the 1980s and 1990s

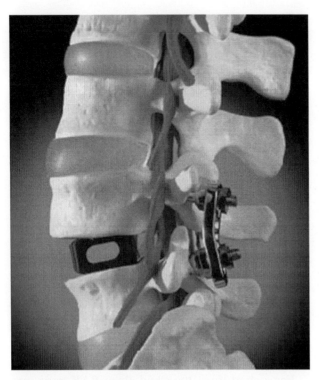

Figure 10.4 CFR-PEEK lumbar fusion cage, used in concert with posterior screws and rods.

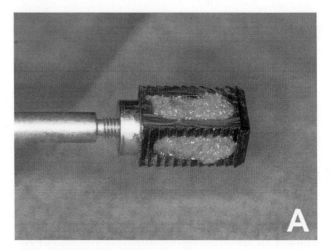

Figure 10.5 CFR-PEEK lumbar fusion cage loaded with fragmented bone graft, prior to implantation. (*Image courtesy of Bill Christianson, DePuy Spine.*)

by AcroMed (Cleveland, OH, now DePuy Spine, Raynham, MA). The CFR-PEEK I/F lumbar fusion cage was approved by the FDA in 2001, following the aftermath of the Cage Rage. By this time, interbody fusion surgery had evolved from the experience with the stand-alone threaded cages. The CFR-PEEK cage has been described in a monograph by John Brantigan M.D., the lead surgeon inventor [25]. In this section, we provide an overview of the development history for the CFR-PEEK cage. Readers interested in a more detailed account are encouraged to read Brantigan's treatise [25].

In contrast with the initial stand-alone design of the threaded cage, the Brantigan cage was typically intended to be used in concert with posterior instrumentation for added stability. A model of a PLIF instrumentation system is illustrated in Figure 10.4. The PLIF procedure is conducted in two phases. In one phase of the surgery, a cage is placed anterolaterally between the vertebral bodies of the treated level. The cage may be packed with bone graft (Figure 10.5) or a sponge containing BMP (e.g., INFUSE bone graft [26]). The cage may be reinforced with an anterior plate, to prevent extrusion. In another phase of the surgery, posterior screws and rods are also typically placed to provide additional stability to the treated level (Figure 10.4).

Due to the mechanical loading requirements for these permanent implants, the surgeons who helped develop the PLIF cage, Arthur Steffee M.D. and John Brantigan M.D., initially conceived of a titanium device that would allow bone to grow through a columnar fenestration in the device [27]. There were two perceived drawbacks with the initial proposed design, the first being the stiffness of the titanium device, which might promote stress shielding and inhibit bone growth, and the second being the radiopacity of the device, which would hinder diagnostic assessment of the bone growth. Carl McMillin, a polymer engineer at AcroMed, was familiar with high-performance thermoplastics and recommended PAEKs for the cage to overcome both limitations [27,28]. The clinical and commercial success of this medical device, which came to be known as the Brantigan cage after its primary surgeon champion, lay the foundation for the current widespread use of PEEK in spine implants.

CFR-PAEK cages were subjected to an extensive in vitro biocompatibility and mechanical testing program, including pull-out tests in cadaver bone, static compression, static compressive shear, static torsion, and dynamic compressive shear testing (Figure 10.6). The mechanical behavior of the cages was found to be more than sufficient for the intended application [29]. Indeed, the mechanical strength of the CFR-PAEK cages, although not as strong as a metal cage, could support the weight of

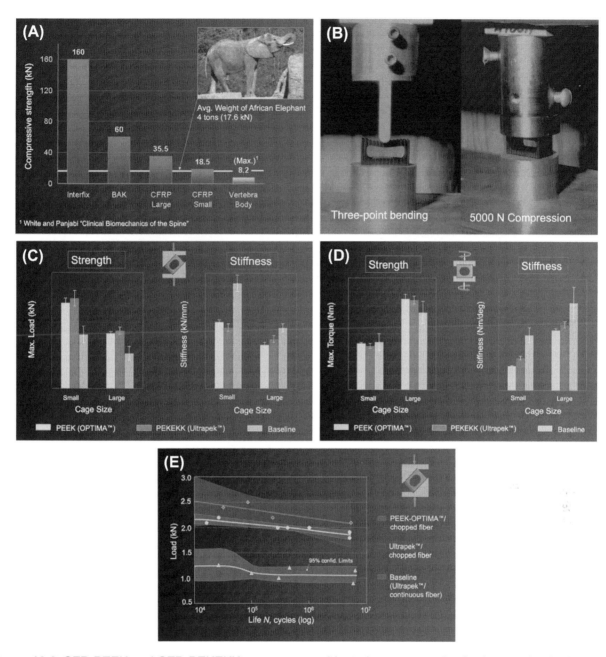

Figure 10.6 CFR-PEEK and CFR-PEKEKK cages were subjected to an extensive in vitro mechanical testing program, including static axial compression (A, B), compressive shear (C), torsion (D), and fatigue testing (E). (*Image courtesy of Bill Christianson, DePuy Spine.*)

a full-grown elephant (Figure 10.6A). Initially, the full suite of biocompatibility testing, prescribed at the time under the Tripartite agreement, was also performed by the manufacturer; these tests were later repeated for PEEK-OPTIMA after the ISO 10993 standard was created [25]. The CFR-PAEK cages passed all of the biocompatibility tests prescribed by the Tripartite agreement and ISO 10993 [25].

Starting in May 1989, PEEK and PEKEKK were evaluated in a 2-year pilot clinical study of the spine cage for PLIF in 26 human patients [30]. Both implant materials were consolidated into plates with continuous 68% by weight carbon fibers for reinforcement, and the cages were subsequently machined from the plates into their final form. In the PLIF procedure, in addition to a cage or bone spacer, the spine is further stabilized by pedicle

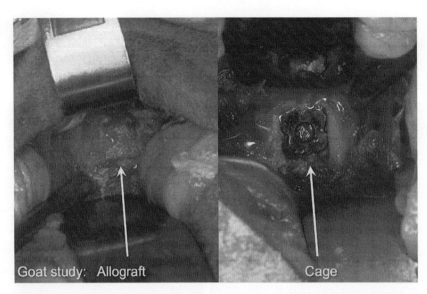

Figure 10.7 PAEK cages were compared with sterilized allografts in a Spanish goat study. (*Image courtesy of Bill Christianson, DePuy Spine.*)

screws and axial rods or plates. In the 26 patients, the initial clinical trial evaluated 32 interbody cages (of two designs and two materials) and 31 alternative interbody fusion therapies, for a total of 63 total fusion levels. Thirty-one of the 32 cages survived 2 years of follow-up. Clinical results were good or excellent in 21 of the 26 patients, and fair or poor results were traced back to problems unrelated to the cage. Because of the radiolucency of the cages, interbody fusion could be identified in 100% (31/31) of the cage levels. Despite the problematic clinical research design, Brantigan's pilot clinical study [30] marks the first implantation of carbon-reinforced PEEK and PEKEKK in the human spine.

These excellent fusion results were also reflected in a 2-year study of reinforced Ultrapek cages in Spanish goats [31]. In this animal study, PAEK cages were compared with sterilized allografts (Figure 10.7). Additional goals of the study were to verify the biocompatibility of the device and potential wear debris in a functional animal model. Fusion was observed radiographically after 2-year follow-ups (Figure 10.8). Histology confirmed extensive growth of trabeculae into the cages (Figure 10.9) and the absence of an inflammatory reaction (Figure 10.10).

Based on the encouraging fusion results from the pilot clinical study and animal study [30,31], a prospective, multicenter IDE study was initiated for the FDA in November 1991 [32]. A total of 221 patients received a carbon-reinforced PEKEKK cage with posterior pedicle screw fixation. The authors reported successful fusion in 176 of the 178 (98.9%) patients who reached 2-year follow-up. Although there were no major device-related complications in the study, 23 major nondevice-related complications occurred (10.4%), including six deaths. These findings underscored the clinical difficulties associated with the PLIF procedure for spinal fusion.

The clinical limitations associated with PLIF were addressed with evolution in surgical technique to explore anterior lumbar interbody fusion (ALIF) with the Brantigan cage, as well as the more extensive "circumferential" or 360° fusion, involving an ALIF procedure and posterior instrumentation with pedicle screws. Two- and 5- to 9-year follow-up data for the ALIF Brantigan cage in a 360° fusion have been reported [33,34], with superior clinical outcomes as compared with posterolateral instrumented fusion.

In the mid 1990s, BASF decided to no longer produce PEKEKK and withdrew the UltraPek resin from the market. Although AcroMed stockpiled sufficient UltraPek to support their products, their cage products were transitioned to PEEK, produced by Invibio, to provide a long-term biomaterial supply [27]. Stockpiled UltraPek continued to be used in Brantigan cages distributed in Japan until February 2007 when DePuy received Japanese approval for a CFR-PEEK OPTIMA cage [27,35].

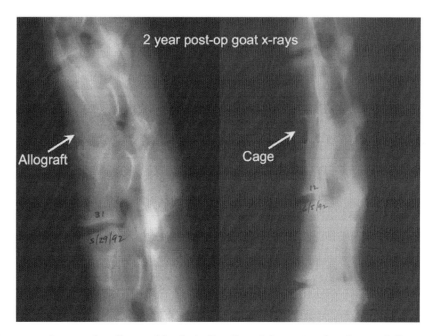

Figure 10.8 Fusion was observed radiographically in the Spanish goats after 2-year follow-up. (*Image courtesy of Bill Christianson, DePuy Spine.*)

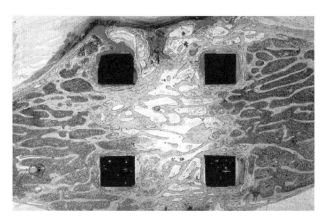

Figure 10.9 Histology confirmed the radiographic findings of fusion in the cages of the Spanish goat study. Extensive growth of trabecular bone was observed through the cages. (*Image courtesy of Bill Christianson, DePuy Spine.*)

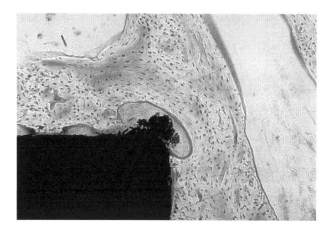

Figure 10.10 Histology confirmed the absence of an inflammatory reaction to the CFR-PAEK in the Spanish goat model. The black particles at the corner of the cage strut may be polishing artifact, rather than wear debris. No foreign body reaction is observed. (*Image courtesy of Bill Christianson, DePuy Spine.*)

Brantigan cages were originally machined from CFR-PAEK plates. Both 30% PEKEKK and 70% continuous carbon fibers, as well as 70% PEKEKK with 30% carbon fiber, were originally used [36]. Today, these cages are fabricated more efficiently by injection molding CFR-PEEK OPTIMA (70% PEEK with 30% chopped carbon fiber) [36].

10.4 Threaded PEEK Lumbar Fusion Cages

Although many articles describe the use of CFR-PEEK for spine implants, many recent studies also involve the use of neat PEEK for both cervical and

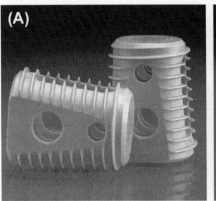
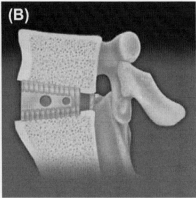

Figure 10.11 Tapered PEEK cage for the lumbar spine (LT-CAGE System: Medtronic Spinal and Biologics, Memphis, TN).

lumbar spinal cages [37–47]. A tapered PEEK cage for the lumbar spine is shown in Figure 10.11. Because the use of neat PEEK for spine is a relatively recent development, the published literature is generally limited to in vitro biomechanical studies [43–45], or short-term outcomes in animal studies or human clinical trials [37–41,46,47]. Recent studies with PEEK cages have looked to improve or accelerate fusion performance by combining the devices with the use of hydroxylapatite [41], 40% β-tricalcium phosphate/60% hydroxylapatite [38], or rhBMP-2 on a collagen sponge [40].

A detailed animal study investigating PEEK interbody cages has recently been reported by Toth et al. [40]. Researchers studied the influence of rhBMP-2 on a collagen sponge (InFuse™: Medtronic Spinal and Biologics, Memphis, TN) on fusion with a PEEK-threaded cage in an ovine model. An autograft group served as a control (Figure 10.12). After 6 months, the biomechanical behavior of the treated level was measured. The cage group treated with InFuse™ was found to be significantly stiffer in flexion and left lateral bending than the control group treated using a PEEK cage filled with autografts. Histology and microradiographs were used to characterize the extent of fusion (Figure 10.13). All the PEEK cages with InFuse™ were diagnosed with fusion at 6 months radiographically and histologically. No evidence of wear debris or damage to the device was noted. Only mild inflammatory response was noted during histological evaluation of tissue adjacent to the PEEK implants, which the authors judged to represent "excellent" biocompatibility for the material.

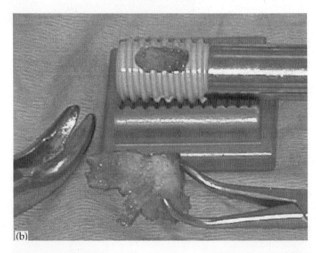

Figure 10.12 Threaded PEEK interbody device filled with autograft prior to implantation into a goal animal model. (*Reproduced with permission from Ref. [40].*)

Intermediate-term clinical reports on the use of unfilled, neat PEEK cages are reported in the spine literature [48]. A retrospective study of neat PEEK cages used for circumferential lumbar fusion was reported by Rousseau et al. [48], who evaluated 57 consecutive patients after a mean follow-up of 5.7 years (range: 4–8 years). They observed fusion in 56 cases, but they were unable to maintain the desired curvature of the spine in 10 patients. They attributed the loss of spinal curvature correction to the order of implantation of the cages, which occurred after the spine was locked in place using a rigid posterior instrumentation system. The authors concluded that "lumbar circumferential arthrodesis using PEEK cages ... provided good clinical results and fusion rate."

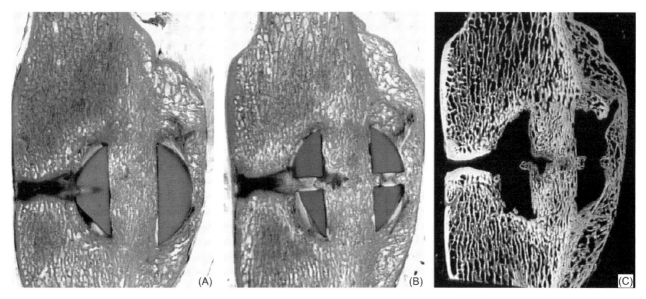

Figure 10.13 Histological section of autograft-treated goats in a prospective study of threaded PEEK cages. (*Reproduced with permission from Ref. [40].*)

10.5 Clinical Diagnostic Imaging of PEEK Spinal Cages and Transpedicular Screws

The compatibility of PAEK polymers with clinical diagnostic imaging has been a major driver for the widespread adoption of this polymer family for spinal applications. Numerous studies have remarked upon the radiolucency of the neat and reinforced spinal implants fabricated from PEKEKK and PEEK, which have been found to greatly facilitate radiographic assessment of fusion in vivo [30–32,40,49]. Computed tomography (CT) generally provides a more reliable assessment of fusion than plane radiographs [49]. Figure 10.14 shows a representative lateral radiograph of a solid fusion in the lumbar spine through the fenestrations of a Brantigan cage.

CFR-PEEK is also used for transpedicular fusion in the cervical spine, where radiographic imaging is crucial to permit safe insertion of the devices using computer-assisted navigation with fluoroscopic guidance (Figure 10.15). The CFR-PEEK screws also contain 0.5% tantalum fibers to provide sufficient visualization using fluoroscopy [50]. In vitro studies have confirmed the feasibility of using CFR-PEEK screws for transpedicular fixation [50],

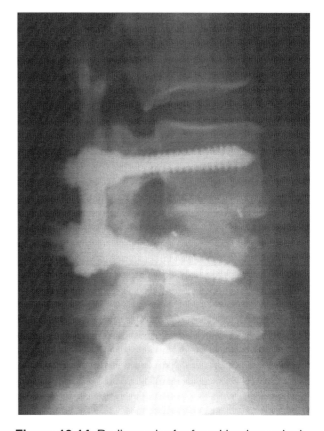

Figure 10.14 Radiograph of a fused lumbar spinal segment using a Brantigan CFR-PEEK cage. (*Image courtesy of DePuy Spine.*)

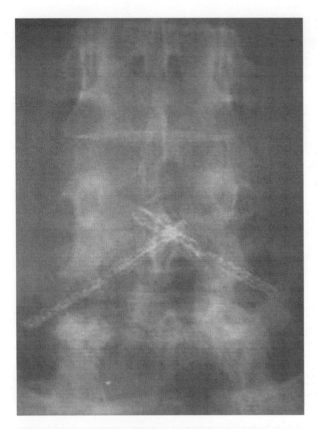

Figure 10.15 CFR-PEEK transpedicular screw and a radiograph of a fused cervical spinal segment. The screws are radiolucent because of the addition of 0.5% tantalum fibers. (*Images courtesy of Invibio.*)

but clinical results using these devices have not yet been reported in the literature.

10.6 Subsidence and Wear of PAEK Cages

Although most of the literature for PAEK biomaterials in the spine focuses on biomechanical stability or clinical outcomes such as fusion, relatively few studies provide insight into the unique limitations of the material when used in cage implants. The potential for some implant complications of PEEK cages, such as subsidence, are shared with metallic cages, and thus are not unique to the use of PEEK [51]. As with any load-bearing implant, wear and fracture are also concerns with PEEK spinal implants. Our experience with these implant-related complications is largely drawn from the Brantigan cage, because of its extensive clinical history. As of 1998, no implant-related complications of carbon fiber cages had been reported in the literature. Tullberg [52] described the fracture of a Brantigan cage in a case study of a failed fusion. Togawa et al. [53] studied biopsy samples from radiologically successful fusions with Ti alloy or Brantigan cages. Researchers noted particles of debris in biopsies from four of the five carbon fiber cages and in one of the four titanium cages, but no evidence of an inflammatory reaction to the particles was seen. The overall clinical significance of particulate debris and fracture is unclear for the Brantigan cage, given the strong evidence of long-term successful fusion using this design and similar findings to those in metal cages.

Nevertheless, due to the loading demands in the spine (especially in the lumbar region) and the competing design goals of strength and thin implant cross-sections to promote internal bone growth, the literature suggests that implant fracture and debris production could be considered important potential failure modes for PEEK biomaterials in the spine. Finite element analysis, in particular, has proven to be an effective tool to evaluate the fracture risk of PEEK implant designs in the spine [45]. The effect of wear debris on the spinal cord has been investigated in a rabbit model [54]. After injecting particle loads into the spinal canal of rabbits, researchers have concluded that PEEK particles appear "harmless" to the spinal cord.

10.7 Posterior Dynamic Stabilization Devices

The continued availability, radiolucency, and biomechanical success of PEEK in spinal fusion applications have stimulated interest in using the biomaterial in posterior dynamic stabilization devices. In contrast with fusion, which aims to stabilize a painful and diseased spinal unit by eliminating motion, the general aim of dynamic stabilization is to restrict motion and forces in directions that cause pain, while allowing motion in the asymptomatic directions [11,55]. Posterior dynamic stabilization devices were developed to treat the degenerated lumbar spine, but the precise indications for treatment are extremely broadly advocated in the literature, ranging from discogenic back pain, spondylesthesis, and spinal stenosis [11,55]. Although the specific biomechanical mechanisms whereby posterior dynamic spinal devices are intended to function vary by design, the devices themselves fall into two general categories depending on whether they are implanted between the spinous processes or are installed as flexible members using pedicle screws. PEEK has been successfully incorporated into both types of spinal dynamic stabilization devices, most notably as a replacement for metallic interspinous process spacers (ISPs) or metallic fusion rods.

10.7.1 Interspinous Process Spacers

Several different designs of ISPs have been developed in recent years and are currently under clinical evaluation [11,55,56], but their gross biomechanical function in the spine appears to be fairly similar [57]. By distracting the posterior elements to insert the ISP, the posterior intervertebral disc is placed into flexion (or local kyphosis), the spinal canal is locally widened, and the pressure on the posterior disc is relieved [57]. Thus, ISPs are intended to stabilize the spine in extension, but provide little to no resistance to flexion, axial rotation, and lateral bending [57]. The posterior distraction created by implanting an ISP also relieves nerve root impingement, one of the causes of low back and leg pain.

ISPs were initially designed and fabricated from Ti alloy, serving as rigid or "static" spacers between the interspinous processes. Examples of rigid ISPs initially fabricated from Ti include the Wallis and X-STOP posterior dynamic stabilization systems [55,56]. As PEEK gained widespread exposure to the spine community through interbody fusion, ISP implant designers developed second-generation devices in which Ti was replaced with PEEK. For example, Senegas [58] noted that the developers of the Wallis devices converted their titanium interspinous component to PEEK in 2004. The St Francis developed X-STOP also converted from Ti alloy to PEEK-OPTIMA as a spacer for its Interspinous Process Decompression System (Figure 10.16) [11]. The X-STOP is currently produced by Medtronic Spinal and Biologics (Memphis, TN).

Among ISPs, the X-STOP has the most extensive track record in the clinical and biomechanical

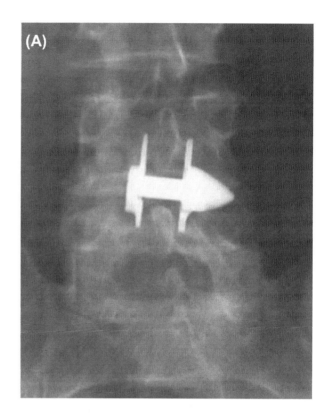

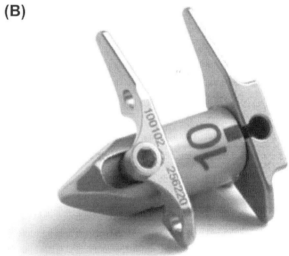

Figure 10.16 Extension-limiting, interspinous device, incorporating a PEEK spacer, and an anterior–posterior radiograph showing the device implanted in the lumbar spine (X-STOP, Medtronic Spinal and Biologics, Sunnyvale, CA).

literature, as summarized recently by Kabir et al. [56], including a 2-year multicenter randomized control trial that was performed as an Investigational Device Exemption study in support of its Premarket Approval (PMA) application for the FDA [59]. At the time of this writing, the X-STOP is the only FDA-approved posterior dynamic stabilization device that can be legally marketed as such in the United States. The approved indications for the X-STOP include treatment of a confirmed diagnosis of lumbar spinal stenosis in patients aged 50 years or older [60].

The designs of ISPs vary from rigid or static devices, like the X-STOP, to so-called "dynamic" designs that are capable of deformation during extension. Examples of dynamic ISPs include the Co-Flex device, fabricated from Ti alloy (Paradigm Spine), and the DIAM device, fabricated from silicone encased within a woven polyethylene terepthalate fiber jacket (DIAM: Medtronic Spinal and Biologics) [11,55,56]. Dynamic ISPs are currently under clinical evaluation in IDE studies for PMA applications for the US FDA [11,55,56].

As the use of ISPs has grown in the United States following FDA approval of the X-STOP in November 2005 [60], reports of complications, including early revision and spinous process fractures, are beginning to surface in the literature [61–63]. For example, Verhoof et al. [63] reported poor results when the X-STOP was implanted in patients with degenerative spondylolisthesis. Using a biplanar radiographic and CT examination protocol, Kim et al. [62] observed a higher spinous process fracture rate (22% of treated levels) than was previously reported (1%) in the randomized clinical trial that was performed for the FDA [59].

The recent reports of complications underscore the importance of better understanding the indications and contraindications for ISP implantation. At present, it still remains under clinical debate which symptomatic spine patients are most likely to obtain lasting pain relief from the targeted benefits of ISPs. Although patient selection criteria for ISP utilization are currently open to debate, the role of PEEK as a suitable biomaterial for this application remains unquestioned.

10.7.2 Pedicle-Based Posterior Stabilization (PEEK Rods)

Pedicle-based systems represent another major design category for posterior dynamic stabilization systems. In this motion-preserving design paradigm, a flexible (or "semiflexible") element is substituted for the metallic rod that is fixed to the posterior spine by pedicle screws. The shift away from rigid instrumentation using metallic rods was driven by the desire to reduce increased stress on adjacent discs and facet joints that were thought to contribute to the degeneration of adjacent levels [64]. In addition, stress shielding of the vertebral column at the level of rigid instrumentation using metal rods was considered to result in decreased stimulus for bone growth during fusion. As a result, there has been growing interest in using flexible or semiflexible posterior fusion constructs to provide increased mobility and allow load sharing while stabilizing the spine [64–68].

10.7.2.1 Early Pedicle-Based Systems: Graf Ligaments and Dynesys

In the 1990s, flexible posterior stabilization systems emerged in Europe. One such device, referred to as the Graf ligament system, consisted of braided polypropylene (PP) bands connected to Ti pedicle screws [69]. Thus, the Graf ligament system was a tension-only device; the PP bands could not support compression. The long-term clinical results of this system were mixed [69–72], and Graf ligaments never gained widespread clinical acceptance, nor were these devices approved for use in the United States.

Another early pedicle-based design developed in the 1990s was the Dynesys system, consisting of polyethylene terepthalate (PET) cord and a cylindrical polycarbonate urethane bumper spanning Ti alloy pedicle screws. In the Dynesys design, the PET cord resists tension and the PCU bumper provides resistance to compressive and lateral loading. Initially commercialized by Sulzer Spine, Dynesys was acquired by Zimmer Spine (Minneapolis, MN) who currently markets the device. The Dynesys system has been widely used in Europe and the United States [73–76].

Dynesys became available on the US market in 2005 after receiving FDA clearance as an adjunct to fusion. However, this 510(k) clearance did not include nonfusion applications of Dynesys, which were included as a PMA application to the FDA. In November 2009, an FDA Panel convened to evaluate Zimmer Spine's PMA did not recommend approval for a variety of reasons, including concern over the proposed indications for use and complications related to screw loosening and breakage.

Since that time, several studies in the clinical literature have reported screw complications with Dynesys [77–80]. Examination of retrieved Dynesys explants has also demonstrated macroscopic creep of the PCU components (on average, 4.3° of angular deformation), and beyond 5 years of implantation evidence of surface degradation was observed on the PCU where it was exposed to bodily fluids [79]. Zimmer Spine developed a modification to Dynesys with the introduction of hydroxyapatite-coated screws. As of this writing, Dynesys has not been granted FDA approval as a dynamic stabilization device, and therefore cannot be legally marketed for nonfusion indications in the United States.

10.7.2.2 PEEK Rods

PEEK rods were developed for both fusion and nonfusion applications [64–68,81], but today only have FDA clearance as adjuncts to fusion. In contrast with the polymers previously considered for posterior spine implants, PEEK exhibits outstanding creep and degradation resistance under in vivo conditions. During cadaver-based biomechanical studies, PEEK rods have been shown to offer comparable stability as Ti rods [65–67]. In addition to radiolucency, the anticipated clinical benefits of PEEK rods are hypothesized to include improved load sharing with bone to promote fusion, as well as decreased stresses at the pedicle screw interface during bone healing [64,67].

PEEK rods are currently available for fusion in the United States from two major manufacturers (CD HORIZON LEGACY: Medtronic Spinal and Biologics, Memphis, TN; EXPEDIUM: DePuy Spine, Raynham, MA). The rods differ in terms of their PEEK formulation and design. EXPEDIUM rods are fabricated from image contrast grade PEEK and have a circular cross-section (Figure 10.17). The CD HORIZON LEGACY is fabricated from unfilled PEEK-OPTIMA and has an elliptical cross-section (Figure 10.18). The LEGACY rods have metallic end caps for visualization in radiographs. If the physician wants to directly visualize the rods, they can be detected using CT scans [82]. A description of the rationale, surgical technique, and case studies of the CD HORIZON LEGACY system have been published [64].

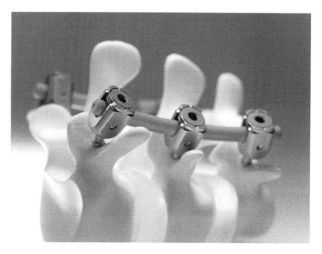

Figure 10.17 PEEK rod system for posterior lumbar fusion (EXPEDIUM System: DePuy Spine, Rayhnam, MA).

Fatigue testing of PEEK rod systems is challenging because of their flexibility and notch sensitivity [83,84]. Care should be taken in the design of the tulip and set screw where the PEEK rod is connected to the pedicle screw. In addition to the tulip and set screw design, the screw tightening torque can also influence the fatigue behavior of PEEK rods [85]. The interaction between the tulip, set screw, and PEEK rod creates a geometric stress concentration and potential initiation site for fatigue failure [67].

Conventional standardized fatigue test methods (i.e., ASTM F1717 [86]) for metallic fusion rod systems need to be modified for flexible fusion constructs incorporating PEEK rods. Specifically, ASTM F1717 provides a basis for both static and dynamic characterization of fusion constructs, but the fatigue test methods specified in the standard recommend load-controlled testing based on static failure. Previous studies suggest that displacement control may be a more relevant method for testing semirigid fusion constructs incorporating PEEK rods [67,68]. Furthermore, while these studies have documented that a PEEK rod construct assembled with traditional titanium polyaxial pedicle screws can survive up to 5 million cycles of loading, the failure location for subendurance limit tests appears to be at the set screw–rod interface.

Thus, current test methods based on ASTM F1717 for PEEK rods appear to challenge the set screw–rod interface and provide limited insight

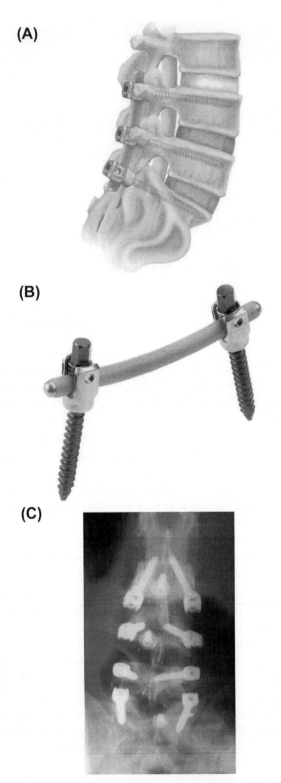

Figure 10.18 (A, B) PEEK rod system for posterior lumbar fusion (CD HORIZON LEGACY System: Medtronic Spinal and Biologics, Memphis, TN). (C) Radiograph of a CD HORIZON LEGACY PEEK rod system, courtesy of Dr. Todd Lanman. Note that PEEK rods are radiolucent and not visible on X-ray, except for the metal end caps.

into the fatigue strength of the PEEK rods themselves. PEEK rod systems currently under development for spinal applications differ considerably in terms of the biomaterials employed (e.g., unfilled vs. radio-opaque grades of PEEK), implant dimensions, and rod cross-sectional geometry. Test method development is currently under way under the auspices of ASTM to create a general test method for evaluating the fatigue strength of PEEK rods that would allow for comparisons of the properties of the rod rather than the set screw–rod interface. By applying greater rotational constraint to the rods at the set screw–rod interface, it is possible to shift the fatigue failure location during the test away from the set screw to the center of the rod [87].

PEEK rod systems are currently evaluated not only in terms of their static and fatigue performance in standardized experimental protocols but also in more clinically relevant biomechanical models, such as cadaver spine and finite element models [65–68]. Both experimental and analytical techniques can thus be used to evaluate load sharing between a PEEK rod system and the thoracolumbar spine. These experimental and analytical techniques are also essential to better understand the ability of the PEEK implant system to resist motion and stabilize the spine.

Clinical data on the performance of PEEK rods are currently very limited [64,67,88], both for fusion and nonfusion applications. A conference poster at Eurospine in 2009 described a clinical series of 120 lumbar fusion patients, in which 60 patients were treated with Ti instrumentation and 60 with PEEK rods [88]. Both groups were only followed up for 6 months and generally comparable outcomes were observed in this preliminary investigation [88]. At present, detailed clinical data for PEEK in these novel and demanding spinal applications are not yet available in the peer-reviewed scientific literature and are eagerly anticipated by the spine implant community.

10.8 Cervical and Lumbar Artificial Discs

All-polymer artificial discs fabricated from PEEK biomaterials have attracted growing interest from the research community as a second-generation alternative to contemporary TDRs, which are now most often fabricated from UHMWPE and CoCr alloys. Polymer bearings are considered promising for artificial discs due to a favorable combination of mechanical strength, wear resistance, radiolucency, biocompatibility, and manufacturability that is unique to the family of PEEK biomaterials [89,90]. Initial investigations of all-polymer PEEK bearings were performed for the lumbar spine [90–96], but recently the focus of scientific and commercial inquiry has shifted to cervical spine applications [89,97,98], which experience lower loads and are biomechanically less demanding. Mirroring the increased interest in all-polymer disc arthroplasty bearings, several basic science, pin-on-disc research studies of PEEK-on-PEEK articulations have also recently been completed [99,100]. In this section, we review the latest advances in all-polymer PEEK bearings for disc arthroplasty.

The first artificial disc fabricated entirely from unfilled, PEEK-OPTIMA LT1 was the NUBAC intradiscal arthroplasty device for the lumbar spine (Pioneer Surgical Technology, Marquette, MI) [90–96]. The design consists of a semiconstrained ball-and-socket joint and is intended to serve as an intradiscal, load-sharing device, analogous to a nucleus replacement (Figure 10.19), with an intact and a competent annulus fibrosus.

The preclinical mechanical testing for the NUBAC has been summarized in a review article [90], as well as in several conference abstracts [92–95]. The purpose of this battery of testing was to confirm the preclinical safety and effectiveness of the lumbar PEEK-on-PEEK artificial disc. Several wear studies of the NUBAC artificial disc have been conducted [93–95]. Initially, the NUBAC was tested for 40 million cycles with unidirectional motion; these tests generated the lowest amount of wear when later compared with multidirectional test conditions, but did not display the marked orientation softening behavior characteristic of UHMWPE tribology [94]. Researchers also conducted three multidirectional, 10 million cycle tests in accordance with ISO/DIS 18192-1, in which the loading was adjusted to account for the load sharing between the annulus and the nucleus in the lumbar spine. In one series of tests, the components were gamma irradiated in air with 200 kGy and accelerated aged in accordance with ASTM F2003 for 40 days [93,94]. ASTM F2003 was developed for gamma-irradiated UHMWPE the protocol is

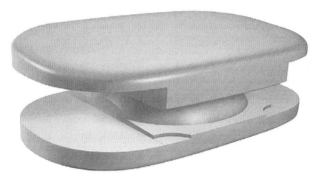

Figure 10.19 PEEK-on-PEEK Lumbar Nucleus Replacement (NUBAC: Pioneer Surgical Technology).

conducted at 70°C and is too low to influence PEEK. Regardless of the testing protocol, and including the standardized UHMWPE oxidative challenge, the average wear rates for the NUBAC experiments were relatively insensitive to changes in testing parameters, and fell within the range of 0.4–1.0 mm^3 per million cycles [94]. Overall, the wear values for the NUBAC were judged by the authors to be comparable with the rates for other metal-on-metal and metal-on-polymer artificial discs [101–103].

An international multicenter prospective clinical trial of the NUBAC is currently under way. At the 2009 meeting of the Spine Arthroplasty Society, it was announced that 225 NUBAC devices had been implanted since December 2004 [91]. The authors reported that "good pain relief and improvement in function" was achieved for up to 2 years [91]. At the time of publication, only 15 of the 225 devices (6.7%) had reached the 2-year milestone of the ongoing clinical study [91].

A cervical all-PEEK TDR, known as the NUNEC, was also developed by Pioneer Surgical Technology [97,98]. According to a recent conference abstract, the cervical TDR was tested for 10 million cycles in accordance with ASTM F2423, followed by an additional 10 million cycles in accordance with ISO 18192 [98]. The wear rates were found to be, on average, 0.3 mm^3 per million cycles for both test methods, and these rates were judged to be comparable with other cervical TDRs. The clinical results of the NUNEC are currently being evaluated by a pilot study. At the 2009 SAS annual meeting, clinical data were reported for 17 patients at 3–6 months of follow-up [97].

In the first full-length journal article dedicated to wear in PEEK cervical discs, researchers from Aesculap AG compared contemporary CoCr/UHMWPE couples with PEEK-OPTIMA LT1, CFR-PEEK (30% PAN fibers), and polyaryletherketone (PEK) all-polymer articulations [89]. The study by Grupp et al. [89] provides the most extensive and detailed peer-reviewed data available to date on the wear test methods, rates, and wear particle characteristics for three groups of all-polymer PEEK and PEK articulations intended for the cervical spine. All the polymer bearings used in this study were based on the design of the Activ-C cervical artificial disc. The UHMWPE was GUR 1020 gamma sterilized in nitrogen (30 kGy). Testing was conducted in accordance with ISO 18192. The PEEK and PEK bearings exhibited comparable wear rates to CoCr/UHMWPE, whereas the CFR-PEEK bearings had significantly lower wear rates (Figure 10.20). The size and morphology of the PEEK and PEK wear particles fell within the range previously observed for CoCr/UHMWPE articulations.

Considered together, recent studies suggest that PEEK biomaterials provide new design opportunities for all-polymer disc arthroplasties. Both cervical and lumbar PEEK artificial discs are currently in clinical trials; however, these studies are still in progress, and final data have yet to be published in peer-reviewed journals. Although the first designs in clinical use were fabricated from unfilled PEEK, there is not yet consensus on the optimal PEEK biomaterial for all-polymer disc bearings. Basic science pin-on-disc studies [99,100] suggest that all polymer CFR-PEEK articulations fabricated with PAN carbon fibers generate less wear than unfilled PEEK articulations and these findings are corroborated by recent cervical TDR tests conducted in a multidirectional spine wear simulator (Figure 10.20) [89]. Similarly, whether evaluated on a pin-on-disc experiment or in a spine wear simulator (Figure 10.20) [89], all-polymer PEK bearings appear to offer relatively modest improvements relative to PEEK. It remains to be seen if all-polymer PEEK bearing performance is design specific, or whether all-polymer disc replacements are equally well suited to the cervical and lumbar spine. Although scientific debate is sure to continue on these topics for years to come, currently available data would suggest that PEEK biomaterials are strong candidates for disc arthroplasty applications.

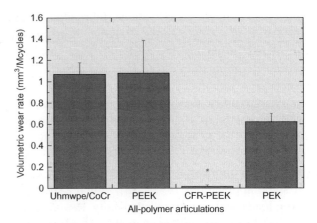

Figure 10.20 Comparison of volumetric wear rates for all-polymer PEEK and PEK articulations with conventional, gamma nitrogen-sterilized UHMWPE/CoCr cervical TDRs. Adapted from Ref. [89]. *CFR-PEEK bearings were significantly lower than the other cervical disc combinations tested ($p < 0.05$).

10.9 Summary

In summary, PEEK biomaterials have over a decade and a half of successful clinical history in load-sharing, fusion applications in the spine. Thus, the clinical history of PEEK biomaterials is heavily weighted by the cage experience from the spine fusion literature. PEEK is playing a growing role in spine implants for a combination of reasons, including the clinical need for improved treatments for operative treatment of persistent low back pain. The radiolucency of PEEK is another key advantage over metals, allowing visualization of the critical soft tissue structures, such as the spinal cord, adjacent to the implant components. Finally, the versatility of PEEK biomaterials allows for spinal devices to be designed with a tailored range of stiffnesses, depending on rigidity desired for a particular spine implant application.

Acknowledgments

The author thanks Marta Villarraga, Exponent, and Frank Chan, Medtronic, for their helpful editorial suggestions; Bill Christianson, DePuy Spine, for assistance with certain figures and many helpful discussions about the history of the Brantigan cage. Thanks are also extended to Brian Murell, Medtronic Spinal and Biologics; Hassan Serhan,

DePuy Spine; Michael Veldman, Invibio; and Dr. Todd Lanman for helpful discussions and editorial feedback about PEEK rod systems.

References

[1] Brown SA, Hastings RS, Mason JJ, Moet A. Characterization of short-fibre reinforced thermoplastics for fracture fixation devices. Biomaterials 1990;11:541–7.

[2] Skinner HB. Composite technology for total hip arthroplasty. Clin Orthop Relat Res 1988;:224–36.

[3] Villarraga ML. Historical review of spinal instrumentation for fusion: rods, screws, and plates. In: Kurtz SM, Edidin AA, editors. Spine technology handbook. New York: Academic Press; 2006. p. 183–208.

[4] Ong K, Lau E, Kurtz SM, Chin K, Ianuzzi A, Villarraga ML. Cervical, thoracic, and lumbar fusion rates in the U.S.: perspective from two health databases, Transactions of the 53rd Orthopedic Research Society; 2007. p. 1016.

[5] Ong K, Lau E, Kurtz SM, Chin K, Ianuzzi A, Villarraga ML. Projections to 2030 of the prevalence of primary and revision spine fusions in the U.S. Transactions of the 53rd Orthopedic Research Society; 2007. p. 1070.

[6] Mendenhall S. 2010 spinal industry update. Orthop Netw News 2010;21:3–6.

[7] Boden SD, Kang J, Sandhu H, Heller JG. Use of recombinant human bone morphogenetic protein-2 to achieve posterolateral lumbar spine fusion in humans: a prospective, randomized clinical pilot trial: 2002 Volvo Award in Clinical Studies. Spine (Phila., PA, 1976) 2002;27:2662–73.

[8] Ong KL, Villarraga ML, Lau E, Carreon LY, Kurtz SM, Glassman SD. Off-label use of bone morphogenetic proteins in the United States using administrative data. Spine 2010;35:1794–800.

[9] Huang RC, Girardi FP, Lim MR, Cammisa Jr. FP. Advantages and disadvantages of nonfusion technology in spine surgery. Orthop Clin North Am 2005;36:263–9.

[10] Singh K, An HS. Motion preservation technologies: alternatives to spinal fusion. Am J Orthop (Belle Mead, NJ) 2006;35:411–6.

[11] Christie SD, Song JK, Fessler RG. Dynamic interspinous process technology. Spine 2005; 30:S73–8.

[12] Kurtz SM. Total disc arthroplasty. In: Kurtz SM, Edidin AA, editors. Spine technology handbook. New York: Academic Press; 2006. p. 303–70.

[13] Albee FH. Transplantation of a portion of the tibia into the spine for Pott's disease. J Am Med Assoc 1911;57:855–8.

[14] Briggs H, Milligan PR. Chip fusion of the low back following exploration of the spinal canal. J Bone Joint Surg Am 1944;26:125–30.

[15] Burns BH. An operation for spondylolisthesis. Lancet 1933;1:1233.

[16] Cloward RB. The treatment of ruptured lumbar intervertebral disc by vertebral body fusion. III. Method of use of banked bone. Ann Surg 1952;136:987–92.

[17] Cloward RB. Vertebral body fusion for ruptured cervical discs. Am J Surg 1959;98:722–7.

[18] McAfee PC. Interbody fusion cages in reconstructive operations on the spine. J Bone Joint Surg Am 1999;81:859–80.

[19] Bagby G. The Bagby and Kuslich (BAK) method of lumbar interbody fusion. Spine (Phila., PA, 1976) 1999;24:1857.

[20] Kuslich SD, Ulstrom CL, Griffith SL, Ahern JW, Dowdle JD. The Bagby and Kuslich method of lumbar interbody fusion. History, techniques, and 2-year follow-up results of a United States prospective, multicenter trial. Spine (Phila., PA, 1976) 1998;23:1267–78. [discussion 79].

[21] McAfee PC, Cunningham BW, Lee GA, Orbegoso CM, Haggerty CJ, Fedder IL, et al. Revision strategies for salvaging or improving failed cylindrical cages. Spine (Phila., PA, 1976) 1999;24:2147–53.

[22] Elias WJ, Simmons NE, Kaptain GJ, Chadduck JB, Whitehill R. Complications of posterior lumbar interbody fusion when using a titanium threaded cage device. J Neurosurg 2000;93:45–52.

[23] Heim SE, Abitbol JJ. Complications and strategies for salvage of intervertebral fixation devices. Orthop Clin North Am 2002;33: 393–402 [vii].

[24] Zdeblick TA, Phillips FM. Interbody cage devices. Spine (Phila., PA, 1976) 2003;28: S2–7.

[25] Brantigan JW, Lauryssen C. Intervertebral fusion using carbon-fiber reinforced polymer implants. St. Louis: Quality Medical Publishing; 2006.

[26] Glassman SD, Carreon L, Djurasovic M, Campbell MJ, Puno RM, Johnson JR, et al. Posterolateral lumbar spine fusion with INFUSE bone graft. Spine J 2007;7:44–9.

[27] Christianson W. Personal communication, 2007.

[28] McMillin CR. Evaluation of PEKEKK composites for spine implants. 38th International SAMPE Symposium; 1993, 591–598.

[29] Brantigan JW, Steffee AD, Geiger JM. A carbon fiber implant to aid interbody lumbar fusion. Mechanical testing. Spine 1991;16: S277–82.

[30] Brantigan JW, Steffee AD. A carbon fiber implant to aid interbody lumbar fusion. Two-year clinical results in the first 26 patients. Spine 1993;18:2106–7.

[31] Brantigan JW, McAfee PC, Cunningham BW, Wang H, Orbegoso CM. Interbody lumbar fusion using a carbon fiber cage implant versus allograft bone. An investigational study in the Spanish goat. Spine 1994;19:1436–44.

[32] Brantigan JW, Steffee AD, Lewis ML, Quinn LM, Persenaire JM. Lumbar interbody fusion using the Brantigan I/F cage for posterior lumbar interbody fusion and the variable pedicle screw placement system: two-year results from a Food and Drug Administration investigational device exemption clinical trial. Spine 2000;25:1437–46.

[33] Christensen FB, Hansen ES, Eiskjaer SP, Hoy K, Helmig P, Neumann P, et al. Circumferential lumbar spinal fusion with Brantigan cage versus posterolateral fusion with titanium Cotrel-Dubousset instrumentation: a prospective, randomized clinical study of 146 patients. Spine 2002;27:2674–83.

[34] Videbaek TS, Christensen FB, Soegaard R, Hansen ES, Hoy K, Helmig P, et al. Circumferential fusion improves outcome in comparison with instrumented posterolateral fusion: long-term results of a randomized clinical trial. Spine 2006;31:2875–80.

[35] Invibio, Press Release. February 14, 2007.

[36] H. Serhan, Personal communication, 2011.

[37] Cho DY, Lee WY, Sheu PC. Treatment of multilevel cervical fusion with cages. Surg Neurol 2004;62:378–85 [discussion 85–86].

[38] Cho DY, Lee WY, Sheu PC, Chen CC. Cage containing a biphasic calcium phosphate ceramic (Triosite) for the treatment of cervical spondylosis. Surg Neurol 2005;63:497–503 [discussion 504].

[39] Cho DY, Liau WR, Lee WY, Liu JT, Chiu CL, Sheu PC. Preliminary experience using a polyetheretherketone (PEEK) cage in the treatment of cervical disc disease. Neurosurgery 2002;51:1343–9 [discussion 9–50].

[40] Toth JM, Wang M, Estes BT, Scifert JL, Seim III HB, Turner AS. Polyetheretherketone as a biomaterial for spinal applications. Biomaterials 2006;27:324–34.

[41] Mastronardi L, Ducati A, Ferrante L. Anterior cervical fusion with polyetheretherketone (PEEK) cages in the treatment of degenerative disc disease. Preliminary observations in 36 consecutive cases with a minimum 12-month follow-up. Acta Neurochir 2006;148:307–12 [discussion 312].

[42] Sekerci Z, Ugur A, Ergun R, Sanli M. Early changes in the cervical foraminal area after anterior interbody fusion with polyetheretherketone (PEEK) cage containing synthetic bone particulate: a prospective study of 20 cases. Neurol Res 2006;28:568–71.

[43] Spruit M, Falk RG, Beckmann L, Steffen T, Castelein RM. The in vitro stabilising effect of polyetheretherketone cages versus a titanium cage of similar design for anterior lumbar interbody fusion. Eur Spine J 2005;14: 752–8.

[44] Kettler A, Schmoelz W, Kast E, Gottwald M, Claes L, Wilke HJ. In vitro stabilizing effect of a transforaminal compared with two posterior lumbar interbody fusion cages. Spine 2005;30:E665–70.

[45] Ferguson SJ, Visser JM, Polikeit A. The long-term mechanical integrity of non-reinforced PEEK-OPTIMA polymer for demanding spinal applications: experimental and finite-element analysis. Eur Spine J 2006;15: 149–56.

[46] Demircan MN, Kutlay AM, Colak A, Kaya S, Tekin T, Kibici K, et al. Multilevel cervical

[47] Kulkarni AG, Hee HT, Wong HK. Solis cage (PEEK) for anterior cervical fusion: preliminary radiological results with emphasis on fusion and subsidence. Spine J 2007;7:205–9.

[48] Rousseau MA, Lazennec JY, Saillant G. Circumferential arthrodesis using PEEK cages at the lumbar spine. J Spinal Disord Tech 2007;20:278–81.

[49] Santos ER, Goss DG, Morcom RK, Fraser RD. Radiologic assessment of interbody fusion using carbon fiber cages. Spine 2003;28:997–1001.

[50] Reinhold M, Magerl F, Rieger M, Blauth M. Cervical pedicle screw placement: feasibility and accuracy of two new insertion techniques based on morphometric data. Eur Spine J 2007;16:47–56.

[51] Bartels RH, Donk RD, Feuth T. Subsidence of stand-alone cervical carbon fiber cages. Neurosurgery 2006;58:502–8 [discussion 508].

[52] Tullberg T. Failure of a carbon fiber implant. A case report. Spine 1998;23:1804–6.

[53] Togawa D, Bauer TW, Brantigan JW, Lowery GL. Bone graft incorporation in radiographically successful human intervertebral body fusion cages. Spine 2001;26:2744–50.

[54] Rivard CH, Rhalmi S, Coillard C. In vivo biocompatibility testing of PEEK polymer for a spinal implant system: a study in rabbits. J Biomed Mater Res 2002;62:488–98.

[55] Bono CM, Vaccaro AR. Interspinous process devices in the lumbar spine. J Spinal Disord Tech 2007;20:255–61.

[56] Kabir SM, Gupta SR, Casey AT. Lumbar interspinous spacers: a systematic review of clinical and biomechanical evidence. Spine (Phila Pa 1976) 2010;35:E1499–506.

[57] Wilke HJ, Drumm J, Haussler K, Mack C, Steudel WI, Kettler A. Biomechanical effect of different lumbar interspinous implants on flexibility and intradiscal pressure. Eur Spine J 2008;17:1049–56.

[58] Senegas J. Mechanical supplementation by non-rigid fixation in degenerative intervertebral lumbar segments: the Wallis system. Eur Spine J 2002;11(Suppl. 2):S164–9.

[59] Zucherman JF, Hsu KY, Hartjen CA, Mehalic TF, Implicito DA, Martin MJ, et al. A multicenter, prospective, randomized trial evaluating the X STOP interspinous process decompression system for the treatment of neurogenic intermittent claudication: two-year follow-up results. Spine (Phila., PA, 1976) 2005;30:1351–8.

[60] United States Food and Drug Administration, X STOP® Interspinous Process Decompression System—P040001, http://www.accessdata.fda.gov/scripts/cdrh/cfdocs/cfTopic/pma/pma.cfm?num = p040001. Approved November 21, 2005 [accessed online March 26].

[61] Tuschel A, Chavanne A, Eder C, Meissl M, Becker P, Ogon M. Implant survival analysis and failure modes of the X STOP interspinous distraction device. Spine (Phila., PA, 1976) 2011.

[62] Kim DH, Tantorski M, Shaw J, Martha J, Li L, Shanti N, et al. Occult spinous process fractures associated with interspinous process spacers. Spine (Phila., PA, 1976) 2011.

[63] Verhoof OJ, Bron JL, Wapstra FH, van Royen BJ. High failure rate of the interspinous distraction device (X-Stop) for the treatment of lumbar spinal stenosis caused by degenerative spondylolisthesis. Eur Spine J 2008;17:188–92.

[64] Highsmith JM, Tumialan LM, Rodts Jr. GE. Flexible rods and the case for dynamic stabilization. Neurosurg Focus 2007;22:E11.

[65] Turner JL, Paller DJ, Murrell CB. The mechanical effect of commercially pure titanium and polyetheretherketone rods on spinal implants at the operative and adjacent levels. Spine (Phila., PA, 1976) 2010;35:E1076–82.

[66] Bruner HJ, Guan Y, Yoganandan N, Pintar FA, Maiman DJ, Slivka MA. Biomechanics of polyaryletherketone rod composites and titanium rods for posterior lumbosacral instrumentation. J Neurosurg 2010;13:766–72.

[67] Ponnappan RK, Serhan H, Zarda B, Patel R, Albert T, Vaccaro AR. Biomechanical evaluation and comparison of polyetheretherketone rod system to traditional titanium rod fixation. Spine J 2009;9:263–7.

[68] Moon SM, Ingalhalikar A, Highsmith JM, Vaccaro AR. Biomechanical rigidity of an all-polyetheretherketone anterior thoracolumbar

spinal reconstruction construct: an in vitro corpectomy model. Spine J 2009;9:330—5.
[69] Rigby MC, Selmon GP, Foy MA, Fogg AJ. Graf ligament stabilisation: mid- to long-term follow-up. Eur Spine J 2001;10:234—6.
[70] Choi Y, Kim K, So K. Adjacent segment instability after treatment with a Graf ligament at minimum 8 years' followup. Clin Orthop Relat Res 2009;467:1740—6.
[71] Kanayama M, Hashimoto T, Shigenobu K, Togawa D, Oha F. A minimum 10-year follow-up of posterior dynamic stabilization using Graf artificial ligament. Spine (Phila., PA, 1976) 2007;32:1992—6 [discussion 7].
[72] Askar Z, Wardlaw D, Muthukumar T, Smith F, Kader D, Gibson S. Correlation between inter-vertebral disc morphology and the results in patients undergoing Graf ligament stabilisation. Eur Spine J 2004;13:714—8.
[73] Bothmann M, Kast E, Boldt GJ, Oberle J. Dynesys fixation for lumbar spine degeneration. Neurosurg Rev 2008;31:189—96.
[74] Welch WC, Cheng BC, Awad TE, Davis R, Maxwell JH, Delamarter R, et al. Clinical outcomes of the Dynesys dynamic neutralization system: 1-year preliminary results. Neurosurg Focus 2007;22:E8.
[75] Schwarzenbach O, Berlemann U, Stoll TM, Dubois G. Posterior dynamic stabilization systems: DYNESYS. Orthop Clin North Am 2005;36:363—72.
[76] Grob D, Benini A, Junge A, Mannion AF. Clinical experience with the Dynesys semi-rigid fixation system for the lumbar spine: surgical and patient-oriented outcome in 50 cases after an average of 2 years. Spine (Phila., PA, 1976) 2005;30:324—31.
[77] Liu CL, Zhong ZC, Shih SL, Hung C, Lee YE, Chen CS. Influence of Dynesys system screw profile on adjacent segment and screw. J Spinal Disord Tech 2010;23:410—7.
[78] Ko CC, Tsai HW, Huang WC, Wu JC, Chen YC, Shih YH, et al. Screw loosening in the Dynesys stabilization system: radiographic evidence and effect on outcomes. Neurosurg Focus 2010;28:E10.
[79] Ianuzzi A, Kurtz SM, Kane W, Shah P, Siskey R, van Ooij A, et al. In vivo deformation, surface damage, and biostability of retrieved Dynesys systems. Spine (Phila., PA, 1976) 2010;35:E1310—6.
[80] Dakhil-Jerew F, Jadeja H, Cohen A, Shepperd JA. Inter-observer reliability of detecting Dynesys pedicle screw using plain X-rays: a study on 50 post-operative patients. Eur Spine J 2009;18:1486—93.
[81] Sarbello JF, Lipman AJ, Hong J, Lawrence J, Bessey JT, Ponnappan RK, et al. Patient perception of outcomes following failed spinal instrumentation with polyetheretherketone rods and titanium rods. Spine (Phila., PA, 1976) 2010;35(17):E843—8.
[82] T. Lanman, Personal communication, 2011.
[83] Sobieraj MC, Murphy JE, Brinkman JG, Kurtz SM, Rimnac CM. Notched fatigue behavior of PEEK. Biomaterials 2010;31:9156—62.
[84] Sobieraj MC, Kurtz SM, Rimnac CM. Notch sensitivity of PEEK in monotonic tension. Biomaterials 2009;30:6485—94.
[85] M. Veldman, Personal communication, 2011.
[86] ASTM F1717-10, Standard test methods for spinal implant constructs in a vertebrectomy model. ASTM International, West Conshohocken, PA, 2010 www.astm.org2010.
[87] Siskey R, Day J, Kurtz SM. Validation of a test method for evaluating the fatigue performance of PEEK spinal fusion rod systems. Transactions of the 56th Orthopedic Research Society, vol. 35; 2010. p. 0274.
[88] Pasciak M, Grzywocz J, Nobis A, Pala A, Wadek T. PEEK plastic rods versus titanium "stiff" rods in transpedicular lumbar stabilization. Clinical comparison of short term results, Transactions of Eurospine; 2009. p. 39.
[89] Grupp TM, Meisel HJ, Cotton JA, Schwiesau J, Fritz B, Blomer W, et al. Alternative bearing materials for intervertebral disc arthroplasty. Biomaterials 2009;31(3):523—31.
[90] Bao QB, Songer M, Pimenta K, Werner D, Reyes-Sanchez A, Balsano M, et al. NUBAC intradiscal arthroplasty: preclinical studies and preliminary safety and efficacy evaluations. SAS J 2007;1:36—45.
[91] Coric D, Songer M, Yuan H, Pimenta L, Reyes-Sanchez A, Werner D, et al. Up to 2-year follow-up results of a novel PEEK-on-PEEK disc arthroplasty: A prospective worldwide multicenter clinical study. Transactions of the 9th Annual Symposium for the International Society for the Advance of Spine Surgery (SAS); 2009.

[92] Brown T, Bao Q. Compressive load sensitivity on the biotribological properties of NUBAC. Transactions of the 9th Annual Symposium for the International Society for the Advance of Spine Surgery (SAS); 2009.

[93] Wimmer M, Schwenke T, Brown T, Kilpela T, Bao Q. The effect of accelerated aging on the wear of PEEK for use in disc arthroplasty. Transactions of the 54th Orthopedic Research Society, vol. 54; 2008. p. 1922.

[94] Brown T, Bao Q, Kilpela T, Schwenke T, Wimmer M. A comprehensive wear assessment of PEEK-OPTIMA for disc arthroplasty applications. Transactions of the World Biomaterials Congress; 2008.

[95] Schwenke T, Brown T, Bao Q, Kilpela T, Wimmer M. Wear assessment of a self mating polymer for nucleus replacement devices. Transactions of the 53rd Orthopedic Research Society, vol. 53; 2007. p. 1125.

[96] Brown T, Bao Q, Kilpela T. A wear assessment of NUBAC under a cross shear motion profile. Transactions of the 7th Annual SAS Global Symposium on Motion Preservation Technology; 2007.

[97] Yuan H, Coric D, Yuan P, Zou D, Ma H, Yang H, et al. Early clinical experience of NuNec, a novel PEEK-on-PEEK artificial cervical disc. Transactions of the 9th Annual Symposium for the International Society for the Advance of Spine Surgery (SAS); 2009.

[98] Brown T, Bao Q, Hallab N. Biotribology assessment of NUNEC, a PEEK on PEEK cervical disc replacement according to ISO and ASTM recommendations. Transactions of the 9th Annual Symposium for the International Society for the Advance of Spine Surgery (SAS); 2009.

[99] Scholes SC, Unsworth A. The wear performance of PEEK-OPTIMA based self-mating couples. Wear 2009; http://dx.doi.org/10.1016/j.wear.2009.08.023.

[100] Austin H, Powell M, Medley J, Langohr D. Exploring the wear of a PEEK all-polymer articulation for spinal applications. Transactions of the Society for Biomaterials; 2009.

[101] Dooris AP, Ares PJ, Gabriel SM, Serhan HA. Wear characterization of an artificial disc using ASTM guidelines. Transactions of the 51st Orthopedic Research Society; 2005. p. 51.

[102] Mummaneni PV, Haid RW. The future in the care of the cervical spine: interbody fusion and arthroplasty. Invited submission from the Joint Section Meeting on Disorders of the Spine and Peripheral Nerves, March 2004. J Neurosurg 2004;(1):155−9.

[103] Nechtow W, Hinter M, Bushelow M, Caddick C. IVD replacement mechanical performance depends strongly on input parameters. Transactions of the 52nd Orthopedic Research Society, vol. 52; 2006. p. 118.

11 Microbubble Applications in Biomedicine

Sana S. Dastgheyb, PhD Candidate and John R. Eisenbrey, PhD

OUTLINE

11.1 Introduction	253	11.4.1 Microbubble-Assisted Delivery of Free Drug	263
11.2 Microbubbles for Ultrasound Imaging	257	11.5 Microbubbles in Gene Delivery	264
11.2.1 Interactions of Microbubbles with Ultrasound	257	11.5.1 Microbubbles as Drug Carriers	264
11.2.2 Microbubble-Specific Ultrasound Modes	259	11.6 Other Emerging Applications	266
11.2.3 Current Clinical Uses of Microbubbles	259	11.6.1 Biofilm Destruction	266
		11.6.2 Noninvasive Pressure Estimation	266
11.3 Targeted Microbubbles	260	11.6.3 Tissue Engineering	267
11.3.1 Ligand/Receptor Targeting	261	11.6.4 Magnetic Resonance Imaging	267
11.3.2 Identification and Quantification of Microbubble Attachment	262	11.6.5 Nanobubbles	267
11.3.3 Active Targeting	262	11.6.6 Lymphosonography	267
11.4 Microbubbles in Drug and Gene Delivery	262	11.7 Conclusion	268
		References	268

11.1 Introduction

Microbubbles are small (<10 μm), gas-containing spheres with a lipid, protein, or polymer shell [1] (Figure 11.1). Microbubbles provide a means for contrast-enhanced ultrasound imaging, targeted drug delivery, and other diagnostic and therapeutic applications.

The developmental history of microbubbles as ultrasound contrast agents is summarized in Figure 11.2. The first indirect mention of the use of microbubbles in medical diagnostics was in 1968, when Gramiak and Shah demonstrated that intracardiac injections of saline-containing small air bubbles significantly increased ultrasound contrast and improved aortic delineation [2]. Given the dissolution time of nonencapsulated air bubbles (dependent on bubble size, but generally a few seconds), the next step was to create a vehicle that would entrap gas and offer enough stability for prolonged ultrasound exposure. In 1984, Feinstein et al. showed that a more stable microbubble could be formed using sonication of various sugar derivatives as a technique to entrap gas within a solid-state shell [3]. From this concept, microbubbles were developed to have protein, polymer, or lipid shells. Variations on the microbubble construction/design increased its utility in the world of ultrasound imaging. In the early 1990s, it was discovered that microbubbles could be targeted by taking advantage of ligand/receptor interactions [4]. By the year 2000, microbubbles had proven to be not only useful contrast agents, but also powerful vehicles for targeted drug and gene delivery. Microbubbles were also proven to have therapeutic applications in thrombus treatment [5]. Currently, the first clinical trials are under way to evaluate the efficacy of VEGFR2-targeted microbubbles (BR55; Bracco, Milan, Italy) in monitoring anti-angiogenic effects of prostate cancer treatment [6].

Microbubbles serve the purpose of providing a relatively inexpensive, bio-inert, and metabolically inert method for increasing ultrasound contrast [7,8]. Both the micron-scale size and the gas core

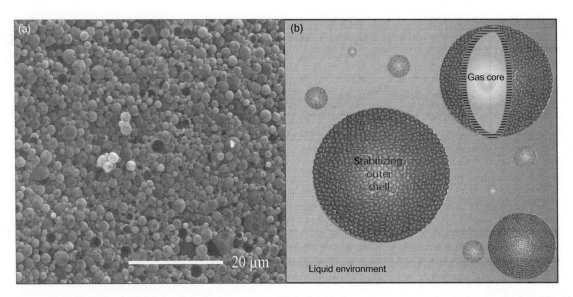

Figure 11.1 Microbubble structure and components. (a) SEM image of polymer-shell microbubbles (PLA) diameter 1–10 μm. (b) The basic structure of microbubbles—outer shell, gas core, liquid environment. *(Courtesy: Dr. Margaret Wheatley, PhD, for providing the SEM image.)*

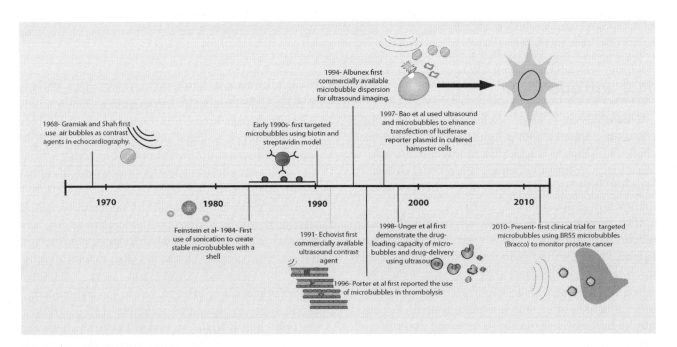

Figure 11.2 Microbubble timeline.

of the microbubbles are key features for their utility in ultrasound imaging. Firstly, microbubbles are small enough to traverse the human circulatory system without causing blockage, or producing physiologic aberrations, but are generally too large to escape out of the vasculature [3]. Second, the difference between the acoustic properties of the gas core of the microbubble and the surrounding medium allows for clinicians to more effectively visualize the cardiovascular system [9].

Microbubbles in solution provide a substantial mismatch in acoustic impedance, which is highly conducive for providing reflection in ultrasound imaging. Soft tissue is nearly homogeneous in acoustic impedance when compared to a gas-phase/filled contrast agent. Ultrasound scanners use a transducer to emit sound energy as well as to collect returning signal [10]. As the sound waves reach the microbubble surface, the microbubble undergoes compression and rarefaction, generating both linear and nonlinear signals which return to the transducer and are processed to form ultrasound images [11].

Microbubbles have been fabricated using several individual gases and may have protein, lipid, surfactant, or polymer shells that are thin (5–10 nm) or thick (up to 250 nm). The microbubble shell provides stability, but also dampens the oscillatory motions of the microbubble when activated. Furthermore, microbubbles can have modified extruding surfaces such as polyethylene glycol (PEG) brushes and ligand attachments [12]. Table 11.1 gives the various microbubble shell types along with the potential benefits each modification imparts.

Clinically, microbubbles are administered via intravenous injection [3]. Once they enter the bloodstream, they can circulate without disrupting normal blood flow. The residence time of microbubbles in circulation is less than 1 h as the shells of the microbubbles are typically removed from the bloodstream by the liver and spleen, while the gas is exhaled [1]. The incorporation of high molecular weight perfluorocarbon gases in microbubbles has ensured that gas exchange is negligible *in vivo* when compared to clearance time of the microbubble injection [18]. Once in circulation, microbubbles may be either imaged using low-power ultrasound (generally with mechanical indexes < 0.4) or burst using localized higher power ultrasound (generally with mechanical indexes > 0.7) to facilitate microbubble

Table 11.1 Table of Microbubble Structure and Function/Use

Microbubble Type	Description
Lipid Shell	Phospholipids, such as phosphatidylethanolamine, spontaneously self-assemble into a spherical monolayer, wherein the hydrophilic polar head groups are oriented towards the liquid environment and the hydrophobic acyl chains face the gaseous core of the microbubble. Lipid-shelled microbubbles are highly echogenic due to the flexibility of the lipid shell, which allows the microbubbles to resonate under ultrasound stimulation with minimal damping [13].
Polymer-Stabilized Lipid Shell	Lipid shells are often stabilized by a thick shell of polymer. A polymer brush, normally polyethylene glycol (PEG), lends rigidity to the microbubble, however it reduces the echogenicity [14]. PEG coatings have also been shown to increase targeting efficacy and decrease complement activation *in vivo* [15].

(Continued)

Table 11.1 Table of Microbubble Structure and Function/Use—Cont'd

Microbubble Type	Description
Polymer Shell	Polymer microbubbles can be made of synthetic polymer such as PLGA, or naturally occurring polymers such as sugar derivatives. At a lower ultrasound pressure intensity, the polymer microbubble has a reduced oscillatory activity when compared with its lipid and albumin counterparts. At higher ultrasound pressure, the polymeric shell will form cracks and disassemble [16].
Protein Shell	Albumin-coated microbubbles were the first commercially available micro-bubbles (Albunex™, GE Healthcare). The albumin shell is stabilized by disulfide bonds between cystein residues in the shell [17].

destruction-based imaging modes or local drug/gene delivery [19].

One particular advantage of microbubbles as a contrast and drug-delivery agent is that microbubbles are highly shelf-stable when the gas headspace is maintained and are manufactured at a relatively low cost and in high quantities [20,21]. Industry has taken advantage of microbubble technologies, making them commercially available and readily accessible by clinicians and researchers alike. Table 11.2 lists current commercially available ultrasound contrast agents which are approved for human use, particularly in left ventricular opacification (LVO) for the diagnosis of coronary artery disease.

It should be noted that the safety of microbubble administration has been questioned at several points in the short history of their clinical use. The bursting of microbubbles has emerged as a double-edged sword. On the one hand, microbubble cavitation is central to microbubble drug-delivery applications. On the other hand, it is known that microbubble destruction as a result of high-powered ultrasound can cause rupturing of microvessel walls and subsequent extravasation of the blood [7]. Though rare, serious adverse reactions generally involve anaphylaxis [22]. A post market study of SonoVue by the European Medicines Agency revealed a nonfatal reaction rate of 0.012% and a fatal reaction rate of 0.002% [22]. Thus, microbubble use in echocardiography was branded as causative for rarely observed cardiopulmonary and hypersensitivity reactions, garnering a Food and Drug Administration (FDA) black box warning. Main et al. demonstrate that it is important to put these rates of adverse reaction in perspective, pointing out the mortality rates of coronary angiography and exercise treadmill testing are 0.1% and 0.04%,

Table 11.2 Table of Commercially Available Microbubble Preparations

Microbubble Preparation	Microbubble Type	Details on Use
Definity (Lantheus Medical Imaging)	Phospholipid Shell octofluoropropane-filled	Available worldwide. Approved for use in the USA (cardiac imaging)
Sonazoid (GE healthcare)	Phospholipid Shell perfluorobutane-filled	Approved and marketed in Japan, South Korea, Taiwan, and China
Sonovue (Bracco)	Phospholipid Shell sulfur hexafluoride-filled	Approved and marketed in European countries, China, South Korea, Hong Kong, and Singapore.
Optison (GE healthcare)	Albumin Shell perfluorobutane-filled	Approved and marketed in European countries. Approved for use in the USA (cardiac imaging)

respectively [23]. This safety issue has also been well addressed by Blomley et al., who point out that the increased enhancement in endocardial border delineation and cardiac perfusion well outweighs the minor side effects (mainly temporary headache and altered sensation at the injection site in roughly 2% of patients) [24]. As a result of the outcry from cardiologists, radiologists, and researchers, as well as the publication of numerous large clinical studies showing both the benefits and safety of microbubbles, the FDA's warning has since been softened [23–25].

In this chapter, microbubble use in medical diagnostics are briefly reviewed as well as additional emerging roles in surface targeting, drug and gene delivery, pressure estimation, and other future potential clinical applications.

11.2 Microbubbles for Ultrasound Imaging

11.2.1 Interactions of Microbubbles with Ultrasound

Clinical ultrasound imaging continues to increase in popularity due to its superior safety (it uses non-ionizing radiation), real-time imaging, cost, and portability relative to other imaging modalities [26]. It is estimated that there are 75,000 ultrasound machines compared to only 5000 magnetic resonance imaging (MRI) machines in the United States and this disparity is expected to increase over time [27]. During an ultrasound scan, acoustic waves are transmitted through the body, some of which are reflected back to the transducer due to differences in acoustic impedance. Reflected waves are then used to generate images. Acoustic impedance (z) is defined as:

$$z = \rho \times c, \quad (11.1)$$

where ρ is the density of the medium (kg/m^3) and c is the speed of sound in the medium (m/s). The degree of reflection an ultrasound wave undergoes when passing from one medium to a second medium is defined by the reflection coefficient (R) as:

$$R = \frac{z_2 - z_1}{z_2 + z_1}, \quad (11.2)$$

where $R = 1$ denotes 100% wave reflection, while $R = 0$ denotes 100% transmission of the wave.

The utility of microbubbles in ultrasound imaging was first discovered incidentally by Gramiak and Shah in 1968 [2]. While injecting indocyanine for an X-ray study of the aorta under ultrasound guidance, the group observed that the small gas bubbles at the syringe tip produced noticeable ultrasound enhancement. Later it was discovered that the gas within the microbubbles provided a substantial impedance mismatch between the blood and gas interface, reflecting the ultrasound waves. For air at atmospheric pressure and 20°C [28]:

$$z_{\text{air}} = 415 \text{ Pa} \cdot \text{s/m} \quad (11.3)$$

while for distilled water (similar to blood and tissue) at 1 atm and 20°C,

$$z_{\text{water}} = 1.48 \times 10^6 \text{ Pa} \cdot \text{s/m} \quad (11.4)$$

Substituting these impedance values into equation (11.2) results in $R \approx 1$, explaining the near perfect reflection of the acoustic wave by gas within the microbubble. Additionally, microbubble scattering or reflection can be categorized by the effective scattering cross section (σ) of the microbubble. The scattering cross section reflects the scattered ultrasound intensity related to the incident intensity and distance from the transducer, and can be calculated as:

$$\sigma = \frac{4\pi}{9} K^4 r^6 \left[\left(\frac{\kappa_s - \kappa_f}{\kappa_f} \right)^2 + \frac{1}{3} \left(\frac{3(\rho_s - \rho_f)}{2(\rho_s + \rho_f)} \right)^2 \right] \quad (11.5)$$

where K is the wave number, r is the bubble radius, κ_s is the compressibility of the scatterer, κ_f is the compressibility of the fluid, ρ_s is the density of the scatterer, and ρ_f is the density of the fluid [29–31]. It is important to note from the bracketed portion of this equation that while the density (and thus impedance) portion of this term plays a central role in the cross scattering area, the difference in compressibilities is more than 10,000 times larger that of the difference in densities [32]. Thus, while the impedance mismatch is important for providing a reflective surface for the ultrasound wave, the differences in compressibility are what truly account for microbubbles having effective backscattering radii several orders of magnitude larger than the bubble itself [31].

As the acoustic wave propagates through the gas microbubble, the gas within the microbubble expands and contracts according to the pressure rarefaction and compression of the sound wave as shown in Figure 11.3. These oscillations result in both a linear and nonlinear response, as shown in the frequency spectrum from an ultrasound contrast agent (Targestar-B; TargesonInc, San Diego, CA) insonated at 4 MHz presented below in Figure 11.4. Note that the strongest frequency response occurs at the fundamental insonation frequency ($f_0 = 4$ MHz), while there are also significant signal components at the subharmonic

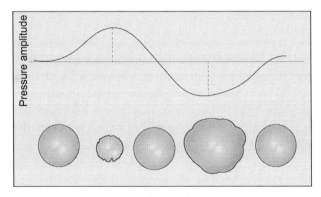

Figure 11.3 Microbubble compression and rarefaction. Illustration of a microbubble undergoing expansion and contraction during the pressure rarefaction and compression phases of the ultrasound pulse.

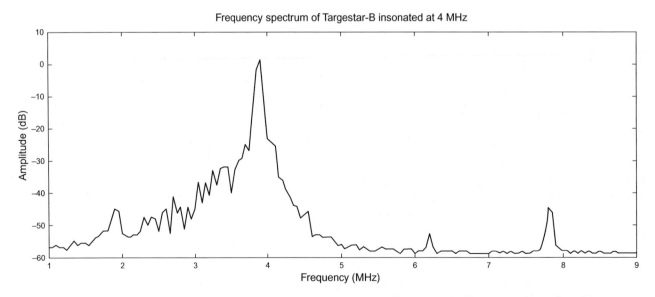

Figure 11.4 Frequency response of the ultrasound contrast agent Targestar-B (Targeson Inc., San Diego, CA). Microbubbles insonated at 4 MHz show a nonlinear response of the microbubble population.

($f_0/2 = 2$ MHz), higher harmonics ($n \cdot f_0$; 8 MHz), and ultraharmonic frequencies (($2n - 1)/2 \cdot f_0$, $n > 1$; 6 MHz). This nonlinearity forms the basis for microbubble-specific imaging modes.

11.2.2 Microbubble-Specific Ultrasound Modes

Microbubbles were initially used with grayscale B-mode ultrasound (i.e., a linear imaging mode) to improve contrast and contour detection [33]. However, these improvements were incremental due to a low detection sensitivity and blood volume relative to tissue [32].

The addition of microbubbles to Doppler imaging (which detects changes in relative movement, generally blood) has proven more advantageous due to this mode's ability to detect microvasculature and has been used for the imaging of a variety of clinical applications [32–37]. In conjunction with Doppler ultrasound, microbubbles are frequently used in echocardiography in the diagnosis and interpretation of cardiac defects such as hypertrophic cardiomyopathy, chest-wall deformities, coronary artery disease, and for the evaluation of heart valves [38–41]. However, the use of contrast microbubbles with Doppler is also associated with significant imaging artifacts such as "blooming" and shadowing of signal below areas of contrast which make smaller, deeper vessels difficult to image [41,42].

Specific microbubble imaging modes have been and are currently being developed to exploit the nonlinearity of these agents. Harmonic imaging relies on the ability of microbubbles to reflect signal at twice the insonation frequency by removing all other frequency components. Additionally, pulse inversion and amplitude modulations can be applied to transmit multiple, inverted pulses which are subsequently summed to further remove linear components and designed to specifically make the microbubbles resonate [43]. Contrast packages involving some variation of these techniques are now commercially available on most scanners and have been shown useful for a variety of applications [44–49].

Despite these advances, tissue itself has also been shown to produce lower amplitude harmonic echoes due to the distortion of the ultrasound wave as it propagates through the tissue, thus limiting the ability of the mode to isolate microbubble signals [50,44]. One emerging attractive alternative to harmonic imaging is subharmonic imaging due to a lack of subharmonic generation in tissue [50]. While still in a research phase, subharmonic imaging has now been implemented on modified commercial scanners [51–55] and used for numerous imaging applications [51,54–58]. Additionally this mode has been implemented in 3D to provide complete visualization of a vascular region [56,59]. Figure 11.5 shows an example of a canine kidney during open abdomen scanning with 3D subharmonic and harmonic imaging [54]. Note the improved levels of tissue suppression in subharmonic mode (evident before contrast arrival at baseline) and the improved visualization of the renal vasculature that this tissue suppression offers relative to the harmonic case. While this mode is still in research phases, this or other improved contrast imaging modes may further improve the utility of microbubbles in contrast ultrasound imaging.

A final class of microbubble imaging modes involves the destruction (using high-intensity ultrasound pulses) of the agent, followed by imaging of the reperfusion into the vasculature. These techniques, such as contrast burst imaging and microflow imaging, have been used to image microvasculature in a variety of applications, particularly in the estimation of blood flow perfusion [60–63] and have also been well reviewed in the literature [32,64].

11.2.3 Current Clinical Uses of Microbubbles

The full extent of microbubbles in clinical imaging (contrast-enhanced ultrasound) is beyond the scope of this chapter but has been well reviewed in the literature [32,65–68]. Additionally, ultrasound and echocardiography professional societies also routinely publish consensus statements on clinical guidelines for the use of ultrasound contrast agents [69–71].

Within the United States, microbubbles are only approved by the FDA for use in echocardiography. Suggested uses include improved visualization for the assessment of cardiac structure and function (particularly in hard to image patients), improved accuracy and decreased variability in stress echocardiography, to assist in the detection and classification of intracardiac masses, and to enhance spectral Doppler signals for the evaluation of diastolic and valvular function [69]. The use of these agents has been demonstrated in large-scale clinical trials. For example, a Phase III study of Optison for left

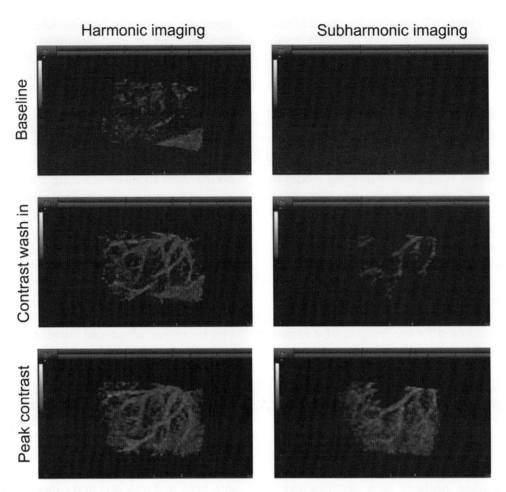

Figure 11.5 Ultrasound image of a canine kidney. Example images obtained from a canine kidney during baseline (top row) and contrast arrivals (bottom row) using 4D harmonic imaging (left column) and 4D subharmonic imaging (right column).

ventricular endocardial border delineation was able to convert 74% of non-diagnostic ultrasound scans to diagnostic, thus providing potentially lifesaving information to physicians [72]. While the initial FDA black box warnings discussed in the introduction section severely dampened the usage of contrast-enhanced echocardiography, usage has increased with the subsequent clarification and abundant published safety studies, and is expected to further increase in the future [73–77].

Microbubble-based ultrasound contrast applications are approved for general vascular imaging in most countries outside the United States and used frequently in abdominal imaging, and clinical guidelines are available [70,71]. The real-time nature of contrast imaging allows detection of microbubble perfusion during the vascular phase within the liver. As a result, one of the largest abdominal applications is for the detection and characterization of focal liver lesions [70,78]. Large clinical trials have shown these techniques to correlate well with contrast-enhanced computed tomography (CT) [32,47,70,79] and this has become the clinical standard of care in many countries. As FDA approval extends to other applications of contrast-enhanced ultrasound, this technology will become a standard clinical tool for both therapeutics and diagnostic applications.

11.3 Targeted Microbubbles

Once microbubbles have entered the circulatory system, they can freely circulate throughout the vasculature with a residence time on the order of 10 min [80] and will typically accumulate in the liver and spleen [1]. Clinically, ultrasound is used on freely circulating microbubbles for contrast imaging purposes (as discussed in the imaging section above) where visualizing physiology is the only objective. In other cases, it might be necessary to direct microbubble accumulation toward a certain pathological manifestation. Once microbubbles have been targeted to the affected area, ultrasound can be used to better image the delineated area. Methods of microbubble targeting include ligand/receptor "pairing" and magnetic guidance [4,81]. Due to the size of the microbubbles, potential targets are currently limited to those expressed within the vasculature. However, the advent of nanobubbles (discussed later in the chapter) may further diversify these targets as smaller bubbles are able to extravasate out of the blood supply.

11.3.1 Ligand/Receptor Targeting

The most common method of targeting microbubbles is through passive targeting, either through ligand-receptor specificity or through organ-specific accumulation.

One of the first reports of targeted microbubbles used biotinylated microbubbles to target a streptavidin-coated surface [4]. Another early study by Unger et al. explored the *in vitro* targeting of microbubbles using a thrombus-specific hexapeptide coupled to microbubbles and showed improved microbubble targeting to blood clots *in vitro* [21,82]. Figure 11.6 depicts the targeting of a biotinylated microbubble onto a streptavidin-coated agar surface.

From these experiments, it became apparent that an antigen-coated surface can be targeted and subsequently imaged with increased microbubble accumulation. It therefore follows that disease states such as inflammation and cancer can potentially be targeted using ligand-conjugated microbubbles.

For example, microbubbles can be targeted to specific inflamed areas within blood vessels allowing for visualization of the diseased state. Most notably, microbubbles have been shown to be able to target atherosclerotic disease markers, such as VCAM-1 using an anti-VCAM-1 antibody that is conjugated to the surface of the microbubble [6]. Once microbubbles have honed in on the inflamed area, ultrasound imaging will reveal the highlighted atherosclerotic plaque. Figure 11.7 illustrates the targeting of microbubbles to atherosclerotic lesions or plaques within the vasculature.

The targeting of neoplasia using microbubbles has become an area of interest in recent years. Pysz et al. developed microbubbles to target human kinase insert domain receptors and/or VEGFR2 receptors using microbubbles conjugated with VEGF [83]. Generic-targeted microbubbles (mainly for angiogenesis or atherosclerosis markers) or kits for preparing microbubbles for specific targets are now commercially available from several companies for research purposes in animals. Recently, the first clinical trial with targeted microbubbles BR55 (Bracco), a VEGFR2-targeted microbubble (which does not use an avidin–biotin linkage, making it suitable for

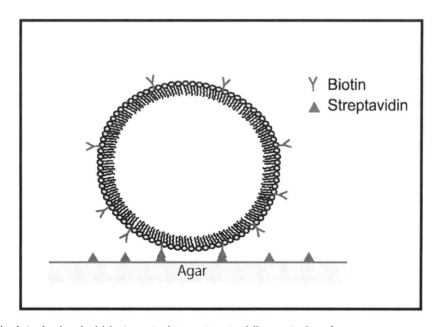

Figure 11.6 Biotinylated microbubble targeted to a streptavidin-coated surface.

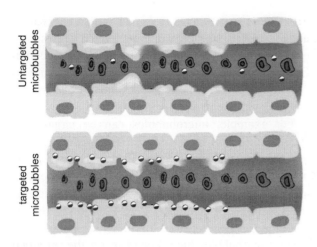

Figure 11.7 Targeting atherosclerosis with microbubbles. Endothelial cells in atherosclerotic areas express up-regulated levels of adhesion molecules such as P-selectin, E-selectin $\alpha 5\beta 3$ integrin, and V-CAM. Targeting microbubbles to these markers allows for enhanced microbubble accumulation as well as identification of specific disease markers.

human use), was employed to evaluate angiogenesis in prostate cancer [6].

Another form of passive targeting is based on the inherent characteristic of microbubbles, wherein they accumulate in the liver and spleen. When those organs are the desired targets for microbubble-assisted drug delivery or contrast-enhanced microbubble imaging, microbubbles can simply be administered and left to self-congregate prior to insonation with low-power imaging [1]. In the liver, contrast-enhanced ultrasound can be particularly useful for the evaluation of hepatic portal vein thrombus, facilitating differentiation between benign and malignant thrombosis [84]. The spleno-specific properties of microbubbles also allow for identification of splenic infarcts and the imaging of splenic abscesses and tumors [85].

These methods of passive targeting provide methods of delineating disease processes that may otherwise not be easily detected and/or evaluated.

11.3.2 Identification and Quantification of Microbubble Attachment

Identifying areas of successful microbubble targeting and accumulation typically involves a "flushing" period wherein unadhered microbubbles are allowed to exit the circulation (generally over 5–10 min). Additionally, before and after, images can be processed in order to determine microbubble attachment following ultrasound-mediated bursting of microbubbles.

For a real-time approach with fewer artifacts, Needles et al. used subharmonic imaging (to identify microbubbles while suppressing tissue) combined with an interframe filtering technique to identify stationary bubbles [55]. Groups have also investigated both the effects of attachment on the acoustic properties of the microbubbles and the strength of these attachments. Attached microbubbles can be characterized *in vitro* under high flow and shear stress, although the strength of adherence is largely related to the ligand receptor pair binding kinetics as well as ligand/receptor concentration [86].

11.3.3 Active Targeting

One method for improving microbubble targeting is through active targeting. Microbubble adhesion can be further improved using acoustic radiation forces, whereby the ultrasound beam pushes microbubbles toward the vasculature wall resulting in more ligand–target interaction [87]. These forces are useful for improving microbubble accumulation, but may also confound identification of receptor attachment.

The use of an external magnetic field has also been shown to redirect modified microbubbles to a desired region in tissues proximal to a magnet. In 2008, Kaminski et al. showed that microbubbles loaded with magnetic nanoparticles can be localized using magnetic guidance in a mouse model [88]. More recently, Wu et al. demonstrated the synergistic effects of targeting when magnetic guidance was used in conjunction with ligand targeting of microbubbles in a mouse model [89].

11.4 Microbubbles in Drug and Gene Delivery

Microbubble-assisted drug and gene delivery has been explored for over 20 years. This research has focused on improving efficacy while also limiting systemic side effects. These approaches utilize the biomechanical effects of both the microbubble as they interact with the ultrasound beam and the physical structure of the agent itself, which allows encapsulation or attachment as a means of drug transport. Microbubble-aided drug delivery has been extensively reviewed in the literature [6,90–92]. In this section, we present a small sample of previous and ongoing research efforts in microbubble-aided drug delivery. These samples are categorized by microbubble-aided delivery of free (unattached) therapeutics or microbubble-transported (attached or encapsulated) drug delivery.

11.4.1 Microbubble-Assisted Delivery of Free Drug

Ultrasound by itself has already been proven as an effective aid for drug delivery through increased drug retention at the tumor site and transient membrane permeability [93]. For example, studies have shown systemic administration of doxorubicin combined with low-intensity ultrasound (0.25–2 W/cm^2) leads to increased drug efficacy *in vivo* [93,94]. The benefits of ultrasound with drug delivery appear to become even more significant in the presence of microbubbles. Several studies have shown that peptides, genes, and other small molecules can be delivered out of the vasculature and into the intracellular space with the help of ultrasound and microbubble cavitation, and that this phenomenon also transiently increases cell permeability [95–97].

Microbubble cavitation can be classified as either stable (repeatable oscillations during insonation) or inertial, in which the bubble violently collapses [98]. Inertial cavitation of a gas bubble produces brief (<1 ms) shock waves, and extreme localized temperatures and pressures (>5000°C and 500 atm) [99]. Linear oscillations of microbubbles during stable cavitation have been shown to be strong enough to rupture lipid-based cellular membranes [97]. Using high-speed imaging of oscillating microbubbles against endothelial cells, van Wamel and colleagues were able to show uptake of propidium iodide and increased membrane permeability as cells became deformed from contact with vibrating phospholipid microbubbles [100]. Additional work using the same high-speed photography setup showed that jetting from inertially cavitating gas microbubbles in the close vicinity (<2 bubble diameters) of a cellular boundary resulted in detachment of roughly 5 cells/localized ultrasound contrast agent *in vitro* [101]. These experiments demonstrate the benefit of using microbubbles to improve drug delivery on a cellular level.

On a more macroscopic level, inertial cavitation of microbubbles within the vasculature has been shown to change the tissue transport properties, allowing transport of large (up to 500 nm) particles out of the vasculature. Price et al. showed they could deliver 200 and 500 nm fluorescent particles out of the capillary vasculature and into the interstitial space when combined with phospholipid ultrasound contrast agent cavitation by 2.3 MHz, 4 cycle pulses of ultrasound at a mechanical index of 0.7 (well within the FDA pressure guidelines for clinical ultrasound scanners) [102]. While the gap junctions within the vasculature are generally quite small (<50 nm in normal tissue) and prevent transport of larger particles, Price was able to show these particles could extrasavate in a time window of up to 5 s after ultrasound contrast agent cavitation [102]. Therefore, ultrasound-triggered destruction of microbubbles may be used to temporarily increase vasculature permeability for increased particle transport as well as increased cellular permeability.

Numerous studies and reviews have been published showing the synergy of these bioeffects when combined with traditional chemotherapy *in vitro* and *in vivo* [20,102–108]. One earlier *in vivo* example of microbubble destruction-aided cancer therapy showed that the cavitation of microbubbles when combined with the anticancer drug bleomycin significantly retarded growth of B-16 melanoma tumors in mice compared to drug alone [109]. Additionally, the group showed that a lower overall dose was required (nearly 10% of the effective dose with ultrasound alone) when combined with microbubble destruction to generate tumor shrinkage [109]. In another cancer therapy application, Sorace et al. showed that ultrasound-triggered microbubble disruption increased delivery and efficacy of Taxol in 2LMP breast cancer tumors in mice [105].

These bioeffects have also been used to deliver drugs and larger particles across the blood–brain barrier, which generally restricts passage of molecules larger than a few nanometers. The cavitation of microbubbles using focused ultrasound near the blood–brain barrier has been shown to transiently increase the gap junctions within this barrier to allow transport of larger therapeutics [110–114]. Potential clinical applications of drug delivery using this technique include treatment of

Alzheimer's, schizophrenia, and other cerebral disorders. In light of the obvious safety concerns, research in this area has progressed incrementally. However, Konofagou's group recently showed that the blood–brain barrier could safely and transiently be opened using microbubble cavitation in primates by monitoring gadolinium perfusion with MRI after cavitation of definity as well as an in house-fabricated agent [115]. While future safety studies will be required, this pilot study was a major milestone toward future human clinical trials.

In cases of blood clots causing blockage to the cerebrovascular system, stroke patients rapidly lose brain function due to ischemia in the brain. Thrombolysis can be performed if the condition is detected recently (generally within 3–6 h) using tissue plasminogen activator (tPA), but this treatment carries major side effects and has varied results. Studies have shown that ultrasound with and without tPA can help disrupt blood clots [116]. This inclusion of microbubbles has been shown to further enhance this phenomenon and spurred an entire field termed "sonothrombolysis" [116–118]. While the majority of results in this field are still at an animal model stage, results have been promising showing that cavitating microbubbles can significantly help clot disruption with and without coadministration of tPA [119–122].

11.5 Microbubbles in Gene Delivery

Gene delivery is another ongoing area of research exploiting the bioeffects of cavitating microbubbles for improved delivery. Previous approaches for delivering genetic material to cells relied on transfection via viral vectors. However, this approach is often associated with low transfection efficiency, immuno-response issues, and may be difficult to pass regulatory approval [123]. Several groups have shown that gene transfection is possible in the presence of cavitating microbubbles without viral vectors [124–128]. Figure 11.8 shows breast cancer cells in the presence of free DNA with and without ultrasound treatment, where ultrasound treatment shows a clear increase in plasmid uptake. Similar to work with the blood–brain barrier, results have progressed gradually due to safety concerns with the technique. Chai et al. recently showed the cavitation of lipid microbubbles can be used to selectively transfect islet cells in the pancreases of rats with rat insulin promoter for potential treatment of type II diabetes [129]. This ongoing work is currently being translated to a baboon model and may ultimately result in future human clinical trials for the treatment of diabetes [130].

11.5.1 Microbubbles as Drug Carriers

The size of microbubbles ($<10\,\mu m$ in diameter) makes them small enough to freely traverse the microcirculation, yet large enough to prevent them from extravasating out into the tissue [32]. Additionally, microbubbles are one of the only medical contrast agents whose destruction can be triggered by the imaging modality [32]. These factors make microbubbles an ideal platform for drug delivery, in that drug can be attached to the microbubble, retained during circulation through the

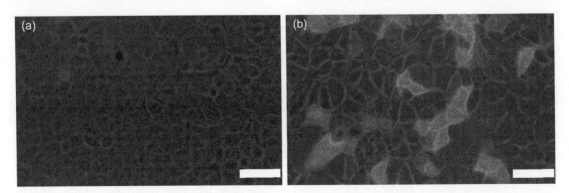

Figure 11.8 MCF 7 cells treated with microbubbles and 10 μg/mL EGFP plasmid. (a) No ultrasound, (b) (1 × treatment) 15 s of ultrasound at 1 MHz (scale bar = 50 μm). (*Courtesy: Dr. Margaret Wheatley, PhD, and Dr. Michael Cochran, PhD.*)

vasculature, and then locally released upon ultrasound-triggered destruction. A great deal of research has been invested in loading strategies and applications for drug-loaded bubbles and this concept has been extensively reviewed [11,19,20,92,131–133]. Figure 11.9 summarizes demonstrated loading strategies for both polymer and lipid microbubbles. Drug payloads can be attached to the microbubble surface, incorporated within the shell itself, encapsulated within the gas core of the microbubble (either in solid or aqueous phase), or encapsulated in nanoparticles and attached to the surface for improving drug payload.

One of the first reports of drug-loaded microbubbles was published by Unger's group who encapsulated paclitaxel in an oil layer within phospholipid-stabilized microbubbles [21]. After fabrication, the group showed that drug could be locally released using 100 kHz pulsed wave therapeutic ultrasound and significantly reduced toxicity in mice relative to unencapsulated drug [21]. Since then, numerous drug-loaded liposomal microbubbles have been fabricated [134–138]. Despite these advances, the relative space within the phospholipid shell or microbubble core (at least some gas is required to maintain acoustic activity) is limited, thus hindering extensive drug payload. One potential solution to this problem is to attach drug-containing nanoparticles to the surface of the microbubble (as illustrated in Figure 11.9(d)) to increase drug payload while still maintaining the required size and acoustic properties [139,140]. As an example, Lentacker et al. formulated microbubbles loaded with nano-sized liposomes-containing doxorubicin and showed that when insonated these particles delivered higher drug concentrations to the nucleus of melanoma cells relative to both nano-liposomal drug and free drug delivered with lipid microbubbles [140]. This may be a useful strategy for increasing the drug payload of microbubbles.

Polymer-shelled microbubbles offer an attractive alternative to lipid-based microbubbles for drug delivery due to their improved stability and thicker shells (which in turn may house/carry more drugs). Similar to previous work by Unger with phospholipid microbubbles, de Jong et al. showed that a paclitaxel/oil mixture can be encapsulated within polylactic acid (PLA) microbubbles and that these can be triggered with ultrasound to slow growth of colon adenocarcinoma in a mouse model [141]. Wheatley's group showed that doxorubicin could either be encapsulated within the shell or electrostatically attached to the surface of PLA microbubbles [142]. These agents were shown to become more toxic to breast cancer cells *in vitro* after ultrasound triggering [143], and that locally triggering these agents *in vivo* led to a 110% increase in drug delivery to a liver tumor model in rabbits via a microbubble fragmentation mechanism [144]. Tumor necrosis factor-related apoptosis-inducing

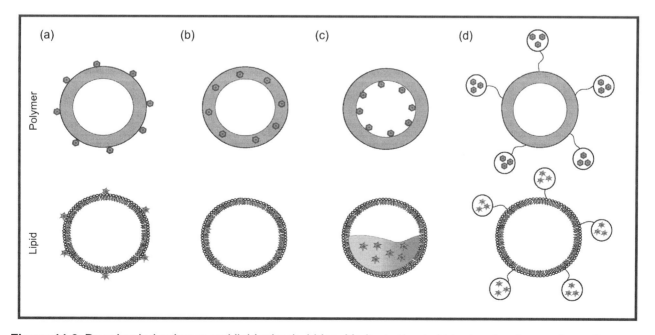

Figure 11.9 Drug loaded polymer and lipid microbubbles. Various microbubble drug-loading conformations.

ligand and genetic material have also been attached to the surface of these agents, demonstrating the flexibility of the platform [145,146].

11.6 Other Emerging Applications

Currently, microbubbles are mainly used as ultrasound contrast agents; however, they have shown utility in several other applications. As previously discussed, targeted drug and gene delivery is a widely recognized emerging microbubble application. Other applications of microbubbles in earlier phases/stages of development include biofilm destruction, pressure estimation techniques, tissue engineering applications, concomitant imaging with MRI through the use of iron-oxide nanoparticles in microbubbles, and lymphosonography [147–151]. As with the general trend in modern science, the scale of technology decreases with time. Accordingly, nanobubbles have emerged as a contrast agent concept with similar (albeit smaller-scale) characteristics and uses as microbubbles. Here, we discuss each of these less developed applications.

11.6.1 Biofilm Destruction

Bacterial infection, particularly of implantable materials, often leads to biofilm formation, which is difficult to treat and can lead to repeated surgical interventions, ultimate removal of the implant, and further health problems [152,153]. Biofilms are inherently resistant to even the most potent antibiotics due to their protective niche, which also evades immune surveillance [154]. Microbubbles have recently been shown to improve biofilm treatment by improving their drug susceptibility. He et al. showed that vancomycin treatment is significantly more effective at decreasing *Staphylococcus epidermidis* biofilm on polyethylene implants, when SonoVue microbubbles insonated in conjunction with free antibiotic over a 10 min ultrasound exposure in a rabbit model (80 KHz, 0.5 W/cm^2, 50% Duty Cycle) [147]. Figure 11.10 depicts increased antibiotic sensitivity of biofilms in the presence of microbubble insonation. Cavitation nuclei formed by microbubble destruction in proximity to a biofilm allow for the entrance of small molecule drugs, such as vancomycin, rendering the biofilm more susceptible to antibacterial activity [155].

11.6.2 Noninvasive Pressure Estimation

Several groups have investigated the use of microbubbles for noninvasive hydrostatic pressure estimation [148,156–159]. Clinically these measurements are currently performed via pressure catheter threaded through the vascular system or a direct wick in needle approach, both of which are moderately invasive and carry significant risk [160–162]. Because applied force will influence the behavior of microbubbles, it was anticipated that a microbubble's response may be useful in evaluating hydrostatic pressures noninvasively. Early efforts focused on measuring changes in bubble resonance frequency [157], microbubble size changes through the use of dual frequency excitations [158], dissolution time of free gas after microbubble rupture [159], and changes in amplitude from single microbubbles [163]. However, these

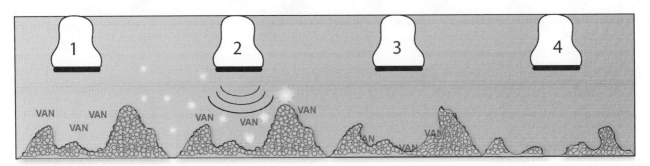

Figure 11.10 Biofilm destruction using microbubbles and ultrasound. 1—Vancomycin (VAN) cannot penetrate biofilm, 2—insonation of microbubbles causes cavitations in the biofilm surface allowing, 3—VAN penetration into the biofilms, and 4—destruction of biofilm architecture.

efforts fell short before reaching *in vivo* trials due to an inability to identify signal from individual bubbles and the inherent polydispersity of microbubble populations. More recent advances have focused on a technique termed subharmonic-aided pressure estimation (SHAPE) in which the subharmonic amplitude at a particular stage (the stage at which point the subharmonic amplitude is most sensitive to changes in applied acoustic pressure) decreases linearly with increases in surrounding hydrostatic pressure [148]. As a result of this technique's *in vitro* validation [164,165], it has successfully been applied *in vivo* to measure left and right ventricle pressures in canines [166,167], intratumoral fluid pressures in swine melanoma (changes of which provide an early indication of treatment response) [168], and hepatic pressures in both canines [169,170] and patients with chronic liver disease [171]. In a recent, first in humans, study, SHAPE was shown to accurately detect portal hypertension (defined as a hepatic-venous pressure gradient > 10 mmHg) in patients with chronic liver disease with a sensitivity of 89% and specificity of 88%, indicating it may be a noninvasive alternative to transjugular catheter-based pressure measurements [171].

11.6.3 Tissue Engineering

Microbubbles have recently been incorporated into tissue engineering technologies. Polymeric tissue engineering scaffolds can be limited in their biomolecular delivery [172]. The use of microbubbles as porogens and growth factor carriers promotes bioactivity in degradable scaffolds [150,173,174]. Nair et al. showed that the incorporation of insulin growth factor-loaded microbubbles in the production of a porous scaffold provides larger pores and a nontoxic biocompatible mode of incorporating growth factors [150]. Microbubbles may therefore result in tissue engineered scaffolds which may foster host in-growth and promote cell survival and proliferation. In another tissue engineering application, microbubbles have shown promise in the targeting of stem cells to areas where regeneration may be required. Toma et al. demonstrated that mesenchymal stem cells conjugated to microbubbles can be targeted and delivered to areas of arterial injury using acoustic radiation force under physiologic flow rates [175].

11.6.4 Magnetic Resonance Imaging

Although microbubbles were originally intended as contrast agents for ultrasound, the potential for microbubbles as contrast agents in MRI has recently been realized. Contrast agents for MRI include gadolinium chelates and superparamagnetic iron oxide particles [176,177]. Microbubbles have been prepared as dual contrast agents for ultrasound and MRI through the incorporation of superparamagnetic iron oxide nanoparticles in polymeric shells [178]. More recently, He et al. demonstrated that polymeric microbubbles with nitrogen gas cores and superparamagnetic iron oxide particles conjugated to the polymeric shell surface rather than incorporated within the shell provided further MRI and ultrasound imaging enhancements [179]. The fusion of MRI and ultrasound imaging could provide more efficient imaging and diagnostics.

11.6.5 Nanobubbles

While technically not microbubbles, several groups have worked to develop nanobubbles using either size separation techniques or modifications to the microbubble fabrication process [180–182]. These bubbles are supposed to offer better penetration into tumor interstitial for drug-delivery purposes, but may not be ideal for imaging purposes (as shown in equation (11.5), the effective cross scattering area is proportional to the bubble radius to the sixth power) [183,184]. Nano-sized ultrasound contrast agents have been fabricated using polymer [181], surfactant [185], and lipid shells [186]. Similar to microbubbles, these agents have also been loaded with drug or had the surface modified with targeting ligands for targeting and drug delivery [183,184,187]. While these agents are still in bench top or early *in vivo* trials, improved tumor penetration is expected to be a major advantage for drug and gene delivery.

11.6.6 Lymphosonography

The identification of sentinel lymph nodes is often required for surgical biopsy or removal and is currently performed using injection of a radioactive tracer or methylene blue dye immediately prior to resection surgery. The ability to noninvasively trace lymphatic channels and identify connected sentinel lymph nodes using microbubbles was first demonstrated by Mattrey et al. [188]. The application has been expanded by Goldberg et al., who showed visualization of these structures using subcutaneous, submucosal, and parenchymal injection of Sonazoid in swine, canines, rabbits, and a monkey [151]. Since then lymphosonography has been shown useful in porcine models for identification of nodes connected to the supraglottis, thyroid, and melanomas [187,189,190]. Sever et al. showed that this technique can be applied to humans by successfully identifying sentinel lymph nodes (with 89% sensitivity in one study) for biopsy and staging in patients with breast cancer prior to surgery [185,191]. Despite these advances, no microbubble is currently approved for subcutaneous injection or use in lymphosonography, but may gain approval in the future.

11.7 Conclusion

The ongoing research on microbubbles continues to result in the discovery of new potential clinical applications. Past research has already established microbubbles as a safe method for contrast-enhanced ultrasound imaging with significant improvement over conventional (non-enhanced) ultrasound imaging.

Polymer, protein, and lipid microbubbles provide a means of increasing contrast within the vasculature, even at the capillary level. As each microbubble undergoes compression and rarefaction upon exposure to ultrasound, the nonlinear oscillations of the microbubble generate signals which return to the transducer, increasing the contrast significantly compared to the surrounding tissue. The pliability of the encapsulating shell allows for microbubble destruction upon an increase in the ultrasound power, creating transient holes in the membranes of neighboring cells and thus potential windows for drug and gene delivery. The engineering of microbubbles as drug carriers either conjugated to or incorporated within the microbubble shell provides a method of more efficient localized drug and gene delivery. Targeted microbubbles may identify specific markers expressed on a desired tissue type as well as a method for increased microbubble accumulation, leading to significantly enhanced contrast in the area.

Microbubble use in medical diagnostics continues to grow and evolve in the United States and is already well established in the majority of other countries. As microbubbles become a more accepted tool for diagnostic imaging, there will be an increase in the ability of ultrasound to aid in the accurate diagnosis and treatment of patients and a more rapid adoption of emerging microbubble applications.

References

[1] Quaia E. Microbubble ultrasound contrast agents: an update. Eur Radiol 2007;17(8):1995–2008.

[2] Gramiak R, Shah PM. Echocardiography of the aortic root. Invest Radiol 1968;3:356–66.

[3] Feinstein SB, Ten Cate FJ, Zwehl W, Ong K, Maurer G, Tei C, et al. Two-dimensional contrast echocardiography. I. In vitro development and quantitative analysis of echo contrast agents. J Am Coll Cardiol 1984;3(1):14–20.

[4] Klibanov A. Targeted delivery of gas-filled microspheres, contrast agents for ultrasound imaging. Adv Drug Deliv Rev 1999;37(1–3):139–57.

[5] Tsutsui JM, Grayburn Pa, Xie F, Porter TR. Drug and gene delivery and enhancement of thrombolysis using ultrasound and microbubbles. Cardiol Clin 2004;22(2):299–312.

[6] Kiessling F, Fokong S, Koczera P, Lederle W, Lammers T. Ultrasound microbubbles for molecular diagnosis, therapy, and theranostics. Journal of nuclear medicine: official publication. Soc Nucl Med 2012;53(3):345–8.

[7] Dijkmans PA, Juffermans LJM, Musters RJP, Van Wamel A, Ten Cate FJ, Van Gilst W, et al. Microbubbles and ultrasound: from diagnosis to therapy. European journal of echocardiography. J Work Group Echocardiogr Eur Soc Cardiol 2004;5(4):245–56.

[8] Stride E, Saffari N. Microbubble ultrasound contrast agents: a review. Proc Inst Mech Eng [H] 2003;217(6):429–47.

[9] Unger EC, Matsunaga TO, McCreery T, Schumann P, Sweitzer R, Quigley R. Therapeutic applications of microbubbles. Eur J Radiol 2002;42(2):160–8.

[10] De Jong N, Emmer M, Van Wamel A, Versluis M. Ultrasonic characterization of ultrasound contrast agents. Med Biol Eng Comput 2009;47(8):861−73.

[11] Ferrara K, Pollard R, Borden M. Ultrasound microbubble contrast agents: fundamentals and application to gene and drug delivery. Annu Rev Biomed Eng 2007;9:415−47.

[12] Yang F, Li Y, Chen Z, Zhang Y, Wu J, Gu N. Superparamagnetic iron oxide nanoparticle-embedded encapsulated microbubbles as dual contrast agents of magnetic resonance and ultrasound imaging. Biomaterials 2009;30 (23−24):3882−90.

[13] Dayton PA, Chomas JE, Lum AF, Allen JS, Lindner JR, Simon SI, et al. Optical and acoustical dynamics of microbubble contrast agents inside neutrophils. Biophys J 2001;80 (3):1547−56.

[14] Duncanson WJ, Oum K, Eisenbrey Jr, Cleveland RO, Wheately MA, Wong JY. Targeted binding of PEG-lipid modified polymer ultrasound contrast agents with tiered surface architecture. Biotechnol Bioeng 2010;106 (3):501−6.

[15] Chen CC, Borden MA. Ligand conjugation to bimodal PEG brush layers on microbubbles. Langmuir 2010;26(16):13183−94.

[16] Kiessling F, Gaetjens J, Palmowski M. Application of molecular ultrasound for imaging integrin expression. Theranostics 2011;1: 127−34.

[17] Grinstaff MW, Suslick KS. Air-filled proteinaceous microbubbles: synthesis of an echo-contrast agent. Proc Natl Acad Sci USA 1991;88(17):7708−10.

[18] Stewart VR, Sidhu PS. New directions in ultrasound: microbubble contrast. Br J Radiol 2006;79(939):188−94.

[19] Sirsi SR, Borden MA. Advances in ultrasound mediated gene therapy using microbubble contrast agents. Theranostics 2012;2 (12):1208−22.

[20] Hernot S, Klibanov A. Microbubbles in ulltrasound-triggered drug and gene delivery. Adv Drug Deliv Rev 2008;60(10):1153−66.

[21] Unger EC, McCreery TP, Sweitzer RH, Caldwell VE, Wu Y. Acoustically active lipospheres containing paclitaxel: a new therapeutic ultrasound contrast agent. Invest Radiol 1998;33(12):886−92.

[22] Camp GV, Droogmans S, Cosyns B. Bioeffects of ultrasound contrast agents in daily clinical practice: fact of fiction? Eur Heart J 2007;28:1190−2.

[23] Main ML, Goldman JH, Grayburn PA. Thinking outside the "Box"—The ultrasound contrast controversy. J Am Coll Cardiol 2007;18(24):34−7.

[24] Blomley M, Claudon M, Cosgrove D. WFUMB safety symposium on ultrasound contrast agents: clinical applications and safety concerns. Ultrasound Med Biol 2007;33 (2):180−6.

[25] Food and Drug administration, USA. <www.fda.gov/cder/drug/infosheet/hcp/microbubble hcp.htm>. 2008

[26] Lewin P. Quo vadis medical ultrasound. Ultrasonics 2004;42:1−7.

[27] Kim JH, Park K, Nam HY, et al. Polymers for bioimaging. Prog Polym Sci 2007;32:1031−53.

[28] Kinsler L, Frey A, Coppens A, Sanders J. Fundamentals of acoustics. Hoboken, NJ: John Wiley & Sons Inc.; 2000.

[29] Morse PM, Ingard KV. Theoretical acoustics. New York: McGraw-Hill; 1968.

[30] Leighton TG. The acoustic bubble. London: Academic Press; 1994.

[31] Hoff L. Acoustic characterization of contrast agents for medical ultrasound imaging. The Netherlands: Kluwer Academic Publishers; 2001.

[32] Goldberg BB, Raichlen JS, Forsberg F. Ultrasound contrast agents; basic principles and clinical applications. 2nd ed. London: Martin Dunitz; 2001.

[33] Forsberg F, Merton DA, Liu JB, et al. Clinical applications of ultrasound contrast agents. Ultrasonics 1998;35:695−701.

[34] Cassano E, Rizzo S, Bozzini A, et al. Contrast enhanced ultrasound of breast cancer. Cancer Imaging 2006;6:4−6.

[35] Choi D, Lim HK, Kim SH, et al. Hepatocellular carcinoma treated with percutaneous radio-frequency ablation: usefulness of power Doppler US with a microbubble contrast agent in evaluating therapeutic response-preliminary results. Radiology 2000;217: 558−63.

[36] Leen E, Angerson WJ, Yarmenitis S, et al. Multi-centre clinical study evaluating the

efficacy of SonoVue (BR1), a new ultrasound contrast agent in Doppler investigation of focal hepatic lesions. Eur J Radiol 2002;41:200–6.
[37] Rickes S, Mönkemüller K, Malfertheiner P. Contrast-enhanced ultrasound in the diagnosis of pancreatic tumors. JOP 2006;7:584–92.
[38] Broillet A, Puginier J, Ventrone R, Schneider M. Assessment of myocardial perfusion by intermittent harmonic power Doppler using SonoVue, a new ultrasound contrast agent. Invest Radiol 1998;33(4):209–15.
[39] Stewart MJ. Contrast echocardiography. Heart 2003;89:342–8.
[40] Wei K, Ragosta M, Thorpe J, et al. Noninvasive quantification of coronary blood flow reserve in humans using myocardial contrast echocardiography. Circulation 2001;29: 2560–5.
[41] Mulvagh SL, DeMaria AN, Feinstein SB, et al. Contrast echocardiography: current and future applications. J Am Soc Echocardiogr 2000;13:331–42.
[42] Forsberg F, Lathia JD, Merton DA, Liu J-B, Le NT, Goldberg BB, et al. Effect of shell type on the in vivo backscatter from polymer-encapsulated microbubbles. Ultrasound Med Biol 2004;30(10):1281–7.
[43] Szabo T. Diagnostic ultrasound imaging: inside out. Invest Radiol 1998;33:209–15.
[44] Choudhry S, Gorman B, Charboneau JW, et al. Comparison of tissue harmonic imaging with conventional US in abdominal disease. Radiographics 2000;20:1127–35.
[45] Burns P. Harmonic imaging with ultrasound contrast agents. Clin Radiol 1996;51:50–5.
[46] Burns PN, Simpson DH, Averkiou MA. Nonlinear imaging. Ultrasound Med Biol 2000;26:S19–22.
[47] Quaia E, Bertolotto M, Forgacs B, et al. Detection of liver metastases by pulse inversion harmonic imaging during Levovist late phase: comparison with conventional ultrasound and helical CT in 160 patients. EurRadiol 2003;13:475–83.
[48] Schmidt T, Hohl C, Haage P, et al. Phase-inversion tissue harmonic imaging compared to fundamental B-mode ultrasound in the evaluation of the pathology of large and small bowel. Eur Radiol 2005;15:2012–30.

[49] Forsberg F, Dicker AP, Thakur ML, et al. Comparing contrast-enhanced ultrasound to immunohistochemical markers of angiogenesis in a human melanoma xenograft model: preliminary results. Ultrasound Med Biol 2002;28:445–51.
[50] Hamilton MF, Blackstone DT. Nonlinear acoustics. San Diego, CA: Academic Press; 1998.
[51] Forsberg F, Piccoli CW, Merton DA, et al. Breast lesions: imaging with contrast-enhanced subharmonic US—initial experience. Radiology 2007;244:718–26.
[52] Dave JK, Halldorsdottir VG, Eisenbrey JR, et al. Noninvasive LV pressure estimation using subharmonic emissions from microbubbles. JACC Cardiovasc Imaging 2012;5:87–92.
[53] Eisenbrey JR, Dave JK, Halldorsdottir VG, et al. Simultaneous grayscale and subharmonic ultrasound imaging on a modified commercial scanner. Ultrasonics 2011;51:890–7.
[54] Eisenbrey JR, Sridharan A, Doyley MM, et al. Parametric subharmonic imaging using a commercial intravascular ultrasound scanner: an in vivo feasibility study. J Ultrasound Med 2012;31:361–71.
[55] Needles A, Couture O, Foster FS. A method for differentiating targeted microbubbles in real time using subharmonic micro-ultrasound and interframe filtering. Ultrasound Med Biol 2009;35:1564–73.
[56] Eisenbrey JR, Dave JK, Merton DA, et al. Parametric imaging using subharmonic signals from ultrasound contrast agents in patients with breast lesions. J Ultrasound Med 2011;30:85–92.
[57] Eisenbrey JR, Joshi N, Dave JK, Forsberg F. Assessment of algorithms for defining vascular architecture from subharmonic images of breast lesions. Phys Med Bio 2011;56:1–12.
[58] Sridharan A, Eisenbrey JR, Machado P, et al. Delineation of atherosclerotic plaque using subharmonic imaging filtering techniques and a commercial intravascular ultrasound scanner. Ultrason Imaging 2013;35:30–44.
[59] Sridharan A., Eisenbrey J.R., Machado P., et al. Perfusion estimation using contrast enhanced three-dimensional subharmonic ultrasound imaging: an in vivo study. Invest Radiol. 2013, In Press.

[60] Linden RA, Trabulsi EJ, Forsberg F, et al. Contrast enhanced ultrasound flash replenishment method for directed prostate biopsies. J Urol 2007;78:2254–8.

[61] Sugimoto K, Shiraishi J, Moriyasu F, Ichimura S, Metoki R, Doi K. Analysis of intrahepatic vascular morphological changes of chronic liver disease for assessment of liver fibrosis stages by micro-flow imaging with contrast-enhanced ultrasound: preliminary experience. Eur Radiol 2010;20(11):2749–57.

[62] Du J, Li FH, Fang H, et al. Microvascular archeticure of breast lesions: evaluation with contrast-enhanced ultrasonographic micro flow imaging. J Ultrasound Med 2007;26:461–7.

[63] Schwenger V, Korosoglou G, Hinkel UP, et al. Real-time contrast-enhanced sonography of renal transplant recipients predicts chronic allograft nephropathy. Am J Transplant 2006;6:609–15.

[64] Qin S, Caskey CF, Ferrara KW. Ultrasound contrast microbubbles in imaging and therapy: physical principles and engineering. Phys Med Biol 2009;54:R27–57.

[65] Barr RG. Off-label use of ultrasound contrast agents for abdominal imaging in the United States. J Ultrasound Med 2013;32(1):7–12.

[66] Correas JM, Bridal L, Lesavre A, et al. Ultrasound contrast agents: properties, principles of action, tolerance, and artifacts. Eur Radiol 2001;11:1316–28.

[67] Blomley MJK, Cooke JC, Unger EC, et al. Microbubble contrast agents: a new era in ultrasound. BMJ 2001;322:1222.

[68] Weskott HP. Emerging roles for contrast-enhanced ultrasound. Clin Hemorheology Microcirc 2008;40:51–71.

[69] Mulvagh SL, Rakowski H, Vannan MA, et al. American society of echocardiography consensus statement on the clinical applications of ultrasonic contrast agents in echocardiography. J Am Soc Echocardiogr 2008;21:1179–201.

[70] Claudon M, Dietrich CF, Choi BI, et al. Guidelines and good clinical practice recommendations for contrast enhanced ultrasound (CEUS) in the liver—update 2012: A WFUMB-EFSUMB initiative in cooperation with representatives of AFSUMB, AIUM, ASUM, FLAUS, and ICUS. Ultrasound Med Biol 2013;39(2):187–210.

[71] Piscaglia F., Nolsøe C., Dietrich C.F., et al. The EFSUMB guidelines and recommendations on the clinical practice of contrast enhanced ultrasound (CEUS): update 2011 on non-hepatic applications. Ultraschall Med. 2012; 33:33–59.

[72] Cohen JL, Cheirif J, Segar DS, et al. Improved left ventricular endocardial border delineation and opacification with Optison (FS069), a new echocardiographic contrast agent. Results of a phase III multicentre trial. J Am Coll Cardiol 1998;32:746–52.

[73] Abdelmoneim SS, Bernier M, Scott CG, Dhoble A, Ness SAC, Hagen ME, et al. Safety of contrast agent use during stress echocardiography in patients with elevated right ventricular systolic pressure: a cohort study. Circ Cardiovasc Imaging 2010;3(3):240–8.

[74] Piscaglia F, Bolondi L. The safety of Sonovue in abdominal applications: retrospective analysis of 23188 investigations. Ultrasound Med Biol 2006;32(9):1369–75.

[75] Ter Haar G. Safety and bio-effects of ultrasound contrast agents. Med Biol Eng Comput 2009;47(8):893–900.

[76] Jakobsen Ja, Oyen R, Thomsen HS, Morcos SK. Safety of ultrasound contrast agents. Eur Radiol 2005;15(5):941–5.

[77] Raisinghani A, Rafter P, Phillips P, Vannan MA, DeMaria AN. Microbubble contrast agents for echocardiography: rationale, composition, ultrasound interactions, and safety. Cardiol Clin 2004;22(2):171–80.

[78] Bartolotta TV, Taibbi A, Midiri M, Lagalla R. Focal liver lesions: contrast-enhanced ultrasound. Abdom Imaging 2009;34:193–209.

[79] Quaia E, Calliada F, Bertolotto M, et al. Characterization of focal liver lesions with contrast-specific US modes and a sulfur hexafluoride-filled microbubble contrast agent: diagnostic performance and confidence. Radiology 2004;232:420–30.

[80] Yang F, Li Y, Chen Z, Zhang Y, Wu J, Gu N. Superparamagnetic iron oxide nanoparticle-embedded encapsulated microbubbles as dual contrast agents of magnetic resonance and ultrasound imaging. Biomaterials 2009;30(23–24):3882–90.

[81] Stride E, Porter C, Prieto AG, Pankhurst Q. Enhancement of microbubble mediated gene delivery by simultaneous exposure to ultrasonic and magnetic fields. Ultrasound Med Biol 2009;35(5):861–8.

[82] Unger EC, McCreery TP, Sweitzer RH, Shen D, Wu G. In vitro studies of a new thrombus-specific ultrasound contrast agent. Am J Cardiol 1998;81(12A):58G–61G.

[83] Pysz MA, Foygel K, Rosenberg J. Antiangiogenic cancer therapy: monitoring with molecular US and a clinically translatable contrast agent (BR55). Radiology 2010;25(2):519–27.

[84] Rossi S, Rosa L, Ravetta V, Cascina A, Quaretti P, Azzaretti A, et al. Contrast-enhanced versus conventional and color Doppler sonography for the detection of thrombosis of the portal and hepatic venous systems. AJR 2006;186(3):763–73.

[85] Catalano O, Sandomenico F. Contrast-enhanced sonography of the spleen. AJR 2005;1:1150–6.

[86] Takalkar AM, Klibanov AL, Rychak JJ, Lindner JR, Ley K. Binding and detachment dynamics of microbubbles targeted to P-selectin under controlled shear flow. J Control Release 2004;96(3):473–82.

[87] Rychak JJ, Klibanov AL, Hossack JA. Acoustic radiation force enhances targeted delivery of ultrasound contrast microbubbles: In vitro verification. IEEE Trans Ultrason Ferroelectr Freq Control 2005;52:421–33.

[88] Li W, Ma N, Ong L, Kaminski A, Skrabal C, Gatzen H, et al. Enhanced thoracic gene delivery by magnetic nanobead-mediated vector. J. Gene Med 2008;10(8):897–909.

[89] Wu J, Leong-poi H, Bin J, Yang L, Liao Y, Liu Y, et al. Effiicacy of contrast-enhanced US and magnetic microbubbles targeted to vascular cell adhesion molecule—1 for molecular imaging of atherosclerosis. Radiology 2011;260(2):463–71.

[90] Geers B, Dewitte H, De Smedt SC, Lentacker I. Crucial factors and emerging concepts in ultrasound-triggered drug delivery. J Control Release 2012;164:248–55.

[91] Geis NA, Katus HA, Bekeredjian R. Microbubbles as a vehicle for gene and drug delivery: current clinical implications and future perspectives. Curr Pharm Des 2012;18:2166–83.

[92] Qin S, Caskey CF, Ferrara KW. Ultrasound contrast microbubbles in imaging and therapy: physical principles and engineering. Phys Med Biol 2009;54:R27–57.

[93] Harrison GH, Balcer-Kubic EK, Eddy HA. Potential of chemotherapy by low-level ultrasound. Int J Radiat Biol 1991;56:1453–66.

[94] Rosenthal I, Sostaric JZ, Riesz P. Sonodynamic therapy—a review of the synergistic effects of drugs and ultrasound. Ultrason Sonochem 2004;11:349–63.

[95] Kinoshita M, Hynynen K. Intracellular delivery of Bak BH3 peptide by microbubble-enhanced ultrasound. Pharm Res 2005;22:716–20.

[96] Miao CH, Braymann AA, Loeb KR, Ye P, Zhou L, Mourad P, et al. Ultrasound enhances gene delivery of human factor IX plasmid. Hum Gene Ther 2005;16:893–905.

[97] Bekeredjian R, Katus HA, Kuecherer HF. Therapeutic use of ultrasound targeted microbubble destruction: a review of non-cardiac applications. Ultraschall Med 2006;27:134–40.

[98] Husseini GA, Diaz de la Rosa MA, Richardson ES, Christensen DA, Pitt WG. The role of cavitation in acoustically activated drug delivery. J Control Release 2005;107:253–61.

[99] Suslick KS. Sonochemistry. Science 1990;247:1439–46.

[100] van Wamel A, Kooiman K, Harteveld M, et al. Vibrating microbubbles poking individual cells: drug transfer into cells via sonoporation. J Control Release 2006;112:149–55.

[101] Ohl CD, Arora M, Ikink R, de Jong N, Versluis M, Delius M, et al. Sonoporation from jetting cavitation bubbles. Biophys J 2006;91:4285–95.

[102] Price RJ, Skyba DM, Kaul S, Skalak TC. Delivery of colloidal particles and red blood cells to tissue through microvessel ruptures created by targeted microbubble destruction with ultrasound. Circulation 1998;98:1264–7.

[103] Geis NA, Katus HA, Bekeredjian R. Microbubbles as a vehicle for gene and drug

[103] delivery: current clinical implications and future perspectives. Curr Pharm Des 2012;18:2166–83.
[104] Nomikou N, McHale AP. Exploiting ultrasound-mediated effects in delivering targeted, site-specific cancer therapy. Cancer Let 2010;296:133–43.
[105] Sorace AG, Warram JM, Umphrey H, Hoyt K. Microbubble mediated ultrasonic techniques for improved chemotherapeurtic delivery in cancer. J Drug Target 2012;20:43–54.
[106] Escoffre JM, Piron J, Novell A, Bouakaz A. Doxorubicin delivery into tumor cells with ultrasound and microbubbles. Mol Pharm 2011;8:799–806.
[107] Castle J, Butts M, Healey A, et al. Ultrasound-mediated targeted drug delivery: recent success and remaining challenges. Am J Physiol Heart Circ Physiol 2013;204:H350–7.
[108] Heath CH, Sorace AG, Knowles J, et al. Microbubble therapy enhances anti-tumor properties of cisplatin and cetuximab in vitro and in vivo. Otolaryngol Head Neck Surg 2012;146:938–45.
[109] Sonoda S, Tachibana K, Uchino E, et al. Inhibition of melanoma by ultrasound-microbubble-aided drug delivery suggests membrane permeabilization. Cancer Biol Ther 2007;6:1276–83.
[110] Baseri B, Choi JJ, Tung YS, Konofagou EE. Multi-modality safety assessment of blood-brain barrier opening using focused ultrasound and definity microbubbles: a short-term study. Ultrasound Med Biol 2010;36:1445–59.
[111] Choi JJ, Pernot M, Brown TR, et al. Spatio-temporal analysis of molecular delivery through the blood-brain barrier using focused ultrasound. Phys Med Biol 2007;33:95–104.
[112] Choi JJ, Wang S, Tung YS, et al. Molecules of various pharmacologically-relevant sizes can cross the ultrasound-induced blood-brain barrier opening in vivo. Ultrasound Med Biol 2010;36:58–67.
[113] Choi JJ, Selert K, Gao Z, et al. Noninvasive and localized blood-brain barrier disruption using focused ultrasound can be achieved at short pulse lengths and low pulse repetition frequencies. J Cereb Blood Flow Metab 2011;31:725–37.
[114] McDannold N, Vykhodtseva N, Hynynen K. Effects of acoustic parameters and ultrasound contrast agent dose on focused-ultrasound induced blood-brain barrier disruption. Ultrasound Med Biol 2008;34:930–7.
[115] Marquet F, Tung YS, Teichert T, et al. Noninvasive, transient and selective blood-brain barrier opening in non-human primates in vivo. PLoS ONE 2011;6(7):e22598.
[116] Meairs S, Alonso A, Hennerici MG. Progress in sonothrombolysis for the treatment of stroke. Stroke 2012;43:1706–10.
[117] Amaral-Silva A, Pineiro S, Molina CA. Sonothrombolysis for the treatment of acute stoke: current concepts and future directions. Expert Rev Neurother 2011;11:265–73.
[118] Bor-Seng-Shu E, Noqueira Rde C, Fiqueiredo EG, et al. Sonothrombolysis for acute ischemic stroke: a review of randomized controlled trials. Neurosurg Focus 2012;32:E5.
[119] Brown AT, Flores R, Hamilton E, et al. Microbubbles improve sonothrombolysis in vitro and decrease hemorrhage in vivo in a rabbit stroke model. Invest Radiol 2011;46:202–7.
[120] Culp WC, Flores R, Brown AT, et al. Successful microbubble sonothrombolysis without tissue-type plasminogen activator in a rabbit model of acute ischemic stroke. Stroke 2011;42:2280–5.
[121] Alonso A, Dempfle CE, Della Martina A, et al. In vivo clot lysis of human thrombus with intravenous abciximab immunobubbles and ultrasound. Thromb Res 2009;124:70–4.
[122] Culp WC, Porter TR, Lowery L, et al. Intracrannial clot lysis with intravenous microbubbles and transcranial ultrasound in swine. Stroke 2004;35:2407–11.
[123] Romano G, Claudio PP, Kaiser HE, Giordano A. Recent advances, prospects and problems in designing new strategies for oligonucleotide and gene delivery in therapy. In vivo 1998;12:56–67.
[124] Chen S, Shohet RV, Bekeredjian R, et al. Optimization of ultrasound parameters for cardiac gene delivery of adenovrial or plasmid deoxyribonucleic acid by ultrasound-targeted microbubble destruction. J Am Coll Cardiol 2003;42:301–8.

[125] Shohet RV, Chen S, Zhou YT, et al. Echocardiographic destruction of albumin microbubbles directs gene delivery to the myocardium. Circulation 2000;101:2554–6.

[126] Lawrie A, Brisken AF, Francis SE, et al. Microbubble-enhanced ultrasound for vascular gene delivery. Gene Ther 2000;7:2023–7.

[127] Rahim A, Taylor SL, Bush NL, et al. Physical parameters affecting ultrasound/microbubble mediated gene delivery efficiency in vitro. Ultrasound Med Biol 2006;32:1269–79.

[128] Passineau MJ, Zourelias L, Machen L, et al. Ultrasound-assisted non-viral gene transfer to the salivary glands. Gene Ther 2010;17:1318–24.

[129] Chai R, Chen S, Ding J, Grayburn PA. Efficient, glucose responsive and islet-specific transgene expression by a modified rat insulin promoter. Gene Ther 2009;16:1202–9.

[130] Benjamin MM. Paul Arthur Grayburn, MD: an interview by Mina Mecheal Benjamin, MD. Proc (Bayl Univ Med Cent) 2012;25:265–70.

[131] Caskey CF, Hu X, Ferrara KW. Leveraging the power of ultrasound for therapeutic design and optimization. J Control Release 2011;156:297–306.

[132] Eisenbrey JR, Forsberg F. Contrast-enhanced ultrasound for molecular imaging of angiogenesis. Eur J Nucl Med Mol Imaging 2010;37:S138–46.

[133] Wheatley MA, Cochran C. Ultrasound contrast agents. J Drug Del Sci Tech. 2013. [In Press].

[134] Huang S, MacDonald RC. Acoustically active liposomes for drug encapsulation and ultrasound-triggered release. Biochim Biophys Acta 2004;665:134–41.

[135] Husseini G, Christensen DA, Rapoport NY, Pitt WG. Ultrasonic release of doxorubicin from pluronic P105 micelles stabilized with an interpenetrating network of N,N-diethylacylamide. J Control Release 2002;83:303–5.

[136] Phillips LC, Klibanov AL, Wamhoff BR, Hossack JA. Localized ultrasound enhances delivery of rapamycin from microbubbles to prevent smooth muscle proliferation. J Control Release 2011;154:42–9.

[137] Tartis MS, McCallan J, Lum AFH, et al. Therapeutic effects of paclitaxel-containing ultrasound contrast agents. Ultrasound Med Biol 2006;32:1771–80.

[138] Tinkov S, Coester C, Serba S, et al. New doxorubicin-loaded phospholipid microbubbles for targeted tumor therapy: in vivo characterization. J Control Release 2010;146:368–72.

[139] Kheirolomoom A, Dayton PA, Lum AFH, et al. Acoustically-active microbubbles conjugated to lipsomes: characterization of a new proposed drug delivery vehicle. J Control Release 2007;118:275–84.

[140] Lentacker I, Geers B, Demeester J, et al. Design and evaluation of doxorubicin-containing microbubbles for ultrasound triggered doxorubicin delivery: cytotoxicicty and mechanisms involved. Mol Ther 2010;18:101–8.

[141] Kooiman K, Böhmer MR, Emmer M, et al. Oil filled polymer microcapsules for ultrasound-mediated delivery of lipophilic drugs. J Control Release 2009;132:109–18.

[142] Eisenbrey JR, Mualem-Burstein O, Kambhampati R, et al. Development and optimization of a doxorubicin loaded poly(lactic acid) contrast agent for ultrasound triggered drug delivery. J Control Release 2010;143:38–44.

[143] Eisenbrey JR, Huang P, Hsu J, Wheatley MA. Ultrasound triggered cell death in vitro with doxorubicin loaded poly lactic-acid contrast agents. Ultrasonics 2009;49:628–33.

[144] Eisenbrey JR, Soulen MC, Wheatley MA. Delivery of encapsulated doxorubicin my ultrasound-mediated size reduction of drug-loaded polymer contrast agents. IEEE Trans Biomed Eng 2010;57:24–8.

[145] Cochran M, Wheatley MA. Polymer ultrasound contrast agents for targeted drug and gene delivery [Drexel University Thesis]. Philadelphia PA; 2012.

[146] Wheatley MA, Cochran MC, Eisenbrey JR, Oum KL. Cellular signal transduction can be induced by TRAIL conjugated to microcapsules. J Biomed Mater Res A 2012;100:2602–11.

[147] He N, Hu J, Liu H, Zhu T, Huang B, Wang X, et al. Enhancement of vancomycin activity against biofilms by using ultrasound-targeted microbubble destruction. Antimicrob Agents Chemother 2011;55(11):5331–7.

[148] Shi W, Forsberg F, Raichlen J, Needleman L, Goldberg B. Pressure dependence of subharmonic signals from contrast microbubbles. Ultrasound Med Biol 1999;25:275–83.

[149] Chow AM, Chan KWY, Cheung JS, Wu EX. Enhancement of gas-filled microbubble R2* by iron oxide nanoparticles for MRI. Mag Reson Med 2010;63(1):224–9.

[150] Nair A, Thevenot P, Dey J, Shen J, Sun M-W, Yang J, et al. Novel polymeric scaffolds using protein microbubbles as porogen and growth factor carriers. Tissue Eng Part C, Methods 2010;16(1):23–32.

[151] Goldberg BB, Merton DA, Liu JB, et al. Contrast-enhanced sonographic imaging of lymphatic channels and sentinel lymph nodes. J Ultrasound Med 2005;24:953–65.

[152] Darouiche RO. Device-associated infections: a macroproblem that starts with microadherence. Clin Infect Dis 2001;33(9):1567–72.

[153] Whitehouse JD, Friedman ND, Kirkland KB, Richardson WJ, Sexton DJ. The impact of surgical-site infections following orthopedic surgery at a community hospital and a university hospital: adverse quality of life, excess length of stay, and extra cost. Infect Control Hosp Epidemiol 2002;23(4):183–9.

[154] Costerton JW. Bacterial biofilms: a common cause of persistent infections. Science 1999;284(5418):1318–22.

[155] Trampuz A, Patel R, Greenleaf JF, Hanssen AD. Microbial Biofilm Removal Methods and Systems. 2007; Patent number US 8,076,117 B2.

[156] Andersen KS, Jensen JA. Impact of acoustic pressure on ambient pressure estimation using ultrasound contrast agent. Ultrasonics 2010;50:294–9.

[157] Fairbank Jr WM, Scully MO. A new noninvasive technique for cardiac pressure measurement: Resonant scattering of ultrasound from bubbles. IEEE Trans Biomed Eng 1977;24:107–10.

[158] Shankar PM, Chapelon JY, Newhouse VL. Fluid pressure measurement using bubbles insonified by two frequencies. Ultrasonics 1986;24:333–6.

[159] Bouakaz A, Frinking PJ, de Jong N, Bom N. Noninvasive measurement of the hydrostatic pressure in a fluid-filled cavity based on the disappearance time of micrometer-sized free gas bubbles. Ultrasound Med Biol 1999;25:1407–15.

[160] Chatterjee K. The Swan-Ganz catheters: past, present and future: a viewpoint. Circulation 2009;119:147–52.

[161] Solomon SD, Stevenson LW. Recalibrating the barometer: is it time to take a critical look at noninvasive approaches to measuring filling pressures? Circulation 2009;119:13–5.

[162] Boody AR, Wongworawat MD. Accuracy in the measurement of compartment pressures: a comparison of three commonly used devices. J Bone Joint Surg Am 2005;87(11):2415–22.

[163] Hok B. A new approach to noninvasive manometry: Interaction between ultrasound and bubbles. Med Biol Eng Comput 1981;19:35–9.

[164] Halldorsdottir VG, Dave JK, Leodore LM, Eisenbrey JR, Park S, Hall AL, et al. Subharmonic contrast microbubble signals for noninvasive pressure estimation under static and dynamic flow conditionses. Ultrason Imaging 2011;33:153–64.

[165] Dave J, Halldorsdottir V, Eisenbrey J, Liu JB, McDonald M, Dickie K, et al. Noninvasive estimation of dynamic pressures in vitro and in vivo using the subharmonic response from microbubbles. IEEE Trans Ultrason Ferroelectr Freq Control 2011;58:2056–66.

[166] Dave JK, Halldorsdottir VG, Eisenbrey JR, Raichlen JS, Liu JB, McDonald ME, et al. Noninvasive LV pressure estimation using subharmonic emissions from microbubbles. JACC Cardiovasc Imaging 2012;5:87–92.

[167] Dave JK, Halldorsdottir VG, Eisenbrey JR, Raichlen JS, Liu JB, McDonald M, et al. Subharmonic microbubble emissions for noninvasively tracing right ventricular pressures. Am J Physiol Heart Circ Physiol 2012;303:H126–32.

[168] Halldorsdottir V, Dave JK, Eisenbrey JR, Machado P, Liu JB, Merton DA, et al. Subharmonic aided pressure estimation for

monitoring interstitial fluid pressure in tumors: in vitro and in vivo proof of concept. J Ultrasound Med 2011;30:S28.

[169] Dave JK, Halldorsdottir VG, Eisenbrey JR, Merton DA, Liu JB, Zhou JH, et al. Investigating the efficacy of subharmonic aided pressure estimation for portal vein pressures and portal hypertension monitoring. Ultrasound Med Biol 2012;38:1784—98.

[170] Dave JK, Halldorsdottir VG, Eisenbrey JR, Merton DA, Liu JB, Machado P, et al. On the implementation of an automated acoustic output optimization for subharmonic aided pressure estimationes.Ultrasonics, [In Press].

[171] Eisenbrey JR, Dave JK, Halldorsdottir VG, Merton DA, Miller C, Gonzalez JM, et al. Noninvasive subharmonic aided pressure estimation of the hepatic venous pressure gradient in patients with chronic liver disease. Radiology, [In Press].

[172] Chen M, Le DQS, Hein S, Li P, Nygaard JV, Kassem M, et al. Fabrication and characterization of a rapid prototyped tissue engineering scaffold with embedded multicomponent matrix for controlled drug release. Int J Nanomed 2012;7:4285—97.

[173] Lima EG, Durney KM, Sirsi SR, Nover AB, Ateshian GA, Borden MA, et al. Microbubbles as biocompatible porogens for hydrogel scaffolds. Acta Biomater 2012;8(12):4334—41.

[174] Nair A, Yang J, Tang L. A novel preparation of degradable scaffolds using BSA microbubbles as Porogen. Engineering In Medicine and Biology Workshop. 2006:31—34. Dallas, TX.

[175] Toma C, Fisher A, Wang J, Chen X, Grata M, Leeman J, et al. Vascular endoluminal delivery of mesenchymal stem cells using acoustic radiation force. Tissue Eng: Part A 2011;17(9 and 10):1457—64.

[176] Rosen BR, Belliveau JW, Buchbinder BR, McKinstry RC, Porkka LM, Kennedy DN, et al. Contrast agents and cerebral hemodynamics. Magnetic resonance in medicine. Soc Magn Reson Med 1991;19(2):285—92.

[177] Simonsen CZ, Ostergaard L, Vestergaard-Poulsen P, Røhl L, Bjørnerud A, Gyldensted C. CBF and CBV measurements by USPIO bolus tracking: reproducibility and comparison with Gd-based values. JMRI 1999;9(2):342—7.

[178] Yang F, Li Y, Chen Z, Zhang Y, Wu J, Gu N. Superparamagnetic iron oxide nanoparticle-embedded encapsulated microbubbles as dual contrast agents of magnetic resonance and ultrasound imaging. Biomaterials 2009;30(23—24):3882—90.

[179] He W, Yang F, Wu Y, Wen S, Chen P, Zhang Y, et al. Microbubbles with surface coated by superparamagnetic iron oxide nanoparticles. Mater Lett 2012;68:64—7.

[180] Oeffinger BE, Wheatley MA. Development and characterization of a nano-scale contrast agent. Ultrasonics 2004;42:343—7.

[181] Wheatley MA, Lewandowski J. Nano-sized ultrasound contrast agent: salting out method. Mol Imaging 2010;9:96—107.

[182] Xing Z, Wang J, Ke H, et al. The fabrication of novel nanobubble ultrasound contrast agents for potential tumor imaging. Nanotechnology 2010;21:145607.

[183] Aoi AM, Watanabe Y, Mori S, et al. Herpes simplex virus thymidine kinase-mediated suicide gene therapy using nano/microbubbles and ultrasound. Ultrasound Med Biol 2008;34:425—34.

[184] Rapoport N, Gao Z, Kennedy A. Multifunctional nanoparticles for combining ultrasonic tumor imaging and targeted chemotherapy. J Natl Cancer Inst 2007;99:1095—106.

[185] Wang Y, Li X, Zhou Y, et al. Preparation of nanobubbles for ultrasound imaging and intracellular drug delivery. Int J Pharm 2009;381:148—53.

[186] Wang CH, Huang YF, Yeh CK. Aptamer-conjugated nanobubbles for targeted ultrasound molecular imaging. Langmuir 2011;27:6971—6.

[187] Goldberg BB, Merton DA, Liu JB, et al. Contrast-enhanced ultrasound imaging of sentinel lymph nodes after peritumoral administration of Sonzaoid in a melanoma tumor animal model. J Ultrasound Med 2011;30:441—53.

[188] Mattrey RF, Kono Y, Baker K, Peterson T. Sentinel lymph node imaging with microbubble ultrasound contrast material. Acad Radiol 2002;9:S231—5.

[189] Curry JM, Grindle CR, Merton DA, et al. Lymphosonographic sentinel node biopsy of

the supraglottis in a swine model. Otolaryngol Head Neck Surg 2008;139:798–804.

[190] Curry JM, Ezzat WH, Merton DA, et al. Thyroid lymphosonography: a novel method for evaluating lymphatic drainage. Ann Otol Rhinal Laryngol 2009;118:645–50.

[191] Sever A, Jones S, Cox K, et al. Preoperative localization of sentinel lymph nodes using intradermal microbubbles and contrast-enhanced ultrasonography in patients with breast cancer. Br J Surg 2009;96:1295–9.

12 Hydrogels in Regenerative Medicine

Justin M. Saul and David F. Williams

OUTLINE

12.1 Introduction: Relevance of Hydrogels to Regenerative Medicine — 279
12.2 Background and Theory — 281
  12.2.1 Classification — 281
  12.2.2 Theory — 281
12.3 Utility in Regenerative Medicine — 282
  12.3.1 Hydrogels as Biomaterials — 283
  12.3.2 Hydrogels for Controlled Release — 284
  12.3.3 Cell Association with Hydrogels — 285
    12.3.3.1 Cell Encapsulation — 285
    12.3.3.2 Spatial Patterning — 287
    12.3.3.3 Hydrogels as Substrates for Promoting Cell Attachment, Growth, and Differentiation — 287
12.4 Applications of Hydrogels in Regenerative Medicine — 290
  12.4.1 Skin and Wound Healing — 290
  12.4.2 Musculoskeletal — 291
  12.4.3 Neural Regeneration — 291
  12.4.4 Liver — 292
  12.4.5 Reproductive Medicine — 292
12.5 Prospects and Conclusions — 293
References — 294

12.1 Introduction: Relevance of Hydrogels to Regenerative Medicine

Hydrogels are crosslinked polymeric networks containing hydrophilic groups that promote swelling due to interaction with water [1]. While hydrogels are heavily used in the field of regenerative medicine, their application to biomedical systems is not new. In fact, it has been suggested that they were truly the first polymer materials to be developed for use in man [2]. They have been in use for clinical applications since the 1960s, initially for use in ocular applications including contact lenses and intraocular lenses due to their favorable oxygen permeability and lack of irritation leading to inflammation and foreign body response, which was observed with other plastics [3]. Before the concept of tissue engineering and regenerative medicine had gained traction, hydrogels were used for cell encapsulation [4]. They have also been utilized extensively in the clinic for wound healing applications due to their oxygen permeability, high water content, and ability to shield wounds from external agents. Perhaps the largest research focus and utility of hydrogels has been found in their use as controlled release systems. This combination of controlled release and cell encapsulation has led to increasing uses of hydrogels in regenerative medicine applications.

Hydrogels used in regenerative applications can be based on naturally or synthetically derived polymers. By most definitions, native tissues, particularly the extra-cellular matrix, are hydrogels and derivatives of these and other naturally based systems are in widespread use. Natural hydrogels are generally regarded as having favorable biodegradation products compared to some synthetic polymers as the monomeric degradation products are typically amino acids or saccharide units. In contrast, synthetics offer wide flexibility in terms of mechanical properties, water swelling, degradation rates, ionic charge, and other important parameters. Table 12.1 describes several prominent synthetic and natural hydrogels. These natural systems are derived from mammals, crustaceans, plants, and bacteria and are typically polypeptides or polysaccharides. Table 12.1, which highlights uses of hydrogels in regenerative

Table 12.1 Hydrogels Used in Regenerative Medicine and Medical Technology Applications

Hydrogel Material [Abbreviation]	Description	Examples of Applications	References
Poly(ethylene glycol) diacrylate [PEG]	Widely used, flexible synthetic polymer with low protein adsorption that is photo-crosslinkable	Neural Cartilage	[5] [6]
Poly(2-hydroxyethyl methacrylate) [pHEMA]	Non-degradable polymer modifiable for degradation [7]	Intraocular lenses Nerve guidance	[3] [8,9]
Oligo-(polypropylene fumarate) [OPF]		Bone Cartilage Nerve	[10] [11] [12,13]
Poly(N-isopropylacrylamide) [pNIPAAM]	Synthetic material with lower critical solution temperature (LCST) near physiological temperature	Corneal sheets	[14]
Collagen	Most prevalent protein in mammals characterized by proline-lysine-glycine repeating units and various isoforms	Bone Tendon	[15] [16]
Fibrin	Protein involved in clot formation and platelet binding in blood coagulation cascade	Surgical glue Neural regeneration Bone Cartilage	[17] [18] [19–21] [22]
Keratin	Protein derived from intermediate filaments of eukaryotes	Neural regeneration Hemostasis	[23] [24]
Silk	Biopolymer derived from spiders, *Bombyx mori*, and other sources	Cartilage Bone	[25] [26]
Agarose	Thermoreversible linear polysaccharide derived from red algae	Cartilage Neural regeneration	[27,28] [29,30]
Alginate	Second most abundant polysaccharide on earth; derived from seaweed and contains β-D-mannuoronate and β-L-guluronate sub-units (1,4 linkage)	Cell encapsulation Bone Ovary follicles	[4] [31] [32]
Chitin	β-(1,4)-N-acetyl glucosamine polysaccharide	Neural regeneration Cartilage	[33] [34]
Chitosan	Deacetylated chitin	Wound dressings	[35,36]
Hyaluronic acid	β-(1,3) glucuronic acid and β(1,4)-N-acetylglucosamine glycosaminoglycan found in connective tissue	Cartilage Vocal cord Bone Wound healing	[37] [38] [39] [40]

(*Continued*)

Table 12.1 Hydrogels Used in Regenerative Medicine and Medical Technology Applications—Cont'd

Hydrogel Material [Abbreviation]	Description	Examples of Applications	References
Methyl cellulose	Cellulose (polysaccharide) with hydroxyl groups substituted with methoxyl groups to disrupt cellulose crysallinity and provide solubility	Neural regeneration Nucleus pulposa	[41] [42]
Bacterial cellulose	Non-degradable cellulosic material produced by *Acetobacter xylinum*	Vascular graft Bone	[43] [44]

medicine, primarily shows the use of single-component systems. However, combinatorial uses of hydrogels to obtain desirable properties of each component are widely investigated.

The diversity and flexibility of natural and synthetic hydrogels makes it impossible to consider every type of hydrogel. The goal of this chapter is to provide an overview of the basic theory of hydrogels, describe important uses and applications in regenerative medicine, and consider their continued importance in research and the clinic.

12.2 Background and Theory

12.2.1 Classification

Several methods can be used to classify hydrogels including network structure or porosity, physical structure, source, and crosslink type [45]. In tissue engineering and regenerative medicine, the porosity of the scaffold materials is often of considerable importance. Hydrogels can be classified according to their *network structure* as macroporous (pores of ~10–200 μm), microporous (pores of ~1–10 μm), and non-porous (pores of <1 μm). Clearly, if used for approaches in which cells must infiltrate the scaffold, macroporous scaffolds must be used. Non-porous scaffolds have low rates of diffusion, making cell viability a significant concern and preventing infiltration of cells not pre-encapsulated in the hydrogel.

Classification by *physical structure* is also fairly intuitive for regenerative applications. Hydrogels can be considered amorphous, semicrystalline, hydrogen bonded, or complexation products. They can be classified according to their *source*, that is, whether they are naturally derived or synthetic. Synthetic systems have a plethora of options and may be homopolymer or copolymer systems. Further, synthetic polymers can also be synthesized to form interpenetrating polymer networks in which the two polymer sheets are physically entangled. Naturally derived systems may be polysaccharide or polypeptide-based and derived from numerous sources.

More common in the polymer chemistry literature is classification according to the *ionic charge* of the hydrogel. The gels may be neutral, anionic, cationic, or ampholytic. The charge properties become crucial in considering their interaction with physiological environments and cells. Ionotropic gels are ionic polymers that contain a balancing multivalent counterion. One example of this is an alginate hydrogel. Alginate in its native form is anionic but is not a hydrogel. In the presence of calcium counterions it forms a physical hydrogel through ionic interactions.

Hydrogels can also be classified according to the type of *crosslink*. The two broadest categorizations are chemical or physical crosslinks. In general, a chemical crosslink is defined as a covalent interaction at a point of overlap or junction (see below). Physical crosslinks may be the physical entanglement of the polymer chains, interpenetrating polymer networks, and other secondary forces (e.g. hydrophobic interactions, hydrogen bonding, ionic interactions, electrostatic interactions) [46].

12.2.2 Theory

An in-depth description of the polymer science theory governing the formation and behavior of hydrogels is beyond the scope of this text. Below we briefly describe several of the key parameters that are of particular importance to scientists working with hydrogels in regenerative medicine applications. More complete descriptions of the theoretical polymer science basis for hydrogels are given in several other locations [1,47]. Nonetheless, the principles that govern their formation are highly relevant to regenerative medicine applications as these properties control (among other things) swelling, interaction with cells, and drug delivery kinetics.

Numerous mathematical models have been developed to estimate the properties of hydrogels and to predict processes related to controlled release (e.g. diffusion parameters and rates of release). Much of the discussion below is taken from review articles on the topic [47].

Three important parameters to consider in defining hydrogels are: (1) the *volume fraction* in the swollen state, (2) the *crosslink density*, and (3) the *porosity of the hydrogel*. These parameters can be described mathematically.

The volume fraction is simply the volume fraction occupied by the polymer and gives a sense of the amount of water in the gel. Mathematically, it has been defined as:

$$v_{2,s} = \frac{\text{Volume of polymer}}{\text{Volume of swollen gel}} = \frac{1}{Q}$$

where Q is another useful parameter known as the volume degree of swelling. Although the polymer volume can be estimated from the density of the polymer, it is sometimes easier to determine the polymer weight. A second set of parameters based on the weights can therefore be defined akin to the volume fractions above:

$$m_{2,s} = \frac{\text{Mass of polymer}}{\text{Mass of swollen gel}} = \frac{1}{q}$$

The effective molecular weight between crosslinks can be inferred from the description in Figure 12.1. This figure shows a schematic of a hydrogel polymer network [48]. Areas of "overlap" in Figure 12.1 are known as junctions and indicate either physical or chemical crosslinks. The average molecular weight between crosslinks is known as the effective molecular weight between crosslinks, M_c. This value can be used to determine the crosslink density based on the known molecular weight of the polymer repeat units, M_o, as:

$$X = \frac{M_c}{M_o}$$

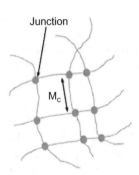

Figure 12.1 Simplified schematic of hydrogel structure. Junctions indicate points of crosslinks, with the distance between the junctions indicating the molecular weight of between crosslinks, M_c. Junctions may be physical entanglements or chemical or ionic crosslinks. *(Adapted from Peppas and Barr-Howell [48], with permission.)*

Several other parameters of interest are those of porosity, tortuosity, and the diffusion coefficients through the gel. Porosity is the volume of the gel that is not physically occupied by the polymer itself. This parameter is often of particular interest to tissue engineers working with macroporous or microporous gels as the porosity is an indication of the volume of the material available for cell infiltration or seeding. Within regenerative medicine, the role that cells play in remodeling a matrix is often important, so materials with higher porosity are viewed as favorable, potentially allowing a larger number of the cellular ("functional") units of the system to be present. Tortuosity is the path that a molecule or cell must navigate in order to penetrate the gel. Both the porosity and tortuosity are important in determining the rate of diffusion within hydrogels. Diffusion is the main transport mechanism of nutrients and oxygen to cells within the gel, of metabolic waste products out of the gel, as well as the release of therapeutic agents from the gel or from cells within the gel.

12.3 Utility in Regenerative Medicine

Hydrogels currently have a wide range of applications from consumer products to electronics and biosensors. Within the biomedical field, the earliest applications of hydrogels were for ocular applications including intraocular lenses [49], soft contact lenses [3,50], and corneal repair [51]. They have also been used as suture, as dental materials, in biosensors, and as coatings for catheters and defibrillators, and for wound care products.

The original use of hydrogels came as stand-alone biomaterials or as devices for controlled release applications. Later, they became the focus of cell-encapsulation approaches. The wedding of these three uses for hydrogels has propelled their use in the field of regenerative medicine as scientists use their properties to direct cell attachment, migration, and differentiation. The application of these individual roles of hydrogels and their combinatorial approaches in regenerative medicine are described in more detail below.

12.3.1 Hydrogels as Biomaterials

Although the field of biomaterials is clearly moving from the use of inert materials that minimize host response to more bioactive and integrative materials, the original use of hydrogels came as stand-alone biomaterials for ophthalmic and blood-contacting applications. Indeed these applications remain important in the biomedical field. At the time of their discovery, one of the appealing aspects of hydrogels was their minimal foreign body response compared to other semi-crystalline polymers (Wichertle and Lim, 1960). This stems from the observation that hydrogels typically have low levels of protein adsorption. For example, poly(ethylene glycol) (PEG) is widely used on drug delivery vehicles due to its ability to provide long circulation times, likely through steric effects on complement proteins. Similarly, PEG-diacrylate gels are known to have low protein adsorption [52], as are various other synthetic-based hydrogels [53] due to steric effects and possibly their hydrophilic surfaces. Low protein adsorption is generally associated with poor cell attachment. Further, synthetic hydrogels and many natural hydrogels (particularly polysaccharides such as alginate and agarose) lack peptidic sequences that would promote cell attachment via integrin binding.

While this lack of biological activity seems counter-intuitive in regenerative medicine, hydrogels are highly labile in terms of chemical and physical modifications that can be used to modulate cellular response in a more bioactive fashion (see below). Thus, while hydrogels remain highly significant as stand-alone biomaterials in minimizing host response, they are also useful for the direction of cell response to materials in a more bioactive fashion.

The method of hydrogel formation is particularly important for maintaining bioactivity of molecules and for minimizing any detrimental effects to cells associated with the gels. Typically, a monomer or non-crosslinked polymer is found in the solution (sol) phase. Upon application of some initiation conditions, the sol phase forms the hydrogel (gel) phase; that is, it undergoes the sol-gel transition. For hydrogels containing bioactive molecules or cells, it is clear that high temperatures and many monomers, solvents, and polymerization initiators cannot be used due to inactivation of bioactives or cytotoxicity. Therefore, approaches that achieve the sol-gel transition with minimal effect on bioactive molecules and cells have been developed and are described here and in other sections of this textbook.

Photopolymerization is commonly used to achieve gelation for regenerative medicine applications. Photopolymerization reactions for hydrogel formation have been performed for poly(vinyl alcohol) [54], polysaccharide-based materials, poly(2-hydroxyethylmethacrylate) [55–57], and modified PEG-collagen [58] among others. Poly(ethylene glycol) or PEG diacrylate gels are the most common gel systems used for the formation of photopolymerized hydrogels [59]. The presence of pi bonds in the diacrylate terminal ends of PEG provides the chemical moieties for the reaction. Photoinitiators used for biomaterial applications have been classified as photolytic or hydrogen abstraction [60]. Photolytic groups include free radical initiators including acetophenone derivatives widely used for hydrogel formation. One advantage of photopolymerizable hydrogels is their ability to be polymerized *in situ*. Materials that spontaneously undergo the sol-gel transition in response to light or physiological temperature can be maintained in solution phase until *in vivo* injection followed by gel formation at the desired location. Other more robust forms of achieving gelation have been described, such as the use of click chemistry [61–63]; however, the effects of this chemistry and the copper initiators on cells have not been established.

Hydrogels have been coupled with most modern approaches to biomaterial scaffold fabrication.

Cell-hydrogel constructs with alginate or poly(ethylene oxide)-pluronic-poly(ethylene oxide) block polymer as the hydrogels have been used with BioPlotter and solid free-form fabrication systems [64,65]. One drawback to hydrogel systems is a lack of mechanical integrity associated with certain applications.

Non-woven electrospun fibers [66] and woven hydrogel/cell mixtures [67] have been reported that may allow for materials of greater mechanical integrity. More complex approaches to achieving spatial regulation of cells within hydrogel biomaterials include photopatterning and photolithographic techniques of cell adhesion and migration molecules to direct cell attachment and material response (see below) [68,69]. The role of topographical cues in cell fate is becoming well established and hydrogels are useful for the creation of three-dimensional topographical cues such as nanopillars [70] to promote cell migration, and recently through the introduction of enzyme-assisted photolithography to achieve spatial functionalization of hydrogels that may provide insight into the topographical designs necessary for larger tissue constructs [71].

12.3.2 Hydrogels for Controlled Release

Over the past 30 years, numerous systems have been developed for delivery of therapeutic agents within the context of the medical device field with the goal of achieving long-term, zero-order release of therapeutic agents. These systems can generally be classified as swelling-controlled, diffusion-controlled, or chemically controlled. Examples include osmotic pumps (swelling-controlled), transdermal patches (diffusion-controlled reservoir matrix), and drug eluting stents (chemically controllable erodible system).

Within the field of regenerative medicine, it desirable to have release of therapeutic agents occur from a system that degrades with time so that secondary retrieval and removal of a device (e.g. osmotic pump) is not required. As such, those systems described above as medical devices are usually not employed within the context of regenerative medicine. Rather, implantable or injectable bulk hydrogels are a preferential alternative. The primary therapeutic agent of interest is the release of growth factors. However, the delivery of small molecules (e.g. antibiotics) and nucleic acids have also been widely employed, often in conjunction with cell therapies.

A drawback to this bulk hydrogel approach is that the complexity provided by a device (e.g. an osmotic pump) is lost, making zero-order release difficult to achieve over the time periods that can be achieved with medical devices. However, in principle, regenerative medicine approaches seek to stimulate a physiological response to a chemical cue such as growth factor release. Following the initial stimulus, the regenerated tissue should move toward normal physiological function, thereby obviating the need for long-term release of the chemical cue as is desirable in the traditional medical device field.

As a controlled release platform, several parameters can be used to modulate the release of the therapeutic agent. Because these systems are examples of diffusion-mediated release, the porosity and tortuosity of the system significantly affect the release of therapeutic agents. The ionic nature of many hydrogel systems also lends itself to the sustained release of counter-charged molecules. More generally, affinity between the hydrogel and therapeutic agent (whether through ionic charge, hydrophobic effects, or protein-protein interactions) can be used to modulate the rates of release.

The ability to modulate the release through external control is also of considerable importance. Examples of these types of systems include increasing binding between the gel and therapeutic, the use of environmental controls such as temperature, pH, or enzymes, or the application of external energy sources such as ultrasound, light, or electrical fields to promote or mitigate release. Such approaches allow for the tunable, responsive, and/or pulsatile release profiles.

The hydrophilic groups of hydrogels that lead to high water content and therefore low protein adsorption or cell binding also provide chemical flexibility for the covalent binding of molecules to the hydrogel backbone. This is described in more detail below for matrix-immobilized ligands. However, this approach can also be used to control the rate of release of therapeutic agents. One example of this approach is in making use of the heparin-binding domains found on many growth factors. By coupling heparin to the hydrogel via these reactive groups, it is possible to maintain the association of heparin-binding growth factors with the hydrogel for a longer timeframe than achieved with diffusion-mediated release [72].

A more sophisticated controlled release system applicable to hydrogels and other polymers is that of cell-demanded liberation and is akin to a pendant-chain system [73]. The premise of this approach is that growth factors can be tethered to the backbone of the hydrogel [19]. The backbone of the hydrogel or the pendant-chain tether itself can contain sequences cleavable by matrix-metalloproteases (MMPs). Diffusion-mediated release from the hydrogel or cleavage of the growth factor from the tether occur only as cells infiltrate the scaffold, hence the term cell-demanded liberation. In one version of this system, the 121 isoform of VEGF was engineered to contain the factor XIII substrate amino acid sequence, for binding to a fibrin hydrogel, and an α2 plasmin-inhibitor that is MMP-cleavable [74]. As cells infiltrate the scaffold, they produce MMPs, leading to cleavage of the VEGF from the hydrogel to promote vascularization of the construct in conjunction with cell infiltration.

The most well known and studied thermally responsive system is the N-isopropylacrylamide or pNIPAAM. pNIPAAM has a lower critical solution temperature (LCST) of approximately 32°C (for the linear form). Therefore, below 32°C the polymer is hydrophilic and promotes cell attachment and adhesion. Above 32°C, the polymer becomes hydrophobic, leading to detachment of cells. This approach has therefore been exploited for use in the creation of cell sheets for various tissue engineering applications including cornea [14,75–77], cardiac grafts [78–80], urothelium [81,82], and skin [83], among others.

In addition to intrinsic physiological control mechanisms such as pH, enzymes, and temperature, release of therapeutic agents can also be controlled through extrinsic mechansisms or energy sources. In one example of these systems, pHEMA has been used as the drug reservoir for the release of small molecules (ciprofloxacin antibiotic, molecular weight ~330 Da) and pHEMA/2-hydroxyethylacrylate PEG-dimethylacrylate has been used to release larger molecules (insulin, molecular weight ~5.8 kDa). This system used a coating of methylene chains to prevent passive diffusion of drug during periods without the application of ultrasound and was compatible with ultrasonic energies that are clinically relevant (43 kHz and 1.1 MHz) [84]. Electrically responsive hydrogels are also an active area of research. Although an important area of research for drug delivery applications, the use of electrically responsive hydrogels has not found widespread use in regenerative medicine due to the need for application of electrical field and/or electrode implantation [85]. Nonetheless, extrinsically mediated systems and feedback-controlled systems provide added control and sophistication that may find utility, particularly in endocrine-related tissues.

In summary, hydrogel systems can provide a mechanism to achieve near zero-order release for finite time periods, which is advantageous as a secondary procedure for device removal is not required. Hydrogels can also be used to achieve on-demand or pulsatile release. Because they can serve as a physical matrix for cells or for cell encapsulation, they can also be considered controlled release systems by slowly releasing therapeutic agents produced by cells.

12.3.3 Cell Association with Hydrogels

12.3.3.1 Cell Encapsulation

Hydrogels have been in use for nearly 30 years as a system to encapsulate cells [86]. For example, endocrine disorders such as diabetes that result from autoimmunity against hormone-secreting cells are intensely studied for regenerative therapies. The ability to achieve a functional effect may be attainable not through whole organ replacement but through delivery of cells microencapsulated in hydrogels (Figure 12.2), which can promote cell viability, controlled release, and protection from immune response to implanted cells. While the spatial distribution of cells is clearly important in the engineering of *de novo* functional tissues, the more general non-spatially controlled encapsulation of cells still provides the potential for a significant clinical impact.

The incorporation of cellular components provides the opportunity to achieve zero-order or physiologically responsive release over prolonged periods of time. Alginate microspheres are among the most studied hydrogel carriers for microencapsulation of cells. The mechanical properties of these gels can be modulated depending on the divalent cation used to achieve crosslinking. For example, the use of barium or strontium instead of calcium leads to more rigid gels. These systems also provide a barrier to immune

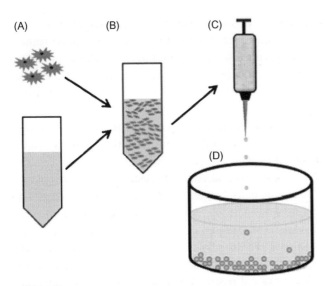

Figure 12.2 Schematic of the process of cell microencapsulation with sol-gel transition of hydrogels. (A) In this process, cultured or isolated cells are dissolved in a solution-phase hydrogel (e.g. alginate) and (B) mixed into a viscous cell suspension. (C) The solution-phase hydrogel/cell mixture is then extruded (e.g. by pressure) from a droplet microencapsulator (typically a syringe, possibly with some electric field applied to regulate droplet size). (D) The droplets are collected in a solution promoting gelation (e.g. calcium-containing solution for alginate). Regulation of drop size allows single or multiple cell encapsulation and mechanical properties can be regulated through the hydrogel precursor concentration or the gelling agent.

Within the last decade, approaches have been developed to provide more control over methods to achieve encapsulation of cells. Two particularly important approaches include *in situ* gelation and photoencapsulation. In situ gelation systems may depend on pH, temperature, or light as the initiating species. Temperature and light are the primary mechanisms of *in situ* gelation initiators used in regenerative medicine with pH systems being used less frequently to avoid exposing cells to caustic environments. Particularly advantageous for regenerative medicine applications are reverse thermogelation compounds that are in solution at low temperatures but gel at higher temperatures, preferably in the physiological range. That is, compounds that undergo the sol-gel transition with increasing temperature. Important natural hydrogels that are reverse thermogelation compounds include collagen, carboxymethylcellulose, and certain combinations of hydrogels. Important synthetic hydrogels known to undergo *in situ* gelation include poly(N-isopropylacrylamide) and block co-polymer systems consisting of poly(ethylene glycol) in combination with Pluronic or PLGA [88]. The ability of hydrogels to undergo sol-gel transitions at increasing temperatures depends on the balance of intermolecular forces including hydrogen bonding and hydrophobic interactions as well as water content and crosslinking density. The applications of these systems are numerous, but include both hard and soft tissues [89,90].

Photo-encapsulation can be a subclass of *in situ* gelling materials. Photo-initiators are widely used in dental applications to cure resins. Photo-initiators have also been used for the formation of hydrogels for approximately 20 years [91] as a solution-phase material can be injected and then cured to the gel phase *in situ*. Various initiators have been employed, but those that are active in the ultraviolet range are most widely reported in part because they are less likely to polymerize in response to ambient light and have higher reported crosslinking efficiencies [92]. The use of polymerization initiators as well as the use of UV-light have been shown to have detrimental effects on cells [93]. However, alternate initiators such as those active in the infrared range may mitigate some of the UV effects, and the ability to achieve spatially controlled encapsulation of cells within hydrogels is clearly important for achieving structure-function relationships [94,95].

response, providing the potential to use autologous stem cells, allogeneic differentiated cells, or even xenografted cells. They can also be coated with polycations such as poly-L-lysine or poly-ornithine for stabilization and to regulate solute release from the capsules [87]. With these semi-permeable membrane coatings, the encapsulated cell/microbead system becomes akin to the traditional reservoir drug delivery systems but with the ability to respond to physiological stimuli. Problems with foreign body response and issues of achieving sufficient nutrient supply and waste removal remain challenges to long-term patency of these systems, but many of the approaches to achieve vascularization currently under investigation may provide more immediate benefit to these types of cell-encapsulation therapies for numerous hormone-related deficiencies.

12.3.3.2 Spatial Patterning

As described above, hydrogels can be utilized to achieve three-dimensional spatial patterning of cells. One important development in the use of hydrogels has been the advent of inkjet printing technology, first described by Boland's group in 2004 [96,97]. Originally used for high-throughput screening of drug compounds [98] and then for the printing of nucleic acids to solid substrates [99], this approach has since garnered more attention for the spatial patterning of cells that may resemble native tissue. In the initial iterations of this work, ink from inkjet printer cartridges was replaced with cells suspended in a non-crosslinked polymer solution. Alginates in the absence of calcium is the most common gel system although there are reports using collagen [97], fibrin [100,101], polyurethanes [102], and polyacrylamide [103]. In each case, the cells are suspended in a non-crosslinked form of the polymer solution and printed into a solution containing the crosslinking agent. In the case of alginate this involves printing into a calcium solution whereas fibrinogen can be printed into a thrombin solution. Cells are printed in a two-dimensional pattern, and three-dimension structures are formed through a layer-by-layer approach. More recently, true three-dimension bioprinters have been developed [104] and the ability to print from an array of cartridges is also under development. The role of gradients in directing migration and/or differentiation is an area of interest in many aspects of regenerative medicine. Inkjet printers provide a medium for the development of these types of gradients [103,105,106]. Current drawbacks to this approach are the lack of mechanical integrity and questions regarding the thermal effects on cells. Although the technology has not shown a noticeable effect on cell viability [107], more subtle effects on gene regulation through the heat shock protein (HSP) family are yet to be fully characterized.

Dielectrophoresis is an approach useful for screening and may also be applicable to the formation of scaffold materials on scales relevant to organ engineering [108]. This approach allows for the patterning of cells within hydrogel constructs via the application of uniform electrical field. One drawback to the approach is that relatively weak hydrogels are required to allow manipulation and patterning of the cells for the dielectrophoretic field. An approach has been described to overcome this, which treats hydrogels as a composite system wherein cells are patterned via electrical field within an agarose or PEG gel and surrounded by a bulk-phase material with the desired mechanical properties, thus providing an approach to scale up this technique to larger-sized constructs [109]. It is unclear whether the application of electrical field or the application of high temperatures in inkjet printing will be less deleterious to cells, but the approach demonstrates the ability to achieve spatial patterning through other approaches.

The ability to spatially pattern cells on or within hydrogels is also important in considering approaches to achieve high-throughput screening of hydrogels to assess the role of hydrogel type, topographical signals, soluble chemical cues, immobilized chemical cues, mechanical properties, and other parameters on cells. Several approaches have been developed toward this end and will likely be important tools in providing more systematic study of the role of hydrogels (and other biomaterials) on cell phenotype and genotype. One approach to high-throughput analysis is the use of the dip pen lithographic technique with hydrogels [110]. This technique allows for the rapid printing of gels with or without cells and is compatible with soluble and matrix-immobilized chemical cues. While this technique is likely limited to screening assays, the knowledge imparted is important for a rational approach to the design of larger-scale constructs.

12.3.3.3 Hydrogels as Substrates for Promoting Cell Attachment, Growth, and Differentiation

It is increasingly clear that both physical (e.g. mechanical properties and topographical cues) as well as chemical cues have a significant impact on cell functions such as attachment, proliferation, migration, and differentiation. As described above, one advantage of hydrogel systems is the ability to achieve three-dimensional constructs of materials and cells that begin to recapitulate the architecture of native tissue. Because their high water content and low protein adsorption typically lead to poor cell attachment (in the absence of native or added binding motifs), these systems also provide the ability to isolate specific effects such as a particular ligand or a range of mechanical properties. That is, they provide the means to conduct systematic evaluations of certain biological ligands, combinations of ligands, or the effects of specific mechanical properties on cell response. Hydrogels have many parameters than can be altered to modulate and study the environmental cues associated with the material. These alterable parameters can generally be divided into chemical and physical parameters. A summary of approaches to modulate these parameters is shown in Figure 12.3.

There are two basic methods to provide chemical cues to cells via hydrogels: soluble factor delivery and matrix-immobilized presentation. Parameters and methods that control soluble factor delivery are described on pages 284–285. The primary function of matrix-bound cues is to promote cell attachment and to provide signaling cues to direct cell behavior. The role of specific ligands is discussed elsewhere in this text, but Table 12.2 lists specific examples of matrix-immobilized molecules on hydrogels.

It is noteworthy that most of the gels shown in Table 12.2 are based on poly(ethylene glycol) or other gels to which cell attachment is poor. One approach to achieving better cell attachment and biological function is to mix hydrogels that have some inherent biological activity with those that do not to provide a type of composite material that has desirable properties [123]. An approach that is slightly more complex but can provide greater control over the presentation of binding molecules is to incorporate cell binding motifs or other cell-guiding peptides via surface immobilization into gels that lack these components. It should be noted, however, that hydrogels based on natural materials that provide good cell attachment (e.g. collagen) can benefit from several of these techniques. For example, the use of gradient techniques should be more broadly applicable to all hydrogels in an effort to direct cell migration, and photolithographic approaches to pattern hydrogels are important for achieving spatial organization of multiple cell type tissue constructs. Lastly, the spatial distribution of specific cell types is an important consideration in attempts to create *de novo* complex tissues due to well-known physiological structure-function relationships. The ability to achieve cell-specific attachment in a spatially defined fashion is key to achieving this physiology. As such, spatial distribution of peptides or proteins that promote the selective (or preferably specific) attachment of certain cell types based on the principles highlighted in Table 12.2 is also of considerable importance [59,124].

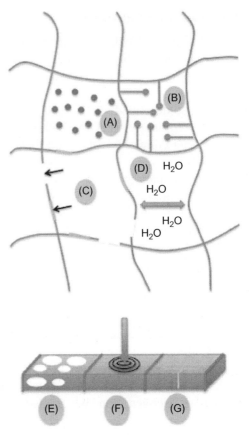

Figure 12.3 Schematic highlighting several key mechanisms and properties of hydrogels important in regenerative medicine applications. Additional details of these are provided in the text. Delivery of growth factors and other compounds may be provided via soluble factors (A) or matrix-bound cues (B). Delivery of soluble factors may also be controlled by the rate of degradation of the hydrogel (C) through hydrolysis of certain regions (arrows) or other specific enzymatic mechanisms. The water content and swelling (D) also affect soluble factor delivery, protein adsorption, and cell attachment. The porosity of the scaffold (E) and mechanical properties (F) such as compressive modulus are known to have significant effects on cellular infiltration. Lastly, hydrogels can be modified through numerous patterning techniques such as photolithography to provide micropatterned substrates to assess and regulate the microenvironment of cells.

Approaches to achieve surface immobilization include selective adsorption and covalent crosslinking. Selective adsorption is difficult to achieve for protein molecules on hydrogels due to their low

Table 12.2 Examples and Applications of Matrix-immobilized Ligands with Hydrogel Systems

Application	Hydrogel Component(s)	Ligand and Immobilization Method	Reference(s)
Cell attachment	Poly(ethylene glycol) (PEG)	Arginine-glycine-aspartic acid (RGD) modified with acryol groups for reaction with poly(ethylene diacrylate) hydrogel	[111]
Vascularization of three-dimensional constructs	Collagenase-degradable PEG	Vascular endothelial growth factor (VEGF) and arginine-glycine-aspartic acid-serine (RGDS) covalently coupled to PEG by attaching acry-moiety to ligand for reaction to PEG during polymerization	[112]
Improve cell adhesion to non-adhesive gels	PEG	Collagen-mimetic peptide co-polymerized into hydrogel	[113]
Delivery of plasmid DNA transgene growth factor expression	Hyaluronic acid/ PEG-collagen	Polyethylenimine-DNA complexes coupled via neutravidin-biotin or non-specific adsorption	[114]
Delivery of plasmid DNA transgene growth factor expression	Fibrin	Polyethylenimine-DNA complexes adsorbed non-specifically with high affinity	[115]
Guided tissue regeneration with focus on bone	Oligo-poly(ethylene glycol)-fumarate	Osteopontin-derived peptide covalently coupled to hydrogel via PEG linker	[116]
Cell attachment to hydrogels	Proteolytically-degradable PEG	RGDS and other cell-adhesive peptides conjugated to PEG linker and photocoupled to hydrogel	[59,117]
Cell attachment for soft tissue constructs in trauma applications	Alginate	RGD covalently coupled to alginate backbone	[118]
Osteoblast adhesion for bone tissue engineering	Poly(propylene fumarate-co-ethylene glycol)	RGDS covalently coupled to hydrogel via PEG linker	[119]
Directing cell attachment and migration	PEG	RGDS or basic fibroblast growth factor (bFGF) covalently immobilized to hydrogel in gradient fashion	[52,120]
Cell adhesion and neurite outgrowth	Agarose	RGDS covalently immobilized to hydrogel via photo-cross-linking	[121]
Cell binding and vascularization of tissue constructs	PEG	RGDS and vascular endothelial growth factor covalently coupled to hydrogel via photo-cross-linker in pattern defined by photo-masking lithography	[122]

protein adsorption. Certain hydrogels may allow adsorption through electrostatic interactions and larger particles (see PEI–DNA complexes in Table 12.2) allow more interactions with the material surface, thereby promoting adsorption through multiple weak interactions. Non-covalent but strong interactions such as avidin-biotin crosslinking has also been used as it is a straightforward process without reaction by-products. However, covalent crosslinking is clearly the most widely used approach to achieving matrix immobilization of bioactive molecules.

For covalent crosslinking, the molecule of interest may be reacted with a chemically labile side group on the hydrogel in the solution phase prior to gelation. Photo-crosslinking is now more widely used, particularly for cellular applications to avoid chemical reaction by products and to prevent loss of activity of the bioactive molecule during the gelation process. Most hydrogels are compatible to some degree with photo-crosslinking as they are somewhat translucent. Thicker constructs, however, may require the use of layered constructs to achieve desired coupling throughout the hydrogel. Photo-crosslinking is also useful as it is compatible with lithographic techniques that allow control over cell spatial distribution. References to representative papers on these approaches are provided in Table 12.2.

In addition to their compatibility with soluble and matrix-bound chemical cues, parameters of hydrogels can be altered to change the mechanical properties of the gel. Table 12.3 lists several of these parameters. Changes in these parameters clearly affect the mechanical properties of the gels, which in turn affect cell systems. For example, low moduli PEG gels have been shown to promote markers of early cardiomyocyte differentiation in an embryonal carcinoma cell model [133]. Proliferation of neural stem cells has been shown to be inversely proportional to the matrix modulus of alginate hydrogels [134]. Matrix modulus in conjunction with mechanical stimulation has been shown to have effects on chondrocyte morphology in PEG gels [6,128]. Other parameters that affect the mechanical properties and the cellular response include the porosity of the hydrogel, which can be modulated through the use of porogens. Effects of the porosity have also been demonstrated to affect mesenchymal stem cell proliferation [135] and mineralization in osteogenic medium [136]. Thus, although chemical regulatory mechanisms are perhaps better understood, it is clear that the mechanical nature of the materials must be given equal consideration.

12.4 Applications of Hydrogels in Regenerative Medicine

As described above, hydrogels are applicable for fundamental studies on the role of topographical patterning, microfluid flow, and high-throughput screening. They are also in use or under investigation as a repair or replacement strategy for virtually all tissues including both hard and soft tissues. It is not possible to describe every tissue and application, but the goal of this section is to highlight several areas in which hydrogels are used in a translational light.

12.4.1 Skin and Wound Healing

The FDA's searchable database (1979 to present) indicates that more than 510,000 applications have

Table 12.3 Effect of Hydrogel Parameters on Mechanical Properties

Parameter	Effect	Relevant Reference(s)
Water content	Inversely correlated with crosslink density. Decreased water content leads to increase in compressive modulus	[125,126]
Crosslink density	Inversely correlated with water content. Increased crosslink density leads to increase in compressive modulus	[6,125,127,128]
Degradation	Decrease in compressive modulus as gel degrades	[126]
Molecular weight	Increase in molecular weight for oligo(polyethylene glycol) leads to decrease in tensile modulus, increase in toughness, and a higher percent elongation	[129]
Charge	For anionic hydrogels, increasing surface charge leads to swelling and decrease in modulus	[130]; [131][a]; [132]
Electrical field	Hydrogel deswells with application of electrical field leading to increase in modulus	[131][a]; [132]

[a][131] is a theoretical model based on experimental results from [130].

been granted for the use of hydrogels in treating wounds than any for other medical device application. This is in part due to the shear number of wound healing products as well as the overlap in mechanical property similarities between skin and most hydrogels. Beyond the mechanical properties, there are numerous advantages to the use of hydrogels in these systems. Namely, hydrogels for wound healing applications are:

- Permeable to oxygen to prevent necrosis of remaining and newly forming tissue.
- Able to retain moisture at the site of injury to promote healing.
- Compatible with therapeutic agents important to wound healing including antimicrobials, steroids, and growth factors.
- Able to stimulate cellular response and infiltration with minimal foreign body response and subsequent scarring.

An FDA-approved dressing that makes use of a number of concepts described earlier is Oxyzyme, and there are other similar market-approved products. This proprietary hydrogel contains glucose oxidase, which, in the presence of oxygen, leads to the formation of gluconic acid and hydrogen peroxide. The hydrogen peroxide decomposes to water and oxygen, thereby further improving the oxygenation of the tissue. This product also contains iodine to inhibit bacterial growth and contamination of the wound [137,138]. Preclinically, bilayered chitosan hydrogels have been used in a third degree porcine burn model [139] and the application of matrix-immobilized fibronectin on hyaluronic acid has been shown to promote fibroblastic wound healing response [40]. These studies indicate that the next generation of clinical hydrogel wound dressings will utilize current-generation research principles.

12.4.2 Musculoskeletal

Some of the earliest-envisioned applications for hydrogels in tissue engineering involved replacements for gel-like tissues such as articular cartilage [140–142]. These tissues have high levels of glycosaminoglycans and therefore have a high water content, making them a type of natural hydrogel. Hydrogels encapsulating chondrogenic cells are a promising approach to cartilage repair. Examples of chondrocyte-encapsulating materials include alginate [143], oligo(polyethylene glycol) fumarate (OPF) with soluble TGFβ1 delivered from gelatin microspheres [144], and fibrin-PEG-poly(lactic acid) hydrogels, which are currently in large animal trials [145]. Indeed, for articular cartilage, an extremely wide range of hydrogels has been used, in part because suitable treatments have not be found. An interesting approach that is applicable to cartilage repair is the use of adhesive hydrogels that contain chondroitin sulfate in combination with methacrylate and aldehydes to bridge the material with native tissue [146].

Hydrogels do not possess the mechanical properties of native bone tissue and are not applied directly for bridging critically sized gaps without fixation. However, the controlled release capabilities of hydrogels have been widely exploited for the delivery of growth factors (and plasmid DNA encoding for growth factors) that promote robust bone formation. For cell-free hydrogels, this generally involves delivery of bone morphogenetic protein 2 (BMP-2) or 7 (BMP-7 also known as OP-1) as these compounds are FDA approved. Recent examples of this approach include delivery of BMP-2 via an *in situ* gelling hyaluronic acid/polyvinyl alcohol hydrogel [147], and BMP-2 delivery from a gelatin hydrogel for a rabbit segmental bone defect model [148] and regeneration of skull tissue in non-human primates [149]. It might be argued that any material that delivers the potent mitogen BMP-2 will lead to successful bone regeneration. However, hydrogels or other materials that minimize ectopic bone formation meet an important criteria for bone regeneration systems. The controlled release of BMP-2 on timescales most beneficial for promoting regeneration is also important. Unfortunately, this timescale is not well defined, though it appears that there exists a threshold level of BMP-2 that can achieve bone regeneration.

12.4.3 Neural Regeneration

Hydrogels are becoming more widely used with encapsulation of Schwann cells and neural progenitor cells to promote neural regeneration via cell-based trophic support. However, hydrogels have been and remain widely investigated as stand-alone materials for neural regeneration applications as well. This is because the regeneration of neuronal axons is different from many other tissues in that the cell body is typically located proximally to the site of injury, requiring migration of a part of the cell (i.e. the axon) to and then through the site of injury.

In the peripheral nervous system, hydrogels are under investigation as fillers for nerve conduits composed of natural materials such as collagen (e.g. Neuragen Nerve Guide) or synthetic materials (e.g. Silastic). Examples of hydrogels used as fillers include agarose, fibrin, and keratin, among others. The role of charge [150] and mechanical properties [151] have been elucidated for peripheral nerve systems. Some natural materials appear to promote regeneration simply through the provision of the physical matrix [23], which allows for Schwann cell infiltration and axonal extension through gels. Others have developed hydrogel scaffolds of higher mechanical integrity that are also promising for neural regeneration through the provision of physical guidance cues [8,152]. Glial and neuronal axon migration through hydrogels has also been enhanced through delivery of soluble growth factors such as NGF from fibrin [153] as well as through the presentation of laminin or laminin-based peptides that are matrix-immobilized [29,154]. Hydrogels have also been created to provide topographical cues in three dimensions alone or in combination with matrix-bound ligands [8,155], indicating the integration of chemical and mechanical properties in guiding neural regeneration.

These principles are also applicable to spinal cord injuries (SCIs). However, injectable gel systems are advantageous in the case of SCIs as complete transection of the spinal cord is rare and materials that can be injected in a less invasive fashion are desirable. Those hydrogels that can gel *in situ* may be particularly appealing as they are injectable yet provide additional mechanical integrity [90].

12.4.4 Liver

The mechanical properties of hydrogels could indicate that they would be best suited to the development of the visceral organs. Indeed, hydrogels are widely used both for fundamental studies at the cell level and in more translational applications toward the development of functional units. As indicated in the previous sections, hydrogels are used extensively as controlled release systems, often for the delivery of factors to promote angiogenesis. Due to diffusional limitations in large tissues, one approach has been the formation of smaller functional constructs. The simplest example of this is the microencapsulation approach described above.

More complex approaches are being developed toward the creation of functional tissues through provision of the correct structural properties of these tissues. In one example of this, hepatocytes encapsulated in thin collagen gel sheets have been shown to be vascularized and demonstrate functional markers [156]. In a more sophisticated approach, PEG hydrogels were functionalized to promote cell adhesion and processed into complex shapes reminiscent of native liver structure, demonstrating functionality [157]. In each case, the hydrogels serve the role of promoting cell engraftment through encapsulation and also likely provide for improved diffusional profiles to allow for bioreactor perfusion [157] and vascularization [156]. These approaches are certainly applicable to other visceral organs. Recently, multi-layered hydrogels have been developed from natural hydrogels such as alginate and hyaluronic acid [158] as well as synthetic materials [159]. Such multi-layer systems provide the opportunity to juxtapose cells in structural orientations that mimic native tissue.

The ideal approach to the generation of complex tissues such as the liver and other visceral organs certainly remains in doubt, but it is clear that hydrogel-based technologies such as these of creating small functional units as well as other encapsulation and printing technologies provide potential solutions alone or in combination with other approaches.

12.4.5 Reproductive Medicine

An area in which the mechanical properties of hydrogels has recently proven useful is in the tissue engineering of ovarian follicles. Females facing radiotherapy or chemotherapy are at increased risk of future infertility. The ability to grow and preserve immature ovarian follicles in culture has been suggested as an approach to minimize the risk of reintroducing cancer cells to patients as may occur with the use of ovarian tissue cryopreservation [160]. Alginate hydrogels have been used to provide three-dimensional context to immature ovarian follicles, allowing growth *in vitro* and also allowing for stable cryopreservation [161]. This approach has resulted in the live birth of fertilized embryos in a mouse model [160]. Early studies have utilized alginate due to its mechanical properties and compatibility with cell encapsulation as described above. Recently, alginate-fibrin hydrogels have shown increased numbers of meiotically competent oocytes [162], indicating that optimization of the hydrogel chemical and mechanical properties may lead to further improvements in this promising technique.

12.5 Prospects and Conclusions

Hydrogels are clearly an important component in the repertoire of biomaterial approaches to regenerative medicine with applications in nearly every organ system currently under exploration. The ability to modify hydrogels with bioactive molecules has proven fortuitous in the era of bioactive compound delivery as it allows for the integration of mechanical properties that mimic native tissue with bound and soluble chemical cues. In looking to the future of hydrogels in regenerative medicine applications, there are several opportunities for the development of these systems.

It should be clear from this chapter that there is a very large number of material parameters that can be altered for numerous applications. While many hydrogels allow a systematic evaluation of these parameters in isolation, the ability to compile a set of parameters that are optimal or near optimal for a particular application is not readily accomplished. The use of statistical analysis and parametric analysis, and the development of sophisticated engineering models in combination with some of the high-throughput screening methods described will be important in the design of regenerative medicine therapies involving hydrogels [163].

The use and characterization of hydrogels for the delivery of therapeutic agents that behave differently from traditionally delivered molecules is also of increasing importance. Examples include the use of hydrogels for the delivery of nucleic acids or gaseous materials. The advent of the gene-activated matrix (GAM) has spurred methods to achieve delivery of DNA, RNA, antisense, siRNA, or other nucleotides from hydrogels. Efficient delivery of these molecules to their cellular site of action has been of interest to the gene delivery community, and recent approaches to promoting viral [164] or non-viral [114] delivery of nucleic acids from hydrogel scaffolds [165] will likely take on increasing importance. The lack of oxygen and nutrient supply to tissue-engineered constructs is also well documented [166]. While delivery of factors promoting vascularization is widely studied, other alternatives such as the direct delivery of oxygen have been investigated more recently [167]. The role of hydrogels in regulating release of these types of molecules will also be an important consideration.

Another challenge in regard to hydrogels is obtaining the mechanical integrity necessary for tissue engineering applications. As described previously, one advantage of hydrogel systems is that they provide a matrix comparable in modulus to native extracellular matrix for many soft tissues. However, the mechanical integrity of many commonly used biodegradable hydrogels diminishes with time and the starting properties may be insufficient to withstand mechanically challenging bioreactor systems that are increasingly used for perfusion as well as mechanical and electrical stimulation. Increasing the polymer concentration within the gels provides additional mechanical support but reduces nutrient and oxygen diffusion, thereby inhibiting cell viability with the material. One approach to providing mechanical stability while promoting cell infiltration into hydrogels is through the use of templating approaches. These approaches include the use of micellar structures [168] and sacrificial polymer beads [169], or other geometries [8,170] that mimic native tissue architecture. This approach promotes cell infiltration or encapsulation throughout the scaffold and allows diffusion to occur in a fashion similar to macroporous hydrogels. This approach may provide the mechanical integrity necessary for bioreactors such as those used for ligament [171,172], tendon [173], and muscle [174]. To date, limited hydrogels have been used in these mechanically challenging systems [175,176]. However, modifications to natural polymers to allow bioreactor pre-conditional in conjunction with their advantageous cell adhesion and differentiation motifs may prove of great utility in regenerative medicine applications.

It is difficult to generalize the host response to hydrogels due to differences in the chemistry of the materials, leachates, processing techniques, and methods of sterilization. However, most experts would agree that the difference in the host response to hydrogels compared to traditional polymer systems was and remains a key point of interest for these materials. Monocyte and macrophage response to traditional polymers involves protein adsorption, monocyte/macrophage response, and (typically) fibrous encapsulation. This is generally considered an acceptable response for a material [177]. However, hydrogels may be well positioned to exploit the body's native machinery to achieve a more desirable host response to the material and cells or tissues associated with it. For example, it has been suggested that certain biological hydrogels and porous hydrogels may promote an alternative macrophage phenotype that is anti-inflammatory and may even lead to recruitment of progenitor cell populations that can transdifferentiate for the promotion of tissue remodeling within and around the hydrogel [178–180]. While further studies are needed to elucidate the mechanisms, the methods described in this chapter provide the tools to harness and manipulate these processes.

References

[1] Peppas NA. Hydrogels in medicine and pharmacy. Boca Raton, FL: CRC Press; 1986.

[2] Kopecek J. Hydrogel biomaterials: a smart future? Biomaterials 2007;28:5185–92.

[3] Wichterle O, Lim D. Hydrophilic gels for biological use. Nature 1960;185:117–8.

[4] Lim F, Sun AM. Microencapsulated islets as bioartificial endocrine pancreas. Science 1980;210:908–10.

[5] Mahoney MJ, Anseth KS. Three-dimensional growth and function of neural tissue in degradable polyethylene glycol hydrogels. Biomaterials 2006;27:2265–74.

[6] Bryant SJ, Anseth KS, Lee DA, Bader DL. Crosslinking density influences the morphology of chondrocytes photoencapsulated in PEG hydrogels during the application of compressive strain. J Orthop Res 2004;22:1143–9.

[7] Atzet S, Curtin S, Trinh P, Bryant S, Ratner B. Degradable poly(2-hydroxyethyl methacrylate)-co-polycaprolactone hydrogels for tissue engineering scaffolds. Biomacromolecules 2008;9:3370–7.

[8] Flynn L, Dalton PD, Shoichet MS. Fiber templating of poly(2-hydroxyethyl methacrylate) for neural tissue engineering. Biomaterials 2003;24:4265–72.

[9] Dalton PD, Flynn L, Shoichet MS. Manufacture of poly(2-hydroxyethyl methacrylate-co-methyl methacrylate) hydrogel tubes for use as nerve guidance channels. Biomaterials 2002;23:3843–51.

[10] Guo X, Park H, Young S, Kretlow JD, van den Beucken JJ, Baggett LS, et al. Repair of osteochondral defects with biodegradable hydrogel composites encapsulating marrow mesenchymal stem cells in a rabbit model. Acta Biomater 2010;6:39–47.

[11] Park H, Temenoff JS, Tabata Y, Caplan AI, Raphael RM, Jansen JA, et al. Effect of dual growth factor delivery on chondrogenic differentiation of rabbit marrow mesenchymal stem cells encapsulated in injectable hydrogel composites. J Biomed Mater Res A 2009;88:889–97.

[12] Hausner T, Schmidhammer R, Zandieh S, Hopf R, Schultz A, Gogolewski S, et al. Nerve regeneration using tubular scaffolds from biodegradable polyurethane. Acta Neurochir 2007;100(Suppl):69–72.

[13] Dadsetan M, Knight AM, Lu L, Windebank AJ, Yaszemski MJ. Stimulation of neurite outgrowth using positively charged hydrogels. Biomaterials 2009;30:3874–81.

[14] Lai JY, Chen KH, Hsiue GH. Tissue-engineered human corneal endothelial cell sheet transplantation in a rabbit model using functional biomaterials. Transplantation 2007;84:1222–32.

[15] Hesse E, Hefferan TE, Tarara JE, Haasper C, Meller R, Krettek C, et al. Collagen type I hydrogel allows migration, proliferation, and osteogenic differentiation of rat bone marrow stromal cells. J Biomed Mater Res A 2010;94:442–9.

[16] Abousleiman RI, Reyes Y, McFetridge P, Sikavitsas V. Tendon tissue engineering using cell-seeded umbilical veins cultured in a mechanical stimulator. Tissue Eng A 2008;15:787–95.

[17] Brennan M. Fibrin glue. Blood Rev 1991;5:240–4.

[18] Kalbermatten DF, Pettersson J, Kingham PJ, Pierer G, Wiberg M, Terenghi G. New fibrin conduit for peripheral nerve repair. J Reconstr Microsurg 2009;25:27–33.

[19] Lutolf MP, Lauer-Fields JL, Schmoekel HG, Metters AT, Weber FE, Fields GB, et al. Synthetic matrix metalloproteinase-sensitive hydrogels for the conduction of tissue regeneration: engineering cell-invasion characteristics. Proc Natl Acad Sci USA 2003;100: 5413–8.

[20] Arrighi I, Mark S, Alvisi M, von Rechenberg B, Hubbell JA, Schense JC. Bone healing induced by local delivery of an engineered parathyroid hormone prodrug. Biomaterials 2009;30:1763–71.

[21] Bian L, Fong JV, Lima EG, Stoker AM, Ateshian GA, Cook JL, et al. Dynamic mechanical loading enhances functional properties of tissue-engineered cartilage using mature canine chondrocytes. Tissue Eng A 2010;16:1781–90.

[22] Ho ST, Cool SM, Hui JH, Hutmacher DW. The influence of fibrin based hydrogels on the chondrogenic differentiation of human bone marrow stromal cells. Biomaterials 2010;31:38–47.

[23] Sierpinski P, Garrett J, Ma J, Apel P, Klorig D, Smith T, et al. The use of keratin biomaterials derived from human hair for the promotion of rapid regeneration of peripheral nerves. Biomaterials 2008;29:118–28.

[24] Aboushwareb T, Eberli D, Ward C, Broda C, Holcomb J, Atala A, et al. A keratin biomaterial gel hemostat derived from human hair: evaluation in a rabbit model of lethal liver injury. J Biomed Mater Res B Appl Biomater 2009;90:45–54.

[25] Aoki H, Tomita N, Morita Y, Hattori K, Harada Y, Sonobe M, Wakitani S, et al. Culture of chondrocytes in fibroin-hydrogel sponge. Biomed Mater Eng 2003;13:309–16.

[26] Fini M, Motta A, Torricelli P, Giavaresi G, Nicoli Aldini N, Tschon M, et al. The healing of confined critical size cancellous defects in the presence of silk fibroin hydrogel. Biomaterials 2005;26:3527–36.

[27] Mauck RL, Soltz MA, Wang CC, Wong DD, Chao PH, Valhmu WB, et al. Functional tissue engineering of articular cartilage through dynamic loading of chondrocyte-seeded agarose gels. J Biomech Eng 2000;122:252–60.

[28] Ng KW, Wang CC, Mauck RL, Kelly TA, Chahine NO, Costa KD, et al. A layered agarose approach to fabricate depth-dependent inhomogeneity in chondrocyte-seeded constructs. J Orthop Res 2005;23:134–41.

[29] Dodla MC, Bellamkonda RV. Anisotropic scaffolds facilitate enhanced neurite extension *in vitro*. J Biomed Mater Res A 2006;78:213–21.

[30] Stokols S, Tuszynski MH. Freeze-dried agarose scaffolds with uniaxial channels stimulate and guide linear axonal growth following spinal cord injury. Biomaterials 2006;27:443–51.

[31] Alsberg E, Kong HJ, Hirano Y, Smith MK, Albeiruti A, Mooney DJ. Regulating bone formation via controlled scaffold degradation. J Dent Res 2003;82:903–8.

[32] Jin SY, Lei L, Shikanov A, Shea LD, Woodruff TK. A novel two-step strategy for *in vitro* culture of early-stage ovarian follicles in the mouse. Fertil Steril 2010;93:2633–9.

[33] Freier T, Montenegro R, Shan Koh H, Shoichet MS. Chitin-based tubes for tissue engineering in the nervous system. Biomaterials 2005;26:4624–32.

[34] Hoemann CD, Sun J, Legare A, McKee MD, Buschmann MD. Tissue engineering of cartilage using an injectable and adhesive chitosan-based cell-delivery vehicle. Osteoarthritis Cartilage 2005;13:318–29.

[35] Neuffer MC, McDivitt J, Rose D, King K, Cloonan CC, Vayer JS. Hemostatic dressings for the first responder: a review. Mil Med 2004;169:716–20.

[36] Wedmore I, McManus JG, Pusateri AE, Holcomb JB. A special report on the chitosan-based hemostatic dressing: experience in current combat operations. J Trauma 2006;60:655–8.

[37] Grigolo B, Roseti L, Fiorini M, Fini M, Giavaresi G, Aldini NN, et al. Transplantation of chondrocytes seeded on a hyaluronan derivative (hyaff-11) into cartilage defects in rabbits. Biomaterials 2001;22:2417–24.

[38] Farran AJ, Teller SS, Jha AK, Jiao T, Hule RA, Clifton RJ, et al. Effects of matrix composition, microstructure, and viscoelasticity on the behaviors of vocal fold fibroblasts cultured in three-dimensional hydrogel networks. Tissue Eng A 2010;16:1247–61.

[39] Kim J, Kim IS, Cho TH, Lee KB, Hwang SJ, Tae G, et al. Bone regeneration using hyaluronic acid-based hydrogel with bone morphogenic protein-2 and human mesenchymal stem cells. Biomaterials 2007;28:1830–7.

[40] Ghosh K, Ren XD, Shu XZ, Prestwich GD, Clark RA. Fibronectin functional domains coupled to hyaluronan stimulate adult human dermal fibroblast responses critical for wound healing. Tissue Eng 2006;12:601–13.

[41] Stabenfeldt SE, Garcia AJ, LaPlaca MC. Thermoreversible laminin-functionalized hydrogel for neural tissue engineering. J Biomed Mater Res A 2006;77:718–25.

[42] Reza AT, Nicoll SB. Characterization of novel photocrosslinked carboxymethylcellulose hydrogels for encapsulation of nucleus pulposus cells. Acta Biomater 2010;6:179–86.

[43] Esguerra M, Fink H, Laschke MW, Jeppsson A, Delbro D, Gatenholm P, et al. Intravital fluorescent microscopic evaluation of bacterial cellulose as scaffold for vascular grafts. J Biomed Mater Res A 2010;93:140–9.

[44] Grande CJ, Torres FG, Gomez CM, Bano MC. Nanocomposites of bacterial cellulose/hydroxyapatite for biomedical applications. Acta Biomater 2009;5:1605–15.

[45] Peppas NA. Hydrogels. In: Ratner BD, Hoffman AS, Schoen FJ, Lemons JE, editors. Biomaterials science: an introduction to materials in medicine. San Diego, CA: Elsevier Academic Press; 2004. p. 100–6.

[46] Hoffman AS. Hydrogels for biomedical applications. Adv Drug Deliv Rev 2002;54:3–12.

[47] Lowman AM, Peppas NA. Hydrogels. In: Mathiowitz E, editor. Encyclopedia of controlled drug delivery. New York: Wiley; 1999. p. 397–418.

[48] Peppas NA, Barr-Howell BD. Characterization of the crosslinked structure of hydrogels. In: Peppas NA, editor. Hydrogels in medicine and pharmacy. Boca Raton, FL: CRC Press; 1986. p. 27–56.

[49] Cavanagh HD, Bodner BI, Wilson LA. Extended wear hydrogel lenses. Long-term effectiveness and costs. Ophthalmology 1980;87:871–6.

[50] Dreifus M, Wichterle O. Clinical experiences with hydrogel contact lenses. Cesk Oftalmol 1964;20:393–9.

[51] Sendele DD, Abelson MB, Kenyon KR, Hanninen LA. Intracorneal lens implantation. Arch Ophthalmol 1983;101:940–4.

[52] DeLong SA, Moon JJ, West JL. Covalently immobilized gradients of bFGF on hydrogel scaffolds for directed cell migration. Biomaterials 2005;26:3227–34.

[53] Horbett TA. Protein adsorption to hydrogels. In: Peppas NA, editor. Hydrogels in medicine and pharmacy. Boca Raton, FL: CRC Press; 1986. p. 127–71.

[54] Bader RA, Rochefort WE. Rheological characterization of photopolymerized poly(vinyl alcohol) hydrogels for potential use in nucleus pulposus replacement. J Biomed Mater Res A 2008;86:494–501.

[55] Bae KH, Yoon JJ, Park TG. Fabrication of hyaluronic acid hydrogel beads for cell encapsulation. Biotechnol Prog 2006;22:297–302.

[56] Ayhan F, Ozkan S. Gentamicin release from photopolymerized PEG diacrylate and pHEMA hydrogel discs and their *in vitro* antimicrobial activities. Drug Deliv 2007;14:433–9.

[57] Faxalv L, Ekblad T, Liedberg B, Lindahl TL. Blood compatibility of photografted hydrogel coatings. Acta Biomater 2010;6:2599–608.

[58] Bayramoglu G, Kayaman-Apohan N, Akcakaya H, Vezir Kahraman M, Erdem Kuruca S, Gungor A. Preparation of collagen modified photopolymers: a new type of biodegradable gel for cell growth. J Mater Sci Mater Med 2010;21:761–75.

[59] Mann BK, West JL. Cell adhesion peptides alter smooth muscle cell adhesion, proliferation, migration, and matrix protein synthesis on modified surfaces and in polymer scaffolds. J Biomed Mater Res 2002;60:86–93.

[60] Nguyen KT, West JL. Photopolymerizable hydrogels for tissue engineering applications. Biomaterials 2002;23:4307–14.

[61] Malkoch M, Vestberg R, Gupta N, Mespouille L, Dubois P, Mason AF, et al. Synthesis of well-defined hydrogel networks using click chemistry. Chem Commun (Camb.) 2006;2774–6.

[62] Crescenzi V, Cornelio L, di Meo C, Nardecchia S, Lamanna R. Novel hydrogels via click chemistry: synthesis and potential biomedical applications. Biomacromolecules 2007;8:1844–50.

[63] Testa G, di Meo C, Nardecchia S, Capitani D, Mannina L, Lamanna R, et al. Influence of dialkyne structure on the properties of new click-gels based on hyaluronic acid. Int J Pharm 2009;378:86–92.

[64] Cohen DL, Malone E, Lipson H, Bonassar LJ. Direct freeform fabrication of seeded hydrogels in arbitrary geometries. Tissue Eng 2006;12:1325—35.

[65] Fedorovich NE, de Wijn JR, Verbout AJ, Alblas J, Dhert WJ. Three-dimensional fiber deposition of cell-laden, viable, patterned constructs for bone tissue printing. Tissue Eng A 2008;14:127—33.

[66] Ji Y, Ghosh K, Li B, Sokolov JC, Clark RA, Rafailovich MH. Dual-syringe reactive electrospinning of crosslinked hyaluronic acid hydrogel nanofibers for tissue engineering applications. Macromol Biosci 2006;6:811—7.

[67] Moutos FT, Freed LE, Guilak F. A biomimetic three-dimensional woven composite scaffold for functional tissue engineering of cartilage. Nat Mater 2007;6:162—7.

[68] Hahn MS, Taite LJ, Moon JJ, Rowland MC, Ruffino KA, West JL. Photolithographic patterning of polyethylene glycol hydrogels. Biomaterials 2006;27:2519—24.

[69] Bryant SJ, Cuy JL, Hauch KD, Ratner BD. Photo-patterning of porous hydrogels for tissue engineering. Biomaterials 2007;28:2978—86.

[70] Kim DH, Kim P, Song I, Cha JM, Lee SH, Kim B, et al. Guided three-dimensional growth of functional cardiomyocytes on polyethylene glycol nanostructures. Langmuir 2006;22:5419—26.

[71] Gu Z, Tang Y. Enzyme-assisted photolithography for spatial functionalization of hydrogels. Lab Chip 2010;10:1946—51.

[72] Sakiyama-Elbert SE, Hubbell JA. Development of fibrin derivatives for controlled release of heparin-binding growth factors. J Control Rel 2000;65:389—402.

[73] Langer R. New methods of drug delivery. Science 1990;249:1527—33.

[74] Ehrbar M, Djonov VG, Schnell C, Tschanz SA, Martiny-Baron G, Schenk U, et al. Cell-demanded liberation of VEGF121 from fibrin implants induces local and controlled blood vessel growth. Circ Res 2004;94:1124—32.

[75] Nishida K, Yamato M, Hayashida Y, Watanabe K, Maeda N, Watanabe H, et al. Functional bioengineered corneal epithelial sheet grafts from corneal stem cells expanded ex vivo on a temperature-responsive cell culture surface. Transplantation 2004;77:379—85.

[76] Nishida K, Yamato M, Hayashida Y, Watanabe K, Yamamoto K, Adachi E, et al. Corneal reconstruction with tissue-engineered cell sheets composed of autologous oral mucosal epithelium. N Engl J Med 2004;351:1187—96.

[77] Hsiue GH, Lai JY, Chen KH, Hsu WM. A novel strategy for corneal endothelial reconstruction with a bioengineered cell sheet. Transplantation 2006;81:473—6.

[78] Shimizu T, Yamato M, Kikuchi A, Okano T. Two-dimensional manipulation of cardiac myocyte sheets utilizing temperature-responsive culture dishes augments the pulsatile amplitude. Tissue Eng 2001;7:141—51.

[79] Shimizu T, Yamato M, Akutsu T, Shibata T, Isoi Y, Kikuchi A, et al. Electrically communicating three-dimensional cardiac tissue mimic fabricated by layered cultured cardiomyocyte sheets. J Biomed Mater Res 2002;60:110—7.

[80] Shimizu T, Yamato M, Isoi Y, Akutsu T, Setomaru T, Abe K, et al. Fabrication of pulsatile cardiac tissue grafts using a novel 3-dimensional cell sheet manipulation technique and temperature-responsive cell culture surfaces. Circ Res 2002;90:e40.

[81] Shiroyanagi Y, Yamato M, Yamazaki Y, Toma H, Okano T. Transplantable urothelial cell sheets harvested noninvasively from temperature-responsive culture surfaces by reducing temperature. Tissue Eng 2003;9:1005—12.

[82] Shiroyanagi Y, Yamato M, Yamazaki Y, Toma H, Okano T. Urothelium regeneration using viable cultured urothelial cell sheets grafted on demucosalized gastric flaps. BJU Int 2004;93:1069—75.

[83] Yamato M, Utsumi M, Kushida A, Konno C, Kikuchi A, Okano T. Thermo-responsive culture dishes allow the intact harvest of multilayered keratinocyte sheets without dispase by reducing temperature. Tissue Eng 2001;7:473—80.

[84] Kwok CS, Mourad PD, Crum LA, Ratner BD. Self-assembled molecular structures as ultrasonically responsive barrier membranes for pulsatile drug delivery. J Biomed Mater Res 2001;57:151—64.

[85] Murdan S. Electro-responsive drug delivery from hydrogels. J Control Rel 2003;92:1—17.

[86] Lim F, Moss RD. Microencapsulation of living cells and tissues. J Pharm Sci 1981;70:351−4.

[87] Orive G, Tam SK, Pedraz JL, Halle JP. Biocompatibility of alginate-poly-l-lysine microcapsules for cell therapy. Biomaterials 2006;27:3691−700.

[88] Jeong B, Kim SW, Bae YH. Thermosensitive sol−gel reversible hydrogels. Adv Drug Deliv Rev 2002;54:37−51.

[89] Chen F, Mao T, Tao K, Chen S, Ding G, Gu X. Injectable bone. Br J Oral Maxillofac Surg 2003;41:240−3.

[90] Jain A, Kim YT, McKeon RJ, Bellamkonda RV. In situ gelling hydrogels for conformal repair of spinal cord defects, and local delivery of BDNF after spinal cord injury. Biomaterials 2006;27:497−504.

[91] Sawhney AS, Pathak CP, Hubbell JA. Interfacial photopolymerization of poly(ethylene glycol)-based hydrogels upon alginate-poly(l-lysine) microcapsules for enhanced biocompatibility. Biomaterials 1993;14:1008−16.

[92] Bryant SJ, Anseth KS. Photopolymerization of hydrogel scaffolds. In: Elisseeff J, Ma PX, editors. Scaffolding in tissue engineering. Boca Raton, FL: CRC Press; 2006. p. 71−90.

[93] Fedorovich NE, Oudshoorn MH, van Geemen D, Hennink WE, Alblas J, Dhert WJ. The effect of photopolymerization on stem cells embedded in hydrogels. Biomaterials 2009;30:344−53.

[94] Elisseeff J, McIntosh W, Anseth K, Riley S, Ragan P, Langer R. Photoencapsulation of chondrocytes in poly(ethylene oxide)-based semi-interpenetrating networks. J Biomed Mater Res 2000;51:164−71.

[95] Williams CG, Kim TK, Taboas A, Malik A, Manson P, Elisseeff J. In vitro chondrogenesis of bone marrow-derived mesenchymal stem cells in a photopolymerizing hydrogel. Tissue Eng 2003;9:679−88.

[96] Roth EA, Xu T, Das M, Gregory C, Hickman JJ, Boland T. Inkjet printing for high-throughput cell patterning. Biomaterials 2004;25:3707−15.

[97] Xu T, Jin J, Gregory C, Hickman JJ, Boland T. Inkjet printing of viable mammalian cells. Biomaterials 2005;26:93−9.

[98] Lemmo AV, Rose DJ, Tisone TC. Inkjet dispensing technology: applications in drug discovery. Curr Opin Biotechnol 1998;9:615−7.

[99] Goldmann T, Gonzalez JS. DNA-printing: utilization of a standard inkjet printer for the transfer of nucleic acids to solid supports. J Biochem Biophys Methods 2000;42:105−10.

[100] Campbell PG, Miller ED, Fisher GW, Walker LM, Weiss LE. Engineered spatial patterns of FGF-2 immobilized on fibrin direct cell organization. Biomaterials 2005;26:6762−70.

[101] Cui X, Boland T. Human microvasculature fabrication using thermal inkjet printing technology. Biomaterials 2009;30:6221−7.

[102] Zhang C, Wen X, Vyavahare NR, Boland T. Synthesis and characterization of biodegradable elastomeric polyurethane scaffolds fabricated by the inkjet technique. Biomaterials 2008;29:3781−91.

[103] Ilkhanizadeh S, Teixeira AI, Hermanson O. Inkjet printing of macromolecules on hydrogels to steer neural stem cell differentiation. Biomaterials 2007;28:3936−43.

[104] Nishiyama Y, Nakamura M, Henmi C, Yamaguchi K, Mochizuki S, Nakagawa H, et al. Development of a three-dimensional bioprinter: construction of cell supporting structures using hydrogel and state-of-the-art inkjet technology. J Biomech Eng 2009;131:035001-1−035001-6.

[105] Cai K, Dong H, Chen C, Yang L, Jandt KD, Deng L. Inkjet printing of laminin gradient to investigate endothelial cellular alignment. Colloids Surf B Biointerfaces 2009;72:230−5.

[106] Miller ED, Phillippi JA, Fisher GW, Campbell PG, Walker LM, Weiss LE. Inkjet printing of growth factor concentration gradients and combinatorial arrays immobilized on biologically relevant substrates. Comb Chem High Throughput Screen 2009;12:604−18.

[107] Xu T, Gregory CA, Molnar P, Cui X, Jalota S, Bhaduri SB, et al. Viability and electrophysiology of neural cell structures generated by the inkjet printing method. Biomaterials 2006;27:3580−8.

[108] Lin RZ, Ho CT, Liu CH, Chang HY. Dielectrophoresis based-cell patterning for tissue engineering. Biotechnol J 2006;1:949−57.

[109] Albrecht DR, Underhill GH, Mendelson A, Bhatia SN. Multiphase electropatterning of cells and biomaterials. Lab Chip 2007;7:702−9.

[110] Baird IS, Yau AY, Mann BK. Mammalian cell-seeded hydrogel microarrays printed via dip-pin technology. Biotechniques 2008;44:249–56.

[111] Hern DL, Hubbell JA. Incorporation of adhesion peptides into nonadhesive hydrogels useful for tissue resurfacing. J Biomed Mater Res 1998;39:266–76.

[112] Leslie-Barbick JE, Moon JJ, West JL. Covalently-immobilized vascular endothelial growth factor promotes endothelial cell tubulogenesis in poly(ethylene glycol) diacrylate hydrogels. J Biomater Sci Polym 2009;20:1763–79.

[113] Lee HJ, Lee JS, Chansakul T, Yu C, Elisseeff JH, Yu SM. Collagen mimetic peptide-conjugated photopolymerizable PEG hydrogel. Biomaterials 2006;27:5268–76.

[114] Segura T, Chung PH, Shea LD. DNA delivery from hyaluronic acid-collagen hydrogels via a substrate-mediated approach. Biomaterials 2005;26:1575–84.

[115] Saul JM, Linnes MP, Ratner BD, Giachelli CM, Pun SH. Delivery of non-viral gene carriers from sphere-templated fibrin scaffolds for sustained transgene expression. Biomaterials 2007;28:4705–16.

[116] Shin H, Zygourakis K, Farach-Carson MC, Yaszemski MJ, Mikos AG. Attachment, proliferation, and migration of marrow stromal osteoblasts cultured on biomimetic hydrogels modified with an osteopontin-derived peptide. Biomaterials 2004;25:895–906.

[117] Mann BK, Gobin AS, Tsai AT, Schmedlen RH, West JL. Smooth muscle cell growth in photopolymerized hydrogels with cell adhesive and proteolytically degradable domains: synthetic ECM analogs for tissue engineering. Biomaterials 2001;22:3045–51.

[118] Halberstadt C, Austin C, Rowley J, Culberson C, Loebsack A, Wyatt S, et al. A hydrogel material for plastic and reconstructive applications injected into the subcutaneous space of a sheep. Tissue Eng 2002;8:309–19.

[119] Behravesh E, Zygourakis K, Mikos AG. Adhesion and migration of marrow-derived osteoblasts on injectable in situ crosslinkable poly(propylene fumarate-co-ethylene glycol)-based hydrogels with a covalently linked RGDS peptide. J Biomed Mater Res A 2003;65:260–70.

[120] DeLong SA, Gobin AS, West JL. Covalent immobilization of RGDS on hydrogel surfaces to direct cell alignment and migration. J Control Release 2005;109:139–48.

[121] Luo Y, Shoichet MS. Light-activated immobilization of biomolecules to agarose hydrogels for controlled cellular response. Biomacromolecules 2004;5:2315–23.

[122] Moon JJ, Hahn MS, Kim I, Nsiah BA, West JL. Micropatterning of poly(ethylene glycol) diacrylate hydrogels with biomolecules to regulate and guide endothelial morphogenesis. Tissue Eng A 2009;15:579–85.

[123] La Gatta A, Schiraldi C, Esposito A, d'Agostino A, de Rosa A. Novel poly(HEMA-co-METAC)/alginate semi-interpenetrating hydrogels for biomedical applications: synthesis and characterization. J Biomed Mater Res A 2009;90:292–302.

[124] Hubbell JA, Massia SP, Desai NP, Drumheller PD. Endothelial cell-selective materials for tissue engineering in the vascular graft via a new receptor. Biotechnology (NY) 1991;9:568–72.

[125] Metters AT, Anseth KS, Bowman CN. Fundamental studies of a novel, biodegradable PEG-b-PLA hydrogel. Polymer 2000;41:3993–4004.

[126] Bryant SJ, Anseth KS. Hydrogel properties influence ECM production by chondrocytes photoencapsulated in poly(ethylene glycol) hydrogels. J Biomed Mater Res 2002;59:63–72.

[127] Kuo CK, Ma PX. Maintaining dimensions and mechanical properties of ionically crosslinked alginate hydrogel scaffolds in vitro. J Biomed Mater Res A 2008;84:899–907.

[128] Villanueva I, Klement BJ, von Deutsch D, Bryant SJ. Cross-linking density alters early metabolic activities in chondrocytes encapsulated in poly(ethylene glycol) hydrogels and cultured in the rotating wall vessel. Biotechnol Bioeng 2009;102:1242–50.

[129] Temenoff JS, Athanasiou KA, LeBaron RG, Mikos AG. Effect of poly(ethylene glycol) molecular weight on tensile and swelling properties of oligo(poly(ethylene glycol) fumarate) hydrogels for cartilage tissue engineering. J Biomed Mater Res 2002;59:429–37.

[130] Beebe DJ, Moore JS, Bauer JM, Yu Q, Liu RH, Devadoss C, et al. Functional hydrogel

structures for autonomous flow control inside microfluidic channels. Nature 2000;404:588–90.

[131] Yew YK, Ng TY, Li H, Lam KY. Analysis of pH and electrically controlled swelling of hydrogel-based micro-sensors/actuators. Biomed Microdev 2007;9:487–99.

[132] Shang J, Shao Z, Chen X. Electrical behavior of a natural polyelectrolyte hydrogel: chitosan/carboxymethylcellulose hydrogel. Biomacromolecules 2008;9:1208–13.

[133] Kraehenbuehl TP, Zammaretti P, van der Vlies AJ, Schoenmakers RG, Lutolf MP, Jaconi ME, et al. Three-dimensional extracellular matrix-directed cardioprogenitor differentiation: systematic modulation of a synthetic cell-responsive PEG-hydrogel. Biomaterials 2008;29:2757–66.

[134] Banerjee A, Arha M, Choudhary S, Ashton RS, Bhatia SR, Schaffer DV, et al. The influence of hydrogel modulus on the proliferation and differentiation of encapsulated neural stem cells. Biomaterials 2009;30:4695–9.

[135] Dadsetan M, Hefferan TE, Szatkowski JP, Mishra PK, Macura SI, Lu L, et al. Effect of hydrogel porosity on marrow stromal cell phenotypic expression. Biomaterials 2008;29:2193–202.

[136] Keskar V, Marion NW, Mao JJ, Gemeinhart RA. *In vitro* evaluation of macroporous hydrogels to facilitate stem cell infiltration, growth, and mineralization. Tissue Eng A 2009;15:1695–707.

[137] Thorn RM, Greenman J, Austin A. An *in vitro* study of antimicrobial activity and efficacy of iodine-generating hydrogel dressings. J Wound Care 2006;15:305–10.

[138] Queen D, Coutts P, Fierheller M, Sibbald RG. The use of a novel oxygenating hydrogel dressing in the treatment of different chronic wounds. Adv Skin Wound Care 2007;20:200–6.

[139] Boucard N, Viton C, Agay D, Mari E, Roger T, Chancerelle Y, et al. The use of physical hydrogels of chitosan for skin regeneration following third-degree burns. Biomaterials 2007;28:3478–88.

[140] Corkhill PH, Trevett AS, Tighe BJ. The potential of hydrogels as synthetic articular cartilage. Proc Inst Mech Eng H 1990;204:147–55.

[141] Oka M, Noguchi T, Kumar P, Ikeuchi K, Yamamuro T, Hyon SH, et al. Development of an artificial articular cartilage. Clin Mater 1990;6:361–81.

[142] Noguchi T, Yamamuro T, Oka M, Kumar P, Kotoura Y, Hyon S, et al. Poly(vinyl alcohol) hydrogel as an artificial articular cartilage: evaluation of biocompatibility. J Appl Biomater 1991;2:101–7.

[143] Elisseeff JH, Lee A, Kleinman HK, Yamada Y. Biological response of chondrocytes to hydrogels. Ann NY Acad Sci 2002;961:118–22.

[144] Park H, Temenoff JS, Holland TA, Tabata Y, Mikos AG. Delivery of TGF-beta1 and chondrocytes via injectable, biodegradable hydrogels for cartilage tissue engineering applications. Biomaterials 2005;26:7095–103.

[145] Lind M, Larsen A, Clausen C, Osther K, Everland H. Cartilage repair with chondrocytes in fibrin hydrogel and MPEG polylactide scaffold: an in vivo study in goats. Knee Surg Sports Traumatol Arthrosc 2008;16:690–8.

[146] Wang DA, Varghese S, Sharma B, Strehin I, Fermanian S, Gorham J, et al. Multifunctional chondroitin sulphate for cartilage tissue-biomaterial integration. Nat Mater 2007;6:385–92.

[147] Bergman K, Engstrand T, Hilborn J, Ossipov D, Piskounova S, Bowden T. Injectable cell-free template for bone-tissue formation. J Biomed Mater Res A 2009;91:1111–8.

[148] Yamamoto M, Takahashi Y, Tabata Y. Enhanced bone regeneration at a segmental bone defect by controlled release of bone morphogenetic protein-2 from a biodegradable hydrogel. Tissue Eng 2006;12:1305–11.

[149] Takahashi Y, Yamamoto M, Yamada K, Kawakami O, Tabata Y. Skull bone regeneration in nonhuman primates by controlled release of bone morphogenetic protein-2 from a biodegradable hydrogel. Tissue Eng 2007;13:293–300.

[150] Dillon GP, Yu X, Sridharan A, Ranieri JP, Bellamkonda RV. The influence of physical structure and charge on neurite extension in a 3D hydrogel scaffold. J Biomater Sci Polym 1998;9:1049–69.

[151] Balgude AP, Yu X, Szymanski A, Bellamkonda RV. Agarose gel stiffness determines rate of DRG neurite extension in 3D cultures. Biomaterials 2001;22:1077−84.

[152] Bozkurt A, Brook GA, Moellers S, Lassner F, Sellhaus B, Weis J, et al. *In vitro* assessment of axonal growth using dorsal root ganglia explants in a novel three-dimensional collagen matrix. Tissue Eng 2007;13:2971−9.

[153] Wood MD, Sakiyama-Elbert SE. Release rate controls biological activity of nerve growth factor released from fibrin matrices containing affinity-based delivery systems. J Biomed Mater Res A 2008;84:300−12.

[154] Yu X, Dillon GP, Bellamkonda RB. A laminin and nerve growth factor-laden three-dimensional scaffold for enhanced neurite extension. Tissue Eng 1999;5:291−304.

[155] Yu TT, Shoichet MS. Guided cell adhesion and outgrowth in peptide-modified channels for neural tissue engineering. Biomaterials 2005;26:1507−14.

[156] Zhao Y, Xu Y, Zhang B, Wu X, Xu F, Liang W, et al. In vivo generation of thick, vascularized hepatic tissue from collagen hydrogel-based hepatic units. Tissue Eng C Methods 2009;16:653−9.

[157] Liu Tsang V, Chen AA, Cho LM, Jadin KD, Sah RL, DeLong S, et al. Fabrication of 3D hepatic tissues by additive photopatterning of cellular hydrogels. Faseb J 2007;21:790−801.

[158] Ladet S, David L, Domard A. Multi-membrane hydrogels. Nature 2008;452:76−9.

[159] Kizilel S, Sawardecker E, Teymour F, Perez-Luna VH. Sequential formation of covalently bonded hydrogel multilayers through surface initiated photopolymerization. Biomaterials 2006;27:1209−15.

[160] Xu M, Kreeger PK, Shea LD, Woodruff TK. Tissue-engineered follicles produce live, fertile offspring. Tissue Eng 2006;12:2739−46.

[161] Amorim CA, van Langendonckt A, David A, Dolmans MM, Donnez J. Survival of human pre-antral follicles after cryopreservation of ovarian tissue, follicular isolation and *in vitro* culture in a calcium alginate matrix. Hum Reprod 2009;24:92−9.

[162] Shikanov A, Xu M, Woodruff TK, Shea LD. Interpenetrating fibrin-alginate matrices for *in vitro* ovarian follicle development. Biomaterials 2009;30:5476−85.

[163] Comisar WA, Kazmers NH, Mooney DJ, Linderman JJ. Engineering RGD nanopatterned hydrogels to control preosteoblast behavior: a combined computational and experimental approach. Biomaterials 2007;28:4409−17.

[164] Schek RM, Hollister SJ, Krebsbach PH. Delivery and protection of adenoviruses using biocompatible hydrogels for localized gene therapy. Mol Ther 2004;9:130−8.

[165] Kasper FK, Jerkins E, Tanahashi K, Barry MA, Tabata Y, Mikos AG. Characterization of DNA release from composites of oligo (poly(ethylene glycol) fumarate) and cationized gelatin microspheres *in vitro*. J Biomed Mater Res A 2006;78:823−35.

[166] Johnson PC, Mikos AG, Fisher JP, Jansen JA. Strategic directions in tissue engineering. Tissue Eng 2007;13:2827−37.

[167] Oh SH, Ward CL, Atala A, Yoo JJ, Harrison BS. Oxygen generating scaffolds for enhancing engineered tissue survival. Biomaterials 2009;30:757−62.

[168] Texter J. Templating hydrogels. Colloid Polym Sci 2009;287:313−21.

[169] Linnes MP, Ratner BD, Giachelli CM. A fibrinogen-based precision microporous scaffold for tissue engineering. Biomaterials 2007;28:5298−306.

[170] Lam MT, Huang YC, Birla RK, Takayama S. Microfeature guided skeletal muscle tissue engineering for highly organized 3-dimensional free-standing constructs. Biomaterials 2009;30:1150−5.

[171] Noth U, Schupp K, Heymer A, Kall S, Jakob F, Schutze N, et al. Anterior cruciate ligament constructs fabricated from human mesenchymal stem cells in a collagen type I hydrogel. Cytotherapy 2005;7:447−55.

[172] Kahn CJ, Vaquette C, Rahouadj R, Wang X. A novel bioreactor for ligament tissue engineering. Biomed Mater Eng 2008;18:283−7.

[173] Saber S, Zhang AY, Ki SH, Lindsey DP, Smith RL, Riboh J, et al. Flexor tendon tissue engineering: bioreactor cyclic strain increases construct strength. Tissue Eng A 2010;16:2085−90.

[174] Moon du G, Christ G, Stitzel JD, Atala A, Yoo JJ. Cyclic mechanical preconditioning improves engineered muscle contraction. Tissue Eng A 2008;14:473−82.

[175] Pfister BJ, Iwata A, Taylor AG, Wolf JA, Meaney DF, Smith DH. Development of transplantable nervous tissue constructs comprised of stretch-grown axons. J Neurosci Methods 2006;153:95–103.

[176] Nicodemus GD, Bryant SJ. The role of hydrogel structure and dynamic loading on chondrocyte gene expression and matrix formation. J Biomech 2008;41:1528–36.

[177] Williams DF. Definitions in biomaterials: proceedings of a consensus conference of the European society for biomaterials. In: Williams DF, editor. European Society for Biomaterials. Chester: Elsevier; 1987. p. 67.

[178] Lee SJ, van Dyke M, Atala A, Yoo JJ. Host cell mobilization for *in situ* tissue regeneration. Rejuvenation Res 2008;11:747–56.

[179] Piterina AV, Cloonan AJ, Meaney CL, Davis LM, Callanan A, Walsh MT, et al. ECM-based materials in cardiovascular applications: inherent healing potential and augmentation of native regenerative processes. Int J Mol Sci 2009;10:4375–417.

[180] Ratner BD, Atzet S. Hydrogels for healing. In: Barbucci R, editor. Hydrogels: biological properties and applications. Milan: Springer; 2009. p. 43–51.

13 Biodegradable Polymers

Zheng Zhang, Ophir Ortiz, Ritu Goyal and Joachim Kohn

OUTLINE

13.1 Introduction 303
13.2 Biodegradable Polymer Selection Criteria 304
13.3 Biologically Derived Polymers 305
   13.3.1 Peptides and Proteins 305
      13.3.1.1 Collagen 305
      13.3.1.2 Gelatin 307
      13.3.1.3 Elastin 308
      13.3.1.4 Keratin 308
      13.3.1.5 Silk 309
      13.3.1.6 Proteoglycans 309
   13.3.2 Biomimetic Materials 310
   13.3.3 Polysaccharides 310
      13.3.3.1 Cellulose 311
      13.3.3.2 Starch 311
      13.3.3.3 Alginate 312
      13.3.3.4 Gellan Gum 312
      13.3.3.5 Glycosaminoglycans 312
      13.3.3.6 Chitosan 313
   13.3.4 Polyhydroxyalkanoates 313
   13.3.5 Polynucleotides 314
13.4 Synthetic Polymers 314
   13.4.1 Aliphatic Polyesters 315
      13.4.1.1 Poly(glycolic Acid), Poly(lactic Acid), and their Copolymers 315
      13.4.1.2 Poly(ε-caprolactone) 318
      13.4.1.3 Poly(p-dioxanone) 318
      13.4.1.4 Poly(ortho Esters) 319
   13.4.2 Biodegradable Polyurethanes 319
   13.4.3 Polyanhydrides (Structure 13.9) 320
   13.4.4 Polyphosphazenes (Structure 13.10) 321
   13.4.5 Poly(amino Acids) and "Pseudo"-poly (amino Acids) 321
13.5 Combinations (Hybrids) of Synthetic and Biologically Derived Polymers 323
13.6 Using Polymers to Create Tissue-Engineered Products 323
   13.6.1 Barriers: Membranes and Tubes 324
   13.6.2 Gels 325
   13.6.3 Matrices 325
13.7 Conclusion 325
References 325

13.1 Introduction

The design and development of tissue-engineered products has benefited from many years of clinical utilization of a wide range of biodegradable polymers. Newly developed biodegradable polymers and modifications of previously developed biodegradable polymers have enhanced the tools available for creating clinically important tissue-engineering applications. Insights gained from studies of cell-matrix interactions, cell-cell signaling, and organization of cellular components, are placing increased demands on medical implants to interact with the patient's tissue in a more biologically appropriate fashion. While in the twentieth century, biocompatibility was largely equated with eliciting no harmful response, the biomaterials of the twenty first century will have to elicit tissue responses that support healing or regeneration of the patient's own tissue.

This chapter surveys the universe of those biodegradable polymers that may be useful in the development of medical implants and tissue-engineered products. Here we distinguish between biologically derived polymers and synthetic polymers. The materials are described in terms of their chemical composition, breakdown products, mechanism of breakdown, mechanical properties, and clinical limitations. Also discussed are product design considerations in processing of biomaterials into a final form (e.g., gel, membrane, matrix) that will effect the desired tissue response.

In this chapter, we follow the official polymer nomenclature conventions adopted by the International Union of Pure and Applied Chemistry (IUPAC). According to these rules, the correct naming of a polymer requires the simple addition of the prefix "poly" in front of the monomer name, *if the monomer name consists of a single word*. For example, the polymer made of ethylene is simply polyethylene. There is no space between poly and ethylene. When the monomer name consists of two or more words, it is important that the entire monomer name be enclosed in parentheses. This is needed to avoid ambiguity. For example, the polymer made of lactic acid is correctly named as poly (lactic acid). Note the absence of a space between the prefix poly and the parenthesis. Polymers made of amino acids are sometimes referred to as peptides, proteins, or poly(amino acid)s. When referring to one polymer that is made of one type of amino acid, IUPAC rules require this material to be named as a poly(amino acid). When referring to several such polymers, the plural of poly(amino acid) is poly(amino acid)s. Note the placement of the plural "s" outside of the parenthesis. When a polymer is made of several different amino acids, then that polymer would be referred to as a poly (amino acids). Note the placement of the plural "s" inside the parenthesis, indicating that this is a single polymer that contains more than one type of amino acid as monomer. Unfortunately, these rules are often violated in the contemporary literature.

13.2 Biodegradable Polymer Selection Criteria

The selection of biomaterials plays a key role in the design and development of medical implants and tissue-engineering products. While the classical selection criterion for a safe, stable implant dictated choosing a passive, "inert" material, it is now understood that any artificial material placed into the body of a patient will elicit a cellular response [1,2]. This means that there are in fact no artificial materials that are totally "inert", and some of the chemically least reactive materials, such as polyethylene or polysiloxane, can cause significant inflammatory responses. Therefore, it is now widely accepted that a biomaterial must interact with tissue in a biologically appropriate manner rather than act simply as an inert body. Consequently, a major focus of biomaterials science centers around harnessing control over cellular interactions with biomaterials. Researchers now tend to explore ways to manipulate the cellular response by including biologically active components in the design of biomaterials. Specific examples of such biologically active components include protein growth factors, anti-inflammatory drugs, and gene delivery vectors [3].

It is important for the tissue-engineering product developer to have many biomaterials options available, as each application calls for a unique environment for cell-cell interactions. Such applications include:

1. Support for new tissue growth (wherein cell-cell communication and cells' access to nutrients, growth factors, and pharmaceutically active agents must be maximized);
2. Prevention of cellular activity (where tissue growth, such as in surgically induced adhesions, is undesirable);
3. Guided tissue response (enhancing a particular cellular response while inhibiting others);
4. Enhancement of cell attachment and subsequent cellular activation (e.g., fibroblast attachment, proliferation, and production of extracellular matrix for dermis repair) [4];
5. Inhibition of cellular attachment and/or activation (e.g., platelet attachment to a vascular graft);
6. Prevention of a biological response (e.g., blocking antibodies against grafted cells used in organ replacement therapies).

Biodegradable polymers are applicable to those tissue-engineering products in which tissue repair or remodeling is the goal, but not where long-term materials stability is required. Biodegradable polymers must also possess:

1. Manufacturing feasibility, including availability of sufficient commercial quantities of the bulk polymer;
2. The capability to form the polymer into the final product design;
3. Mechanical properties that adequately address short-term function and do not interfere with long-term function;

4. Low or negligible toxicity of degradation products, in terms of both local tissue response and systemic response;
5. The capability to be formulated as a drug delivery system in applications that call for prolonged release of pharmaceutically active compounds.

13.3 Biologically Derived Polymers

Biologically derived polymers are materials created by living organisms, as opposed to synthetic materials which are man-made. This distinction divides the universe of medically useful, biodegradable polymers into two large subgroups. However, the delineation between these groups is not always clear-cut. For example, glycolic acid is a natural metabolite and poly(glycolic acid) is naturally produced by many organisms. However, glycolic acid can also be created synthetically from oil-derived starting materials. Currently, poly(glycolic acid) is produced commercially by both fermentation and synthetic processes. Both production pathways result in the same final product, making poly(glycolic acid) either a biologically derived polymer or a synthetic polymer. A similar situation exists in regard to polymers derived from hydroxybutyric acid and hydroxyvaleric acid. Commonly referred to as polyhydroxyalkanoates, these polymers can be derived from bacterial fermentation, as well as purely synthetic processes. In this chapter, polyhydroxyalkanoates are included among the biologically derived polymers (since the most prevalent mode of commercial production is based on bacterial fermentation), while poly(glycolic acid) and the closely related poly(lactic acid) are introduced to the reader as synthetic polymers (since the predominant mode of commercial production is currently based on oil-derived starting materials and synthetic polymerization reactions).

The biologically derived polymers can be further classified into peptides and proteins, polysaccharides, polyhydroxyalkanoates, and polynucleotides. Each of these subgroups will be discussed separately.

13.3.1 Peptides and Proteins

Peptides and proteins are polymers derived from naturally occurring α-L-amino acids. Peptides are usually shorter chains of dozens of amino acids linked together via amide bonds, while proteins are longer chains of hundreds of individual amino acids. The amino acids are connected via hydrolytically stable amide bonds. Therefore, these materials are usually degraded via enzymatic mechanisms. The major shortcoming of peptides and proteins as starting materials for the fabrication of any medical implant is their lack of "processibility". This term refers to the ability of creating a shaped device by any of the conventional polymer processing methods used in the plastics industry: compression molding, extrusion, injection molding and fiber spinning. Another important limitation of peptides and proteins as biomaterials is their inherent immunogenicity. Any peptide or protein carries the risk of being recognized as foreign by the patient's immune system. For example, for many years, the safety of using bovine collagen was a hotly debated topic because of fears that the implantation of bovine collagen could provoke an immune response and predispose the patient to autoimmune diseases.

On the other hand, peptides and proteins can have outstanding biological properties and can help the tissue engineer in designing a polymer with desirable biological activities. This fact has been the driving force behind the long-standing interest in using peptides and proteins as starting materials for medical implants or tissue-engineering products. Unfortunately, most peptides and proteins have mechanical properties that are not conducive for their use in medical implants, resulting in the utilization of only a very small number of proteins as biomaterials (Table 13.1).

13.3.1.1 Collagen

Collagen is the major component of mammalian connective tissue, accounting for approximately 30% of all protein in the human body. It is found in every major tissue that requires strength and flexibility. Fourteen types of collagens have been identified, the most abundant being type I [5]. Because of its abundance and its unique physical and biological properties, type I collagen has been used extensively in the formulation of biomedical materials [6]. Type I collagen is found in high concentrations in tendon, skin, bone and fascia, which are consequently convenient and abundant sources for isolation of this natural polymer.

Table 13.1 Proteins Used as Degradable Biomaterials in Medical Implants

Type of protein	Source	Function
Collagen	Isolated from cattle, fish, and other species	Key component of tissue architecture, provides mechanical strength, supports cell attachment and growth, provides a biocompatible matrix for cell transplantation. Used extensively as a tissue expander and bulking agent in cosmetic products
Gelatin	Partially hydrolized collagen	Used in food industry, widely explored by researchers as a matrix for three-dimensional cell culture and as a component of tissue-engineering scaffolds
Elastin	Isolated from elastic tissues of cattle and birds	Key component of tissue architecture, provides elasticity to tissues
Keratin	Isolated from skin, hair and nails of cattle and birds	Key structural component of outer skin, hair and nails. Used as a matrix for cell growth and as a component in wound dressings and skin care products
Silk	Isolated from insect larvae	Used in the textile industry because of its extraordinaty strength. Also studied as a component of tissue-engineering scaffolds and as a cell culture substrate
Proteoglycans	Various tissue extracts	Used in research of cell-matrix interactions, matrix-matrix interactions, cell proliferation, cell migration

Table 13.2 Widely Investigated Polysaccharides

Type of polysaccharide	Source	Function
Cellulose	Cell wall of green plants	Main structural component of plants which keeps the stems, stalks and trunks rigid
Starch (amylose and amylopectin)	Present in all staple foods	Important in plant energy storage
Alginate	Found in the cell walls of bacteria	Protects bacteria from engulfment by predatory protozoa or white blood cells (phagocytes)
Glycosaminoglycans	Widely distributed	Cell-matrix interactions, matrix-matrix interactions, cell proliferation, cell migration
Chitin/chitosan	Major component of the exoskelton of insects, shells of crustaceans, cell walls of fungi	Structural component

The structure, function, and synthesis of type I collagen has been thoroughly investigated [7]. Because of its phylogenetically well-conserved primary sequence and its helical structure, collagen is only mildly immunoreactive [8]. However, many human recipients of medical or cosmetic products containing bovine collagen have anti-bovine collagen antibodies. The clinical significance of this finding is not yet fully understood.

The individual collagen molecules will spontaneously polymerize to form strong fibers that form larger organized structures. Collagen exists in tissue in the form of collagen fibers, fibrils, and macroscopic bundles [9]. For example, tendon and ligaments are comprised mainly of oriented type I collagen fibrils, which are extensively crosslinked in the extracellular space.

In vitro, collagen crosslinking can be enhanced after isolation through a number of well-described physical or chemical techniques [10]. Increasing the intermolecular crosslinks:

1. Increases biodegradation time, by making collagen less susceptible to enzymatic degradation;
2. Decreases the capacity of collagen to absorb water;
3. Decreases its solubility; and
4. Increases the tensile strength of collagen fibers.

The free amines on lysine residues on collagen can be utilized for crosslinking, or can similarly be modified to link or sequester active agents. These simple chemical modifications provide a variety of processing possibilities and consequently the potential for a wide range of tissue-engineering applications using type I collagen.

It has long been recognized that substrate attachment sites are necessary for growth, differentiation, replication, and metabolic activity of most cell types in culture. Collagen and its integrin-binding domains (e.g., RGD sequences) assist in the maintenance of such attachment-dependent cell types in culture. For example, fibroblasts grown on collagen matrices appear to differentiate in ways that mimic *in vivo* cellular activity and to exhibit nearly identical morphology and metabolism [11]. Chondrocytes can also retain their phenotype and cellular activity when cultured on collagen [12]. Such results suggest that type I collagen can serve as tissue-regeneration scaffolds for any number of cellular constructs.

The recognition that collagen matrices could support new tissue growth was exploited to develop the original formulations of artificial extracellular matrices for dermal replacements [1,2,13–15]. Yannas and Burke were the first to show that the rational design and construction of an artificial dermis could lead to the synthesis of a dermis-like structure whose physical properties "would resemble dermis more than they resembled scar" [15].

They created a collagen–chondroitin sulfate composite matrix with a well-described pore structure and crosslinking density that optimizes regrowth while minimizing scar formation [16]. The reported clinical evidence and its simplicity of concept make this device an important potential tool for the treatment of severely burned patients [17].

The advantageous properties of collagen for supporting tissue growth have been used in conjunction with the superior mechanical properties of synthetic biodegradable polymer systems to make hybrid tissue scaffolds for bone and cartilage [18,19]. These hybrid systems show good cell adhesion, interaction and proliferation compared to the synthetic polymer system alone. Collagen has also been used to improve cell interactions with electrospun nanofibers of poly(hydroxy acids) such as poly(lactic acid), poly(glycolic acid), poly(ε-caprolactone) and their copolymers [18–22].

In recent years, the combination of collagen scaffolds with active biological entities, such as cells, growth factors, platelet rich plasma [23] and various autologous or allogenic cell types [24] have provided significant opportunities for researchers to achieve tendon and ligament regeneration.

13.3.1.2 Gelatin

Gelatin is commonly used for pharmaceutical and medical applications because of its enzymatic biodegradability and biocompatibility in physiological environments [25–27]. Of the two types, acidic and alkaline gelatin, the former has an isoelectric point similar to collagen. The isoelectric point depends on its extraction procedure from collagen, and variations in it allow gelatin to bind with either positively or negatively charged therapeutic agents. Based on this, the acidic gelatin, with an isoelectric point of 5.0, could be used as a carrier for basic proteins *in vivo*, while basic gelatin, with an isoelectric point of 9.0, could be used for the sustained release of acidic proteins under physiological conditions. The advantage of gelatin as a carrier for controlled drug release is that the therapeutic agent can be loaded into the gelatin matrix under mild conditions. Gelatin hydrogels have been used as controlled release devices for a variety of growth factors known to enhance bone formation. Yamada et al. successfully incorporated bFGF (basic fibroblast growth factor) into acidic gelatin hydrogels, which were implanted into a rabbit skull defect to allow for the localized release over 12 weeks [28,29].

13.3.1.3 Elastin

Elastin is an extracellular matrix protein and is most abundant in tissues where elasticity is of major importance, such as blood vessels (50% of dry weight), elastic ligaments (70% of dry weight), lungs (30% of dry weight) and skin (2–4% of dry weight) [30,31].

The incorporation of elastin into biomaterials was a major topic of research in the 1970s and 1980s. The basic structure-function-activity correlations of various elastin sequences were discovered by Urry and his associates [32]. It is important to note that elastin is not a single, well-defined molecule. Rather, the name "elastin" is associated with a wide range of elastic peptide and protein sequences that exist in different lengths and with different compositions. A common feature of all elastin sequences is that they are rich in glycine, proline, and lysine. In humans, elastin is synthesized early in life. By age 40 (approximately) elastin biosynthesis in humans slows down to a trickle. The appearance of skin wrinkles and other aging processes are directly related to the loss of elastin biosynthesis. This fact has been exploited as a marketing gimmick by cosmetic companies, who add elastin to a wide range of anti-aging products. However, there is overwhelming evidence that externally applied elastin is not able to pass through the skin and is not able to slow the loss of elastin from aging tissues.

When elastin was used as a component in heart valve prosthetic devices, the deposition of calcium-rich precipitates was a significant problem. This process, often referred to as "calcification", limited the utility of elastin-containing biomaterials in cardiovascular prosthetic implants [33]. This experience illustrates that the use of natural substances is not necessarily a guarantee for clinically successful device performance.

Another important point is that not all biologically derived polymers are good cell growth substrates. While collagen is highly cell adhesive, elastin tends to discourage cell attachment and growth. This has been a concern in the biomedical community, since many potential applications of elastin (for example in blood vessel and ligament regeneration) would require a highly cell adhesive surface. This challenge can be addressed using the tools of protein engineering to incorporate cell adhesive peptide sequences within the elastin structure [32].

Overall, elastin is a highly versatile biomaterial that continues to inspire the imagination and curiosity of biomedical engineers. Recently, the ability of elastin to self-assemble into large supramolecular structures was used to fabricate sponges, scaffolds, sheets and tubes from human tropoelastin [34]. These promising studies are still ongoing.

13.3.1.4 Keratin

Keratin is the name for a family of structural proteins which are abundant in the outer layer of human skin, in hair, and in nails. Keratin is rich in the amino acid cysteine, and it has the ability to self-assemble into bundles of fibers. Within these fiber bundles, individual strands are further cross-linked through S-S (sulfur-sulfur) bonds involving the cysteine side chains. In this way, keratin forms particularly tough, insoluble structures that are among the strongest non-mineralized tissues found in nature. The only other non-mineralized tissue that resembles the toughness of keratin is chitin (the material found in the exoskeleton of insects and the outer shell of shellfish).

Since human hair is rich in keratin, this protein is added to many hair care products. However, as in the case of the misleading marketing claims made for elastin-containing anti-aging skin products, there is no evidence that externally applied keratin can penetrate into the hair structure. While keratin was mostly studied for use in cosmetic (hair care) products, the exploration of keratin's properties also led to the development of keratin-based biomaterials for use in biomedical applications. The unusual mechanical properties and strength of keratin and its ability to self-assemble were the driving force for these biomedical studies.

The history of keratin research illustrates another major challenge when using biologically derived polymers as biomaterials. Based on the animal source used, and depending on the exact extraction procedure employed, individual keratin preparations can differ significantly from each other. The variability and irreproducibility of individual preparations is a general feature of most biologically derived polymers. Early research, mostly by Yamauchi's laboratory, focused on the preparation of protein films from keratin extracted from wool and human hair. These pure protein films were brittle and weak. The researchers could not reproduce in the laboratory the outstanding strength of keratin formed *in vivo*. Only when glycerol was added as a plasticizer, could keratin films be obtained that were relatively strong and flexible [35]. Fujii et al. also demonstrated that hair keratins were useful for preparing protein films and described a rapid casting method [36]. This research also revealed the feasibility of incorporating bioactive molecules such as alkaline phosphatase into the keratin films for controlled release applications. The films, however, had poor strength and flexibility [36]. Recently, significant progress was made by researchers at Wake Forest University, where keratin extracted from human hair was used as a matrix for the regeneration of peripheral nerves. This is currently one of the most advanced applications of keratin as a biomaterial [37].

13.3.1.5 Silk

On a weight basis, natural silk fibers can be stronger than high-grade steel. However, the strength of natural silk fibers is difficult to reproduce in the laboratory once pure silk has been extracted from the cocoons of silkworm larvae or from spider's webs. Still, the unique mechanical properties of natural silk fibers have fascinated scientists for more than a century. Recent work has demonstrated the biocompatibility of various silk protein preparations [38]. Another very interesting fact is that the degradation rate of laboratory-made silk fibers can be tailored to be from months to years after implantation *in vivo*, based on the processing procedure employed during the material's formation [39]. Finally, the thermal stability of silk biomaterials allows processing over a wide range of temperatures up to about 250°C, as evidenced by the ability to autoclave silk biomaterials without loss of functional integrity. Min and colleagues investigated the potential of electrospun silk matrices for accelerating early stages of wound healing [40]. In another study, chitin was blended with silk fibroin to fabricate composite fibrous scaffolds for skin tissue engineering. The rationale of these experiments was to combine the good mechanical properties of silk fibers with the wound healing effects of chitin [41]. The chitin/silk fibroin blends were electrospun to form nanofibrous matrices and evaluated for initial cell attachment and spreading [42]. *In vitro*, increased adhesion of keratinocytes was observed on chitin/silk blend matrices compared to pure chitin matrices, but the significance of these results for wound healing *in vivo* has not yet been established.

Overall, the exploration of silk as a biomaterial has not yet produced any commercially available medical products. While silk is a fascinating material, the studies performed so far have not discovered truly compelling reasons for the use of silk as a medical implant material.

13.3.1.6 Proteoglycans

Proteoglycans (PGs) are a major component of the extracellular matrix (ECM). They consist of one or more glycosaminoglycan (GAG) chains that are attached, via a tetrasaccharide link, to serine residues within a core protein [43,44]. GAGs are long chains of repeating disaccharide units that are variably sulfated. There are four main classes of GAGs—hyaluronan (HA), chondroitin sulfate (CS) and dermatan sulfate (DS), heparan sulfate (HS), and keratan sulfate (KS). PGs exhibit great structural diversity because each type of PG may contain different kinds of GAGs, different numbers and lengths of GAG chains, modifications in the repeating patterns of the disaccharides by a complex pattern of sulfate groups, and a different core protein structure. PGs can be present in monomeric form or can form very large aggregates. Both the core protein and the GAG chains of PGs play key roles in tissue remodeling, intracellular signaling, uptake of proteins, cell migration, and many other crucial functions in native tissues [43,44]. The fact that PGs seem to be involved in so many crucial cell signaling pathways is the main reason for the intense interest of biomedical engineers in understanding their properties.

To replicate the biological functions of PGs in tissue scaffolds, PGs or their GAG chains have frequently been grafted to the polymers used in fabricating tissue scaffolds, or they have been grafted onto the surface of tissue-engineering scaffolds. Most notably, chondroitin sulfate GAGs have been used to create collagen–GAG hybrid materials which seem to be particularly effective in skin regeneration.

PGs are sometimes used alone or in combination with other matrix proteins such as fibrin, collagen, or chitosan to create hybrid materials [45–47]. The rationale for exploring such complex mixtures is usually an attempt to "mix and match" biological properties with appropriate mechanical properties. For example, a mixture of PGs and extracellular matrix proteins are part of the widely used Matrigel™ scaffold. Among the various combinations, collagen–GAG scaffolds are often preferred for tissue-engineering applications, because collagen provides a very cell friendly matrix environment and the specific GAG used can affect (and regulate) cell behavior. Collagen–GAG hybrids can be readily sterilized using heat, and can be manufactured with a variety of pore structures and a wide range of degradation rates [48]. The first commercially used tissue-engineered product, an artificial skin scaffold, developed by Integra LifeSciences, a New Jersey company, is a collagen–GAG hybrid.

13.3.2 Biomimetic Materials

Biomimetic materials are synthetic (man-made) materials that mimic natural materials or that follow a design motif derived from nature. In the previous section, a number of peptides and proteins were discussed. In general, peptides and proteins are isolated from natural sources and are therefore listed among the biologically derived polymers. However, significant research breakthroughs were made when scientists started to create mimics of natural polymers by semi-synthetic or totally synthetic means. An excellent example for this type of research approach is the work of Urry and coworkers, who used peptide synthesis methods to create artificial variants of elastin [49,50]. Using a combination of solid-phase peptide chemistry and genetically engineered bacteria, they synthesized several polymers which contained homologies of the elastin repeat sequences valine-proline-glycine-valine-glycine (VPGVG). These biomimetic polymers had better engineering properties than their natural equivalents, making it possible to create films and fibers that could then be further modified by cross-linking. The resultant films had intriguing mechanical responses, such as a reverse phase transition which results in contraction with increasing temperature [50], resembling the action of muscles. The exact transition temperature could be varied by variations in the polymer's amino acid composition [50]. Several medical applications are under consideration for this system, including musculoskeletal repair mechanisms, ophthalmic devices, and mechanical and/or electrically stimulated drug delivery.

Other investigators, notably Tirrell and Cappello, have combined techniques from molecular and fermentation biology to create novel protein-based biomaterials [51–54]. These researchers had the remarkably innovative idea of creating genetically-engineered microorganisms that would produce exactly those polymers that the researchers liked to study. In this way, completely new variations of biologically derived peptides and proteins could be prepared. These protein polymers were based on repeat oligomeric peptide units, which were controlled via the genetic information inserted into the producing bacteria. It has been shown that the mechanical properties and the biological activities of these protein polymers can be pre-programmed, suggesting a large number of potential biomedical applications [55].

Another approach to elicit an appropriate cellular response to a biomaterial is to graft active peptides to the surface of a biodegradable polymer. For example, peptides containing the RGD sequence have been grafted to various biodegradable polymers to provide active cell-binding surfaces [56]. Similarly, Panitch et al. incorporated oligopeptides containing the REDV sequence to stimulate endothelial cell binding for vascular grafts [57].

13.3.3 Polysaccharides

Polysaccharides are polymers made of various sugar (saccharide) units. The most common monosaccharides are glucose and fructose. Sucrose is the chemical name of the widely used table sugar. Sucrose is a disaccharide composed of glucose and fructose. Scientists who are not experts in sugar chemistry are often unaware of the exquisite structural variability of these molecules. For example, the important human food, *starch*, and the structural polymer of all plants, *cellulose*, are both polymers of glucose. The only difference between starch and cellulose is the way in which the individual glucose units are linked together. Considering the many different isomeric variations possible for saccharides, and the different chemical bonds that can be used to link individual saccharide units together, the number of structurally different polysaccharides is extremely large. In fact, the chemistry of polysaccharides is as rich in diversity and variability as protein chemistry. It is therefore not surprising that various saccharides and polysaccharides play an important role in fine-tuning the responses of cells to their environment. As outlined above, proteoglycans (PGs) and glucosaminoglycans (GAGs) are critical in regulating key cell functions. In contrast, the industrially used polysaccharides (such as starch and cellulose) are polymers comprising exclusively various sugar (saccharide) units as monomers. These polysaccharides can be extremely large polymers containing millions of monomers, and they are mostly used in nature for cellular energy storage or as a structural material. As a general rule, most of the natural polysaccharides are not biodegradable when implanted in any mammalian species due to the lack of digestive enzymes. Therefore, without further chemical modification, most polysaccharides are not obvious material choices for use in biomedical applications.

13.3.3.1 Cellulose

Cellulose is the most abundant polymeric material in nature. In its most common form, it is a fibrous, tough, water-insoluble material that is mostly found in the cell walls of plants, mainly in stalks, stems or trunks. Cellulose is the major ingredient of wood. Cellulose is composed of D-glucose units that are linked together by β-$(1\rightarrow 4)$ glycosidic bonds. In nature, cellulose is formed by a simple polymerization of glucose residues from a substrate such as UDP-glucose [58]. Cellulose possesses high strength in the wet state [59]. The major commercial applications of cellulose are in the paper, wood, and textile industries [60] where millions of tons of cellulose are processed annually worldwide.

The major limitation of cellulose as a biomaterial is that it is not biodegradable, due to the lack of digestive enzymes for cellulose in the human organism [61,62]. However, a number of cellulose derivatives, such as methylcellulose, hydroxypropylcellulose and carboxymethylcellulose are used as biomaterials, due to the useful material properties exhibited by these synthetically created derivatives [63].

Cellulose is not an obvious choice for biomedical applications and there is no scientific rationale to expect cellulose to have unique or useful properties as a cell growth substrate or tissue-regeneration scaffold. This, however, has not prevented a number of laboratories from exploring cellulose or cellulose derivatives as a drug delivery implant, as a barrier for the prevention of surgical adhesions, or as a scaffold in cartilage tissue engineering [64,65]. *In vivo* studies have been performed to assess the biocompatibility of a bacterial cellulose scaffold by subcutaneous implantation in rats. While there were no macroscopic or microscopic signs of inflammation around the implants, and no fibrotic capsule or giant cells were observed, the limited biodegradability of cellulose will most probably prevent the use of this material in most biomedical applications [65].

13.3.3.2 Starch

Whereas cellulose is composed of D-glucose units that are linked together by β-$(1\rightarrow 4)$ glycosidic bonds, starch is composed of D-glucose units that are linked together by α-$(1\rightarrow 4)$ glycosidic bonds. This change makes starch digestible, allowing its use as a major human nutrient. The chemistry of starch is complicated by the fact that starch consists of linear and branched chains, referred to as amylose and amylopectin respectively [66]. The relative abundance of these two natural ingredients can significantly influence the material properties of starch. Consequently, literally hundreds of different starches exist, each with its own particular composition of amylose and amylopectin.

Starch can be totally water insoluble, or partially soluble at room temperature, depending on the proportions of amylose and amylopectin present. Water-soluble starches can be dispersed in water, forming clear solutions upon heating. Upon cooling, soluble starch forms a highly viscous solution at low concentrations and a stiff hydrogel at higher concentrations. This is the basis of the thickening action of soluble corn starch, which is used extensively in the food industry.

Although enzymes present in the human gut can digest starch, it is not readily biodegradable when implanted into human tissues. The cellular energy storage polymer in humans is glycogen and not starch. Consequently, starch is not an obvious choice for biomedical applications. However, some starch-based polymers are biodegradable in human tissues and biocompatible. Among many potential applications, starch-based polymers were used to prepare scaffolds for cartilage regeneration [67].

These scaffolds did not perform better than other types of scaffolds. Starch was also used for the design of implantable drug delivery systems. In spite of the research conducted by several laboratories worldwide, starch-based polymers are not likely to find major biomedical applications in the near future.

13.3.3.3 Alginate

Alginate is a natural anionic polysaccharide found in seaweed, which is composed of β-(1−4) linked D-mannuronic acid and α-L-guluronic acid units. Along its polymer chain, alginate has regions rich in sequential mannuronic acid units, guluronic acid units and regions in which both monomers are equally prevalent.

The most important use of alginate in biomedicine is as a cell-compatible hydrogel. Alginate can form strong hydrogels in the presence of divalent cations (such as Ca^{2+} or Ba^{2+}) that interact with the carboxylic groups present in the alginate backbone to form ionic crosslinks. In a typical experiment, a solution of alginate is added to cells suspended in physiologic buffer solution. This mixture is then dropped slowly into a solution of calcium chloride. As each drop of the cell suspension touches the calcium chloride solution, the alginate forms a hydrogel that encapsulates and captures the suspended cells. This process has been used in vitro to encapsulate human articular chondrocytes in the presence of recombinant human BMP-2 [68].

Alginate has a well-characterized structure, which allows for a range of comparative studies to be performed. Cells do not readily attach and grow on or within alginate hydrogels. This is a common feature of most unmodified polysaccharides. However, the carboxylic groups in its guluronic acid residues provide an easy handle for the chemical modification of alginate [69]. This feature makes it possible to attach biologically active ligands (such as the important RGD peptide) to the alginate backbone [69].

Alginate's major disadvantage is the difficulty of its isolation from contaminated seaweed, which leads to the presence of mitogenic, cytotoxic and apoptosis inducing impurities in the final processed material. Although such molecules can be removed by further purification steps, it is a time consuming and costly process [70].

13.3.3.4 Gellan Gum

Gellan gum is another anionic polysaccharide, similar in utility profile to alginate. Gellan gum can be easily processed into transparent gels that are resistant to heat. Gellan gum is not cytotoxic [71]) and can be injected into tissues. It has been used in vivo in humans as an ocular drug delivery vehicle [4]. Gellan gum is still relatively unknown in the biomedical community and only a few studies have explored this material for tissue engineering [72]. Like alginate, gellan gum can be used for the encapsulation and in vitro culture of cells [71]. Gellan gum hydrogels were able to support the development of nasal chondrocytes, and injectable gellan gum hydrogels were efficient in the encapsulation and support of human articular chondrocytes, while also enabling active synthesis of ECM components.

13.3.3.5 Glycosaminoglycans

Glycosaminoglycans (GAGs), which consist of repeating disaccharide units in linear arrangement, usually include a uronic acid component (such as glucuronic acid) and a hexosamine component (such as N-acetyl-D-glucosamine). The predominant types of GAGs attached to naturally occurring core proteins of proteoglycans include chondroitin sulfate, dermatan sulfate, keratan sulfate, and heparan sulfate [73,74]. The GAGs are attached to the core protein by specific carbohydrate sequences containing three or four monosaccharides.

The largest GAG, hyaluronic acid (hyaluronan), is an anionic polysaccharide with repeating disaccharide units of N-acetylglucosamine and glucuronic acid, with many unbranched units ranging from 500 to several thousand. Hyaluronic acid can be isolated from natural sources (e.g., rooster combs) or via microbial fermentation [75]. Because of its water-binding capacity, dilute solutions of hyaluronic acid form viscous solutions.

Like collagen, hyaluronic acid can be easily chemically modified, for instance by esterification of the carboxyl moieties, which reduces its water solubility and increases its viscosity [75,76]. Hyaluronic acid can be crosslinked to form molecular weight complexes in the range 8 to 24×10^6 or to form an infinite molecular network (gel). In one method, hyaluronic acid is crosslinked using aldehydes and small proteins to form bonds between the C—OH groups of the polysaccharide and the amino or imino groups of the protein, thus yielding high molecular weight complexes [77]. Other crosslinking techniques include the use of vinyl sulfone, which reacts to form an infinite network through sulfonyl-bis-ethyl crosslinks [78]. The resultant infinite network gels can be formed into sheaths, membranes, tubes, sleeves, and particles of various shapes and sizes. No species variations have been found in the chemical and physical structure of hyaluronic acid. The fact that it is not antigenic, eliciting no inflammatory or foreign body reaction, makes it desirable as a biomaterial. Its main drawbacks in this respect are its residence time and the limited range of its mechanical properties.

Because of its relative ease of isolation and modification and its superior ability in forming solid structures, hyaluronic acid has become the preferred GAG in medical device development. It has been used as a viscoelastic during eye surgery since 1976, and has undergone clinical testing as a means of relieving arthritic joints [79]. In addition, gels and films made from hyaluronic acid have shown clinical utility in preventing formation of post-surgical adhesions [80–82].

The benzyl ester of hyaluronic acid, sold under the trade name HYAFF-11, has been studied for use in vascular grafts [83–88].

13.3.3.6 Chitosan

Chitosan is a biosynthetic polysaccharide that is the deacylated derivative of chitin. Chitin is a naturally occurring polysaccharide that can be extracted from crustacean exoskeletons or generated via fungal fermentation processes. Chitosan is a β-1,4-linked polymer of 2-amino-2-deoxy-D-glucose; thus it carries a positive charge from amine groups [89]. It is hypothesized that the major path for chitin and chitosan breakdown *in vivo* is through lysozyme, which acts slowly to depolymerize the polysaccharide [90]. The biodegradation rate of the polymer is determined by the amount of residual acetyl content, a parameter that can easily be varied. Chemical modification of chitosan produces materials with a variety of physical and mechanical properties [91–93]. For example, chitosan films and fibers can be formed utilizing crosslinking chemistries adapted from techniques for altering other polysaccharides, such as treatment of amylose with epichlorohydrin [94]. Like hyaluronic acid, chitosan is not antigenic and is a well-tolerated implanted material [95].

Chitosan has been formed into membranes and matrices suitable for several tissue-engineering applications [96–99] as well as conduits for guided nerve regeneration [100,101]. Chitosan matrix manipulation can be accomplished using the inherent electrostatic properties of the molecule. At low ionic strength, the chitosan chains are extended via the electrostatic interaction between amine groups, whereupon orientation occurs. As ionic strength is increased, and chain-chain spacing diminishes; the consequent increases in the junction zone and stiffness of the matrix result in increased average pore size. Chitosan gels, powders, films, and fibers have been formed and tested for such applications as encapsulation, membrane barriers, contact lens materials, cell culture, and inhibitors of blood coagulation [102].

13.3.4 Polyhydroxyalkanoates

Polyhydroxyalkanoates (PHA) are a group of copolymers of hydroxybutyric acid and hydroxyvaleric acid. These linear polyesters are intracellular energy storage polymers whose function is to provide a reserve of carbon and energy [103] in certain microorganisms. These polyesters are slowly biodegradable, biocompatible, thermoplastic materials [104,105]. Depending on growth conditions, bacterial strain, and carbon source, the molecular weights of these polyesters can range from tens into the hundreds of thousands. Although the structures of PHA can contain a variety of *n*-alkyl side chain substituents (see Structure 13.1), the most extensively studied PHA is the simplest: poly(3-hydroxyburtyrate) (PHB).

ICI developed a biosynthetic process for the manufacture of PHB, based on the fermentation of sugars by the bacterium *Alcaligenes eutrophus*. PHB homopolymer, like all other PHA homopolymers, is highly crystalline, extremely brittle, and relatively hydrophobic. Consequently, the PHA homopolymers have degradation times *in vivo* on the order of years [106,104]. The copolymers of PHB with hydroxyvaleric acid are less crystalline, more flexible, and more readily processable, but suffer from the same disadvantage of being too hydrolytically stable to be useful in short-term applications, in which resorption of the degradable polymer within less than one year is desirable.

hydroxybutyric acid (HB)   hydroxyvaleric acid (HV)

Structure 13.1 Poly(b-hydroxybutyrate) and copolymers with hydroxyvaleric acid. For a homopolymer of HB, Y = 0; commonly used copolymer ratios are 7, 11, or 22 mole percent of hydroxyvaleric acid.

PHB and its copolymers with up to 30% of 3-hydroxyvaleric acid are now commercially available under the trade name Biopol, and are mostly used as environmentally friendly polymers that degrade slowly when disposed of in a landfill. It was previously found that a PHA copolymer of 3-hydroxybutyrate and 3-hydroxyvalerate, with a 3-hydroxyvalerate content of about 11%, may have an optimum balance of strength and toughness for a wide range of possible applications. PHB has been found to have low toxicity, in part due to the fact that it degrades *in vivo* to D-3-hydroxybutyric acid, a normal constituent of human blood. Applications of these previously tested polymers, and others now under development, include controlled drug release, artificial skin, and heart valves, along with industrial applications such as paramedical disposables [107–109]. Among the biomedical applications, sutures are the main product where polyhydroxyalkanonates are used, although a number of clinical trials for other applications may still be ongoing [110].

13.3.4 Polynucleotides

Gene delivery from the surfaces of tissue scaffolds represents a new approach to manipulating the local environment of cells [111]. Gene therapy approaches can be employed to increase the expression of tissue inductive factors or block the expression of factors that would inhibit tissue formation [112]. A biomaterial can enhance gene transfer by localized expression of the genetic material and by protecting the genetic material against degradation by nucleases and proteases. Sustained delivery of DNA from a polymer matrix may transfect large numbers of cells at a localized site and lead to the production of a therapeutic protein that could enhance tissue development. The work by Yao [113] serves as a specific example for this approach: Yao investigated the potential of chitosan/collagen scaffolds with pEGFP-TGFβ1 as a gene vector candidate in cartilage tissue engineering.

13.4 Synthetic Polymers

The concept of a "polymer" evolved from the study and commercial development of biologically derived macromolecules such as cellulose derivatives (celluloid, cellulose acetate) and vulcanized rubber in the nineteenth century. In 1907, the first totally synthetic polymer, Bakelite, was invented. At that time, the macromolecular structure of Bakelite and all other polymers was still not understood. It was only in 1922 that Hermann Staudinger proposed that the properties of polymers can be best explained by assuming that they consist of long chains of monomers linked together via regularly repeating bonds. The shortage of natural materials (in particular rubber) during World War II was the driving force behind the development of totally synthetic polymers. During World War II, Nylon, Teflon, various polyesters, and synthetic rubber emerged. The tremendous improvements in virtually all consumer products since 1945 would not have been possible without the development of hundreds of specialized polymers.

World War II left an additional legacy: the medical needs of millions of injured war fighters across the globe stimulated the development of new surgical procedures and innovative medical devices. Often, advances in the material sciences produced and enabled commensurate advances in medical practice. A new polymer, referred to as "Vinyon N", was developed during World War II for use in parachutes. In 1952, vascular surgeons noticed the stretchiness and elasticity of this material and developed the first vascular graft using Vinyon N. This effort became the starting point for the development of polymer-based medical implants and devices.

The systematic development of polymers for medical implants started with a focus on inert, biostable materials to be used in implants that lasted for the lifetime of the patient. It was only in 1969 that the first biodegradable polymer, poly (glycolic acid), was used to create the first, synthetic degradable suture line—a breakthrough that ended the use of suture lines made from the intestines of animals. Due to the efforts of many research groups, a number of different polymeric structures and compositions have been explored as degradable biomaterials. However, commercial efforts to develop these new materials for specific medical applications have been limited. Thus, detailed toxicological studies *in vivo*, investigations of degradation rate and mechanism and careful evaluations of the physicomechanical properties have so far been published for only a very small fraction of those polymers. This leaves the tissue engineer with just a relatively limited number of promising polymeric compositions to choose from. The following section is focused on a review of the most commonly investigated classes of biodegradable, synthetic polymers.

13.4.1 Aliphatic Polyesters

Aliphatic polyesters made of hydroxy acids, such as glycolic acid, lactic acid, and ε-hydroxy-caproic acid, have been utilized for a variety of medical product applications. As an example, bioresorbable surgical sutures made from poly(α-hydroxy acids) have been in clinical use since 1969 [114–116]. Other implantable devices made from these versatile polymers (e.g., internal fixation devices for orthopedic repair) are now part of standard surgical protocol [56,117,118].

Although polyesters can be synthesized by polycondensation of hydroxy acids such as lactic acid [119], it is difficult to achieve high molecular weights and control the molecular weight, molecular weight distribution, and architecture of the polymer in this process. In most cases, biodegradable polyesters are synthesized in a two-step procedure: first, the hydroxy acids are transformed into intramolecular lactones (see Structure 13.2), which are then used as monomers in ring-opening polymerizations.

The ester bond of the aliphatic polyesters is cleaved by hydrolysis, which results in a decrease in the polymer molecular weight of the implant [120]. This initial degradation occurs until the molecular weight of the resulting oligomers is less than 5000 Da, at which point the oligomers become water soluble and the degrading implant starts to lose mass as well. The final degradation and

Structure 13.2 Cyclic esters used in ring-opening polymerizations. *Lactide has two optically active carbon atoms in the ring.

resorption of the polyester implants may also involve inflammatory cells (such as macrophages, lymphocytes, and neutrophils). Although this late-stage inflammatory response can have a deleterious effect on some healing events, these polymers have been successfully employed as matrices for cell transplantation and tissue regeneration [121,122]. The useful lifetime of implants made from these polymers is determined by the initial molecular weight, exposed surface area, crystallinity, and (in the case of lactide-glycolide copolymers) by the ratio of the monomers.

Aliphatic polyesters have a modest range of thermal and mechanical properties and a correspondingly modest range of processing conditions. The polymers can generally be formed into films, tubes, and matrices using such standard processing techniques as molding, extrusion, solvent casting, and spin casting. Ordered fibers, meshes, and open-cell foams have been formed to fulfill the surface area and cellular requirements of a variety of tissue engineering constructs [56,117,123]. The aliphatic polyesters have also been combined with other components, e.g., poly(ethylene glycol), to modify the cellular response elicited by the implant and its degradation products [124].

13.4.1.1 Poly(glycolic Acid), Poly(lactic Acid), and their Copolymers

Poly(glycolic acid) (PGA), poly(lactic acid) (PLA), and their copolymers poly(lactic acid-co-glycolic acid) (PLGA) are the most widely used synthetic degradable polymers in medicine (see Structure 13.3). Of this family of linear aliphatic polyesters, PGA has the simplest structure and is more hydrophilic than PLA. Since PGA is highly

Structure 13.3 Poly(glycolic acid), poly(lactic acid) and their copolymer.

Structure 13.4 Lactide enantiomers: d-lactide, l-lactide and meso-lactide.

crystalline, it has a high melting point and low solubility in organic solvents. PGA was used in the development of the first totally synthetic absorbable suture [114]. The crystallinity of PGA in surgical sutures is typically in the range 46–52% [125]. Due to the hydrophilic nature and quick water uptake, surgical sutures made of PGA lose their mechanical strength typically over a period of 2 to 4 weeks post implantation [126].

In order to adapt the materials properties of PGA to a wider range of possible applications, researchers undertook an intensive investigation of copolymers of PGA with the more hydrophobic poly(lactic acid) (PLA) (see Structure 13.3). Alternative sutures composed of copolymers of glycolic acid and lactic acid are currently marketed under the trade names Vicryl.

Due to the presence of an extra methyl group in lactic acid, PLA is more hydrophobic than PGA. The hydrophobicity of high molecular weight PLA limits the water uptake of thin films to about 2% [125] and results in a rate of backbone hydrolysis lower than that of PGA [126]. In addition, PLA is more soluble in organic solvents than PGA.

It is noteworthy that there is no linear relationship between the ratio of glycolic acid to lactic acid and the physicomechanical properties of their copolymers. Whereas PGA is highly crystalline, crystallinity is rapidly lost in PGA-PLA copolymers. These morphological changes lead to an increase in the rates of hydration and hydrolysis. Thus, copolymers tend to degrade more rapidly than either PGA or PLA [125,126].

Since lactic acid is a chiral molecule, it exists in two stereoisomeric forms that give rise to four morphologically distinct polymers. D-PLA and L-PLA are the two stereoregular polymers, D,L-PLA is the racemic polymer obtained from a mixture of D- and L-lactic acid, and meso-PLA can be obtained from D,L-lactide. The polymers derived from the optically active d and l monomers are semi-crystalline materials, while the optically inactive D,L-PLA is always amorphous (Structure 13.3).

The differences in the crystallinity of D,L-PLA and L-PLA have important practical ramifications: Since D,L-PLA is an amorphous polymer, it is usually considered for applications such as drug delivery, where it is important to have a homogeneous dispersion of the active species within a monophasic matrix. On the other hand, the semi-crystalline L-PLA is preferred in applications where high mechanical strength and toughness are required—for example, sutures and orthopedic devices [127–129].

L-PLA (PLLA) and D-PLA (PDLA) are semi-crystalline polymers with a glass transition temperature (Tg) of approximately 60°C, and a peak melting temperature (Tm) of approximately 180°C. D,L-PLA (PDLLA) is amorphous with a Tg of approximately 55°C. Both semi-crystalline PLLA and amorphous PDLLA polymers are rigid materials. Their Young's modulus and stress at break values are close to 3.5 GPa and 65 MPa, respectively. However, these polymers are relatively brittle with an elongation at break of less than 6% [130–132].

These polymers degrade by hydrolysis in which naturally occurring lactic acid is formed. Degradation of the polymers starts with water uptake, followed by random cleavage of the ester bonds in the polymer chain. The degradation is throughout the bulk of the material [133]. Upon degradation, the number of carboxylic end groups increases, which leads to a decrease in pH and an autocatalytic acceleration of the rate of degradation [134]. During the degradation of semi-crystalline PLLA, crystallinity of the residual material increases as hydrolysis preferentially takes place in the amorphous domains [135]. In general, the rate of degradation and erosion of amorphous PDLLA is faster than that of PLLA [136].

Ikada et al. were the first to report on the stereocomplexation of enantiomeric PLLA and PDLA polymers during co-precipitation of mixed polymer solutions in non-solvents [222]. Since then, they have shown that stereocomplexation of PLLA and PDLA can take place in dilute and concentrated solutions, during solvent evaporation and spinning, and during annealing of their mixtures prepared in the melt [137]. Other groups have also reported the formation of poly(lactic acid) stereocomplexes [138,139].

Upon stereocomplexation, the melting temperature of the poly(lactide) stereocomplexes increases to about 230°C. This is 50°C higher than the melting temperature of the enantiomeric PLLA and PDLA polymers. Stereocomplexation influences the mechanical properties of poly(lactide) films [133]. When stereocomplexes were formed from PLLA and PDLA their films were stiffer, stronger, and tougher than films prepared from the enantiomeric polymers. In addition, under hydrolytic degradation conditions, the degradation of thin films of stereocomplexes of PLLA and PDLA is slower than that of the enantiomeric PLLA and PDLA homopolymers [140]. These findings are of great interest to biomedical engineers as they provide a simple way to increase the mechanical strength of these polymers with a concomitant increase in hydrolytic stability.

Recently, PLA, PGA, and their copolymers have been combined with bioactive ceramics, such as Bioglass particles or hydroxyapatite, that stimulate bone regeneration while greatly improving the mechanical strength of the composite material [141]. It was also reported that composites of polymer and Bioglass are angiogenic (e.g., they supported the growth of blood vessels), suggesting a novel approach for providing a vascular supply to implanted devices [142].

Some controversy surrounds the use of these materials for orthopedic applications. According to one review of the clinical outcomes for over 500 patients treated with resorbable pins made from either PGA or PGA:PLA copolymer, 1.2% required reoperation due to device failure, 1.7% suffered from bacterial infection of the operative wound, and 7.9% developed a late noninfectious inflammatory response that warranted operative drainage [143]. This delayed inflammatory reaction represents the most serious complication of the use of PGA or PLA in orthopedic applications. The mean interval between device implantation and the clinical manifestation of this reaction is 12 weeks for PGA and can be as long as three years for the more slowly degrading PLA [143]. Whether avoiding reoperation to remove a metal implant outweighs an approximately 8% risk of severe inflammatory reaction is a difficult question; in any event, an increasing number of trauma centers have suspended the use of these degradable fixation devices. It has been suggested that the release of acidic degradation products (glycolic acid for PGA, lactic acid for PLA, and glyoxylic acid for polydioxanone) contributes to the observed inflammatory reaction. Thus, the late inflammatory response appears to be a direct consequence of the chemical composition of the polymer degradation products [143]. The incorporation of alkaline salts or antibodies to inflammatory mediators may diminish the risk of a late inflammatory response [144]. A more desirable solution to these problems for orthopedic (and perhaps other) applications requires the development of new polymers that do not release acidic degradation products upon hydrolysis.

Using biodegradable PGA mesh scaffolds and a biomimetic perfusion system, Niklason et al. have successfully engineered small-diameter vessel grafts using either endothelial cells (ECs) and smooth muscle cells (SMCs) obtained from vessels in various species, or mesenchymal stem cells derived from adult human bone marrow [145,146]. In this approach, *ex vivo* culture resulted in the formation of a tissue-engineered vascular structure composed of cells and ECM while the PGA degraded during the same period. Cellular material was removed with detergents to render the grafts non-immunogenic. Tested in a dog model, grafts demonstrated excellent patency and resisted dilatation, calcification, and intimal hyperplasia [147].

13.4.1.2 Poly(ε-caprolactone)

Poly(ε-caprolactone) (PCL) (Structure 13.5) is an aliphatic polyester that has been intensively investigated as a biomaterial. The discovery that PCL can be degraded by microorganisms led to evaluation of PCL as a biodegradable packaging material; later, it was discovered that PCL can also be degraded by a hydrolytic mechanism under physiological conditions [148–150]. Under certain circumstances, crosslinked PCL can be degraded enzymatically, leading to what can be called enzymatic surface erosion [148,149]. Low molecular weight fragments of PCL are reportedly taken up by macrophages and degraded intracellularly, with a tissue reaction similar to that of the other poly(hydroxy acids) [150]. Compared with PGA or PLA, the degradation of PCL is significantly slower. PCL is therefore most suitable for the design of long-term, implantable systems such as Capronor, a one-year implantable contraceptive device [151].

Poly(ε-caprolactone) exhibits several unusual properties not found among the other aliphatic polyesters. Most noteworthy are its exceptionally low glass transition temperature of about −60°C and its low melting temperature of 57°C. Another unusual property is its high thermal stability. Whereas other tested aliphatic polyesters had decomposition temperatures (Td) between 235 and 255°C, poly(ε-caprolactone) has a Td of 350°C, which is more typical of poly(ortho esters) than aliphatic polyesters [152].

A useful property of PCL is its propensity to form compatible blends with a wide range of other polymers [153]. In addition, ε-caprolactone can be copolymerized with numerous other monomers (e.g., ethylene oxide, chloroprene, THF, δ-valerolactone, 4-vinylanisole, styrene, methyl methacrylate, vinylacetate). Particularly noteworthy are copolymers of ε-caprolactone and lactic acid, which

Structure 13.5 Poly(ε-caprolactone).

have been studied extensively [149,154]. PCL and copolymers with PLA have been electrospun to create nanofibrous tissue-engineered scaffolds that show promise for vascular applicaions [155,20–22]. The toxicology of PCL has been extensively studied as part of the evaluation of Capronor. Based on a large number of tests, the monomer ε-caprolactone, and the polymer PCL, are currently regarded as non-toxic and tissue compatible materials. Early clinical studies [156] of the Capronor system were started around the year 2000 and resulted in a commercial implant used in Europe, but not in the USA.

13.4.1.3 Poly(p-dioxanone)

Poly(p-dioxanone) (PDS) is prepared by the ring-opening polymerization of p-dioxanone (Structure 13.6). It is a relatively weak, rapidly biodegrading polymer that was introduced into the market in the 1980s as a new degradable suture material. When compared on a weight basis (for example per 1 gram of implant), poly(p-dioxanone) releases degradation products that are less acidic than the degradation products released by PGA or PLA. This is a potential advantage for orthopedic applications, which led to the development of small bone pins for the fixation of fractures in non-load bearing bones. Bone pins based on poly(p-dioxanone) are marketed under the trade name Orthosorb in the USA and under the name Ethipin in Europe. Poly(p-dioxanone) is also found in suture clips.

Unfortunately, poly(p-dioxanone) is relatively weak and lacks the stiffness and strength required for most orthopedic applications. Its range of applications is therefore limited. Academic laboratories have investigated poly(p-dioxanone) mostly as a polymer for implantable drug delivery applications. Little work has been done to explore this polymer as a scaffold for tissue engineering, probably because the polymer offers no clear advantages in terms of cell attachment and tissue compatibility over the widely used poly(lactic acid) and the copolymers of lactic and glycolic acid.

Structure 13.6 p-Dioxanone and polydioxanone.

Structure 13.7 Poly(orthoesters). The specific composition shown here is a terpolymer of hexadecanol (1,6-HD), trans-cyclohexyldimethanol (t-CDM), and DETOSU.

13.4.1.4 Poly(ortho Esters)

Poly(ortho esters) are a family of synthetic degradable polymers that have been under development since 1970 [157,158]. Devices made of poly(ortho esters) can be formulated in such a way that the device undergoes surface erosion—that is, the polymeric device degrades at its surface only and will thus tend to become thinner over time rather than crumbling into pieces. Since surface-eroding, slab-like devices tend to release drugs embedded within the polymer at a constant rate, poly(ortho esters) appear to be particularly useful for controlled release drug delivery [159]; this interest is reflected by the many descriptions of these applications in the literature [160].

There are two major types of poly(ortho esters). Originally, poly(ortho esters) were prepared by the condensation of 2,2-diethoxytetrahydrofuran and a dialcohol [161]) and marketed under the trade names Chronomer and Alzamer. Upon hydrolysis, these polymers release acidic by-products that autocatalyze the degradation process, resulting in degradation rates that increase with time. More recently, Heller et al. [162]) synthesized a new type of poly(ortho ester) based on the reaction of 3,9-bis(ethylidene 2,4,8,10-tetraoxaspiro {5,5} undecane) (DETOSU) with various dialcohols (Structure 13.7). These poly(ortho esters) do not release acidic by-products upon hydrolysis and thus do not exhibit autocatalytically increasing degradation rates. By selecting diols having different degrees of chain flexibility, polymers can be obtained that range from hard, brittle materials to materials that have a gel-like consistency. A drug release system for mepivacaine (a treatment for post-operative pain), was tested in Phase 2 clinical trials between 2000 and 2005 [158], and as of 2012, a fourth generation, poly(ortho ester)-based drug delivery system for prevention of chemotherapy-induced nausea and vomiting was in Phase 3 clinical trials.

13.4.2 Biodegradable Polyurethanes

Polyurethanes, polymers in which the repeating unit contains a urethane moiety, were first produced by Bayer in 1937. These polymers are typically produced through the reaction of a diisocyanate with a polyol. Conventional polyols are polyethers or polyesters. The resulting polymers are segmented block copolymers with the polyol segment providing a low glass transition temperature (i.e., $<25°C$) soft segment and the diisocyanate component, often combined with a hydrocarbon chain extender, providing the hard segment (Structure 13.8). A wide range of physical and mechanical properties have been realized with commercial polyurethanes.

Polyurethanes have been used for nearly 50 years in biomedical applications, particularly as blood-contacting material in cardiovascular

Structure 13.8 General structure of a segmented poly(urethane) prepared from diisocyanate, OCN-R-NCO; chain extender, HO-R'-OH; and polyol building blocks.

devices. Intended as non-biodegradable coatings, polyurethanes fell out of favor with the failure of pacemaker leads and breast implant coatings. Subsequent studies, as reviewed by Santerre et al., have clarified much about the behavior of polyurethanes in biological systems [163]. Elucidation of the biodegradation mechanism and its dependence on the polyurethane structure and composition have led to the development of biodegradable polyurethanes for a variety of tissue-engineering applications such as meniscal reconstruction [164], myocardial repair [165] and vascular tissues [166]. Design of biodegradable polyurethanes has required alternative diisocyanate compounds. The traditional aromatic diisocyanates are putative carcinogenic compounds. Biodegradable polymers are made from biocompatible diisocyanates such as lysine-diisocyanate or hexamethylene diisocyanate that release non-toxic degradation products.

The urethane bond is essentially non-degradable under physiological conditions. Therefore, biodegradable poly(urethane)s can only be obtained when the employed soft polyol segments are degradable [163]. As an example, aliphatic poly(ester urethane)s containing random 50/50 ε-caprolactone/L-lactide copolymer segments, 1,4-butanediol and 1,4-butanediisocyanate were synthesized and used to prepare porous structures for meniscus reconstruction [167]. In these polymers, the biodegradation mechanism involves the hydrolytic cleavage of the ester bonds in the ε-caprolactone/L-lactide copolymer segments, resulting in the formation of low molecular weight blocks of the non-degradable hard segments which are ultimately excreted from the body via the liver and/or kidney.

An interesting application of polyurethanes was developed by Santerre et al. where fluoroquinolone antimicrobial drugs were incorporated into the polymer as hard-segment monomers [163]. This led to the design of drug polymers (trade name: Epidel)

Structure 13.9 Poly(SA-HDA anhydride). This composition represents one of many polyanhydrides that were explored. The clinically relevant polyanhydrides are copolymers of sebacic acid and p-carboxy-phenoxypropane.

that release the drug when degraded by enzymes generated by an inflammatory response. This is an example of a "smart" system in that antibacterial agents are released only while inflammation is present. Once healing occurs, the enzyme level drops and the release of drug diminishes.

13.4.3 Polyanhydrides (Structure 13.9)

Polyanhydrides were first investigated in detail by Hill and Carothers [168] and were considered in the 1950s for possible applications as textile fibers [169]. Their low hydrolytic stability, the major limitation for their industrial applications, was later recognized as a potential advantage by Langer et al. [170], who suggested the use of polyanhydrides as degradable biomaterials. A study of the synthesis of high molecular weight polyanhydrides has been published by Domb et al. [171].

A comprehensive evaluation of the toxicity of the polyanhydrides showed that, in general, they possess excellent *in vivo* biocompatibility [172]. Their most immediate applications are in the field of drug delivery, although tissue-engineering applications are also being developed. Drug loaded devices are best prepared by compression molding or microencapsulation [173]. A wide variety of drugs and proteins, including insulin, bovine growth factors, angiogenesis inhibitors (e.g., heparin and cortisone), enzymes (e.g., alkaline phosphatase and b-galactosidase) and anesthetics have been incorporated into polyanhydride matrices, and their *in vitro* and *in vivo* release characteristics have been evaluated [174]. One of the most aggressively-investigated uses of the polyanhydrides is for the delivery of chemotherapeutic agents. An example of this application is the delivery of BCNU (bis-chloroethylnitrosourea) to the brain for the treatment of glioblastoma multiformae, a universally fatal brain cancer [175]. For this application, polyanhydrides derived from bis-p-(carboxyphenoxy propane) and sebacic acid received Food and Drug Administration (FDA) regulatory clearance in the fall of 1996 and are currently being marketed under the name Gliadel®.

13.4.4 Polyphosphazenes (Structure 13.10)

Polyphosphazenes consist of an inorganic phosphorous-nitrogen backbone, in contrast to the commonly employed hydrocarbon-based polymers [176a]. Consequently, the phosphazene backbone undergoes hydrolysis to phosphate and ammonium salts, with the concomitant release of the side group. Of the numerous polyphosphazenes that have been synthesized, those that have some potential use for medical products are substituted with amines of low pKa, and those with activated alcohol moieties [177–179]. Singh and colleagues have modified the side groups to tune polyphophazine properties such as glass transition temperature, degradation rate, surface wettability, tensile strength and elastic modulus, enabling these polymers to be considered for a wider range of biomedical applications [180]. The most extensively studied polyphosphazenes are hydrophobic, having fluoroalkoxy side groups. In part, these materials are of interest because of their expected minimal tissue interaction, which is similar to Teflon.

Aryloxyphosphazenes and closely related derivatives have also been extensively studied. One such polymer can be crosslinked with dissolved cations such as calcium to form a hydrogel matrix because of its polyelectrolytic nature [181]. Using methods similar to alginate encapsulation, microspheres of aryloxyphosphazene have been used to encapsulate hybridoma cells without affecting their viability or

Structure 13.10 Polyphosphazene. Shown here is a polymer containing an amino acid ester attached to the phosphazene backbone.

their capacity to produce antibodies. Interaction with poly(L-lysine) produced a semi-permeable membrane. Similar materials have been synthesized that show promise in blood contacting and with novel drug delivery applications.

13.4.5 Poly(amino Acids) and "Pseudo"-poly(amino Acids)

Since proteins are composed of amino acids, many researchers have tried to develop synthetic polymers derived from amino acids to serve as models for structural, biological and immunological studies. In addition, many different types of poly (amino acids) have been investigated for use in biomedical applications [176]. Poly(amino acids) are usually prepared by the ring-opening polymerization of the corresponding *N*-carboxy anhydrides, which are in turn obtained by reaction of the amino acid with phosgene [182].

Poly(amino acids) have several potential advantages as biomaterials. A large number of polymers and copolymers can be prepared from a variety of amino acids. The side chains offer sites for the attachment of small peptides, drugs, crosslinking agents, or pendant groups that can be used to modify the physicomechanical properties of the polymer. Since these polymers release naturally occurring amino acids as the primary products of polymer backbone cleavage, their degradation products may be expected to show a low level of systemic toxicity.

Poly(amino acids) have been investigated as suture materials [178], as artificial skin substitutes [183] and as drug delivery systems [184]. Various drugs have been attached to the side chains of poly(amino acids), usually via a spacer unit that

Structure 13.11 A poly(amide carbonate) derived from desaminotyrosyl tyrosine alkyl esters. This is an example for a group of new, amino acid derived polymers.

distances the drug from the backbone. Combinations of poly(amino acid)s and drugs that have been investigated include poly(L-lysine) with methotrexate and pepstatin [185], and poly(glutamic acid) with adriamycin and norethindrone [186]. Short amino acid sequences such as RGD and RGDS, strong promotors of specific cell adhesion, have been linked to the polymer backbone to promote cell growth in tissue-engineering applications [187,188].

Despite their apparent potential as biomaterials, poly(amino acids) have actually found few practical applications. *N*-carboxy anhydrides, the starting materials, are expensive to make and difficult to handle because of their high reactivity and moisture sensitivity. Most poly(amino acids) are highly insoluble and non-processible materials. Since poly(amino acids) degrade via enzymatic hydrolysis of the amide bond, it is difficult to reproduce and control their degradation *in vivo,* because the level of relevant enzymatic activity varies from person to person. Furthermore, the antigenicity of poly(amino acids) containing three or more amino acids limits their use in biomedical applications [176]. Because of these difficulties, only a few poly(amino acids), usually derivatives of poly(glutamic acid) carrying various pendent chains at the γ-carboxylic acid group, have been identified as promising implant materials [189].

As an alternative approach, Kohn et al. have replaced the peptide bonds in the backbone of synthetic poly(amino acids) by a variety of "nonamide" linkages such as ester, iminocarbonate, urethane, and carbonate bonds [190,191]. The term *pseudo-poly(amino acid)* is used to denote this new family of polymers in which naturally occurring amino acids are linked together by nonamide bonds (Structure 13.11).

The use of such backbone-modified pseudo-poly(amino acids) as biomaterials was first suggested in 1984 [192]. The first pseudo-poly(amino acids) investigated were a polyester from *N*-protected trans-4-hydroxy-L-proline and a poly(iminocarbonate) from tyrosine dipeptide [193,194]. Several studies indicate that the backbone modification of conventional poly(amino acids) generally improves their physicomechanical properties [190,195,196]. This approach is applicable to, among other materials, serine, hydroxyproline, threonine, tyrosine, cysteine, glutamic acid, and lysine; it is only limited by the requirement that the nonamide backbone linkages give rise to polymers with desirable material properties. Additional pseudo-poly(amino acids) can be obtained by considering dipeptides as monomeric starting materials. Hydroxyproline-derived polyesters [194,197], serine-derived polyesters [198], and tyrosine-derived polyiminocarbonates

[199] and polycarbonates [200] represent specific embodiments of these synthetic concepts.

13.5 Combinations (Hybrids) of Synthetic and Biologically Derived Polymers

Biologically derived polymers have important advantages over synthetic materials. These advantages often include reduced toxicity, since they generally originate from molecules that occur naturally in the body and biodegrade under physiological conditions [201,202], and they also exhibit improved *bioactivity*. In this context, the term bioactivity refers to the ability of a material to elicit specific cellular responses. Collagen, for example, is a bioactive material because of its ability to support cell attachment, growth and differentiation. However, the usefulness of biologically derived polymers is often limited by their poor engineering properties. Important disadvantages of biologically derived polymers are:

1. High batch-to-batch variability due to complex isolation procedures from inconsistent sources,
2. Poor solubility and processibility, preventing the use of industrial manufacturing processes,
3. Risk of contamination by pyrogens or pathogens,
4. Poor or limited materials properties such as strength, ductility, elasticity, or shelf life, and
5. Their high cost.

In overall terms, synthetic materials offer a wider range of useful engineering properties (polymer composition, architecture, mechanical properties, etc.) but they generally fail to promote cell growth and differentiation to the same degree as some of the biologically derived polymers [203]. To address these shortcomings, it is an obvious idea to combine biologically derived polymers with synthetic materials. As a general rule, the purpose of such hybrid materials is to combine the bioactivity of biologically derived polymers with the superior engineering properties of synthetic materials.

As an example, a clinically useful cornea replacement material was obtained when collagen was incorporated into a synthetic, polyacrylate-based hydrogel [204]. Another example of this approach is provided by a hybrid material derived from silk fibroin (as the hydrophobic, bioactive material) and poly(vinyl alcohol) (as the hydrophilic, synthetic component) [205]. Poly(vinyl alcohol) (PVA) can be crosslinked under mild conditions by exposure to UV (ultraviolet) radiation. This crosslinking method allows PVA and fibroin to form a highly biocompatible hydrogel with adjustable engineering properties [205].

A final example of this approach is provided by a hybrid material composed of poly(N-isopropylacrylamide) (pNIPAM) as the synthetic component and various natural polysaccharides as the biologically derived component. pNIPAM undergoes a thermally induced phase transition around 32°C that causes the soluble material to precipitate. This property allows the design of a product that is liquid and injectable at room temperature and that precipitates and forms a hydrogel at body temperature, facilitating the formation of a solid implant while eliminating the need for surgical insertion. The disadvantage of pNIPAM as a biomaterial is its inability to support cell growth and its lack of biodegradability. This can be overcome by crosslinking pNIPAM with natural polysaccharide precursors, leading to cell-permissive formulations that will biodegrade *in vivo*.

13.6 Using Polymers to Create Tissue-Engineered Products

The medical implant of the future will not be an artificial prosthetic device that replaces tissue lost due to trauma, disease, or aging, but a tissue scaffold that integrates with the surrounding healthy tissue and assists in the regeneration of lost or damaged tissue. As one possible implementation of this concept, the biomedical literature currently envisions such tissue scaffolds as consisting of bioactive polymers that may be shaped as porous sponge-like structures. These tissue scaffolds may either be preseeded with specific cell populations outside of the body of the patient prior to implantation into the patient, or the tissue scaffolds may be implanted into the body of the patient first, and then be colonized by the patient's own cells, leading to the regeneration of the desired tissue. In either case, one can formulate several design criteria that can guide the biomedical engineer in the process of selecting an appropriate biomaterial for the intended application.

First and foremost, one must be concerned with the bulk polymer properties. The biomaterial must have an appropriate range of physicomechanical properties, biodegradation rates, and biocompatibility appropriate for the intended application. Next, it must be possible to create the desired tissue scaffold. This requires that the desired device shape and architecture can actually be created by cost-effective fabrication methods. For example, electrospinning may be the preferred fabrication method to create an ECM-like scaffold that consists of nano-sized fibers. Since electrospinning requires that the biomaterial is soluble in non-toxic solvents, any insoluble biomaterial would not meet a key design requirement. Finally, it is important to consider the biological properties of the biomaterial. Tissue-engineering products require specific cellular responses. For example, in a bone regeneration scaffold, the ability to support the attachment and growth of osteoblasts in combination with the ability to adsorb and concentrate endogenous bone morphogenic protein on the polymer surface may be important design requirements (Figure 13.1). There is a wide range of additional requirements that impose further limitations on the selection of the biomaterial and/or the architecture of the implant. For example, whenever functional tissue has to form within the tissue-engineering scaffold, a lack of proper vascularization will impede a favorable tissue response. For encouraging angiogenesis within the scaffold, details such as pore size, pore structure and pore connectivity are often critical [206].

Once an appropriately shaped tissue scaffold has been conceptionalized, it is time to consider a wide range of secondary design criteria relating to device shelf life, ability of the device to be sterilized and packaged for clinical use, and overall cost. Here, being able to create a terminally sterilized device is a factor often overlooked by academic researchers, who fail to consider the fact that most FDA-recognized sterilization methods cannot be applied to products that contain living cells. Thus, the requirement to ensure device sterility has been a major hurdle in translating research concepts from the laboratory to clinical practice.

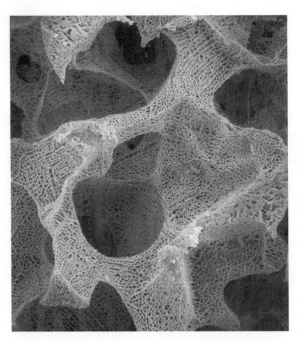

Figure 13.1 Bone regeneration scaffold from the New Jersey Center for Biomaterials. The scaffold has a delicate and carefully optimized pore structure consisting of large macropores (200–400 μm) and linearly aligned micropores (5–20 μm). This particular pore architecture is believed to facilitate the regeneration of bone *in vivo*. (Photo: Courtesy of the Laboratory of Professor Joachim Kohn, Rutgers-the State University of New Jersey)

13.6.1 Barriers: Membranes and Tubes

Design formats requiring cell activity on one surface of a device while precluding transverse movement of surrounding cells onto that surface calls for a barrier material. For example, peripheral nerve regeneration must allow for axonal growth, while at the same time precluding fibroblast activity that could produce neural-inhibiting connective tissue. Structures such as collagen tubes can be fabricated to yield a structure dense enough to inhibit connective tissue formation along the path of repair while allowing axonal growth through the lumen [207]. More recently, conduits composed of a silk fibroin scaffold coupled with biologics have shown improvement in performance [208]. Similarly, collagen membranes for periodontal repair provide an environment for periodontal ligament regrowth and attachment while preventing epithelial ingrowth into the healing site [209]. Anti-adhesion formulations using hyaluronic acid, which prevent ingrowth of connective tissue at a surgically repaired site, also work in this way [80].

13.6.2 Gels

Gels are used to provide a hydrogel scaffold, encapsulate, or provide a specialized environment for isolated cells. For example, collagen gels for tissue engineering were first used to maintain fibroblasts, which were the basis of a living skin equivalent [210]. Gels have also been used for the maintenance and immunoprotection of xenograft and homograft cells such as hepatocytes, chondrocytes, and islets of Langerhans used for transplantation [211–213]. Semi-permeable gels have been created to limit cell-cell communication and interaction with surrounding tissue, and to minimize movement of peptide factors and nutrients through the implant. Injectable biodegradable gel materials that form through crosslinking *in situ* show promise for regeneration of bone and cartilage. Temenoff and Mikos review a number of injectable systems that demonstrate appropriate properties for these applications [214]. Lee and colleagues discuss the use of biodegradable polyester dendrimers (highly branched, synthetic polymers with layered architectures) to form hydrogels for tissue-engineering applications such as corneal wound sealants [215]. In general, non-degradable materials are used for cell encapsulation to maximize long-term stability of the implant. In the future, however, it may be possible to formulate novel "smart" gels in which biodegradation is triggered by a specific cellular response instead of simple hydrolysis.

13.6.3 Matrices

It has been recognized since the mid-1970s that three-dimensional structures are an important component of engineered tissue development [13,14]. Yannas and his coworkers were the first to show that pore size, pore orientation, and fiber structure are important characteristics in the design of cell scaffolds. Several techniques have subsequently been developed to form well-defined matrices from synthetic and biologically derived polymers, and the physical characteristics of these matrices are routinely varied to maximize cellular and tissue responses [216–219]. Examples of engineered matrices that have led to several resorbable templates are oriented pore structures designed for regeneration of trabecular bone [220,221].

13.7 Conclusion

Research using currently available biomaterials and research aimed at developing novel biodegradable polymers has helped to advance the field of tissue engineering. Throughout most of the twentieth century, most research and development efforts relied on a small number of biodegradable polymers that had a history of regulatory approval, making poly(lactic acid) the most widely used biodegradable polymer. Research in the twenty first century aims to develop advanced biodegradable polymers that elicit predictable and useful cellular responses. To achieve this goal, current research efforts focus on creating bioactive materials that combine the superior engineering properties of synthetic polymers with the superior biological properties of natural materials. The extremely complex material requirements of tissue scaffolds pose significant challenges and require a continued research effort toward the development of new bioresorbable polymers.

References

[1] Peppas NA, Langer RL. New challenges in biomaterials. Science 1994;263(5154):1715–20.

[2] Langer R, Tirrell DA. Designing materials for biology and medicine. Nature 2004;428(6982): 487–92.

[3] Murphy WL, Mooney DJ. Controlled delivery of inductive proteins, plasmid DNA and cells from tissue engineering matrices. J Periodontal Res 1999;34(7):413–9.

[4] Shedden A, Laurence J, Tipping R, Timoptic XE. Efficacy and tolerability of timolol maleate ophthalmic gel-forming solution versus timolol ophthalmic solution in adults with open-angle glaucoma or ocular hypertension: a six-month, double-masked, multicenter study. Clin Ther 2001;23(3):440–50.

[5] Vanderrest M, Dublet B, Champliaud MF. Fibril-associated collagens. Biomaterials 1990;11(1):28–31.

[6] Pachence JM. Collagen-based devices for soft tissue repair. J Appl Biomater 1996;33(1): 35–40.

[7] Tanzer ML, Kimura S. Phylogenetic aspects of collagen structure and function. Collagen 1988; M. E. Nimni. Boca Raton, FL, CRC Press. 2: 55–98.

[8] Anselme K, Bacques C, Charriere G, Hartmann DJ, Herbage D, Garrone R. Tissue reaction to subcutaneous implantation of a collagen sponge—a histological, ultrastructural, and immunological study. J Biomed Mater Res 1990;24(6):689–703.

[9] Nimni ME, Harkness RD. Molecular structure and functions of collagen. In: N. M. E., editor. Collagen, vol. 1. Boca Raton, FL: CRC Press; 1988. p. 10–48.

[10] Pachence JM, Berg RA, Silver FH. Collagen: its place in the medical device industry. Med Device Diagn Ind 1987;9:49–55.

[11] Silver FH, Pins G. Cell-growth on collagen—a review of tissue engineering using scaffolds containing extracellular-matrix. J Long Term Eff Med Implants 1992;2(1):67–80.

[12] Toolan BC, Frenkel SR, Pachence JM, Yalowitz L, Alexander H. Effects of growth-factor enhanced culture on a chondrocyte-collagen implant for cartilage repair. J Biomed Mater Res 1996;31(2):273–80.

[13] Yannas IV, Burke JF. Design of an artificial skin: basic design principles. J Biomed Mater Res 1980;14(1):65–81.

[14] Yannas IV, Burke JF, Gordon PL, Huang C, Rubenstein RH. Design of an artificial skin: control of chemical composition. J Biomed Mater Res 1980;14(2):107–31.

[15] Burke JF, Yannas IV, Quinby WC, Bondoc CC, Jung WK. Successful use of a physiologically acceptable artificial skin in the treatment of extensive burn injury. Ann Surg 1981;194(4):413.

[16] Dagalakis N, Flink J, Stasikelis P, Burke JF, Yannas IV. Design of an artificial skin: control of pore structure. J Biomed Mater Res 1980;14(4):511–28.

[17] Heimbach D, Luterman A, Burke J, Cram A, Herndon D, Hunt J, et al. Artificial dermis for major burns—a multi-center randomized clinical-trial. Ann Surg 1988;208(3):313–20.

[18] Chen GP, Sato T, Tanaka J, Tateishi T. Preparation of a biphasic scaffold for osteochondral tissue engineering. Mater Sci Eng C-Biomim Supramol Syst 2006;26(1):118–23.

[19] Hsu SH, Chang SH, Yen HJ, Whu SW, Tsai CL, Chen DC. Evaluation of biodegradable polyesters modified by type II collagen and Arg-Gly-Asp as tissue engineering scaffolding materials for cartilage regeneration. Artif Organs 2006;30(1):42–55.

[20] He W, Ma ZW, Yong T, Teo WE, Ramakrishna S. Fabrication of collagen-coated biodegradable polymer nanofiber mesh and its potential for endothelial cells growth. Biomaterials 2005;26(36):7606–15.

[21] He W, Yong T, Teo WE, Ma Z, Ramakrishna S. Fabrication and endothelialization of collagen-blended biodegradable polymer nanofibers: Potential vascular graft for blood vessel tissue engineering. Tissue Eng 2005;11 (9–10):1574–88.

[22] Venugopal J, Zhang YZ, Ramakrishna S. Fabrication of modified and functionalized polycaprolactone nanofiber scaffolds for vascular tissue engineering. Nanotechnology 2005;16(10):2138–42.

[23] Murray MM, Spindler KP, Ballard P, Welch TP, Zurakowski D, Nanney LB. Enhanced histologic repair in a central wound in the anterior cruciate ligament with a collagen-platelet-rich plasma scaffold. J Orthop Res 2007;25(8):1007–17.

[24] Butler DL, Juncosa-Melvin N, Boivin GP, Galloway MT, Shearn JT, Gooch C, et al. Functional tissue engineering for tendon repair: A multidisciplinary strategy using mesenchymal stem cells, bioscaffolds, and mechanical stimulation. J Orthop Res 2008;26 (1):1–9.

[25] Tabata Y, Ikada Y. Protein release from gelatin matrices. Adv Drug Deliv Rev 1998;31 (3):287–301.

[26] Kawai K, Suzuki S, Tabata Y, Ikada Y, Nishimura Y. Accelerated tissue regeneration through incorporation of basic fibroblast growth factor-impregnated gelatin microspheres into artificial dermis. Biomaterials 2000;21(5):489–99.

[27] Balakrishnan B, Jayakrishnan A. Self-crosslinking biopolymers as injectable in situ forming biodegradable scaffolds. Biomaterials 2005;26(18):3941–51.

[28] Yamada K, Tabata Y, Yamamoto K, Miyamoto S, Nagata I, Kikuchi H, et al. Potential efficacy of basic fibroblast growth

factor incorporated in biodegradable hydrogels for skull bone regeneration. J Neurosurg 1997; 86(5):871–5.

[29] Yamamoto M, Ikada Y, Tabata Y. Controlled release of growth factors based on biodegradation of gelatin hydrogel. J Biomater Sci Polym Ed 2001;12(1):77–88.

[30] Faury G. Function-structure relationship of elastic arteries in evolution: from microfibrils to elastin and elastic fibers. Pathol Biol (Paris) 2001;49(4):310–25.

[31] Martyn CN, Greenwald SE. A hypothesis about a mechanism for the programming of blood pressure and vascular disease in early life. Clin Exp Pharmacol Physiol 2001;28(11): 948–51.

[32] Urry DW, Pattanaik A, Xu J, Woods TC, McPherson DT, Parker TM. Elastic protein-based polymers in soft tissue augmentation and generation. J Biomater Sci Polym Ed 1998;9(10):1015–48.

[33] Nimni ME, Myers D, Ertl D, Han B. Factors which affect the calcification of tissue-derived bioprostheses. J Biomed Mater Res 1997;35(4):531–7.

[34] Mithieux SM, Rasko JEJ, Weiss AS. Synthetic elastin hydrogels derived from massive elastic assemblies of self-organized human protein monomers. Biomaterials 2004; 25(20):4921–7.

[35] Yamauchi K, Yamauchi A, Kusunoki T, Kohda A, Konishi Y. Preparation of stable aqueous solution of keratins, and physiochemical and biodegradational properties of films. J Biomed Mater Res 1996;31(4):439–44.

[36] Fujii T, Ogiwara D, Arimoto M. Convenient procedures for human hair protein films and properties of alkaline phosphatase incorporated in the film. Biol Pharm Bull 2004;27(1):89–93.

[37] Lin YC, Ramadan M, Van Dyke M, Kokai LE, Philips BJ, Rubin JP, et al. Keratin Gel Filler for Peripheral Nerve Repair in a Rodent Sciatic Nerve Injury Model. Plast Reconstr Surg 2012;129(1):67–78.

[38] Minoura N, Aiba SI, Higuchi M, Gotoh Y, Tsukada M, Imai Y. Attachment and growth of fibroblast cells on silk fibroin. Biochem Biophys Res Commun 1995;208(2):511–6.

[39] Wang Y, Rudym DD, Walsh A, Abrahamsen L, Kim HJ, Kim HS, et al. In vivo degradation of three-dimensional silk fibroin scaffolds. Biomaterials 2008;29(24–25):3415–28.

[40] Min BM, Jeong L, Lee KY, Park WH. Regenerated silk fibroin nanofibers: water vapor-induced structural changes and their effects on the behavior of normal human cells. Macromol Biosci 2006;6:285–92.

[41] Okamoto Y, Watanabe M, Miyatake K, Morimoto M, Shigemasa Y, Minami S. Effects of chitin/chitosan and their oligomers/monomers on migrations of fibroblasts and vascular endothelium. Biomaterials 2002;23(9): 1975–9.

[42] Park KE, Jung SY, Lee SJ, Min BM, Park WH. Biomimetic nanofibrous scaffolds: preparation and characterization of chitin/silk fibroin blend nanofibers. Int J Biol Macromol 2006;38(3–5):165–73.

[43] Kreis T, Vale R. Guidebook to the extracellular matrix, anchor, and adhesion proteins. 2nd ed. New York, NY: Oxford University Press; 1999.

[44] Alberts B, Johnson A, Lewis J, Raff M, Roberts K, Walter P. Molecular biology of the cell. 4th ed. New York: Garland Science; 2002.

[45] Gerard C, Catuogno C, Amargier-Huin C, Grossin L, Hubert P, Gillet P, et al. The effect of alginate, hyaluronate and hyaluronate derivatives biomaterials on synthesis of non-articular chondrocyte extracellular matrix. J Mater Sci-Mater Med 2005;16(6):541–51.

[46] Hahn SK, Hoffman AS. Preparation and characterization of biocompatible polyelectrolyte complex multilayer of hyaluronic acid and poly-L-lysine. Int J Biol Macromol 2005;37(5): 227–31.

[47] Allison DD, Grande-Allen KJ. Review. Hyaluronan: a powerful tissue engineering tool. Tissue Eng 2006;12(8):2131–40.

[48] O'Brien FJ, Harley BA, Yannas IV, Gibson LJ. The effect of pore size on cell adhesion in collagen-GAG scaffolds. Biomaterials 2005; 26(4):433–41.

[49] Nicol A, Gowda DC, Urry DW. Cell Adhesion and growth on synthetic elastomeric matrices containing Arg-Gly-Asp-Ser$_3$. J Biomed Mater Res 1992;26(3):393–413.

[50] Urry D. Elastic biomolecular machines. Sci Am 1995;64–9.

[51] Cappello J. Genetic production of synthetic protein polymers. MRS Bulletin 1992;17:48–53.

[52] Anderson JP, Cappello J, Martin DC. Morphology and primary crystal structure of a silk-like protein polymer synthesized by genetically engineered E. coli bacteria. Biopolymers 1994;34(8):1049–58.

[53] Tirrell JG, Fournier MJ, Mason TL, Tirrel DA. Biomolecular materials. Chem Eng News 1994;72(51):40–51.

[54] van Hest JCM, Tirrell DA. Protein-based materials, toward a new level of structural control. Chem Commun 2001;19:1897–904.

[55] Krejchi MT, Atkins ED, Waddon AJ, Fournier MJ, Mason TL, Tirrell DA. Chemical sequence control of beta-sheet assembly in macromolecular crystals of periodic polypeptides. Science 1994;265(5177):1427–32.

[56] Hubbell JA. Biomaterials in tissue engineering. Biotechnology 1995;13(6):565–76.

[57] Panitch A, Yamaoka T, Maurille JF, Thomas LM, David AT. Design and biosynthesis of elastin-like artificial extracellular matrix proteins containing periodically spaced fibronectin CS5 domains. Macromolecules 1999; 32(5):1701–3.

[58] OSullivan AC. Cellulose: the structure slowly unravels. Cellulose 1997;4(3):173–207.

[59] Bosch T, Schmidt B, Samtleben W, Gurland HJ. Biocompatibility and clinical performance of a new modified cellulose membrane. Clin Nephrol 1986;26:S22–9.

[60] Princi E, Vicini S, Pedemontea E, Gentileb G, Coccab M, Martuscellib E. Synthesis and mechanical characterisation of cellulose based textiles grafted with acrylic monomers. Eur Polym J 2006;42(1):51–60.

[61] Miyamoto T, Takahashi S, Ito H, Inagaki H, Noishiki Y. Tissue biocompatibility of cellulose and its derivatives. J Biomed Mater Res 1989;23(1):125–33.

[62] Hayashi T. Biodegradable polymers for biomedical uses. Prog Polym Sci 1994;19(4):663–702.

[63] Bodin A, Concaro S, Brittberg M, Gatenholm P. Bacterial cellulose as a potential meniscus implant. J Tissue Eng Regen Med 2007;1(5):406–8.

[64] Svensson A, Nicklasson E, Harrah T, Panilaitis B, Kaplan DL, Brittberg M, et al. Bacterial cellulose as a potential scaffold for tissue engineering of cartilage. Biomaterials 2005;26(4):419–31.

[65] Helenius G, Backdahl H, Bodin A, Nannmark U, Gatenholm P, Risberg B. In vivo biocompatibility of bacterial cellulose. J Biomed Mater Res Part A 2006;76A(2):431–8.

[66] Funami T, Kataoka Y, Omoto T, Goto Y, Asai I, Nishinari K. Food hydrocolloids control the gelatinization and retrogradation behavior of starch. 2b. Functions of guar gums with different molecular weights on the retrogradation behavior of corn starch. Food Hydrocolloids 2005;19(1):25–36.

[67] Mano JF, Reis RL. Osteochondral defects: present situation and tissue engineering approaches. J Tissue Eng Regen Med 2007; 1(4):261–73.

[68] Grunder T, Gaissmaier C, Fritz J, Stoop R, Hortschansky P, Mollenhauer J, et al. Bone morphogenetic protein (BMP)-2 enhances the expression of type II collagen and aggrecan in chondrocytes embedded in alginate beads. Osteoarthritis Cartilage 2004;12(7): 559–67.

[69] Rowley JA, Madlambayan G, Mooney DJ. Alginate hydrogels as synthetic extracellular matrix materials. Biomaterials 1999;20(1): 45–53.

[70] Zimmermann U, Klock G, Federlin K, Hannig K, Kowalski M, Bretzel RG, et al. Production of mitogen-contamination free alginates with variable ratios of mannuronic acid to guluronic acid by free-flow electrophoresis. Electrophoresis 1992;13(5):269–74.

[71] Oliveira JT, Martins L, Picciochi R, Malafaya PB, Sousa RA, Neves NM, et al. Gellan gum: a new biomaterial for cartilage tissue engineering applications. J Biomed Mater Res Part A 2010;93A(3):852–63.

[72] Smith AM, Shelton RM, Perrie Y, Harris JJ. An initial evaluation of gellan gum as a material for tissue engineering applications. J Biomater Appl 2007;22(3):241–54.

[73] Heinegard D, Paulsson M. Proteoglycans and matrix proteins in cartilage. In: Lennarz WJ, editor. The biochemistry of glycoproteins and proteoglycans. New York, NY: Plenum Press; 1980. p. 297–328.

[74] Naeme PJ, Barry FP. The link proteans. Experimentia 1993;49:393–402.

[75] Balazs EA. Sodium hyaluronate and viscosurgery. In: Miller D, Stegmann R, editors. Healon (Sodium Hyaluronate): a guide to its

use in ophthalmic surgery. 1st ed. New York, NY: John Wiley and Sons; 1983. p. 5–28.

[76] Sung KC, Topp EM. Swelling properties of hyaluronic acid ester membranes. J Memb Sci 1994;92(2):157–67.

[77] Balazs EA, Leshchiner A. Cross-linked gels of hyaluronic acid and products containing such gels. 1986; US 4582865A.

[78] Balazs EA, Leshchiner A. Hyaluronate modified polymeric articles. 1985; US 4500676A.

[79] Weiss C, Balazs EA. Arthroscopic viscosurgery. Arthroscopy 1987;3(2):138.

[80] Urmann B, Gomel V, Jetha N. Effect of hyaluronic acid on post-operative intraperitoneal adhesion prevention in the rat model. Fertil Steril 1991;56(3):563–7.

[81] Holzman S, Connolly RJ, Schwaitzberg SD. Effect of hyaluronic acid solution on healing of bowel anastomoses. J Invest Surg 1994;7(5):431–7.

[82] Medina M, Paddock HN, Connolly RJ, Schwaitzberg SD. Novel anti-adhesion barrier does not prevent anastomotic healing in a rabbit model. J Invest Surg 1995;8(3):179–86.

[83] Turner NJ, Kielty CM, Walker MG, Canfield AE. A novel hyaluronan-based biomaterial (Hyaff-11) as a scaffold for endothelial cells in tissue engineered vascular grafts. Biomaterials 2004;25(28):5955–64.

[84] Lepidi S, Grego F, Vindigni V, Zavan B, Tonello C, Deriu GP, et al. Hyaluronan biodegradable scaffold for small-caliber artery grafting: Preliminary results in an animal model. Eur J Vasc Endovasc Surg 2006;32(4):411–7.

[85] Solchaga LA, Yoo JU, Lundberg M, Dennis JE, Huibregtse BA, Goldberg VM, et al. Hyaluronan-based polymers in the treatment of osteochondral defects. J Orthop Res 2000;18(5):773–80.

[86] Grigolo B, Lisignoli G, Piacentini A, Fiorini M, Gobbi P, Mazzotti G, et al. Evidence for redifferentiation of human chondrocytes grown on a hyaluronan-based biomaterial (HYAFF (R) 11): molecular, immunohistochemical and ultrastructural analysis. Biomaterials 2002;23(4):1187–95.

[87] Giordano C, Sanginario V, Ambrosio L, Silvio LD, Santin M. Chemical-physical characterization and in vitro preliminary biological assessment of hyaluronic acid benzyl ester-hydroxyapatite composite. J Biomater Appl 2006;20(3):237–52.

[88] Sanginario V, Ginebra MP, Tanner KE, Planell JA, Ambrosio L. Biodegradable and semi-biodegradable composite hydrogels as bone substitutes: morphology and mechanical characterization. J Mater Sci-Mater Med 2006;17(5):447–54.

[89] Kaplan DL, Wiley BJ, Mayer JM, Arcidiacono S, Keith J, Lombardi SJ, et al. Biosynthetic polysaccharides. Biomedical polymers. 1st ed. Munich Vienna New York: Hanser Publishers; 1994; 189–212.

[90] Taravel MN, Domard A. Relation between the physicochemical characteristics of collagen and its interactions with chitosan: I. Biomaterials 1993;14(12):930–8.

[91] Muzzarelli R, Baldassara V, Conti F, Ferrara P, Biagini G. Biological activity of chitosan: ultrastructural study. Biomaterials 1988;9(3):247–52.

[92] Wang E, Overgaard SE, Scharer JM, Bols NC, Young MM. Occlusion immobilization of hybridoma cells in chitosan. Biotechnol Tech 1988;2(2):133–6.

[93] Laleg M, Pikulik I. Wet-web strength incease by chitosan. Nordic Pulp Paper Res J 1991;6(3):99–103.

[94] Wei JC, Hudson SM, Mayer JM, Kaplan DL. A novel method for crosslinking carbohydrates. J Polym Sci 1977;30:2187–93.

[95] Malette W, Quigley M, Quigley Jr. HJ, Adickes ED. Chitosan effect in vascular surgery, tissue culture and tissue regeneration. In: Muzzarelli R, Jeuniaux C, Gooday G, editors. Chitin in nature and technology. 1st ed. New York, NY: Plenum Press; 1986. p. 435–42.

[96] Hirano S. Chitosan wound dressings. In: Skjak-Braek G, Anthonsen T, Sandford P, editors. Chitin and Chitosan. London, England: Elsevier; 1989. p. 1–835.

[97] Sandford PA. Chitosan chemistry. In: Skjak-Braek G, Anthonsen T, Sandford P, editors. Chitin and Chitosan. London, England: Elsevier; 1989. p. 51–69.

[98] Byrom D. Chitosan and chitosan derivatives. In: Byron D, editor. Biomaterials: novel materials from biological sources. New York, NY: Stockton Press; 1991. p. 333–59.

[99] Madihally SV, Matthew HWT. Porous chitosan scaffolds for tissue engineering. Biomaterials 1999;20(12):1133–42.

[100] Bini TB, Gao SJ, Wang S, Ramakrishna S. Development of fibrous biodegradable polymer conduits for guided nerve regeneration. J Mater Sci Mater Med 2005;16(4):367–75.

[101] Huang YC, Huang YY, Huang CC, Liu HC. Manufacture of porous polymer nerve conduits through a lyophilizing and wire-heating process. J Biomed Mater Res Part B-Appl Biomater 2005;74B(1):659–64.

[102] East GC, McIntyre JE, Qin Y. Medical use of chitosan. In: Skjak-Braek G, Anthonsen T, Sandford P, editors. Chitin and Chitosan. London, England: Elsevier; 1989. p. 757–64.

[103] Dawes EA, Senior PJ. The role and regulation of energy reserve polymers in microorganisms. Adv Microb Physiol 1973;10:135–266.

[104] Miller ND, Williams DF. On the biodegradation of poly-b-hydroxybutyrate (PHB) homopolymer and poly-b-hydroxybutyrate-hydroxyvalerate copolymers. Biomaterials 1987;8(2):129–37.

[105] Gogolewski S, Jovanovic M, Perren SM, Dillon JG, Hughes MK. Tissue response and in vivo degradation of selected polyhydroxyacids: Polylactides (PLA), poly (3-hydroxybutyrate) (PHB), and poly(3-hydroxybutyrate-co-3-hydroxyvalerate) (PHB/VA). J Biomed Mater Res 1993;27(9):1135–48.

[106] Holland SJ, Jolly AM, Yasin M, Tighe BJ. Polymers for biodegradable medical devices II. Hydroxybutyrate- hydroxyvalerate copolymers: hydrolytic degradation studies. Biomaterials 1987;8(4):289–95.

[107] Yasin M, Holland SJ, Jolly AM, Tighe BJ. Polymers for biodegradable medical devices VI. Hydroxybutyrate-hydroxyvalerate copolymers: accelerated degradation of blends with polysaccharides. Biomaterials 1989;10(6):400–12.

[108] Doi Y, Kanesawa Y, Kunioka M, Saito T. Biodegradation of microbial copolyesters: Poly(3-hydroxybutyrate-co-3-hydroxyvalerate) and poly(3-hydroxybutyrate-co-4-hydroxyvalerate). Macromolecules 1990;23(1):26–31.

[109] Sodian R, Hoerstrup SP, Sperling JS, Martin DP, Daebritz S, Mayer Jr. JE, et al. Evaluation of biodegradable, three-dimensional matrices for tissue engineering of heart valves. Asaio J 2000;46(1):107–10.

[110] Ueda H, Tabata Y. Polyhydroxyalkanonate derivatives in current clinical applications and trials. Adv Drug Deliv Rev 2003;55(4):501–18.

[111] Pannier AK, Shea LD. Controlled release systems for DNA delivery. Mol Ther 2004;10(1):19–26.

[112] Bumcrot D, Manoharan M, Koteliansky V, Sah DW. RNAi therapeutics: a potential new class of pharmaceutical drugs. Nat Chem Biol 2006;2(12):711–9.

[113] Tong JC, Yao SL. Novel scaffold containing transforming growth factor-®1 DNA for cartilage tissue engineering. J Bioact Compat Polym 2007;22(2):232–44.

[114] Frazza EJ, Schmitt EE. A new absorbable suture. J Biomed Mater Res Biomed Mater Symp 1971;5(2):43–58.

[115] Rosensaft MN, Webb RL. Synthetic Polyester Surgical Articles. A. C. Company. 1981; US Patent. 4243775.

[116] Pillai CKS, Sharma CP. Review paper: absorbable polymeric surgical sutures: chemistry, production, properties, biodegradability, and performance. J Biomater Appl 2010;25(4):291–366.

[117] Helmus MN, Hubbell JA. Materials selection. Cardiovasc Pathol 1993;2(3):53S–71S.

[118] Shalaby SW, Johnson RA. Synthetic absorbable polyesters. In: Shalaby S, editor. Biomedical polymers. Munich Vienna New York: Hanser Publishers; 1994. p. 2–34.

[119] Ajioka M, Enomoto K, Suzuki K, Yamaguchi A. The basic properties of poly(lactic acid) produced by the direct condensation polymerization of lactic-acid. J Env Polym Degradation 1995;3(4):225–34.

[120] Vert M, Li SM. Bioresorbability and biocompatibility of aliphatic polyesters. J Mater Sci-Mater Med 1992;3(6):432–46.

[121] Freed LE, Grande DA, Lingbin Z, Emmanual J, Marquis JC, Langer R. Joint resurfacing using allograft chondrocytes and synthetic biodegradable polymer scaffords. J Biomed Mater Res 1994;28(8):891–9.

[122] Freed LE, Vunjak-Novakovic G, Biron RJ, Eagles DB, Lesnoy DC, Barlow SK, et al. Biodegradable polymer scaffolds for tissue engineering. Bio/Technology 1994;12(7): 689−93.

[123] Wintermantel E, Mayer J, Blum J, Eckert KL, Luscher P. Tissue engineering scaffolds using superstructures. Biomaterials 1996;17(2):83−91.

[124] Sawhney AS, Pathak CP, Hubbell JA. Bioerodible hydrogels based on photopolymerized poly(ethylene glycol)-co-poly (α-hydroxy acid) diacrylate macromers. Macromolecules 1993;26(4):581−7.

[125] Gilding DK, Reed AM. Biodegradable polymers for use in surgery—poly(glycolic)/poly (lactic acid) homo and copolymers. Polymer 1979;20(12):1459−64.

[126] Reed AM, Gilding DK. Biodegradable polymers for use in surgery—poly(glycolic)/poly (lactic acid) homo and copolymers: 2. *In vitro* degradation. Polymer 1981;22(4): 494−8.

[127] Christel P, Chabot F, Leray JL, Morin C, Vert M. Biodegradable composites for internal fixation in biomaterials. Winter GO, Gibbons DF, Pienkj H, editors. New York, NY: Wiley & Sons; 1982. p. 271−280.

[128] Leenstag JW, Pennings AJ, Bos RRM, Roxema FR, Boenng G. Resorbable materials of polyl-lactides VI. Plates and screws for internal fracture fixation. Biomaterials 1987;8(1):70−3.

[129] Vainionpaa S, Kilpukart J, Latho J, Heleverta P, Rokkanen P, Tormala P. Strength and strength retention *in vitro*, of absorbable, self-reinforced polyglycolide (PGA) rodes for fracture fixation. Biomaterials 1987;8(1):46−8.

[130] Grijpma DW, Nijenhuis AJ, Vanwijk PGT, Pennings AJ. High-impact strength as-polymerized PLLA. Polym Bull 1992;29(5): 571−8.

[131] Fambri L, Pegoretti A, Fenner R, Incardona SD, Migliaresi C. Biodegradable fibers of poly(L-lactic acid) produced by melt spinning. Polymer 1997;38(1):79−85.

[132] Pego AP, Poot AA, Grijpma DW, Feijen J. Physical properties of high molecular weight 1,3-trimethylene carbonate and D, L-lactide copolymers. J Mater Sci-Mater Med 2003;14 (9):767−73.

[133] Tsuji H, Ikada Y. Stereocomplex formation between enantiomeric poly(lactic acid)s. XI. Mechanical properties and morphology of solution-cast films. Polymer 1999;40(24): 6699−708.

[134] Fu K, Pack DW, Klibanov AM, Langer R. Visual evidence of acidic environment within degrading poly(lactic-co-glycolic acid) (PLGA) microspheres. Pharm Res 2000;17(1): 100−6.

[135] Chu CC. Degradation phenomena of 2 linear aliphatic polyester fibers used in medicine and surgery. Polymer 1985;26(4):591−4.

[136] Li SM, Garreau H, Vert M. Structure property relationships in the case of the degradation of massive aliphatic poly-(alpha-hydroxy acids) in aqueous-media. 1. Poly (DL-Lactic Acid). J Mater Sci-Mater Med 1990;1(3):123−30.

[137] Tsuji H, Ikada Y. Stereocomplex Formation between Enantiomeric Poly(Lactic Acid)S .9. Stereocomplexation from the Melt. Macromolecules 1993;26(25):6918−26.

[138] Yui N, Dijkstra PJ, Feijen J. Stereo block copolymers of L-Lactides and D-Lactides. Makromolekulare Chemie-Macromol Chem Phys 1990;191(3):481−8.

[139] Spinu M, Jackson C, Keating MY, Gardner KH. Material design in poly(lactic acid) systems: block copolymers, star homo- and copolymers, and stereocomplexes. J Macromol Sci-Pure Appl Chem 1996;A33(10): 1497−530.

[140] Tsuji H. *In vitro* hydrolysis of blends from enantiomeric poly(lactide)s Part 1. Well-stereo-complexed blend and non-blended films. Polymer 2000;41(10):3621−30.

[141] Rezwan K, Chen QZ, Blaker JJ, Boccaccini AR. Biodegradable and bioactive porous polymer/inorganic composite scaffolds for bone tissue engineering. Biomaterials 2006;27(18):3413−31.

[142] Day RM, Maquet V, Boccaccini AR, Jerome R, Forbes A. *In vitro* and *in vivo* analysis of macroporous biodegradable poly(D, L-lactide-co-glycolide) scaffolds containing bioactive glass. J Biomed Mater Res Part A 2005;75A(4):778−87.

[143] Böstman OM. Absorbable implants for the fixation of fractures. J Bone Joint Surgery 1991;73(1):148−53.

[144] Bostman O, Pihlajamaki H. Clinical biocompatibility of biodegradable orthopaedic implants for internal fixation: a review. Biomaterials 2000;21(24):2615−21.

[145] Niklason LE, Gao J, Abbott WM, Hirschi KK, Houser S, Marini R, et al. Functional arteries grown in vitro. Science 1999;284(5413): 489−93.

[146] Gong ZD, Niklason LE. Small-diameter human vessel wall engineered from bone marrow-derived mesenchymal stem cells (hMSCs). FASEB J 2008;22(6):1635−48.

[147] Dahl SLM, Kypson AP, Lawson JH, Blum JL, Strader JT, Li YL, et al. Readily available tissue-engineered vascular grafts. Sci Trans Med 2011;3(68): 68ra9

[148] Pitt CG, Chasalow FI, Hibionada YM, Klimas DM, Schindler A. Aliphatic polyesters 1. The degradation of poly-e-caprolactone in vivo. J Appl Polym Sci 1981;28 (11):3779−87.

[149] Pitt CG, Gratzl MM, Kimmel GL, Surles J, Schindler A. Aliphatic polyesters II. The degradation of poly-d, l-lactide, poly-ε-caprolactone, and their copolymer in vivo. Biomaterials 1981;2(4):215−20.

[150] Pitt CG, Hendren RW, Schindler A, Woodward SC. The enzymatic surface erosion of aliphatic polyesters. J Control Release 1984;1(1):3−14.

[151] Pitt CG. Poly-ε-caprolactone and its copolymers. In: Chasin M, Langer R, editors. Biodegradable polymers as drug delivery systems. New York, NY: Marcel Dekker; 1990. p. 71−119.

[152] Engelberg I, Kohn J. Physico-mechanical properties of degradable polymers used in medical applications: a comparative study. Biomaterials 1991;12(3):292−304.

[153] Koleske JV. Blends containing poly-ε-caprolactone and related polymers. In: Paul OR, Newman S, editors. Polymer blends. New York, NY: Academic Press; 1978. p. 369−89.

[154] Feng XD, Song CX, Chen WY. Synthesis and evaluation of biodegradable block copolymers of e-caprolactone and D, L-lactide. J Polym Sci Polym Lett Ed 1983;21(8): 593−600.

[155] Xu CY, Inai R, Kotaki M, Ramakrishna S. Aligned biodegradable nanofibrous structure: a potential scaffold for blood vessel engineering. Biomaterials 2004;25(5):877−86.

[156] Kovalevsky G, Barnhart K. Norplant and other implantable contraceptives. Clin Obstet Gynecol 2001;44(1):92−100.

[157] Heller J, Sparer RV, Zentner GM. Poly(ortho esters) for the controlled delivery of therapeutic agents. J Bioact Compat Polym 1990; 3(2):97−105.

[158] Heller J, Barr J. Poly(ortho esters)—from concept to reality. Biomacromolecules 2004;5(5):1625−32.

[159] Heller J. Synthesis and use of poly(ortho esters) for the controlled delivery of therapeutic agents. J Bioact Compat Polym 1988;3(2):97−105.

[160] Heller J, Daniels AU. Poly(ortho esters). In: Shalaby S, editor. Biomedical polymers. Munich Vienna New York: Hanser Publishers; 1994. p. 35−67.

[161] Cho NJ, Heller J. Drug delivery devices manufactured from polyorthoesters and polyorthocarbonates. 1978; US Patent 4078038.

[162] Heller J, Penhale DWH, Helwing RF. Preparation of poly(ortho esters) by the reaction of diketen acetals and polyolis. J Polym Sci (Polymer Letters Edition) 1980;18: 619−24.

[163] Santerre JP, Woodhouse K, Laroche G, Labow RS. Understanding the biodegradation of polyurethanes: from classical implants to tissue engineering materials. Biomaterials 2005;26(35):7457−70.

[164] deGroot JH, deVrijer R, Pennings AJ, Klompmaker J, Veth RP, Jansen HW. Use of porous polyurethanes for meniscal reconstruction and meniscal prostheses. Biomaterials 1996;17(2):163−73.

[165] McDevitt TC, Woodhouse KA, Hauschka SD, Murry CE, Stayton PS. Spatially organized layers of cardiomyocytes on biodegradable polyurethane films for myocardial repair. J Biomed Mater Res Part A 2003;66A(3):586−95.

[166] Guan J, Fujimoto KL, Sacks MS, Wagner WR. Preparation and characterization of highly porous, biodegradable polyurethane scaffolds for soft tissue applications. Biomaterials 2005;26(18):3961−71.

[167] Spaans CJ, Belgraver VW, Rienstra O, de Groot JH, Veth RP, Pennings AJ. Solvent-free fabrication of micro-porous polyurethane amide and polyurethane-urea scaffolds for repair and replacement of the knee-joint meniscus. Biomaterials 2000;21(23): 2453–60.

[168] Hill JW, Carothers WH. Studies of polymerizations and ring formations (XIV): a linear superpolyanhydride and a cyclic dimeric anhydride from sebacic acid. J Am Chem Soc 1932;54(4):1569–79.

[169] Conix A. Aromatic polyanhydrides, a new class of high melting fiber-forming polymers. J Polym Sci 2003;29(120):343–53.

[170] Rosen HB, Chang J, Wnek GE, Linhardt RJ, Langer R. Bioerodible polyanhydrides for controlled drug delivery. Biomaterials 1983;4(2):131–3.

[171] Domb AJ, Amselem S, et al. Polyanhydrides as carriers of drugs. In: Shalaby S, editor. Biomedical polymers. Munich Vienna New York: Hanser Publishers; 1994. p. 69–96.

[172] Laurencin C, Domb A, Langer R, Maniar M. Poly(anhydride) administration in high doses in vivo: Studies of biocompatibility and toxicology. J Biomed Mater Res 1990;24: 1463–81.

[173] Mathiowitz E, Saltzman WM, Domb A, Dor P, Langer R. Polyanhydride microspheres as drug carriers. II. Microencapsulation by solvent removal. J Appl Polym Sci 1988;35(3): 755–74.

[174] Chasin M, Domb A, Ron E, Mathiowitz E, Leong K, Laurencin C, et al. Polyanhydrides as drug delivery systems. In: Chasin M, Langer R, editors. Biodegradable polymers as drug delivery systems. New York, NY: Marcel Dekker, Inc.; 1990. p. 43–69.

[175] Langer R. Novel drug delivery systems. Chem Britain 1990;26(3):232–6.

[176] Anderson JM, Spilizewski KL, Hiltner A. Poly-α-amino acids as biomedical polymers. In: Williams DF, editor. Biocompatibility of tissue analogs, vol. 1. Boca Raton, FL: CRC Press Inc.; 1985. p. 67–88.

[176a] Scopelianos AG. Polyphosphazenes as new biomaterials. In: Shalaby S, editor. Biomedical polymers. Munich Vienna New York: Hanser Publishers; 1994. p. 153–71.

[177] Allcock HR. Polyphosphazenes as new biomedical and bioactive materials. In: Chasin M, Langer R, editors. Biodegradable polymers as drug delivery systems. New York, NY: Marcel Dekker; 1990. p. 163–93.

[178] Crommen JHL, Schacht EH, et al. Biodegradable polymers. II. Degradation characteristics of hydrolysis-sensitive poly [(organo)phosphazenes]. Biomaterials 1992; 13(9):601–11.

[179] Laurencin CT, Norman ME, Elgendy HM, el-Amin SF, Allcock HR, Pucher SR, et al. Use of polyphosphazenes for skeletal tissue regeneration. J Biomed Mater Res 1993;27(7):963–73.

[180] Singh A, Krogman NR, Sethuraman S, Nair LS, Sturgeon JL, Brown PW, et al. Effect of side group chemistry on the properties of biodegradable L-alanine cosubstituted polyphosphazenes. Biomacromolecules 2006;7(3): 914–8.

[181] Allcock HR, Kwon S. An ionically-crosslinkable polyphosphazene: Poly[bis-(carboxylatophenoxy)phosphazene] and its hydrogels and membranes. Macromolecules 1989;22(1):75–9.

[182] Bamford CH, Elliot A, Hanby WE. Synthetic polypeptides—preparation, structure and properties. In: Hutchinson E, editor. Physical chemistry—a series of monographs. New York, NY: Academic Press; 1956. p. 5.

[183] Aiba S, Minoura N, Fujiwara Y, Yamada S, Nakagawa T. Laminates composed of polypeptides and elastomers as a burn wound covering. Physicochemical properties. Biomaterials 1985;6(5):290–6.

[184] McCormick-Thomson LA, Duncan R. Poly (amino acid) copolymers as a potential soluble drug delivery system. 1. Pinocytic uptake and lysosomal degradation measured in vitro. J Bioact Compat Polym 1989;4(3): 242–51.

[185] Campbell P, Glover GI, Gunn JM. Inhibition of intracellular protein degradation by pepstatin, poly(L-lysine) and pepstatinyl-poly(L-lysine). Arch Biochem Biophys 1980;203(2): 676–80.

[186] van Heeswijk WAR, Hoes CJT, Stoffer T, Eenink MJD, Potman W, Feijen J. The

synthesis and characterization of polypeptide-adriamycin conjugates and its complexes with adriamycin. Part 1. J Control Release 1985;1(4):301−15.
[187] Masuko T, Iwasaki N, Yamane S, Funakoshi T, Majima T, Minami A, et al. Chitosan-RGDSGGC conjugate as a scaffold material for musculoskeletal tissue engineering. Biomaterials 2005;26(26):5339−47.
[188] Yang F, Williams CG, Wang DA, Lee H, Manson PN, Elisseeff J. The effect of incorporating RGD adhesive peptide in polyethylene glycol diacrylate hydrogel on osteogenesis of bone marrow stromal cells. Biomaterials 2005;26(30):5991−8.
[189] Lescure F, Gurny R, Doelker E, Pelaprat ML, Bichon D, Anderson JM. Acute histopathological response to a new biodegradable, polypeptidic polymer for implantable drug delivery system. J Biomed Mater Res 1989;23(11):1299−313.
[190] James K, Kohn J. Pseudo-poly(amino acid)s: examples for synthetic materials derived from natural metabolites. In: Park K, editor. Controlled drug delivery: challenges and strategies. Washington, DC: American Chemical Society; 1997. p. 389−403.
[191] Kemnitzer J, Kohn J. Degradable polymers derived from the amino acid L-tyrosine. In: Domb AJ, Kost J, Wiseman DM, editors. Handbook of biodegradable polymers, vol. 7. Amsterdam, The Netherlands: Harwood Academic Publishers; 1997. p. 251−72.
[192] Kohn J, Langer R. A new approach to the development of bioerodible polymers for controlled release applications employing naturally occurring amino acids. Polym Mater, Sci Eng 1984;51:119−21. Washington, DC, American Chemical Society
[193] Kohn J, Langer R. Non-peptide poly(amino acids) for biodegradable drug delivery systems. In: Peppas NA, Haluska RJ, editors. 12th International symposium on controlled release of bioactive materials, Geneva, Switzerland. Lincolnshire, IL: Controlled Release Society; 1985. p. 51−2.
[194] Kohn J, Langer R. Polymerization reactions involving the side chains of a-L-amino acids. J Am Chem Soc 1987;109(3):817−20.
[195] Ertel SI, Kohn J. Evaluation of a series of tyrosine-derived polycarbonates as degradable biomaterials. J Biomed Mater Res 1994;28(8):919−30.
[196] Fiordeliso J, Bron S, Kohn J. Design, synthesis, and preliminary characterization of tyrosine-containing polyarylates: new biomaterials for medical applications. J Biomater Sci Polym Ed 1994;5(6):497−510.
[197] Yu-Kwon H, Langer R. Pseudopoly(amino acids): a study of the synthesis and characterization of poly(trans-4-hydroxy-N-acyl-L-proline esters). Macromolecules 1989;22(8): 3250−5.
[198] Zhou QX, Kohn J. Preparation of poly(L-serine ester): A structural analogue of conventional poly(L-serine). Macromolecules 1990; 23(14):3399−406.
[199] Pulapura S, Li C, Kohn J. Structure-property relationships for the design of polyiminocarbonates. Biomaterials 1990;11(9):666−78.
[200] Pulapura S, Kohn J. Tyrosine derived polycarbonates: Backbone modified, "pseudo"-poly(amino acids) designed for biomedical applications. Biopolymers 1992;32(4): 411−7.
[201] Joy MB, Dodgson KS, Olavesen AH, Gacesa P. The purification and some properties of Pig-Liver hyaluronidase. Biochimica Et Biophysica Acta 1985;838(2):257−63.
[202] Ferreira L, Gil MII, Cabrita AM, Dordick JS. Biocatalytic synthesis of highly ordered degradable dextran-based hydrogels. Biomaterials 2005;26(23):4707−16.
[203] Shin H, Nichol JW, Khademhosseini A. Cell adhesive and mechanically tunable glucose-based biodegradable hydrogels. Acta Biomaterialia 2011;7(1):106−14.
[204] Patenaude M, Hoare T. Injectable, mixed natural-synthetic polymer hydrogels with modular properties. Biomacromolecules 2012;13(2):369−78.
[205] Kundu J, Poole-Warren LA, Martens P, Kundu SC. Silk fibroin/poly(vinyl alcohol) photocrosslinked hydrogels for delivery of macromolecular drugs. Acta Biomaterialia 2012;8(5):1720−9.
[206] Curtis A, Riehle M. Tissue engineering: the biophysical background. Phys Med Biol 2001;46(4):R47−65.
[207] Li ST, Archibald SJ, Krarup C, Madison RD. Peripheral nerve repair with collagen conduits. Clin Mater 1992;9(3-4):195−200.

[208] Tang X, Xue C, Wang Y, Ding F, Yang Y, Gu X. Bridging peripheral nerve defects with a tissue-engineered nerve graft composed of an *in vitro* cultured nerve equivalent and a silk fibroin-based scaffold. Biomaterials 2012;33(15):3860–7.

[209] van Swol RL, Ellinger R, Pfeifer J, Barton NE, Blumenthal N. Collagen membrane barrier therapy to guide regeneration in class II furcations in humans. J Periodontol 1993;64(7):622–9.

[210] Parenteau N. Skin: the first tissue-engineered products. Sci Am 1999;280(4):83–4.

[211] Sullivan SJ, Maki T, Borland KM, Mahoney MD, Solomon BA, Muller TE, et al. Biohybrid artificial pancrease: long-term implantation studies in diabetic, pancreatectomized dogs. Science 1991;252(5006): 718–21.

[212] Chang TMS. Artificial liver support based on artificial cells with emphasis on encapsulated hepatocytes. Artificial Organs 1992;16(1):71–4.

[213] Lacy PE. Treating diabetes with transplanted cells. Sci Am 1995;51–8.

[214] Temenoff JS, Mikos AG. Injectable biodegradable materials for orthopedic tissue engineering. Biomaterials 2000;21(23):2405–12.

[215] Lee CC, MacKay JA, Fréchet JMJ, Szoka FC. Designing dendrimers for biological applications. Nat Biotechnol 2005;23(12): 1517–26.

[216] Langer R, Vacanti J. Tissue Engineering. Science 1993;260(5110):920–6.

[217] Fenkel SR, Toolan B, Menche D, Pitman MI, Pachence JM. Chondrocyte transplantation using a collagen bilayer matrix for cartilage repair. J Bone Joint Surgery (British Volume) 1997;79(5):831–6.

[218] Hodde J. Naturally occurring scaffolds for soft tissue repair and regeneration. Tissue Eng 2002;8(2):295–308.

[219] Salem AK, Stevens R, Pearson RG, Davies MC, Tendler SJ, Roberts CJ, et al. Interactions of 3T3 fibroblasts and endothelial cells with defined pore features. J Biomed Mater Res 2002;61(2):212–7.

[220] Borden M, El-Amin SF, Attawia M, Laurencin CT. Structural and human cellular assessment of a novel microsphere-based tissue-engineered scaffold for bone repair. Biomaterials 2003;24(4): 597–609.

[221] Lin ASP, Barrows TH, Cartmell SH, Guldberg RE. Microarchitectural and mechanical characterization of oriented porous polymer scaffolds. Biomaterials 2003;24(3):481–9.

[222] Ikada Y, Jamshidi K, Tsuji H, Hyon SH. Stereocomplex formation between enantiomeric poly(lactides). Macromolecules 1987; 20(4):904–6.

14 Regulations for Medical Devices and Application to Plastics Suppliers: History and Overview

Vinny R. Sastri

OUTLINE

14.1 History and Introduction	337	14.4.3 Australia	343
14.2 United States Regulations	338	14.4.4 India	344
14.2.1 FDA Master Files	340	14.4.5 South America	344
14.3 ISO 13485 (European and Global Standard)	340	14.5 Global Harmonization Task Force (GHTF)	344
14.3.1 European Union Medical Device Directive	341	14.6 Applicability of the Regulations to Material Suppliers	345
14.4 Other Countries	343	14.7 Conclusion	345
14.4.1 Japan	343	References	346
14.4.2 China	343		

14.1 History and Introduction

Over the past 2000 years, many devices have been developed and used in the mitigation and diagnosis of diseases. The materials used in these devices have ranged from stone, wood, metal, ceramics, and most recently plastics. Medical devices have also evolved in sophistication and complexity over time. With the formalization of the scientific method in the seventeenth century such devices became more prevalent [1]. Many medical devices were manufactured by doctors or small companies and sold directly to the public with no government standards or oversight. With the explosion of medical technology in the early twentieth century, several intermediaries had evolved between the medical device industry and the public. In 1879, Dr E.R. Squibb, in an address to the Medical Society of the State of New York, proposed the enactment of a national statute to regulate food and drugs [2]. It was not until 27 years later that the Food and Drug Act of 1906 was introduced into the Congress and signed into law by President Theodore Roosevelt [3]. At that time, devices that were harmful to human safety and health proliferated the market but regulation of medical devices by the Bureau of Chemistry (the precursor to the Food and Drug Administration—FDA) was limited to challenging commercial products only *after* they had been released into the market. Devices in the marketplace that were defective, adulterated, or misbranded were seized and the device manufacturers were prosecuted in a court of law, but only *after* the products were sold in the market and caused harm to the end users. Thus, there was a strong need for regulating the devices *before* they entered the marketplace. An FDA report [4], issued in September 1970, detailed as many as 10,000 injuries and 731 deaths from ineffective medical devices. The report recommended the formation of a regulatory system and body that would enforce the production and sale of safe and effective devices to the public. All medical devices already on the market would be inventoried and classified into a three-tiered system based on their criticality of end use. It also detailed requirements for records and reports, registration and inspection of establishments, and uniform quality assurance programs called good manufacturing practices (GMP). After much lobbying by the FDA, Senate bill SR 510,

"The Medical Device Amendments of 1973" was introduced by Senator Edward M. Kennedy and was passed by the Senate in 1975. House bill HR 11124, introduced by Representative Paul Rogers, was passed by the House in 1976. These bills eventually became the Medical Device Amendments of 1976, and were signed into law by President Nixon. The Medical Device Amendments of 1976 became the basis for the medical device regulation in the United States to control and regulate the production of finished devices and thus the device manufacturers themselves.

The GMP requirements for medical devices came into effect on December 18, 1978. This regulation was designed to specify general requirements for all manufacturers as well as special requirements for what were termed "critical devices." Yet, between 1978 and 1990 a number of studies and data from recalls of medical devices [5,6] indicated that a significant number of recalls were due to improper, faulty, or ineffective designs. On November 28, 1990, Congress passed the Safe Medical Device Act (SMDA), providing the FDA with the authority to add pre-production design controls to the GMP regulation. This meant that device manufacturers would need to have controls over their design and development processes including strict controls of the raw materials and components used to manufacture the finished device. It also incorporated a provision to include the oversight of foreign countries selling products into the United States. Quality System Regulation 21 CFR Parts 820 [7] was then drafted. Efforts were made to harmonize this regulation with both the ISO 9001:1994 entitled "Quality systems: Model for quality assurance in design, development, production, installation and servicing" and with ISO 13485:1996 entitled "Quality Systems—Medical Devices—Particular requirements for the application of ISO 9001." This new regulation removed the term "critical devices" and allowed manufacturers to tailor their quality systems commensurate with the risk associated with their device during end use. For example, an implantable device will need more stringent (design, development, and production) controls compared to a simple tongue depressor and these will differ in the level of detail and complexity of their respective quality system requirements.

The purpose of the regulations is to ensure that manufacturers of medical devices have the appropriate procedures and processes in place to design, develop, and produce consistent, safe, and effective devices for their intended use. The regulations are a framework for manufacturers and are flexible enough to allow them to formulate and implement those parts of the regulation that are applicable to their products and processes and the risk of their products.

14.2 United States Regulations

The design, development, production, distribution, and use of medical devices in the United States of America are regulated by the Federal Drug and Cosmetics Act in the Code of Federal Regulations (CFR)—21 CFR Parts 820 [7]. This regulation is entitled "The Quality System Regulation." To sell medical devices in the United States of America, all (domestic or international) finished medical device manufacturers must register with the Federal Drug Administration (FDA), must be willing to comply with the regulation, and must be willing to let the FDA inspect their facilities.

The intent of 21 CFR Parts 820 is that "quality must be designed and built into components through the application of proper quality systems" [8]. The regulation requires that medical device manufacturers establish and implement an appropriate quality system that encompasses the design, manufacture, packaging, labeling, storage, installation, and servicing of the finished device intended for commercial use and distribution in the United States. Effective quality systems will ensure that manufacturers are in a "state of control" and produce consistent, safe, and effective devices for their intended use. The FDA monitors and inspects the complaints, data, and records from both end users and manufacturers to track and determine the safety and efficacy of a device.

Table 14.1 details the various sections of the regulation with a brief description of each section. This regulation pays particular attention to the design controls that were added to the latest (1997) version.

Suppliers of raw materials or components do not have to comply with the regulations, but are subject to the *purchasing controls* of the regulations. Finished device manufacturers must establish procedures and controls with their suppliers for essential raw materials that include quality metrics, material performance and purity specifications, assurance of supply, and notification of any formulation or process changes.

Table 14.1 FDA 21 CFR Part 820 and Its Subsystems

Section	Title	Description
Subpart A	General requirements	Defines the scope and applicability requirements for the quality system. Who needs to comply?
Subpart B	Quality System requirements	Outlines the methods of formulating, implementing an effective quality system via management reviews, quality audits, and appropriate personnel.
Subpart C	Design controls	Describes the process and controls during the various stages in design and development of a medical device from design inputs, design outputs, design verification and validation, design reviews, and effective design transfers.
Subpart D	Document controls	Review, approval, retention, accuracy, and accessibility of appropriate documents.
Subpart E	Purchasing controls	Controls and processes all raw materials, components, products, and services.
Subpart F	Identification and traceability	Documentation and process to identify and trace incoming, in process, and finished device products and components, especially those of high-risk devices.
Subpart G	Production and process controls	The development, monitoring, and control of all processes used in production of the finished device.
Subpart H	Acceptance activities	Establishing and using acceptance criteria for the control of incoming, in-process and finished device performance, quality, and consistency.
Subpart I	Nonconforming product	Developing and implementing procedures to assess and control all products and processes that do not meet specified requirements.
Subpart J	Corrective and preventive action	Establishing and implementing procedures and processes for sustainable corrective and preventive action of identified issues.
Subpart K	Labeling and packaging	Ensuring that there are procedures and processes in place to include the requirements, design, production, and control of device packaging and labeling into the quality system.
Subpart L	Handling, storage, distribution, and installation	Having procedures for the handling and storage of all incoming, in-process, and finished device products. Ensuring proper distribution procedures for finished devices and if applicable, procedures and processes for the installation of finished devices at the end user's facility.
Subpart M	Records	Documents specific to this regulation include the Design History File (DHF), the Device Master Record (DMR), the Device History Record (DHR), and complaint files.
Subpart N	Servicing	If needed, maintenance and servicing procedures and processes must be included to continue and to ensure safety and efficacy of devices at the end user.
Subpart O	Statistical techniques	The regulation encourages the use of statistical techniques (like sampling, data analysis, design of experiments) where appropriate.

14.2.1 FDA Master Files

For the submission of a Premarket Approval (PMA) [9], a 510(k) [10] for substantially equivalent devices or an Investigational Device Exemption (IDE) [11] a finished device manufacturer submits an application to the FDA containing substantive data of the finished device including performance, chemical resistance, biocompatibility, toxicity, and clinical data. In many cases, the finished device or components are made from a supplier's product or raw materials. In order that a sound scientific evaluation may be made of the PMA, 510(k) or the IDE, a review of data and other information related to the supplier's product, facility, or manufacturing procedures is required. While suppliers may be willing to have the FDA review this information, they may not want their proprietary information in the hands of their customers (the finished device manufacturers). A system for the submission of Master Files was developed by the FDA to permit the suppliers of the materials to provide confidential product information directly to the FDA for its review without disclosing the confidential information to the customer or manufacturer. If the same raw material is used in various applications, components, or devices, only one Master File is required.

There are various types of master files depending upon the intended use.

- Device master files (MAF)—Supporting data on material used in medical devices (information for pre-manufacturing notices, 510(k)s and Investigational Device Exemptions);
- Drug Master File (DMF)—Supporting data on material used in drugs; (information for Investigational New Drug Applications (IND), New Drug Applications (NDA), and Abbreviated New Drug Applications (ANDA));
- Biologics Master Files—Supporting data for material used in applications contacting blood or blood products (information for notices of claimed Investigational Exemption for an Investigational New Drug (IND) for biologics and biologic licenses);
- Food Master Files (FMF)—Supporting data material used in food applications (information for Food Additive and Color Additive Petitions); and
- Veterinary Medicine Master Files—Supporting data for materials used in animal drug and devices (Investigational New Animal Exemptions (INAD) and New Animal Drug Applications (NADA)).

The content of a Master File includes the following:

- Company Name,
- Product Name,
- Manufacturing Address,
- Statement of Commitment,
- Product Formulation,
- Product Specification, and
- Test methods and results (physical, chemical, biocompatibility, and toxicity).

The information provided in the master file gives the device manufacturer and the FDA a level of comfort that the raw material being used in the device will pass the specific physical, chemical, biocompatibility, and toxicity tests. The FDA must be notified of any changes to the formulation and subsequent properties of the material and the Master File must be updated. Failure to notify and comply will render the finished device "adulterated" and may not be subjected for sale or use.

MAFs may be submitted for various types of operations and products and can be grouped by the following types:

- facilities and manufacturing procedures and controls;
- synthesis, formulation, purification, and specifications for chemicals, materials (e.g., an alloy, plastic, etc.), or subassemblies for a device;
- packaging materials;
- contract packaging and other manufacturing (e.g., sterilization);
- nonclinical study data; and
- clinical study data.

14.3 ISO 13485 (European and Global Standard)

The international standard for medical devices is ISO 13485:2003 entitled "Medical devices—Quality management systems—Requirements for regulatory purposes" [12]. Though geared specifically toward medical device manufacturers, the ISO 13485 standard is harmonized with ISO 9001:2000 with some differences. ISO 13485:2003 includes particular requirements for medical devices and excludes some of the requirements of ISO 9001:2000 that are not appropriate as regulatory requirements with respect to medical devices. Thus, organizations which conform to ISO 13485:2003 cannot claim that they conform to ISO 9001:2000 or vice versa unless their quality management systems conform to *all* the requirements of ISO 9001:2000. Risk management is a key part of ISO 13485 [13]. Terms like customer satisfaction and continuous improvement have been removed from this document (compared to ISO 9001:2000). The regulation consists of the sections as described in Table 14.2. An ISO technical report (ISO/TR 14699) [14] provides guidance for the application of ISO 13485.

The primary objective of the regulation is to provide harmonized guidelines to organizations so that they can consistently meet end user and regulatory requirements. Compliance with ISO 13485 is recognized as a first step in achieving compliance with European regulatory compliance. Certification of the Quality Management System allows the manufacturer to sell medical devices in the European Union.

14.3.1 European Union Medical Device Directive

There are three directives for medical devices in the European Union.

Table 14.2 ISO 13485:2003 Sections and their Descriptions

Section	Title	Description
1	Scope	Defines the scope of the regulation, describes the requirements for exclusion to design and development where appropriate, and the applicability of the regulations
2	Normative references	References ISO 9001:2000
3	Terms and definitions	Provides the terms and definitions used in the regulation
4	Quality management system	Focuses on procedures and processes for the implementation of an effective quality management system including the review, approval, and control of records and documents
5	Management responsibility	Emphasizes the involvement of management in the entire process, from customer needs, to product planning and product realization. Use of effective reviews, communication to ensure implementation and effectiveness of the quality system
6	Resource management	Ensures that there are adequate resources that include personnel, infrastructure, and the work environment
7	Product realization	A significant part of the regulation, includes product planning, product design and development, purchasing process and controls, production and service validation and controls, and, the identification and traceability of all products and components used in the production of devices
8	Measurement analysis and improvement	A separate section is devoted to the importance of good measurement systems, monitoring products and processes, controlling nonconforming products, analysis of data, and corrective and preventive action
9	Annex A	Differences between ISO 13485:2003 and ISO 13485:1996
10		Differences between ISO 13485:2003 and ISO 9001:2000
11	Bibliography	References

- The Active Implantable Medical Device (AIMD) Directive—90/385/EEC;
- The Medical Device Directive (MDD)—93/42/EEC; and
- The In Vitro Diagnostic Directive (IVD)—98/79/EC.

After June 14, 1998, medical devices could not be offered for sale in the European Union without "CE marking" and a "declaration of conformity." The letters CE stand for "Conformité Europêene" in French literally meaning "European Conformity." For many products CE marking and a declaration of conformity may only be affixed with proof of a certified quality system and/or product testing based on its end use. The quality systems certification, the CE marking, and the declaration of conformity are provided by a "Notified Body" which is an organization appointed by the national accreditation authorities and which "notifies" the European Commission to approve products covered by the Medical Devices Directive. All medical device manufacturers must designate a notified body to certify and register their products. For all classes of devices, a detailed technical file must be submitted providing objective evidence demonstrating compliance with the Medical Device Directive's essential requirements and with appropriate harmonized standards which include ISO 13485:2003 and ISO 10993 standards [8].

Products shipped must bear the CE marking to show compliance with the directive (Figure 14.1). If a Notified Body is involved in the approval, the number of the Notified Body must also appear adjacent to the CE marking.

Additionally, the product must be shipped with a Declaration of Conformity, an example of which is shown in Figure 14.2.

Documentation can include the following:

- Evidence demonstrating compliance with essential requirements detailed in the directive for the particular product's end use;
- Demonstration of design verification and validation;
- Risk assessment and analysis;
- Clinical evidence demonstrating effectiveness of the device;
- Procedures for post-market surveillance;

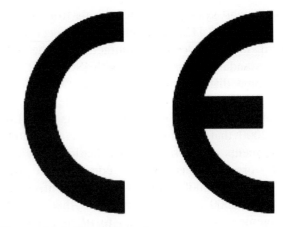

Figure 14.1 The CE mark.

EC Declaration of Conformity

Council Directive 93/42/EEC concerning medical devices

We <u>(Name and address of manufacturer)</u>

Certify that the product described is in conformity with the applicable provisions of Council Directive 93/42/EEC concerning medical devices.

<u>(Name, type or model, lot, batch or serial no. etc.)</u>

<u>(Description)</u>

<u>(Name of Responsible Person) (Signature of Responsible Person)</u>

<u>(Date)</u>

Figure 14.2 CE marking declaration of conformity.

- Complete declaration of conformity;
- Technical information of the finished device—including toxicity and biocompatibility studies;

- Accurate product identification, labels, procedures, and user instructions; and
- CE mark or label on product or packaging.

14.4 Other Countries

14.4.1 Japan

The Japanese government, through the Ministry of Health, Labor, and Welfare (MHLW), regulates all medical devices, whether manufactured in Japan or imported from other countries. In Japan, the term "medical device" is used for any instrument, apparatus, or material as designated by the Japanese government that is used in diagnosing, treating, and/or preventing diseases in humans or animals and which can be used to affect the structure and functions of humans or animals. The Pharmaceutical Affairs Law (PAL) is the primary governing law for medical devices in Japan. Medical devices must undergo thorough safety examinations and demonstrate medical efficacy before they are granted approval, or "shonin," to be sold in Japan. PAL regulations specify very detailed requirements for companies that manufacture or import medical devices for sale in Japan, ranging from infrastructure and facilities to personnel and processes. For new medical devices for which there are no equivalent products already approved in Japan or for devices that have been improved or modified that might affect device safety and efficacy, clinical trials are required. Clinical trials must be conducted to demonstrate the safety and efficacy of the product under strict Good Clinical Practice (GCP) standards, and must be followed by standard Post-Marketing Assessment (PMA) reporting and a follow-up program.

In April 2004, the Pharmaceuticals and Medical Devices Agency (PMDA) was established in an effort to create a more efficient and transparent medical device registration review process. The PMDA was formed by merging three already existing organizations: (1) the Pharmaceuticals and Medical Devices Evaluation Center (PMDEC), (2) the Organization of Pharmaceutical Safety and Research (OPSR), and (3) the Japan Association for the Advancement of Medical Equipment (JAAME). Two of these three agencies (PMDEC and JAAME) were previously involved in the medical device approval process, including the review of product registration applications and clinical trial consultations. Prior to the creation of the PMDA, the application and review process for *new* devices could take as long as 2 years. Over the next several years, the PMDA intends to shorten this process, although it has not had success in doing so thus far.

Under the New PAL, the Quality Assurance Controller will be responsible for ensuring compliance with the new Good Manufacturing Practice (GMP) requirement, based on Japan's own adaptation of ISO 13845:2003, as well as Good Quality Practice Ordinance (GQP) standards [15]. The Standard Operating Procedures (SOPs) for GQP include product storage controls, the release of products into the market, quality control at local offices, ensuring the maintenance of all quality assurance documents and reports, the handling of product recalls, and audits.

Necessary Governmental Authorizations (for sale of devices into Japan):

- Manufacturing (or import) approval ("*Shonin*") which guarantees the safety and efficacy of the device, obligatory for every product;
- Manufacturing (or import) license ("*Kyoka*") of a device, which the Japanese manufacturer and importer hold, renewable every 5 years; and
- Reimbursement listing approval.

14.4.2 China

There are two main agencies in China that regulate medical devices, the State Food and Drug Administration (SFDA) and the Department of Medical Devices. The State Food and Drug Administration (SFDA) is the Chinese equivalent of the FDA in the United States. All imported medical devices must be registered with the SFDA. The Department of Medical Devices under the SFDA is responsible for the standardization, product registration, safety, and supervision of all imported devices into China. Some of the standards used by the agency are ISO 10993 (Biologic Evaluation of Materials and Medical Devices), ISO 14971 (Risk Management), and ISO 13485 (Medical Devices—Quality Management Systems).

14.4.3 Australia

The medical device legislation has been established by the Therapeutic Goods Act 1989 as amended by the Therapeutic Goods Amendment (Medical Devices) Bill 2002 and the Therapeutic Goods (Medical Devices) Regulations 2002. The new framework also adopts the philosophies of the Global Harmonization Task Force on medical devices.

The new regulatory system has the following features:

- a device classification scheme based on different levels of risk for each class of device;
- essential principles for the quality, safety, and performance of the medical device that must be complied with before the product can be supplied;
- options as to how compliance with the essential principles can be satisfied and assessed;
- manufacturer quality systems, type testing, and design evaluation;
- the use of recognized standards to satisfy the requirements of the essential principles;
- a comprehensive post-market surveillance and adverse incident reporting program;
- appropriate regulatory controls for the manufacturing processes of medical devices;
- the continued use of the Australian Register of Therapeutic Goods as the central point of control for the legal supply of medical devices in Australia; and
- chemical, physical, and biological properties.

14.4.4 India

The Central Drugs Standards Control Organization (CDSCO) under the Ministry of Health and Family Welfare regulates the licensing, import, manufacture, and sale of medical devices into the country. Approvals can be facilitated by evidence of approval from the US FDA, the EU MDD (CE certificate), and approvals from Australia, Canada, Japan, and other countries. ISO certification for specific manufacturing facilities (ISO 13485) is also accepted. Device master files must contain details of good manufacturing practices including components and materials used in the device. It must also include the manufacturing and quality assurance processes, risk assessment, design verification, sterilization, stability, biocompatibility, and toxicological data associated with the materials and production of the finished device.

14.4.5 South America

For most companies the access point to South America is Brazil. Brazil has the second largest healthcare market in the Americas (bigger than Canada and second only to the United States). It is a member of Mercosur—the South American Free Trade Area that includes Brazil, Argentina, Uruguay, and Paraguay. Separate submissions have to be made in each country. Registration of products or product families must contain information on the manufacturer, the materials and composition used, and the intended use.

Mexico has patterned its regulations after the US FDA and ISO requirements under the Secretaría de Salud.

14.5 Global Harmonization Task Force (GHTF)

The GHTF was conceived in 1992 and is an informal grouping that was formed to respond to the growing need for the international harmonization of regulations in medical devices. The members of the GHTF include government and industry officials from the European Union, Japan, Canada, Australia, and the United States. These representatives working with medical device manufacturers and other organizations related to medical devices try to harmonize global approaches to the safety, efficacy, clinical performance, and quality of medical devices with the goal of protecting public health, promoting innovation, and facilitating international trade. Global harmonization is the aligning of the different regulatory systems of the world making them globally on par with each other to manufacture and sell safe and effective devices. The GHTF is committed to developing guidelines accepted in all GHTF countries and gives technical guidance toward a more coherent approach on the interpretation of technical and quality requirements for medical devices. It has four study groups, dealing with product approval-related issues, post-market surveillance, quality system requirements, and audits of quality systems.

14.6 Applicability of the Regulations to Material Suppliers

The regulations (FDA 21 CFR Parts 820 and ISO 13485:2003) are applicable to the manufacturers of "finished devices." Suppliers of raw materials are not expected to comply with these regulations but must meet acceptable material requirements set forth by the device manufacturers (as per their purchasing controls). Finished device or component manufacturers expect their material suppliers to have consistently good quality and process control in their facilities.

In July 1998 in the United States, the Biomaterials Access Assurance Act—BAAA (HR 872) was signed into law by President Bill Clinton. The purpose of the act was to "establish rules governing product liability actions against raw materials and bulk component suppliers to medical device manufacturers, and for other purposes" [16]. This was a very important bill, as it protects the suppliers of biomaterials or components of implanted devices from liability if an entire device results in injury or death, provided it was not the fault of the material or component. This act was in response to a very serious concern expressed by suppliers following many expensive lawsuits where it was found that the eventual cause of the problem was not with the material but with the finished device itself. Many plastics suppliers are willing to supply materials as long as their materials are used in devices that are in contact with the human body for less than 29 days (minimal contact with and minimal residence time within the body). A few plastics suppliers are willing to recommend their products for implants and devices that are in the body for more than 29 days (implantable devices) based on the extensive studies and data that show their materials pass all physical, chemical, biocompatibility, hemocompatibility, and toxicity tests required for implantable devices.

Finished device manufacturers are expected to establish purchasing controls [17], providing material suppliers with acceptance criteria and material specifications and requirements needed for their specific devices and applications. Such requirements might include the following:

- Raw material performance specifications,
- Biocompatibility,
- Sterilization requirements,
- Material purity,
- Chemical resistance,
- Toxicity requirements,
- Product quality and consistency,
- Notification of formula changes,
- Adherence to good manufacturing practices, and
- Assurance of supply.

14.7 Conclusion

The purpose of regulations for medical devices is to ensure that the products are consistent, safe, and effective for their intended use. The two major regulations are the 21 CFR Parts 820 Quality Systems Regulations enforced by the Food and Drug Administration in the United States and the global standard by the International Organization of Standards ISO 13485:2003 "Medical devices—Quality management systems—Requirements for regulatory purposes" enforced by the European Union. Most countries have adopted modified versions of the ISO 13485 and/or the FDA regulations. Finished device manufacturers need to comply with the regulations. Suppliers of raw materials and components do not need to comply with the regulations, but are subject to the purchasing controls of the finished device manufacturers. Finished device manufacturers must have stringent supplier qualification procedures that include supplier audits, incoming raw material and component specifications, and quality metrics. Plastic material suppliers must provide appropriate data and information about their products that the regulatory bodies and the finished device manufacturers can use to assess the performance and viability of the raw materials for their specific devices. This is only required for high-risk devices. Such information includes the formulation, the performance specifications, the test methods and release criteria, the quality metrics, material characteristics (physical, chemical, biocompatibility, and toxicity), the assurance of supply, and the notification of any formulation changes. This information is typically maintained by the regulatory bodies in master files, is kept confidential, and is accessible only to the regulatory bodies but not to the finished device manufacturers or the public at large.

References

[1] Estrin NF. The medical device industry. New York: CRC Press: Marcel Dekker Inc; 1990.

[2] Squibb ER. The collected papers of Edward Robinson Squibb, M.D., 1819–1900. In: Porter D, Earl R, editors. Food labeling: toward national uniformity. Washington DC, USA: National Academies Press; 1992. p. 39.

[3] Federal food and drugs act of 1906 (The "Wiley Act") Public Law Number 59–384 34 Stat. 768 (1906) 21 U.S.C. Sec 1–15 (1934) (Repealed in 1938 by 21 U.S.C. Sec 329 (a)).

[4] Study Group on Medical Devices. Medical devices: a legislative plan. Washington, D.C.: Department of Health Education and Welfare; 1970.

[5] FDA office of compliance and surveillance. Device recalls: a study of quality problems. HHS Publication FDA-90-4235: Washington DC, USA; 1990.

[6] FDA medical device regulation from premarket approval to recall—department of health and human services inspector general's study; 1990.

[7] 21 CFR Part 820—Quality Systems Regulation.

[8] 21 CFR Parts 808, 812, 820 Medical Devices; Current Good Manufacturing Practices (CGMP); Final Rule; October 7, 1996, p. 52606, response #7.

[9] Premarket Approval (PMA)—is the FDA process of scientific and regulatory review of devices "that support or sustain human life, are of substantial importance in preventing impairment of human health, or which present a potential, unreasonable risk of illness or injury."

[10] 510(k) application and submission—is the FDA scientific and regulatory approval process of devices that a manufacturer thinks is "substantially equivalent" to a similar device that was on the market prior to May 28, 1976. This is less involved than the premarket approval defined in reference 9.

[11] Investigational Device Exemption (IDE) is issued by the FDA to allow the use of investigational devices in human subjects for clinical trials and investigation in order to evaluate the safety and effectiveness of the investigational medical device.

[12] ISO 13485:2003, Medical devices—Quality management systems—Requirements for regulatory purposes.

[13] ISO 14971:2007, Medical devices—Application of risk management to medical devices.

[14] ISO/TR 14969:2004, Medical devices—Quality management systems—Guidance to the application of ISO 13485:2003.

[15] Ministerial Ordinance on Standards for Quality Assurance for Drugs, Quasi-drugs, Cosmetics, and Medical Devices MHLW. Ordinance Number 136; September 22, 2004.

[16] Public Law 105–230, sect. 1, 112 Stat. 1519 codified in 21 U.S.C. 1601–1606, 1999.

[17] Quality Management System—Medical Devices—Guidance on the Control of Products and Services Obtained from Suppliers.

Index

Note: Page numbers followed by "*f*", "*t*", and "*b*" refer to figures, tables, and boxes, respectively.

A

Abdominoplasty, 119
AbioCor, 156
Acoustic wave propagation, 258–259
4-Acryloyloxyethyl trimellitate anhydride (4-AETA), 123
Adhesives, uses
  cyanoacrylate adhesives
    benefits and limitations of, 106*t*
    polymerization reaction of, 105*f*
  cyanoacrylate monomers, structures of, 104*f*
  cyanoacrylic adhesives, 104–110
  medical/dental applications, 111–119
  in medicine and dentistry, 103–104
  natural adhesives, 104
  for skin closure, 112
  suture and tissue, 112–114
  synthetic/semisynthetic, 104
  tissue adhesives, case studies of, 112–119
Aintree intubation catheter, 199*f*
Airway evaluation
  difficult airway, predicting, 200–201
  esophageal bulb detector, 201*f*
  esophageal intubation, detection, 201–203
  homemade syringe device, 201*f*
  identifying proper position, 201–206
  supraglottic devices, 200*f*
Airway exchange catheters, 199*f*, 210
Airway resistance, 196
algC, 80–81
Alkoxysilane, 136–137
Anterior lumbar interbody fusion (ALIF), 236
Antibiofilm properties, of biomaterials, 89–91
Antibiotics, bioelectric effect, 92–94
Appendectomies, 11
Appropriate depth, confirmation of, 203–204

Artificial heart, 154–155
Artificial organs RoboticallyAssisted surgery (AORobAS) system, 184–185, 184*f*
Aryloxyphosphazenes, 321
Asclepiades, 192
ASTM Method E 2196-02, 91
Atactic polypropene, 23
Atrial fibrillation, technology, 174–175
  cryoablation, 175
  laser ablation, 175
  microwave ablation, 175
  radiofrequency used in ablation, 174–175
  ultrasound ablation, 175
Audible cuff leak, evaluation, 204–205
Autoclave sterilization, 35, 41
Automated endoscopic system for optimal positioning (AESOP)
  disadvantages for, 181
  robots replacing, 178
  Zeus system, 180–181
Automatic tube compensation (ATC), 217–218
Avalve, simplest configuration of, 166*f*

B

Bacterial adherence, 85–87
Bacterial biofilms
  extracellular polymeric substance, 78
  in orthopedic prosthetic joint infection, 87–89
  phenotypic heterogeneity, 78
  on surgical mesh, 87
  on sutures, 85–87
Bacterial counts, for contaminated lacerations, 113*t*
Bacterial infection, 266
Bacteriostatic behavior, 113
Baekeland, Leo, 3*f*
Bagby and Kuslich (BAK) technique, 233
Balloon angioplasty, 172–173
Balloon valvotomy, 164
Basic local alignment search tool (BLAST), 84–85

Berlin heart, 158
Berlin Heart Excor, 160–161
Biodegradable polymers, 33, 303–305
  biologically derived polymers, 305–314
  design/development of, 303
  selection criteria, 304–305
Bioelectric effect, 92–93
  to antibiotics, 92–94
  treating *S. epidermidis*, 92–93
Biofilm bacteria, 78
  cell-cell communication, 78
  resistance of, 79
Biofilm destruction, 266
Biofilm development, key processes, 78*f*
Biofilm formation
  nucleic acid-based detection methods, 84–85
  orthopedic screws, 84*f*
  processes of, 80–81
  by staphylococci, 82–83
Biofilm infected sutures, 86*f*
Biofilm infections
  clinical examples of, 85–89
  surgical repair materials, 85
Biofilm microbiology
  bacterial adhesion, to surfaces, 79–80
  biofilm formation, processes of, 80–81
  infectious disease, 79–81
Biofilm-resistant biomaterials, prevention/treatment, 89–94
Biofilm structure, adaptation of, 78–79
Bioinspiration, 94
Biologically derived polymers, 305–314, 323
  alginate, 312
  aliphatic polyesters, 315–319
    copolymers, 315–318
    poly(glycolic acid), 315–318
    poly(lactic acid), 315–318
  barriers, 324–325
  biodegradable polyurethanes, 319–320
  biomimetic materials, 310
  cellulose, 311

Biologically derived polymers (*Continued*)
  chitosan, 313
  collagen, 305–307
  elastin, 308
  gelatin, 307–308
  gellan gum, 312
  gels, 325
  glycosaminoglycans (GAGs), 312–313
  hybrids of, 323
  in vitro, 307
  keratin, 308–309
  lactide enantiomers, 316f
  matrices, 325
  peptides and proteins, 305–310
  poly(amide carbonate), 322f
  poly(amino acids), 321–323
  polyanhydrides, 320–321
  poly(ε-caprolactone) (PCL), 318, 318f
  polyhydroxyalkanoates (PHA), 313–314
  polynucleotides, 314
  poly(orthoesters), 319, 319f
  poly(*p*-dioxanone) (PDS), 318
  polyphosphazenes, 321
  polysaccharides, 310–313
  proteins uses, as degradable biomaterials, 306t
  proteoglycans (PGs), 309–310
  'pseudo'-poly(amino acids), 321–323
  segmented poly(urethane), general structure of, 320f
  silk, 309
  starch, 311–312
  synthetic polymers, 314–323
  widely investigated polysaccharides, 306t
Biomaterials
  antibiofilm properties of, 89–91
  microbial colonization control, 91–92
  polymeric. See Polymeric biomaterials
  resist bacterial attachment/biofilm formation, 93–94
  surfaces, biofilm control agents, 92
Biomedicine, microbubble applications. See Microbubble applications, in biomedicine
Biomimicry, 94
Bioresorbable polymer, 37
Biotinlylated microbubble targete to streptavidin-coated surface, 261f
Bisphenol A (BPA), 17–18
Blalock-Taussig (B-T) shunt, 185
Blood pump support, in palliative surgery study, 185
B-16 melanoma tumors, 263
Bone adhesives, 119
  characteristics of, 120t
  development of, 119
Bone glue, 119

Bone regeneration scaffold, 324f
Bronchodilators, inhaled, 219
Bronchospasm, 220
Butyl cyanoacrylate, 107–108
N-Butyl-2-cyanoacrylate, 110
Bypass system aortic connector, 176

C

Cannot intubate, cannot ventilate (CICV), 210
Capnography yields quantifiable measurements, 201–202
CarboMedics, 170
Carbon fibers, 29
Carcinogenesis, 33
Cardiac devices, evolution, 146t
Cardiac surgery, 151, 181–182
Cardiopulmonary bypass (CPB), 66
Cardiopulmonary resuscitation (CPR), 201
Cardiovascular devices
  artificial heart, 154–155
    schematic diagram, 154f
  blood pumps, 151–162
  in open-heart surgery, 151–171
  POLTAH design process, steps, 153f
  William Kolff, in Kampen, 155f
Cardiovascular surgeons, 11
Carel's techniques, 4–5
Carpentier-Edwards pericardial valve, 169–170
Carpentier-Edwards PERIMOUNT pericardial bioprosthesis, 170
Carpentier-Edwards prostheses, 167
Catheter-lock solutions (CLS), 82
CE marking declaration, 342f
Cell microencapsulation, schematic of, 286f
Center for Biofilm Engineering (CBE), 80
Central Drugs Standards Control Organization (CDSCO), 344
Central nervous system (CNS), 67
Centrifugal pumps, 152–153
Chemical sterilants, 43
Chest physiotherapy, 215–216
  high-frequency chest wall compression, 216
  intrapulmonary percussive ventilation (IPV), 216
  percussion/postural drainage, 216
  positive end-expiratory pressure therapy, 216
Coatings, 92–93
Coefficient of friction (COF), 26
Collagen, 305–307
  adhesives, 104
  advantageous properties, 307
  in vitro, 307
  in vivo, 307–308
Colorimetric capnometric device, 203f

Comparative tracking index (CTI), 31
Complete airway management (CAM), 214
Compression molding, 139
Computational fluid dynamics (CFD), 171
Confocal microscopy, 89–90
Continuous positive airway pressure (CPAP), 217
Conventional endoscopic instruments, 181
Coronary artery bypass graft (CABG) surgery, 10–11
Coronary artery disease, 176
Cryoablation, 175
Crystalline polymers, 49
Cuff pressure monitoring, 204
Cyanoacrylate monomer, 104–105
Cyanoacrylates, 105, 115–116
  polymerization of, 106
  tissue adhesives, 104–105
    benefits and limitation, 106t
    commercial grades, 109–110
    cured loctite, typical performance of, 107t
    manufacturers of, 109
    medical grade, 107–109
  topical adhesives, 116
Cyanoacrylic acid butyl ester, 112
Cyclic di-GMP, 91–92
Cystic fibrosis (CF) lung, 79
Cytotoxicity, 33

D

da Vinci S model, 182
Delrin disk, 168–169
Denaturing gel gradient electrophoresis (DGGE), 84–85
Dental adhesives, 119–120
  applications, 119–124
  capability of, 120
  ingredients of, 122t
  methacrylic acid (MA), 121–122
  resin monomers, 121
Derjaguin, Landau, Verwey, and Overbeek (DLVO) theory, 79–80
Dermabond (2-octylcyanoacrylate), 110
Device-related infection, 81–85
  biofilm formation, 81
  detection, 83–84
  surgical repair materials, 85
Dielectrophoresis, 287
Double-lumen endotracheal tube (DLT), 199
Dry heat sterilization, 43
Dynesys, 242–243

E

Edwards-Tekna valve, 168–169
Eicosamethylnonasiloxane three-dimensional representation, 141f

Index

Electrohydraulic artificial heart (EHTAH), 155–156
Electromagnetic interference shielding (EMI), 29
EndoAssist, 181
Endothelial cells (ECs), 317–318
Endotracheal tube (ETT), in medicine, 192
   airway adjuncts, 195–200
      choice of, 195–196
   airway emergencies, rapid response cart, 209–210
   airway evaluation
      difficult airway, predicting, 200–201
      esophageal bulb detector, 201*f*
      esophageal intubation, detection, 201–203
      homemade syringe device, 201*f*
      identifying proper position, 201–206
      supraglottic devices, 200*f*
   airway resistance, 195–196
   American Society of Anesthesiologists difficult airway algorithm, 211*f*
   anatomy of, 192–194
   anticholinergics, 219–220
   automatic tube compensation, 217–218
   ballard closed endotracheal tube suctioning system, 213*f*
   biofilm accumulation, 214*f*
   biofilm management, 214–215
   bronchoscopy, 213–214
   clinical pearls, 221–222
   continuous positive airway pressure (CPAP), 217
   corticosteroids, 220
   cuff leaks, causes/solutions, 205*t*
   development/properties of, 194
   difficult airway cart
      contents of, 212*b*
   double-lumen endotracheal tubes, 199–200
   heat and moisture exchanger, 212*f*
   inhalation
      antibiotics, 220
      bronchodilators, 219
   inhalation drug delivery, 218–219
      metered-dose inhalers, 218–219
      nebulizers, 218
   intubated patient, respiratory therapies, 215–221
      chest physiotherapy, 215–216
      mucolytic agents, 215
      secretion clearance, 215–216
   intubating laryngeal mask airway (ILMA)
      structural comparison of, 193*f*
   large tubes and trauma, 196
   laser tubes, 197–198
   maintenance of, 210–215
      inspired gas, heat/humidity of, 210–212
   Mallinckrodt endobronchial tube, 198*f*, 199*f*
   overcoming work of, 217–218
   patient, positioning of, 220–221
   pilot balloon of, 193–194
   placement
      complications of, 195
      physiologic effects of, 194–195
   potentially beneficial alternatives, 196–200
   preformed/reinforced tubes, 196–197
   pressure support, 217
   proper position, identification, 201–206
      appropriate depth, 203–204
      audible cuff leak, 204–205, 205*t*
      cuff pressure monitoring, 204
      placement, documentation of, 205–206
   properties of, 192–195
   Rusch Lasertubus laser-safe endotracheal tube, 198*f*
   stabilization of, 206–209
      AnchorFast system, 209*f*
      commercially available devices, 209
      emergency intubations, airway record for, 208*f*
      facial burns, stapling, 209
      split-tape method, 208*f*
      taping, 206–209
   subglottic care, 213
   subglottic suctioning evac endotracheal tubes, 198–199
   suctioning, 212–213
   supraglottic airways, 200
   taperguard endotracheal tube cuff, 193*f*
   ventilator circuits, 217–218
Endotracheal tube placement, 202*b*
Enterococcus faecium, 110
Enzyme-linked immunosorbent array (ELISA), 83–84
Escherichia coli, 110
Esophageal variceal bleeding, 115
Ester bond, of aliphatic polyesters, 315
Ethylene oxide (EtO), 31
   resistance, 41
   sterilization, 38
Exopolysaccharide (EPS) fibers, 79–80
Extracellular bacterial DNA (eDNA), 79
Extracorporeal membrane oxygenation (ECMO), 152

F

Facial burns, stapling, 209
Fatigue tests
   conventional standardized methods, 243
   nanocrystalline diamond and steel coronary stents, 174*f*
   of PEEK rod systems, 243
Fiberoptic bronchoscopy
   to aid therapy, 195
   use of, 213–214
Fibrin, 111
Fibrin sealants, 104
Fibrinogen, 104, 111
Finger-printing method, 84–85
Fluorescence, 28
Fluorescence *in situ* hybridization (FISH), 84*f*
Foundation of cardiac surgery development (FCSD), 178–179

G

Gamma radiation resistance, 35, 37, 40–41, 43, 46
Gastrointestinal (GI) endoscopy, 115–116
   bleeding from other sources, 115
   closure of fistula, 115–116
   esophageal variceal bleeding, 115
   gastric variceal bleeding, 115
   peptic ulcer bleeding, 115
Gelatin hydrogels, 307–308
Gelatine-resorcinol-formaldeyde (GRF), 104
Gellan gum, 312
Gene delivery, 264
Gene-activated matrix (GAM), 293
Generic-targeted microbubbles, 261–262
Genetic testing, 12
Genotoxicity testing, 33
Glass transition temperatures, 141–142
Glenn procedure, 185
Global harmonization task force (GHTF), 344
Glubran 2, 116
Glyceryl methacrylate (GMA), 56–58
Glycosaminoglycans (GAGs), 312–313
Gold
   marker lines, 173–174
   self-assembled monolayers (SAMs), 93
   standard, resistance of biomaterials, 90–91
Good Clinical Practice (GCP), 343
Good manufacturing practices (GMP), 337–338, 343
   critical devices, 338
   quality assurance programs, 338
Good Quality Practice Ordinance (GQP) standards, 343
Green heart, 155–156

H

Health-care industry, 9
Health-care trends, 10–12
   alternate site treatment, 11–12
   minimally invasive surgeries, 10–11
   prevention *vs.* treatment, 12
Heart diseases, 150–151
   ischemic heart disease, 151
   valvular heart disease, 151
Heart failure, congestive, 150–151

Heart pacemaker, 171
Heart prostheses, 169f
HeartSaver VAD, 158
Heart-lung machines, 151
Heat and moisture exchanger (HME), 210–212
Heat shock protein (HSP) family, 287
Hemocompatibility, 33, 66
Hemolysis test, 165f
Hexafluoropropylene (HFP), 65
High consistency rubber (HCR), 139
High-consistency silicone rubbers (HCRs), 136
High-density polyethylene (HDPE), 34
High-frequency chest wall compression, 216
High pressure, low volume (HPLV), 192–193
   ILMAs risky, 197
   silicone ETTs, 192–193
   structural comparison of, 193f
High volume and low pressure (HVLP) cuff, 192–193, 197
Homopolymers, 35–36
Homo sapiens, 145
Hospital acquired infections (HAIs), 12
Hydrogels, in regenerative medicine, 42, 279–281
   applications of, 290–293
      hydrogel parameters, effect of, 290t
      skin and wound healing, 290–291
   as biomaterials, 283–284
   cell association
      cell encapsulation, 285–286
      promoting cell attachment, substrates, 287–290
      schematic diagram of, 288f
      spatial patterning, 287
   characterization of, 293
   classification, 281
   for controlled release, 284–285
   liver, 292
   matrix-immobilized ligands, 289t
   and medical technology applications, 280t
   musculoskeletal, 291
   neural regeneration, 291–292
   poly(ethylene oxide), 4t
   prospects, 293–294
   regenerative medicine, utility in, 282–290
   relevance of, 279–281
   reproductive medicine, 292–293
   theory, 281–282
Hydroxy ethyl methacrylate (HEMA), 56, 123
   of artificial heart, 154f
   homopolymer of, 123
   hydrolysis of, 122–123, 123f
Hypoperfusion, 151
Hypoxemia, 212–213

I

IgG human antibodies, 79
Impact copolymers, 35–36
Impact modifiers, 27–28
Implant materials, in rats, 91–92
Incor device, 161
Injection molding, 139
Interpenetrating polymer networks (IPNs), 60
   dimethylacrylate, 285
   poly(dimethylsiloxane) (PDMS), 60
   poly(ethylene glycol) (PEG), 60
Intra-aortic balloon pump (IABP), 152–153
Intraocular lenses (IOLs), 56
Intrapulmonary percussive ventilation (IPV), 216
Intubating laryngeal mask airway (ILMA)
   difficult airway cart, 212b
   structural comparison, 193f
Investigational device exemption (IDE) clinical trial, 233
Investigational new animal exemptions (INAD), 340
Irritation tests, 33
Ischemic heart disease, 151
Isomers, 22–24
   geometric, 22–23
   stereosiomers, 23–24
   structural, 22, 22f
Isotactic polypropene, 23

K

Knotting instruments, 176

L

Labile catalysts, 135
Lactide dimer
   to remove water molecule, 37
   stereoisomeric structures of, 38f
Laminar gas flow, 195–196
Langerhans, for transplantation, 325
Laparoscopic, 176
Laryngeal structures, 196
Laryngoscopy, 210
Laser ablation, 175
Left ventricular assist devices (LVADs), 62
   HeartMate II, 158
   intermediate-to-chronic, 159–160
   short-term circulatory support, 161
Left ventricular assist system (LVAS), 160
Left ventricular opacification (LVO), 256
Linear low-density polyethylene (LLDPE), 13, 34
Lipopolysaccharide (LPS), 79–80
Liquid crystalline polymer, 37
Liquid silicone rubber (LSR), 13, 139–140
Low-density polyethylene (LDPE), 34
Lung
   cystic fibrosis (CF), 79
   isolation, endobronchial blocking devices, 199f
Lysine diisocyanate, 62

M

Magnetic resonance imaging (MRI) machines, 21
Magnetic vascular positioner (MVP), 177
Mallampati score, 200–201
Material suppliers, regulations applicability of, 345
Medical devices—material selection process
   chemical resistance, 31
   common medical device polymers, 34–49
   electrical properties, 31
   FDA device class, 29t
   joining and welding, 33
   leachables and extractables, 32–33
   long-term durability, 31–32
   medical grade plastics, 33
   physical and mechanical properties, 29–30
   shelf life and aging, 33
   steam sterilization, effect of, 31f
   sterilization capability, 31
   supplemental tests, 33
   thermal properties, 31
   USP classification, 30t
Medical devices, USP classification of, 30t
Medical plastic
   in common use, 4t
   development, timeline of, 2f
   device industry overview, 9–10
   historical example, 4–5
   plastics application, 9
Medical robotic systems, 178–179
Medium density polyethylene (MDPE), 34
Medium vessels, sutureless anastomoses, 114
Medos-HIA VAD, 158
Medtronic intact, 170
Metered-dose inhalers (MDIs), 218
Methacrylate-based adhesives, use of, 111
Methacrylic acid (MA), 121–122
10-Methacryloyloxydecyl dihydrogenphosphate (10-MDP), 123–124
11-Methacryloyloxy-1, 10-undecanedicarboxylic acid (MAC-10) monomers, 124
4-Methacryloyloxyethyl trimellitic acid (4-MET), 123

Methicillin-resistant *S. epidermidis* (MRSE), 82
Methicillin-resistant *Staphylococcus aureus* (MRSA), 18–19, 82, 84–85
Methyl ester (methyl-2-cyanoacrylate), 105–106
Methyl/ethyl cyanoacrylate adhesive, bond strength of, 108*t*
Methyl methacrylate (MMA), 111, 122–123
Microbial colonization control, biomaterials, 91–92
Microbubble applications, in biomedicine
  biofilm destruction, 266, 266*f*
  canine heart, ultrasound image of, 260*f*
  components, 254*f*
  compression and rarefaction, 258*f*
  current clinical uses of, 259–260
  developmental history of, 253
  emerging applications, 266–268
  Food and Drug Administration (FDA), 256–257
  in gene delivery, 264–266
    as drug carriers, 264–266
  gene delivery/drug, 262–264
  identification/quantification, 262
  left ventricular opacification (LVO), 256
  lymphosonography, 267–268
  magnetic resonance imaging, 267
  microbubble-specific ultrasound modes, 259–260
  nanobubbles, 267
  noninvasive pressure estimation, 266–267
  overview of, 253–257
  preparations table, 257*t*
  structure/function/use, table of, 255*t*
  targeting, 260–262
    active, 262
    atherosclerosis, 262*f*
    biotinlylated microbubble, 261*f*
    ligand/receptor, 261–262
    timeline, 254*f*
  tissue engineering, 267
  ultrasound contrast agent Targestar-B, frequency response of, 258*f*
  ultrasound imaging, interactions of, 257–259
Microbubble cavitation, 263
Microbubble-assisted drug, gene delivery, 262–264
Microbubble-based ultrasound contrast applications, 260
Micromolding, 16
Microwave ablation, 175
Mild tissue reaction, 114
Minimally invasive cardiology tools, 171–174

Minimally invasive surgery (MIS), 151, 175–185
  CardioVations, 176
  classical thoracoscopic tools, 176–177
  Coalescent Surgical, 176
  coronary surgery, anastomotic devices for, 176
  laparoscopic suturing, 176
  Passport, 176
  robot daVinci, 180*f*
  robots replacing, 178
  Spyder device, 177
  surgical robots, 177–182
  symmetry bypass system aortic connector, 176
Minimally invasive valve implantation, 185–186
Ministry of Health, Labor, and Welfare (MHLW), 343
Mitral valve area (MVA), 162
Mitral valve, physical percutaneous balloon valvuloplasty simulation, 173*f*
Mitral valve replacement (MVR), 167
  heterograft tissue valves, 167
  with mechanical prostheses *vs.* bioprostheses, 170–171
Mitral valvuloplasty, hemodynamic improvement, 173
Monocyte, 293–294
Motion preservation spine technology, 232–233
Multi-locus strain typing (MLST), 80
Murphy eye, 192
Myocardial infarction (MI), 151

N
Natural antibiofilm strategies, 91
Natural orifice transluminal endoscopic surgery (NOTES), 11
Natural polymers, 61–62
Neoplasia, targeting, 261–262
Nerve guidance, 68
Neuragen nerve guide, 292
Neural stem cells, proliferation of, 290
New animal drug applications (NADA), 340
Nexaband liquid, 113
Non-woven electrospun fibers, 284
Nucleic acid-based detection methods, 84–85
N-vinyl-2-pyrrolidone (NVP), 56

O
Octylcyanoacrylate, 108–109
Octyl-2-cyanoacrylate (2-OCA), 108
Off-pump coronary artery bypass (OPCAB)
  anastomotic devices, 177
  lateral wall grafting, 177

Oligo(polyethylene glycol) fumarate (OPF), 291
Organization of Pharmaceutical Safety and Research (OPSR), 343
Orthopedic implant infections, 87–88
Orthopedic implant materials, 93
Orthopedic procedures, 11
Oxygen transmission
  hydrophilic monomers, 56–58
  silicone hydrogel lenses and conventional hydrogel lenses, 42

P
P. aeruginosa, 80–81
Pacemaker, 171
Parkes, Alexander, 3*f*
Parylene, 47
  coatings, 47
  polymer molecules, structures of, 47*f*
PennState LionHeart, 157
Peptic ulcer bleeding, 115
Percutaneous balloon dilation, 173
Percutaneous balloon valvuloplasty, 173
Percutaneous transluminal coronary angioplasty (PTCA), 172–173
Percutaneous valve, 185–186
Peripheral nervous system (PNS), 67
Permeant molecule, tortuous path of, 27*f*
Pharmaceutical Affairs Law (PAL), 343
Pharmaceuticals and Medical Devices Agency (PMDA), 343
Photo-encapsulation, 286
Photopolymerization, 283
Pill Cam, 14
Pilot balloon repair device, 194*f*
Pittsburgh-Thermo cardiosystems, 159–160
Planktonic bacteria, 79–80, 92
Plastic compositions, 22–29
  additives, 25–29
  antistats, 29
  atactic polypropene, structure, 23*f*
  catalysts, 27
  coupling agents, 28
  impact modifiers, 27–28
  isomers, 22–24
    cis/trans-isomers, 23*f*
    geometric, 22–23
    structural, 22, 22*f*
  isotactic polypropene, structure, 24*f*
  linear/branched/crosslinked polymers, 22
  molecular weight, 24
  optical brighteners, 28
  pigments/extenders/dyes/mica, 28
  plasticizers, 28
  polymer blends, 24–25
  polymer properties, 22–24
  radiation stabilizers, 28
  reinforcing fillers, 25–26

Plastic compositions (*Continued*)
  release agents, 26
  slip additives/internal lubricants, 26–27
  stereoisomerism, 23
  stereosiomers, 23–24
  syndiotactic polypropene, structure of, 24f
  thermal stabilizers, 28
  tougheners, 27–28
Plastics, in medical devices
  bisphenol A (BPA), 17–18
  compatibility, 14–15
  construction, commoditizing materials, 15–16
  diethyl hexyl phthalate (DEHP) plasticized PVC, 17
  ecological/environmental concerns, 16–17
  energy costs, 18
  functionality, 13–14
  global influences, 18–19
    economic pressures, 19
    manufacturing, 18
    markets, 18
    SARS (severe acute respirator syndrome), 18–19
  light weighting, 15
  market factors affecting, 17–19
  material costs/process improvements, 15
  need for "green," 18
  technology innovations, 16
  trends, 13–17
Plastics production, timeline of, 2f
Plastics, story, 2–3
Plastics suppliers
  Australia, 343–344
  CE marking declaration, 342f
  China, 343
  European Union medical device directive, 341–343
  FDA 21 CFR Part 820, 339t
  FDA master files, 340
  history, 337–338
  India, 344
  ISO 13485, 340–343, 341t
  Japan, 343
  South America, 344
  United States regulations, 338–340
Plastic-to-rubber bonds, 106
Platelet additives, 26
Pneumatic pulsatile VADs, 160
Pneumatically driven artificial heart (POLTAH)
  artificial heart, schematic diagram of, 154f
  design process, 153f
  in vivo, 165f
Pneumatically driven ventricular assist device (POLVAD)
  implantation, semiautomatic tools, 153f
  Polish ventricle assist devices, 158–159
Pneumomediastinum, 219
Pneumoperitoneum, 219
Pneumothorax, 219
Polyamides (nylon), 4t
Poly glycolic acid (PGA), 15, 66, 305, 315–316
Poly(amino acids), 321
Polyaryletheretherketone (PEEK), 231–232
  applications. *See* Spinal implants, polyaryletheretherketone (PEEK) applications
  carbon fiber-reinforced (CFR), 233
Polyaryletherketone (PAEK)
  all-polymer articulations, 246
  biomaterials, 231
Polybutadiene, 25
Polybutylene terephthalate (PBT), 24
Polycaprolactone (PCL) polymers, 15
Polycarbonate (PC), 4t, 24
  steam sterilization, effect of, 31f
Polydimethylmethylhydrogenosiloxane, 135
Polydimethylsiloxane (PDMS), 131–132, 141
  see also Silicone rubber
Poly-*p*-dioxanone (PDS), 66
Polyester-based TPUs, 45
Polyether ether ketone (PEEK), 43–44
  applications and uses, 44, 46
  EtO resistance, 43, 46
  gamma radiation resistance, 43, 46
  polymers, 13
  rod system, 244f
  steam sterilization resistance, 43–44
  structure of, 43f
Polyether imide (PEI), 13
  PEI-DNA complexes, 288–289
Polyethersulfone (PES), 41
Polyethylene (PE), 13, 34
  polyvinyl chloride (PVC), 22
Poly(ethylene glycol) (PEG), 283
  brushes, 255
  interpenetrating polymer networks (IPNs), 60
Polyethylene terephthalate (PETE), 4t, 5, 13, 24, 62
Polyhydroxyalkanoates (PHA), 38, 313–314
Poly(2-hydroxyethyl methacrylate) (PHEMA), 56–58
Polyhydroxyhexanoate (PHH), 38
Polyhydroxyvalerate (PHV), 38
Polylactic acid (PLA), 15, 64, 315–316
  electron beam sterilization, effect of, 32f
  lactic acid, conversion of, 37f
  microbubbles, 265–266
Poly(lactic-co-glycolic acid) (PLGA), 64
Poly-L-lysine, 285–286
Polymerase chain reaction (PCR)
  detection techniques, 84–85
Polymer-shelled microbubbles, 265–266
Polymeric biomaterials
  applications of, 55
  artificial cornea, 58–60
  in cardiovascular diseases, 62–64
    expanded PTFE, 63–64
    polyethylene terephthalate, 63
    polyurethanes, 62–63
    for wound closure, 64–66
  common monomers, chemical structures of, 57f
  contact lens, 56–58
  extracorporeal artificial organs, 66–67
  glyceryl methacrylate (GMA), 56–58
  intraocular lens, 58
  for IOLs, 59t
  natural polymers, 61–62
  for nerve regeneration, 67–68
  in ophthalmology, 56–60
  in orthopedics, 60–62
  polyacrylates, 61
  polyethylene, 60–61
Polymeric coatings, self-assembled monolayers (SAMs), 93
Polymers, 323
  common medical device
    fluoropolymers, 47–49
    hydrogel (acrylate), 42
    polyacrylate (acrylic, PMMA), 41–42
    polycarbonate, 38–40
    polyester, 36–37
    polyethersulfone, 41
    polyethylene, 34–35
    polypropylene, 35–36
    poly-*p*-xylylene (Parylene), 47
    polystyrene, 36
    polysulfone (PSU), 42–43
    polyvinyl chloride, 40–41
    schematic of, 44f
    sterilization matrix of, 50t
    thermoplastic elastomers (TPE, TPU), 44–46
    thermoset elastomers—silicone, 46
  devices, legacy materials, 12–13
  molecular weight, 24
  natural, 61–62
  tissue-engineered products, 323–325
Poly(methyl methacrylate) (PMMA), 4t, 56, 92
  application of, 61
Polynucleotides, gene delivery, 314
Poly(*p*-dioxanone) (PDS), 318
Polypropylene (PP), 4t, 13
Polysaccharide teichoic acid fibers, 79–80

Polysaccharides, 310–311
Polysialic acid, 68
Polysiloxanes, structure, 46f
Polystyrene (PS), 13, 25, 36
Polysulfone (PSU), structure of, 43f
Polytetrafluoroethylene (PTFE), 3
    chemical structure of, 49f
    gamma sterilization, effect of, 32f
Poly(tetramethylene ether) glycol
        terephthalate (PTMG), 65–66
Poly(tetramethylene ether terephthalate)
        copolymers of, 65–66
Polyurethane (PU), 4t, 59–60
    bioresistant, 62–63
    mechanisms responsible for, 62–63
    physical percutaneous balloon
        valvuloplasty simulation, 173f
Poly(vinyl alcohol) (PVA), 323
    homopolymer of, 59–60
Polyvinyl chloride (PVC), 5, 192
Polyvinylidene fluoride (PVDF), 65
Positive end-expiratory pressure therapy
        (PEEP) therapy, 216
Postanesthesia care unit (PACU),
        204–205
Posterior capsular opacification (PCO), 58
Posterior lumbar interbody fusion (PLIF),
        233–234
Premarket approval (PMA), 340
PressureEasy device, 204
Prostate specific antigen (PSA), 12
    silicone PSAs, 140–141
Proteoglycans (PGs), 309–310
Pseudomonas aeruginosa, 110
Pulmonary artery axial blood pump,
        185f
Pulmonary artery stenosis, 173
Pulmonary toilet bronchoscopy, 213–214

R
Radiation sterilization, 38
Radiofrequency, 174–175
Random copolymers, 35–36
Rats, implant materials, 91–92
Reproductive, 33
Restriction fragment length polymorphism
        (RFLP), 84–85
Reverse transcriptase PCR (RT-PCR), 83
Rigid gas-permeable (RGP), 56
Risk management, 340
RNAIII-activating protein (RAP), 91–92
RNAIII-inhibiting peptide (RIP), 91–92
Robotic surgery, 146
Robotic systems, 178–179
Robotics, potential applications of,
        182
Room temperature vulcanization (RTV),
        136–137
    elastomers, 140
Rubber-to-rubber bonds, 106

S
S. epidermidis, 92–93
Safe Medical Device Act (SMDA), 338
Schwann cells, 291–292
Self-assembled monolayers (SAMs), 93,
        93f
Self-etch adhesives (SEAs), 120–121
Severe acute respiratory syndrome (SARS),
        18–19
Short-term circulatory support, 162–171
Silicone elastomers, 138–139
Silicone gel adhesives, 141
Silicone materials, 131
    basic steps, 134t
    chemical structure/nomenclature,
        131–142
    development, key milestones, 132t
    elastomers, 136–140
        cross-linking by addition, 137–138
        cross-linking by condensation,
            136–137
        cross-linking with radicals, 136
        filler, 138
        processing of, 138–140
        silica network, 138f
        silicone film-in-place, 141
    gels, 140
    high consistency rubber (HCR), 139
    historical milestones, 132
    liquid silicone rubber (LSR), 139–140
    nomenclature, 132–133
    olymers, preparation, 133
    physico-chemical properties, 141–142
    polycondensation, 133–136
    polymerization, 133–136
    silicone adhesives, 140–141
        bonding adhesives, 140
        gel adhesives, 141
        pressure-sensitive adhesives, 140
    Silicone Shorthand Notation, 133t
Silicone organic copolymers, 141
Silicone polymers, 136
Silicone preparation, catalyst removal, 135
Silicone rubber, 4t, 46
Single use disposables (SUDs), 12
Skin wrinkles, 308
Smooth muscle cells (SMCs), 317–318
SonarMed airway monitoring device, 214
Sorin Bicarbon mechanical prosthesis, 170
Spinal cord injuries (SCIs), 292
Spinal implants, polyaryletheretherketone
        (PEEK) applications, 232f
    autograft-treated goats
        histological section of, 239f
    cervical/lumbar artificial discs,
        244–246
    CFR-PEEK
        and CFR-PEKEKK cages, 235f
        lumbar cages, 233–237, 234f
        transpedicular screw, 240f
    early pedicle-based systems, 242–243
    fused lumbar spinal segment,
        radiograph of, 239f
    fusion, 237f
        radiographic findings, 237f
    graf ligaments/dynesys, 242–243
    inflammatory reaction to CFR-PAEK,
        237f
    interbody fusion
        and cage rage, 233
        devices, 232f
    motion preservation spine technology,
        232–233
    overview of, 231–233
    pedicle-based posterior stabilization
        rods, 242–244, 243f, 244f
    PEEK spinal cages, clinical
        diagnostic imaging, 236f, 239–240
    PEEK-on-PEEK lumbar nucleus
        replacement (NUBAC), 245f
    posterior dynamic stabilization devices,
        240–244
    interspinous process spacers,
        241–242
    spacer, extension-limiting, 241f
    spinal fusions, incidence of, 232f
    subsidence/wear cages, 240
    threaded PEEK
        interbody device, 238f
        lumbar fusion cages, 237–238, 238f
    transpedicular screws, 239–240
    volumetric wear rates, comparison of,
        246f
Spyder device, 177
Stainless steel (SS) materials, 14–15
Staphylococci, biofilm formation, 82–83
Staphylococcus aureus, 110
Staphylococcus epidermidis
    adheres, 110, 112
    biofilm, 214–215, 266
Staphylococcus mucoidy, 81
Starfish2 heart positioner, 177
Starr-Edwards ball valve design, 168
State Food and Drug Administration
        (SFDA), 343
Steam sterilization resistance, 37, 41,
        43–44
Stentless bioprosthetic porcine aortic
        valves, 169–170
Sterilization methods, 34
    with hot air, 39
    on parylene, 48t
    with peracetic acid, 39
    resistance, 35
Subglottic suctioning, 213
Subharmonic-aided pressure estimation
        (SHAPE), 266–267
Supraglottic airways, 200
Surgery planning
    medical applications, 187

Surgery planning (*Continued*)
  remote-control manipulators, 186
  RobinHeart robot, 188*f*
  robots, 186
Syncardia systems, 155
Syndiotactic polypropene, 23–24
Synthetic polymer, 5

T
Taperguard endotracheal tube cuff, 193*f*
Thermoplastic polyurethane elastomer, molecular structure, 45*f*
Thoracoscopic surgery, 176
Thoratec PVAD (paracorporeal ventricular assist device), 158
Thrombin, 104
Ti-cron braided polyester suture, 86*f*
Tissue adhesives
  characterize strength, test methods, 110
  classification of, 121*f*
  dental applications, 119–124
  in gastrointestinal endoscopic procedures, 115–116
    bleeding from other sources, 115
    closure of fistula, 115–116
    esophageal variceal bleeding, 115
    gastric variceal bleeding, 115
    peptic ulcer bleeding, 115
  hernia incisions, closure of, 116–119
  open pediatric urological procedures, 114–115
  plastic surgery, uses, 119
  potential cyanoacrylate pitfalls, 118*t*
  in topical skin wounds, 116
  wound closure devices, 117*t*
Tissue valves, 167
Tortuous path effect, 26
Total disc replacements (TDRs), 232–233
Total endoscopic coronary artery bypass (TECAB), 177
Total joint replacement (TJR), 88
Tracheostomy tubes, pressure support, 217
Transfer molding, 139

U
U-CLIP anastomotic device technology, 176–177
Ultrahigh molecular weight polyethylene (UHMWPE) chains, 24
Ultra-low-density polyethylene (ULDPE), 34
Ultrasound ablation, 175
Unfixed biofilms, confocal microscope images of, 90*f*
Unique identification (UID), for devices, 14
Urethane bond, 320
Urethanes, 45
Urinary catheters, 77–78

V
Valine-proline-glycine-valine-glycine (VPGVG)
  elastin repeat sequences, 310
Valve prostheses, 162–171
Valve repair, 164
Valve test tester, 166*f*
Valve-related problems, 168
  bioprosthetic valves, 168
  mechanical valves, 168
Valvular heart disease, 151, 162–171
VEGFR2-targeted microbubble, 261–262
Ventilator-associated pneumonia (VAP), 193
Ventilator circuits, pressure support, 217
Ventricular assist devices (VADs), 145
  implantation, types of, 160–161
Vinci S model, 182
Vinci telemanipulator, 181
Vision systems, 16

W
Water uptake adversely influences, 123
Wistar rats, 116–118
Wongworawat, 114
WorldHeart, 160
Wound bacterial counts, 113
Woven hydrogel/cell mixtures, 284

Y
Young's modulus, 316–317

Z
Zeus surgical system, 180

THE NEW
CRAFT COLLECTION

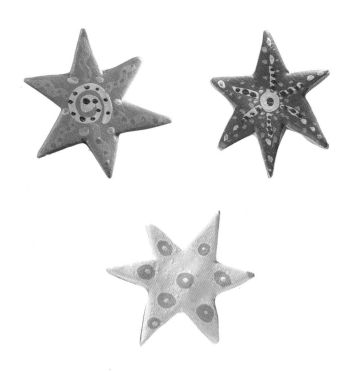

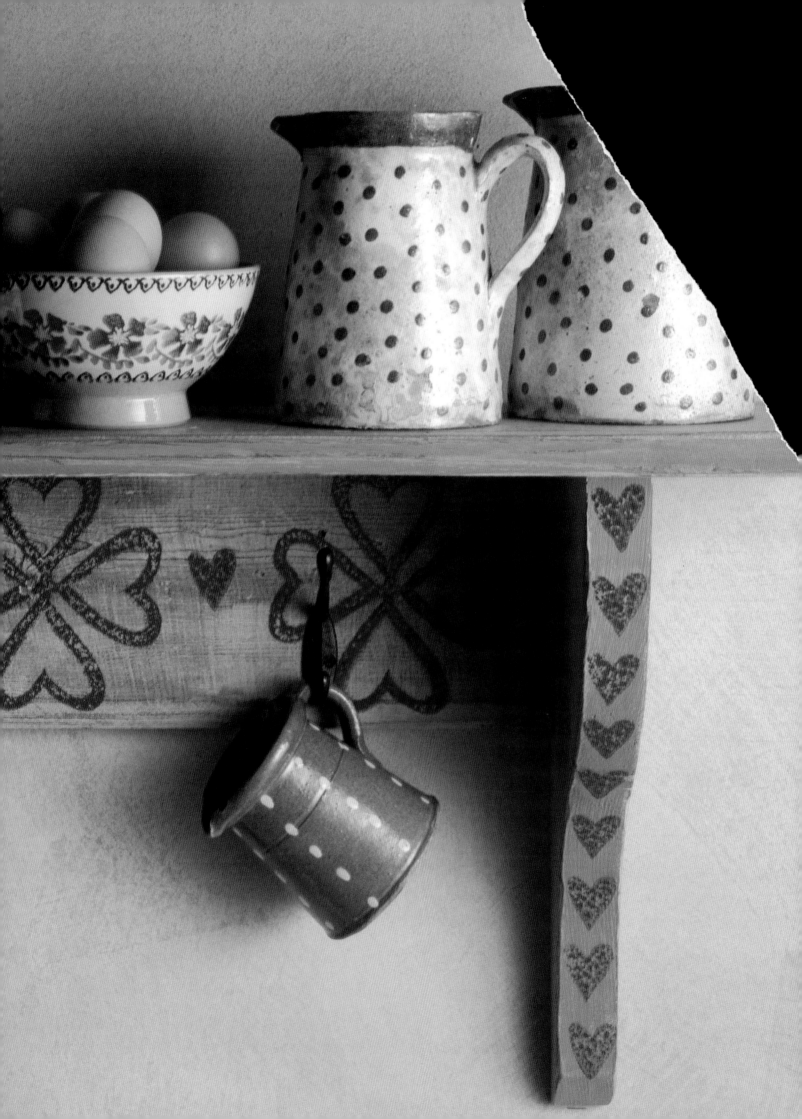

THE NEW
CRAFT COLLECTION

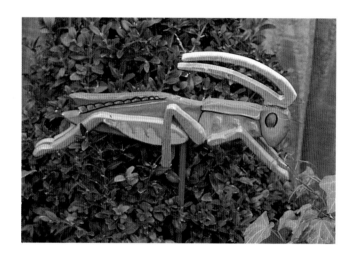

HERMES HOUSE

This edition first published in 1997 by
Hermes House
27 West 20th Street, New York, NY 10011

HERMES HOUSE books are available for bulk purchase for
sales promotion and for premium use. For details, write or call
the sales director, Hermes House, 27 West 20th Street, New York,
NY 10011; (800) 354-9657

© Anness Publishing Limited 1997

Hermes House is an imprint of Anness Publishing Limited

All rights reserved. No part of this publication may be reproduced,
stored in a retrieval system, or transmitted in any way or by any means,
electronic, mechanical, photocopying, recording or otherwise, without
the prior written permission of the copyright holder.

ISBN 1 901289 14 1

Printed and bound in China

10 9 8 7 6 5 4 3 2 1

Acknowledgments *Projects* Ofer Acoo, Madeleine Adams, Dinah Alan-Smith, Deborah Alexander, Michael Ball, Evelyn Bennett, Amanda Blunden, Petra Boase, Penny Boylan, Janet Bridge, Al Brown, Louise Brownlow, Esther Burt, Judy Clayton, Gill Clement, Lilli Curtiss, Sophie Embleton, Lucinda Ganderton, Louise Gardam, Lisa Gilchrist, Andrew Gilmore, Dawn Gulyas, David Hancock, Jill Hancock, Lesley Harle, Stephanie Harvey, Bridget Hinge, Labeena Ishaque, Sameena Ishaque, Paul Jackson, Mary Maguire, Rachel Howard Marshall, Abigail Mill, Terence Moore, Izzy Moreau, Jack Moxley, Oliver Moxley, Cleo Mussie, Sarbjitt Natt, Cheryl Owen, Emma Petitt, Lizzie Reakes, Kim Rowley, Deborah Schneebeli-Morrell, Debbie Siniska, Isabel Stanley, Thomasina Smith, Adele Tipler, Kellie-Marie Townsend, Karen Triffitt, Liz Wagstaff, Sally Walton, Stewart Walton, Emma Whitfield, Josephine Whitfield, Melanie Williams, Dorothy Wood
Photography Steve Dalton, James Duncan, Michelle Garrett, Lucy Mason, Gloria Nicol, Debbie Patterson, Peter Williams

Publisher: Joanna Lorenz
Project Editor: Christopher Fagg
Editor: Harriette Lanzer
Designer: Patrick McLeavey, Hannah Attwell, Dean Hollowood

FRONTISPIECE *This country-style shelf decoration is easy to do: the perfect way to cheer up the dullest kitchen.*

Contents

Introduction	6
Papercrafts and Papier-mâché	10
Stencilling, Stamping and Printing	44
Embroidery	78
Appliqué, Patchwork and Cross Stitch	112
Modelling and Salt Dough	146
Wood, Wire and Tinwork	180
Decorating Glass and Ceramics	214
Templates	246
Index	256

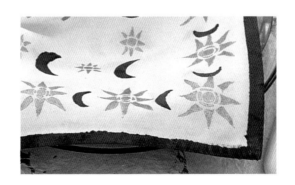

INTRODUCTION

*T*his book contains over 160 step-by-step projects using a variety of exciting crafts, both traditional and new. You can select a project at any level of skill, from the simplicity of paper cut-outs to the more detailed art of soldering tin. Or, use a needlework craft to create soft furnishings for the home and complement them with some beautiful painted glassware. Children, in particular, will love the salt dough ideas, and anyone wanting to cheer up walls and furniture should look no further than the stamping projects.

Whatever your preferred style of craft, you're bound to find inspiration in this collection. You could also try out a craft new to you and discover hidden talents. Just pick your project, experiment with the materials, follow the clear instructions and enjoy the result.

USING TEMPLATES

There are easy-to-use templates at the back of the book for a lot of the projects. For tracing templates, you will need tracing paper, a pencil, card or paper and a pair of scissors. The templates can be traced on to tracing paper and cut out to use as pattern guides. If a pattern is to be used a number of times, the template tracing should be transferred to thin card. To do this, trace the template on to tracing paper, using a pencil, then place the tracing paper face down on the card. Re-draw the motif on the back of the tracing and it will appear on the card.

To enlarge the templates to the required size, either use a grid system or a photocopier. For the grid system, trace the template and draw a grid of evenly spaced squares over your tracing. To scale up, draw a larger grid on to another piece of paper. Copy the outline on to the second grid by taking each square individually and drawing the relevant part of the outline in the larger square.

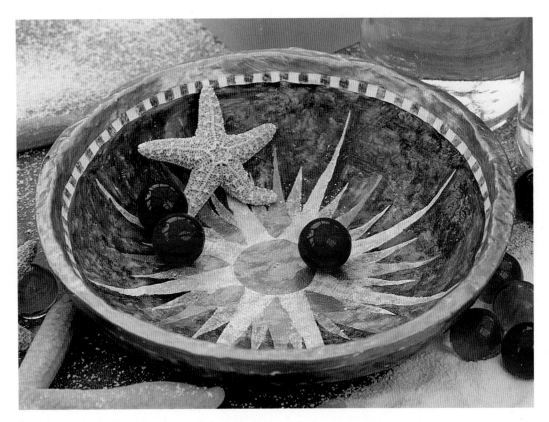

PAPERCRAFTS AND PAPIER-MACHE

Experiment with paper to create some memorable gifts, such as this charming Sunburst Bowl.

· INTRODUCTION ·

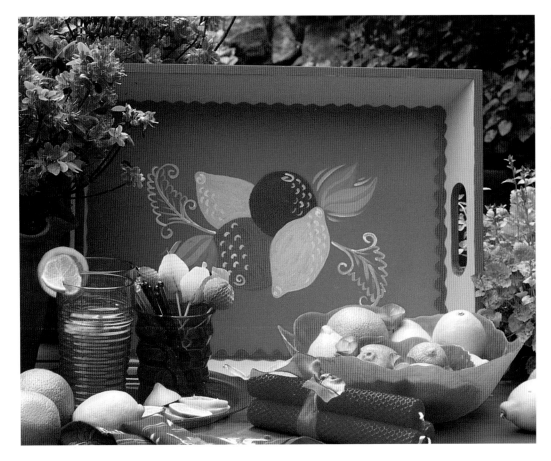

STENCILLING, STAMPING AND PRINTING

A marvellously easy and effective method to make individual pieces, such as this Mexican Citrus Tray.

EMBROIDERY

Embroider beautiful effects on to fabrics, as is illustrated in this Underwater Picture.

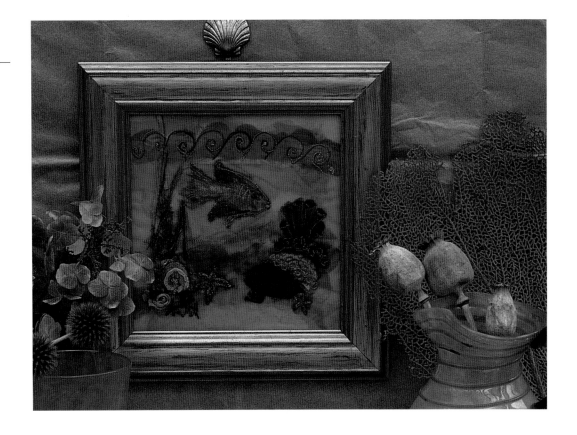

Applique, Patchwork and Cross Stitch

Follow the step-by-step instructions to make exciting projects, such as this pretty Seashell Beach Bag.

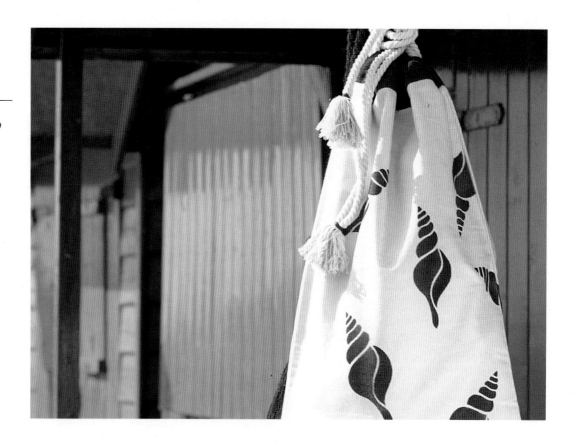

Modelling and Salt Dough

Get stuck into the wonderful texture of salt dough and clay, and create some amazing end results, such as these Salt and Pepper Pots.

• INTRODUCTION •

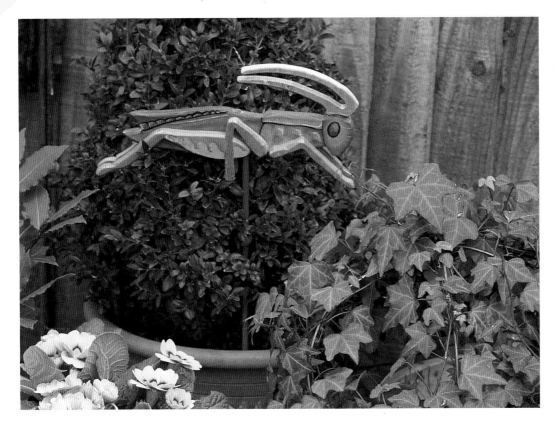

WOOD, WIRE AND TINWORK

This section includes fun ideas such as this wood Grasshopper on a Stick, as well as exciting wire and tin projects.

DECORATING GLASS AND CERAMICS

Re-vamp old china and glass and your crockery cupboard will soon be transformed with projects such as this Fruit Bowl.

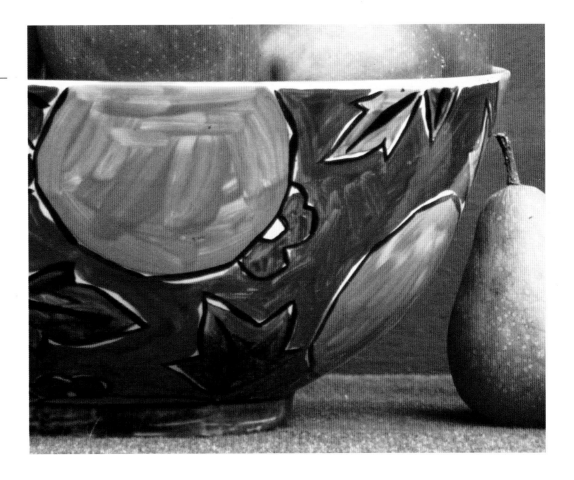

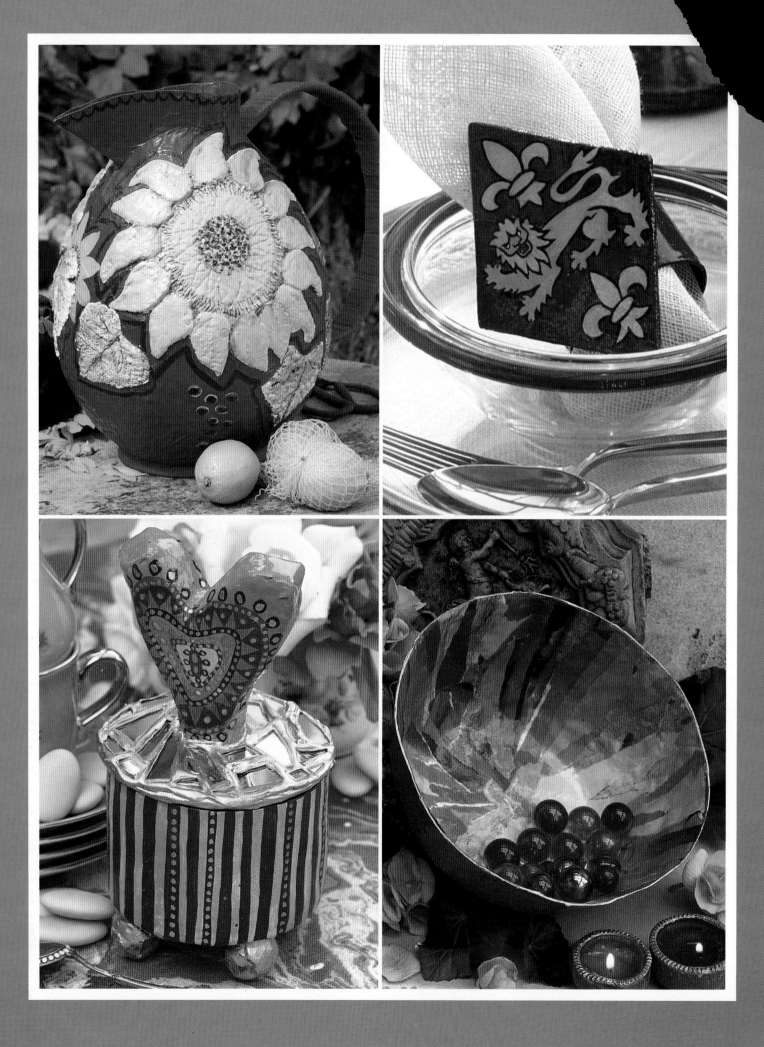

PAPERCRAFTS AND PAPIER-MACHE

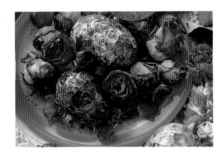

*W*orking with paper is a truly satisfying and creative craft, and the bonus is that it can also be good for the environment, if you recycle old and used papers in your projects. There is such a wealth of colours, textures and sizes available in paper that the scope for producing wonderful decorations and gifts really is endless.

The projects in this book should inspire you to experiment with paper whatever your tastes and ability. Steps are provided to take you through the process of creating a traditional paper cut-out, which you can easily adapt to make as simple or intricate as you like. Or, if you prefer a more weighty project, you could get involved in the art of papier-mâché – and explore the delights you can make from the simplest of materials.

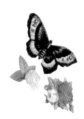

• PAPERCRAFTS AND PAPIER-MACHE •

Materials and Equipment

Paper comes in many different weights, textures, patterns and colours. Before you embark on the projects here, explore some possible paper sources. Art and hobby shops, printers, office stationers and specialist suppliers are all good starting points. And don't forget to look around your own home – you'll be amazed at how many pieces of paper and card you have got already. You just need to view the material in a different light, and recognize that those old newspapers on the coffee table can be transformed into an exciting new creation.

A craft knife and a cutting mat or a pair of paper scissors are vital when working with paper, and so too is masking tape as it won't tear the paper. Paper glue or spray adhesive are also useful to have at hand if you want to attach pieces of paper to each other.

Painting and colouring your paper projects presents no problem, and there is a wide range of crayons, pens, paints and varnishes available that are suitable for paper. Just check the manufacturer's instructions before you apply the material to paper, and if you like, you can always do a test run on a scrap of paper first, just to make sure.

RIGHT *The equipment necessary for papercrafts is very simple and straightforward.*

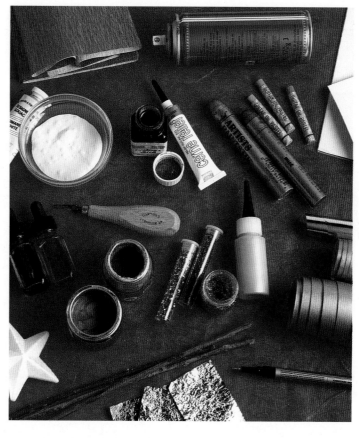

Working with different papers

There are so many varieties of paper available that you will have to let your personal taste dictate what you use for your projects. Here are a few of the more exciting papers you could try.

Tissue and crepe paper are cheap papers sold at stationers and craft suppliers. Tissue paper needs to be layered to build up intense colour. Crepe paper is thicker and crinkly and its only drawback is that adhesive tape doesn't stick to it well.

Hand-printed paper is the perfect way to personalize gift wrap. All you need is plain paper and a spark of inspiration. Potato cuts, rubber stamps, stencils, rollers or brushstrokes will all produce unique patterned papers. Use lightweight paper, or cheap brown wrapping paper for the best results.

Corrugated card gives projects a unique texture and depth, and it is also very cheap to buy.

Natural papers are environmentally friendly handmade papers usually imported from the East; the selection really is enormous. It is possible to buy paper made from banana skins or recycled Bombay newsprint inlaid with rose petals. The colours are often hotter and spicier than home-produced papers, so it is well worth seeking out a specialist paper outlet and stocking up for future use.

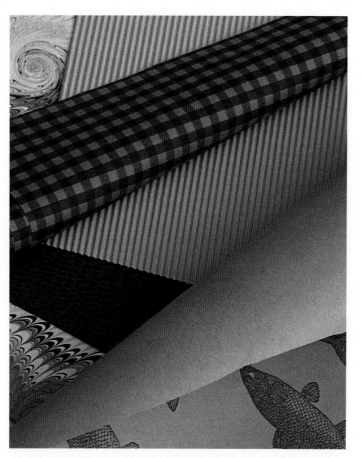

LEFT *Papers are available in every kind of colour and texture from art suppliers and craft shops.*

Basic Techniques

Tearing newspaper

Sheets of newsprint are laid and have a definite grain, usually running from the top to the bottom of the newspaper.

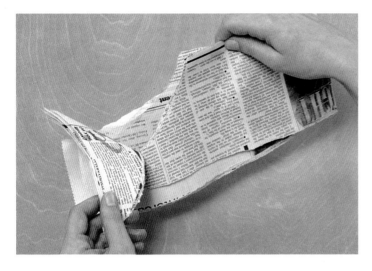

1 If you try to tear a sheet of newspaper against the grain – from side to side – it is impossible to control.

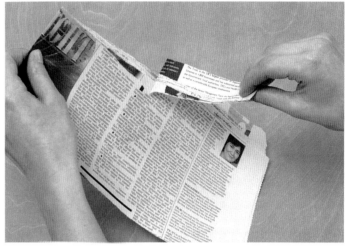

2 If newspaper is torn along the grain it is possible to produce very regular strips, as wide or narrow as you need.

Making papier-mâché pulp

Materials

5 sheets newspaper
45 ml/3 tbsp PVA (white) glue
20 ml/4 tsp wallpaper paste
10 ml/2 tsp plaster of Paris
10 ml/2 tsp linseed oil

1 Tear the newspaper into pieces about 2.5 cm/1 in square and put them in an old saucepan with water to cover. Simmer for about half an hour.

2 Spoon the paper and any water into a blender or food processor and liquidize it. Pour it into a suitable container with a lid.

3 Add the PVA (white) glue, wallpaper paste, plaster of Paris and linseed oil. Stir vigorously and the pulp is ready to use.

Preparing the surface for papier-mâché painting

The surface of the papier-mâché should be primed before painting to conceal the newsprint and to provide a good ground for decoration.

Materials

fine sandpaper
paintbrush
white emulsion (latex) paint

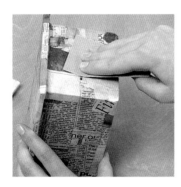

1 Gently smooth the surface of the papier-mâché using fine sandpaper.

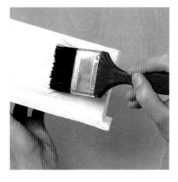

2 Apply a coat of white emulsion (latex) paint and leave the object to dry.

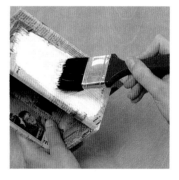

3 Rub down the dry paint lightly using fine sandpaper, and apply a second coat of paint. Once this has dried, the papier-mâché may be decorated.

• PAPERCRAFTS AND PAPIER-MACHE •

Paper Cut-outs

*G*emini – the twins – is the chosen motif for this effective paper card decoration: the two halves of the card are identical in design, yet one is the negative image of the other. These cut-outs are a traditional skill in Poland, where they are usually deftly cut freehand using a pair of scissors.

You Will Need

MATERIALS
*tracing paper
thin card or paper in two
colours, plus a large sheet
for backing
all-purpose glue*

EQUIPMENT
*pencil
craft knife
cutting mat
scissors*

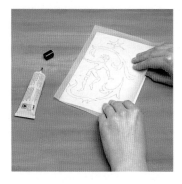

1 Trace the template from the back of the book, enlarging if necessary. Attach the tracing to the wrong side of one piece of coloured card with a few dabs of glue.

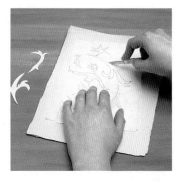

2 Using a craft knife, cut out through the template and reserve all the shapes.

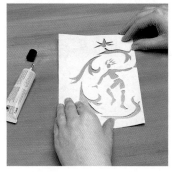

3 Remove the tracing paper, turn the card over and then back it with some card in a contrasting colour.

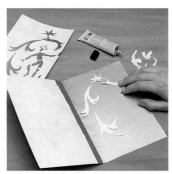

4 Cut the backing card twice the size of the cut-out card and fold down the centre. Stick a piece of the contrast card or paper to one side of the fold and arrange cut-out pieces on it to match the original design. Stick the cut-out card on the opposite side.

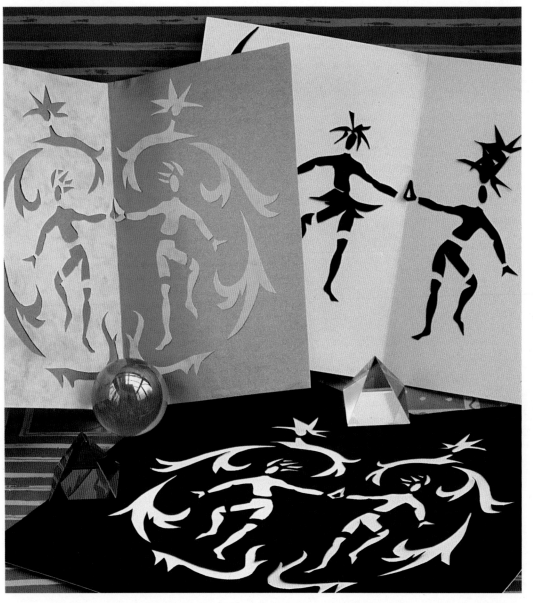

Decoupage Rose Eggs

Re-use old wrapping paper when you are making these patterned eggs.

You Will Need

Materials
*rose scrapbook motifs or rose-decorated wrapping paper
PVA (white) glue
wooden or blown eggs
clear nail varnish*

Equipment
*small scissors
paintbrush*

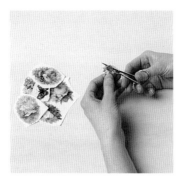

1 Cut out a selection of small rose motifs. You may find other motifs you can use, such as butterflies or forget-me-nots. Look out for interesting shapes and cut them out carefully around the outlines.

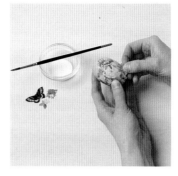

2 Using PVA (white) glue, stick the cut-out flowers to the wooden or blown eggs, making sure you overlap the edges to give a densely patterned surface. Make sure that all the wood or shell is covered.

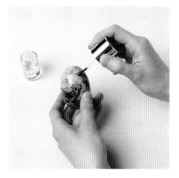

3 Once the glue is dry, coat the eggs with three or four coats of clear nail varnish, allowing each coat to dry thoroughly before adding the next one.

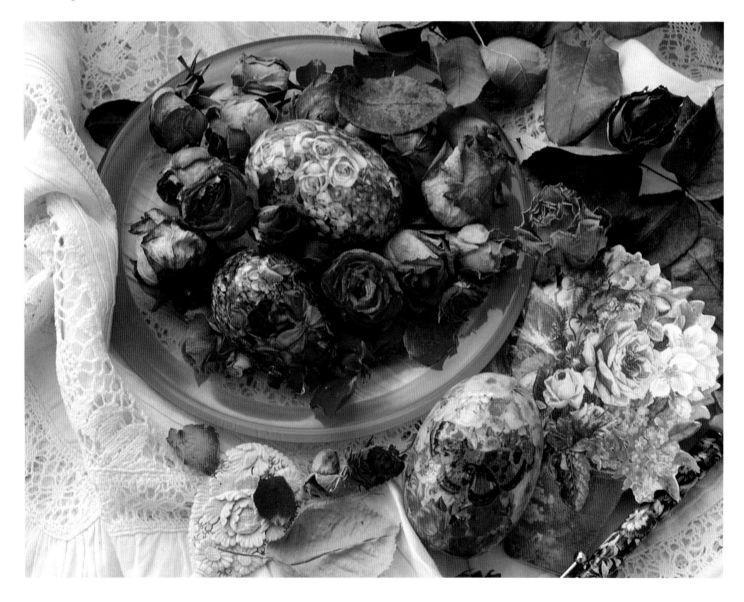

• PAPERCRAFTS AND PAPIER-MACHE •

CHRISTMAS TREE STAR

Persuade the fairy to take a well-earned rest this year, and make a magnificent gold star to take pride of place at the top of the Christmas tree.

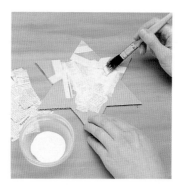

YOU WILL NEED

MATERIALS	EQUIPMENT
tracing paper	pencil
thin card or paper	scissors
corrugated card	craft knife
newspaper	cutting mat
PVA (white) glue	metal ruler
gold spray paint	bowl
gold relief or puff paint	paintbrush
gold glitter	
thin gold braid	

1 Trace the template from the back of the book, enlarging if necessary, then transfer it to thin card or paper. Cut it out and draw around it on the corrugated card. Cut it out using a craft knife and metal ruler. Tear the newspaper into small strips. Thin the PVA (white) glue with some water and brush it on to both sides of the newspaper, coating it thoroughly. Stick it on the star, brushing it down with more glue to get rid of any air bubbles. Work all over the star in a single layer, covering the edges and points neatly. Allow the star to dry thoroughly, then apply a second layer.

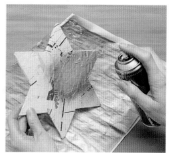

2 If the star begins to buckle, place it under a heavy weight. When it is thoroughly dry, spray both sides of it gold and allow to dry.

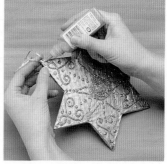

3 Draw the design on one side of the star in gold relief paint and sprinkle it with glitter while it is still wet. Allow to dry thoroughly before repeating the design on the other side. Attach thin gold braid with which to hang the star from the top of the Christmas tree.

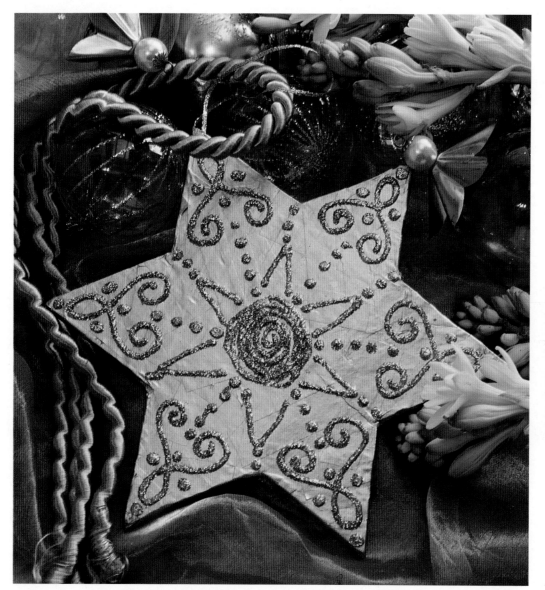

Papier-Mache Plate

For this papier-mâché plate, the colour is incorporated into the paper pulp before it is moulded. This would be a wonderful project for a whole family to do together, with each person making his or her own sign for the plate.

You Will Need

Materials	Equipment
acrylic paints	fork
paper pulp (see Basic Techniques)	pencil
strong card	plate
PVA (white) glue	craft knife
crepe paper	cutting mat
wallpaper paste	paintbrush (optional)
tracing paper	
thin card or paper	
chalk or white pencil	
black emulsion (latex) paint and gold paint (optional)	

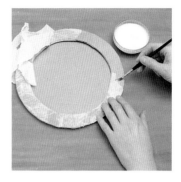

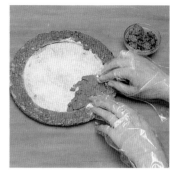

1 Using a fork, mash acrylic paint into the paper pulp until the colour is evenly mixed. Cut out two circles of card the same size, using an old plate as a template. Cut a smaller circle from one and glue the rim to the front of the other circle and the centre to the back. Cover with crepe paper soaked in wallpaper paste.

2 Press coloured pulp on to the edge of the plate, building it up in thin layers, and adding more when dry. Trace the template from the back of the book, enlarging if necessary. Transfer to thin card or paper. Cut it out and draw around it with chalk or white pencil on to the plate. Build up the body with pulp, covering the outline.

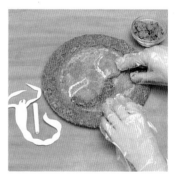

3 Add finer details such as legs and claws with more thin layers of paper pulp. Allow to dry thoroughly. To add some definition, take a dry brush with some black emulsion (latex) paint and wipe lightly over the scorpion and the rim of the plate. Repeat with gold paint.

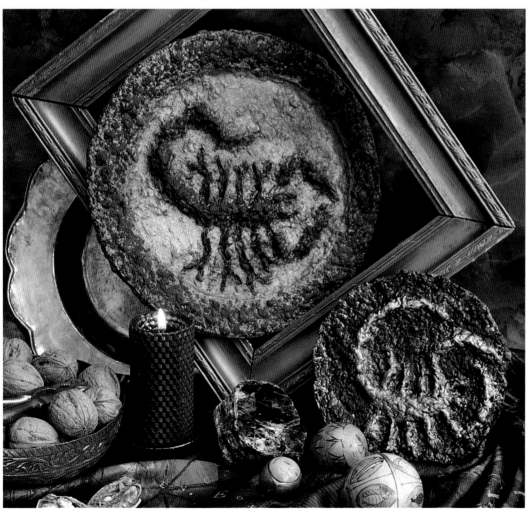

Gilded Bookmark

Look for pictures of old engravings and heraldic devices for this découpage: the clearly defined images will photocopy perfectly and look great once they've been cunningly aged with tea. Use stiff card so that the bookmark isn't too bulky.

YOU WILL NEED

MATERIALS	EQUIPMENT
stiff card	craft knife
acrylic gesso	cutting mat
acrylic paints: red, orange and green	metal ruler
gold paint	paintbrush
tea bags	bowl
photocopied images	scissors
PVA (white) glue	
velvet ribbon	

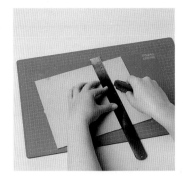

1 Using a craft knife and metal ruler, cut a rectangle of card 15 x 5 cm/6 x 2 in, and cut off the corners diagonally.

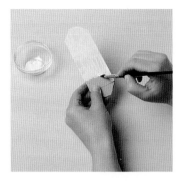

2 Paint it with acrylic gesso. Mix a red oxide colour using red, orange and green acrylics and paint this all over the bookmark. When dry, cover with gold paint, leaving some of the red oxide showing through.

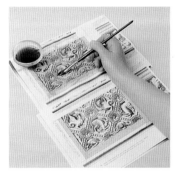

3 Make a very strong solution of tea and paint the photocopies with this to create an aged appearance. Allow to dry, then cut out.

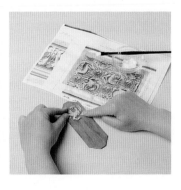

4 Stick on the cut-outs with PVA (white) glue and varnish with diluted PVA (white) to seal. Glue a length of velvet ribbon to the back of the bookmark.

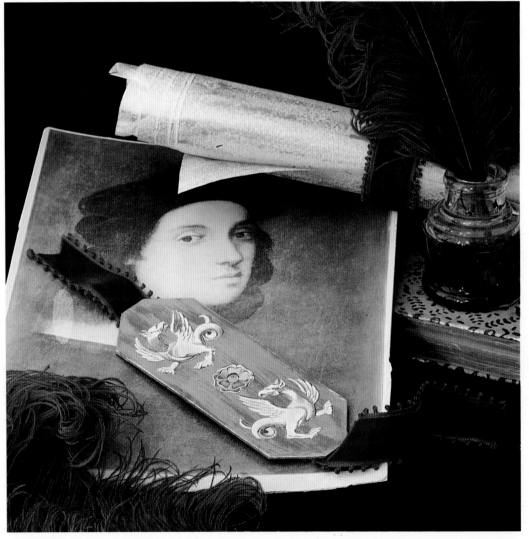

Garland Tray Cut-outs

*T*he simple leaf design for this pretty découpage tray is folded and cut out like a row of dancing paper dolls. When drawing the design, make sure that your outline continues to the folds so that your paper garland stays in one piece when it is opened out.

You Will Need

Materials	Equipment
wooden tray	paintbrushes
yellow emulsion (latex) paint	pencil
large sheet of green paper	scissors
PVA (white) glue	scrap paper
clear gloss acrylic varnish	

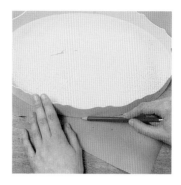

1 Paint the tray with two coats of yellow emulsion (latex) paint and allow to dry. Place the tray on the green paper and draw around it. Cut out the shape just inside the line.

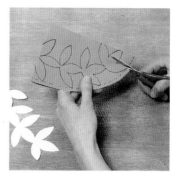

2 Fold the paper in half, then in half again. Draw a series of connecting leaf shapes on to scrap paper and cut them out. When you are happy with the design, draw around it on to the green paper, making sure that it reaches the folded edges. Cut along the pencil line.

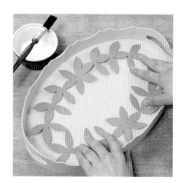

3 Open out the garland carefully and glue it on to the tray. Allow to dry.

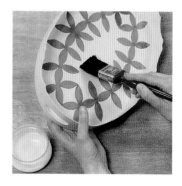

4 Protect the tray with up to four coats of varnish.

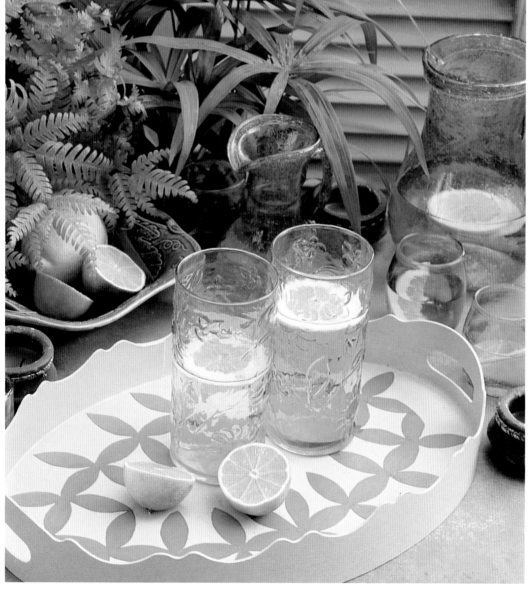

Beaming Sun Wall Plaque

A cheerful sunny face looking down at you is sure to cheer you up, so put this wall plaque where it will do you most good – perhaps over the breakfast table! The plaque is made from sandwiched layers of corrugated card and mounted on card in the same way, so it is very easy to make. There is also an alternative idea, using papier-mâché pulp to mould the face.

You Will Need

Materials
corrugated card
PVA (white) glue
masking tape
white undercoat paint
acrylic paints: red, yellow and blue
matt varnish

Equipment
pair of compasses
pencil
craft knife
scissors
paintbrushes

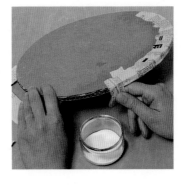

1 Draw and cut out five equal circles of card to the size required. Glue together three circles. Bind the edges with masking tape.

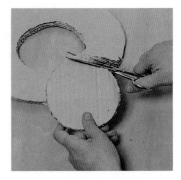

2 Glue the remaining two circles together and cut out a circle from the centre. Trim this smaller circle so that there will be a gap all around it when it is replaced.

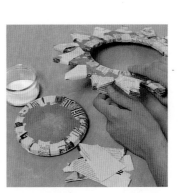

3 On the circle with the hole, draw the rays of the sun and cut them out. Bind the edges inside and out and also the edges of the small circle.

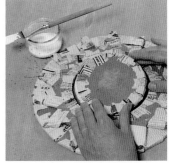

4 Glue the prepared sun rays and the face on to the backing circle, centralizing the face in the slightly larger area left for it.

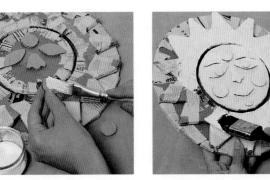

5 Draw the features on card freehand and cut them out. Glue them on to the face.

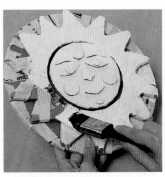

6 Prime the whole of the plaque with white undercoat and allow to dry.

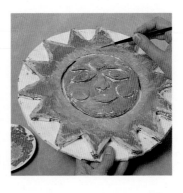

7 Decorate with acrylic paints. When dry, apply two coats of varnish.

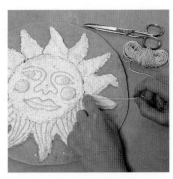

8 Alternatively, make the sun shape from papier-mâché pulp (see Basic Techniques), moulding it by hand on the backing circle. Use fine string to delineate the features and give relief detail to the rays. Coat the face in primer and paint as before.

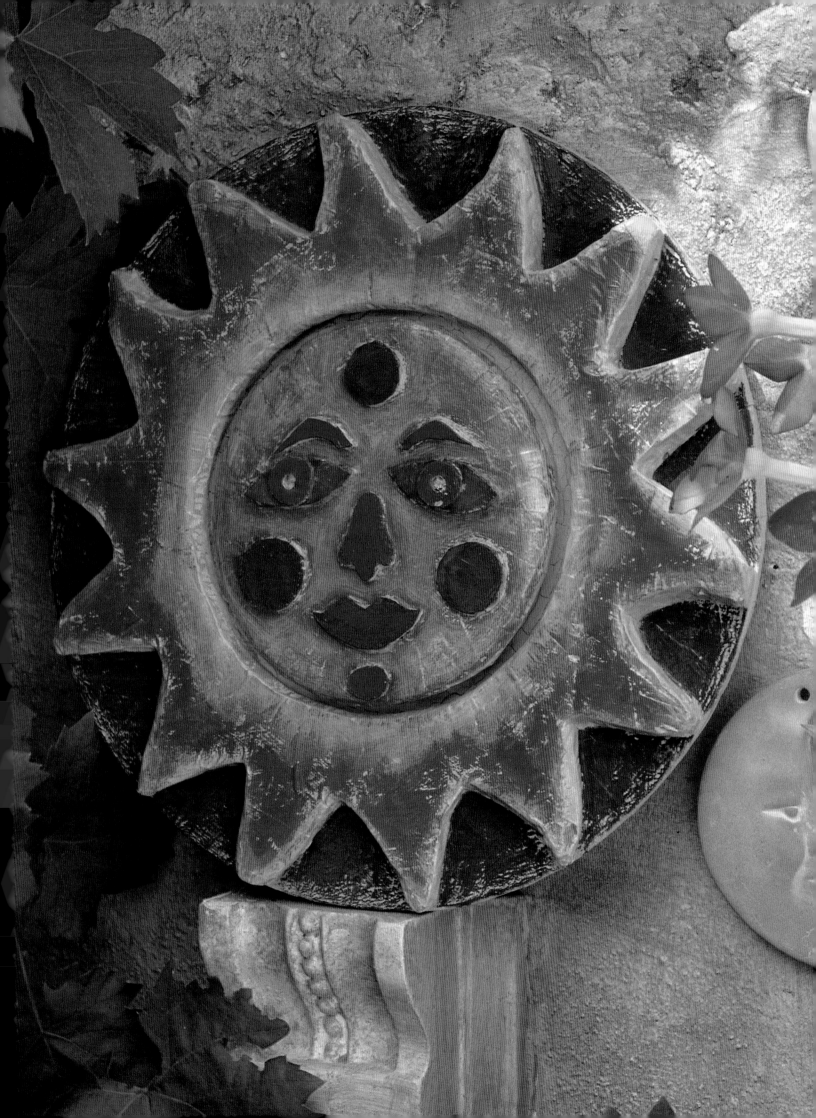

• PAPERCRAFTS AND PAPIER-MACHE •

DECORATIVE NAPKIN RING

This practical project recycles old card to create something special for the dinner table. You could decorate the ring with a design of your choice, or use this stylish heraldic motif.

YOU WILL NEED

MATERIALS	EQUIPMENT
tracing paper	*hard and soft pencils*
thick card	*craft knife*
poster tube	*cutting mat*
newspaper	*bowl*
wallpaper paste	*fine and medium*
acrylic gesso	*paintbrushes*
acrylic paints: blue, red, yellow, light gold, black and white	*glue gun or epoxy resin glue*
gloss acrylic varnish	

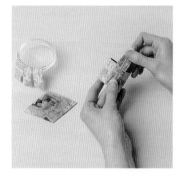

1 Trace the template from the back of the book, enlarging if necessary. Cut out a card diamond. Cut a 4 cm/1½ in section from the poster tube. Coat strips of newspaper with wallpaper paste. Cover the ring, with the edges, with several layers. Cover the diamond with about ten layers.

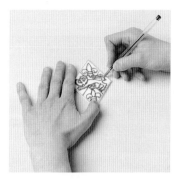

2 When the papier-mâché is dry, prime it with three coats of acrylic gesso. Transfer the traced design on to the diamond by rubbing over the back with a soft pencil, then drawing over the outlines.

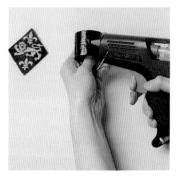

3 Paint the background diamonds in blue and red and the lion and fleur-de-lys in yellow. Highlight the design in light gold paint and outline the shapes in black. Pick out details in red and white. Paint the ring with two coats of blue. Seal the diamond and ring with acrylic varnish and, when dry, glue the two parts together.

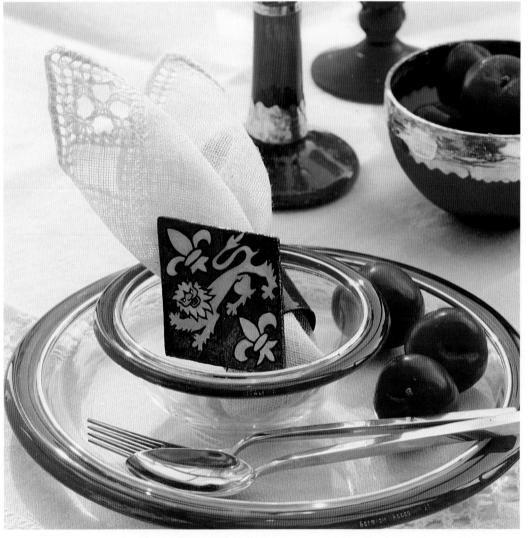

• PAPERCRAFTS AND PAPIER-MACHE •

ORANGE BOWL

Hoard your old magazines so that you can assemble a good collection of orange and yellow papers for this papier-mâché bowl. It is designed to look like half an orange – plain on the outside and beautifully textured inside.

YOU WILL NEED

MATERIALS

*petroleum jelly
newspaper
wallpaper paste
old magazine pages that are predominantly orange and yellow
orange wrapping paper
gloss varnish
gold paint*

EQUIPMENT

*large bowl
scissors
medium and fine paintbrushes*

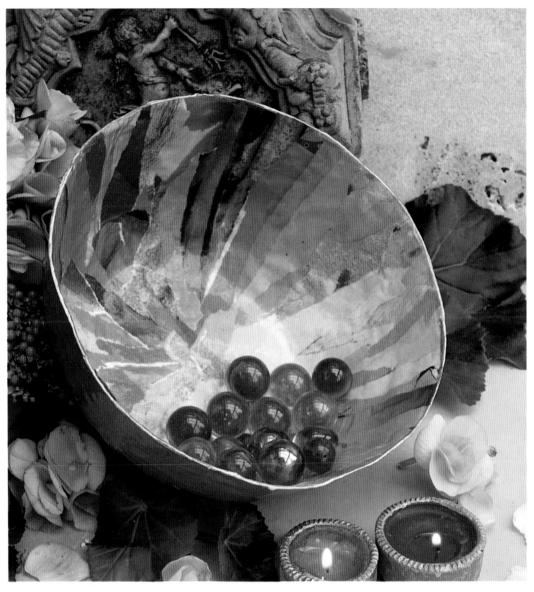

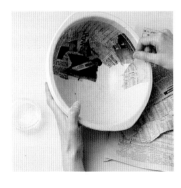

1 Coat the inside of the bowl with a layer of petroleum jelly. Soak strips of newspaper in wallpaper paste. Cover the inside of the bowl with at least ten layers of strips. Allow to dry thoroughly, then gently ease the bowl from the mould.

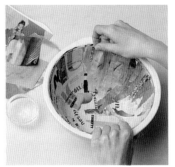

2 Tear the magazine pages into long, narrow triangles and paste them around the inside of the bowl so that they taper towards the bottom.

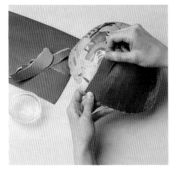

3 Cover the outside of the bowl with torn strips of plain orange and yellow wrapping paper, carefully overlapping the edges.

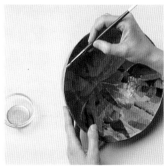

4 Leave the bowl to dry thoroughly, then trim the top edge with scissors. Coat the bowl with a protective layer of varnish. Paint a thin line of gold paint along the top edge to complete the bowl.

Sunburst Bowl

This spectacular sun seems to burst out of the bowl towards you. Use all your creativity to make the design as exuberant as possible. Papier-mâché gives you the ability to make graceful vessels without the skill and equipment needed for making ceramics. This bowl is ideal for fruit, nuts or small display items, but you might well want to leave it empty to show it off.

YOU WILL NEED

MATERIALS
petroleum jelly
newspaper
paper pulp (see Basic Techniques)
PVA (white) glue
white undercoat paint
gouache or acrylic paints: yellow, blue and red
gold "liquid leaf" paint or gold gouache paint
fixative spray
gloss varnish

EQUIPMENT
bowl
medium and fine paintbrushes
paint-mixing container
pair of compasses
pencil

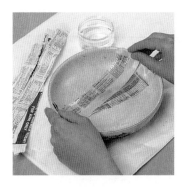

1 Coat the inside of the bowl with a layer of petroleum jelly. Dip strips of newspaper in water, then lay them over the inside of the bowl.

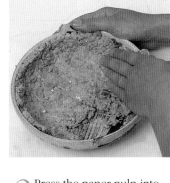

2 Press the paper pulp into the mould so that it is about 1 cm/½ in thick. Allow to dry in an airing cupboard, for about five days.

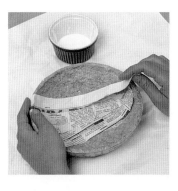

3 Release the dried paper pulp from the mould and cover it in strips of newspaper dipped in PVA (white) glue. Allow to dry thoroughly.

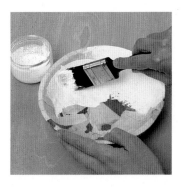

4 Give the bowl two coats of white undercoat, allowing each coat to dry.

5 Use the pair of compasses to locate the sun shape accurately, then draw a small circle for the centre and a larger one to contain the rays. Draw the rays freehand.

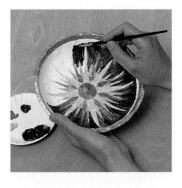

6 Fill in the yellow and gold areas first of all. Then paint the rim in gold. Fill in the blue background, leaving a white band below the gold rim.

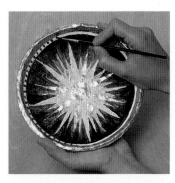

7 Paint the red border and allow to dry. Seal the bowl with fixative spray and protect it with a coat of varnish.

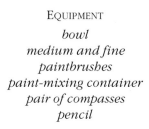

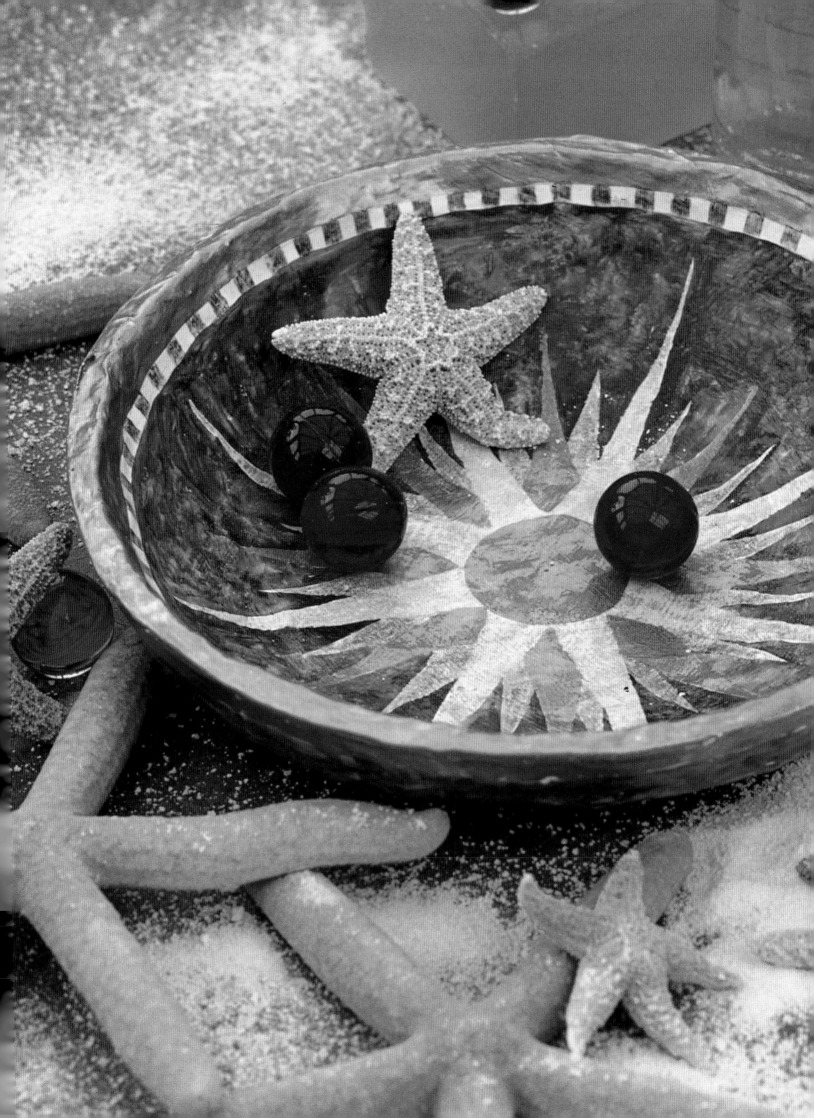

TWISTED PAPER FRAME

This frame is made from unravelled twisted paper, which is available from most gift shops. It is simple to make, and provides the ideal frame for your favourite photo or picture.

YOU WILL NEED

MATERIALS	EQUIPMENT
card	plate and saucer
twisted paper	pencil
PVA (white) glue	scissors
emulsion (latex) paints:	craft knife
white and gold	cutting mat
fabric star motifs	old toothbrush
backing card (optional)	paint-mixing containers

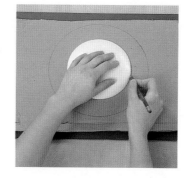

1 Draw around the plate on to the card. Place the saucer in the centre of the circle and draw around it. Cut out the outer circle with scissors and then the inner circle using a craft knife, so you are left with a card ring.

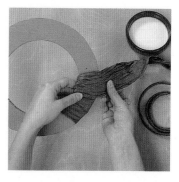

2 Unwind the twisted paper and wind it carefully around the ring until it is fully covered. Stick the end down with PVA (white) glue.

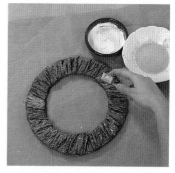

3 Dip an old toothbrush into the white paint and run your finger along the bristles so that a fine spray of paint lands on the card frame. Repeat with the gold paint.

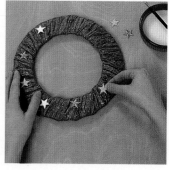

4 Stick the star motifs all over the frame with PVA (white) glue. If you like, stick a card backing circle on the back, leaving a gap in which to insert a picture.

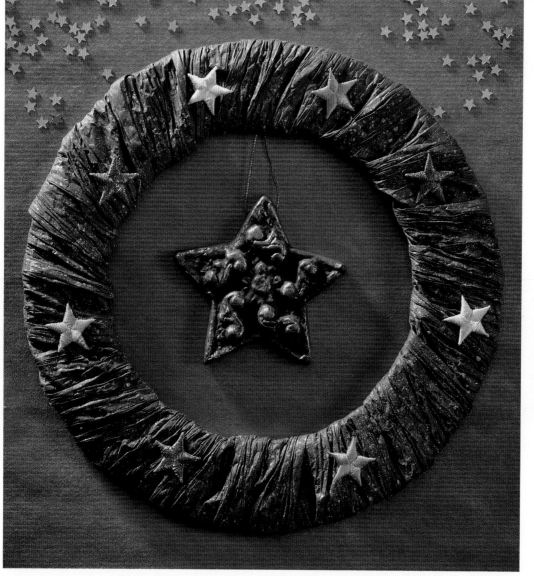

• PAPERCRAFTS AND PAPIER-MACHE •

PAPIER-MACHE JUG

This jug looks like a modern Italian ceramic, with its elegant shape and brilliant colours, but in fact it is made from papier-mâché shaped round a blown-up balloon. A sunflower moulded from paper pulp makes a relief decoration.

YOU WILL NEED

MATERIALS
*balloon
newspaper
wallpaper paste
thin card
masking tape
round margarine container
fine string
paper pulp (see Basic Techniques)
acrylic paints: blue, yellow, red and green
clear varnish*

EQUIPMENT
*scissors
medium and fine paintbrushes
paint-mixing container*

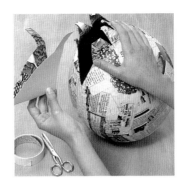

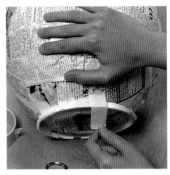

1 Blow up the balloon and tie a knot in it. Soak strips of newspaper in wallpaper paste, and cover the balloon with at least eight layers of them. Allow to dry. Cut slits in the top of the balloon at the knot end and remove the balloon. Cut out a V-shape in one side. Cut a piece of card to form a spout and tape in position.

2 Tape the rim of a margarine container to the bottom for the base. For the handle, roll up some glued newspaper sheets and curve them to fit the jug. Allow to dry. Cover the handle with string, leaving about 1–2.5 cm/½–1 in at each end uncovered. Cut two slits in the side and insert the handle.

3 Model the paper pulp on the side of the jug in the shape of sunflowers and leaves. Allow to dry overnight. Paint the background, flowers and details and allow to dry, before giving the jug a coat of varnish.

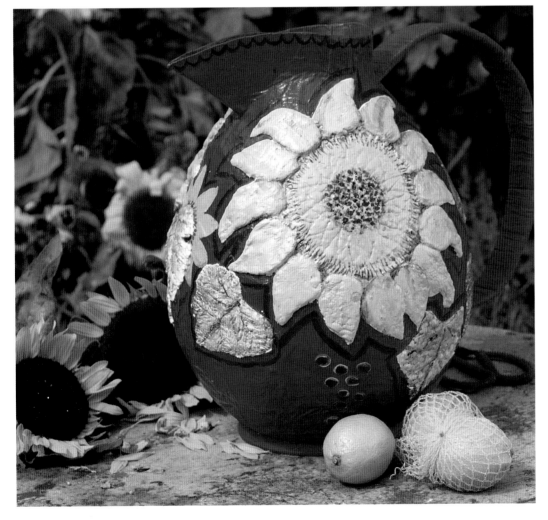

27

Papier-Mache Frame

This frame provides a beautiful three-dimensional background to a picture or painting. You can experiment as much as you like with the frame: try using softer colours instead of the strong ones here, or replace the heart motifs with a design of your choosing to create a truly individual frame.

You Will Need

Materials
tracing paper
card
masking tape
wire
newspaper
wallpaper paste
white emulsion (latex) paint
self-hardening clay
poster paints: royal-blue, violet and yellow
clear varnish
photo or picture
PVA (white) glue (optional)

Equipment
pencil
craft knife
cutting mat
paintbrushes
clay modelling tool

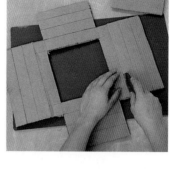

1 Trace the template from the back of the book, enlarging if necessary. Cut out the centre square. Score along the dotted lines using a craft knife, taking care not to cut right through.

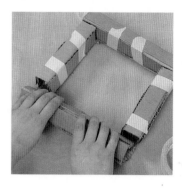

2 Fold each flap inwards along the scored edges and tape the frame together with masking tape.

3 Fix a piece of wire to the back, using masking tape.

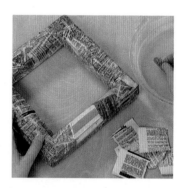

4 Tear the newspaper in small squares, measuring about 2.5 x 2.5 cm/ 1 x 1 in. Dip them in wallpaper paste and stick them on to the frame until both the front and the back of the frame are well covered.

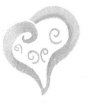

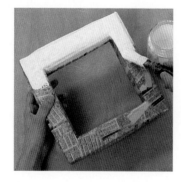

5 Prime the covered frame with a coat of white paint and allow to dry. Apply a second coat of paint to make sure that the surface is opaque. Allow to dry thoroughly.

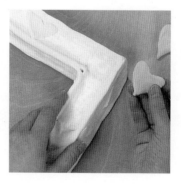

6 Form heart shapes out of clay by hand and push these on to the front of the frame for decoration. Fix the hearts in place by smoothing down the sides with a clay modelling tool.

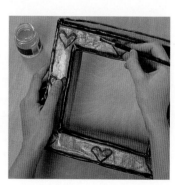

7 Paint the frame with poster paints and allow to dry. Seal with a coat of varnish. Once dry, stick your chosen photo or picture on to the card (set aside in step 1) and glue or tape it in place.

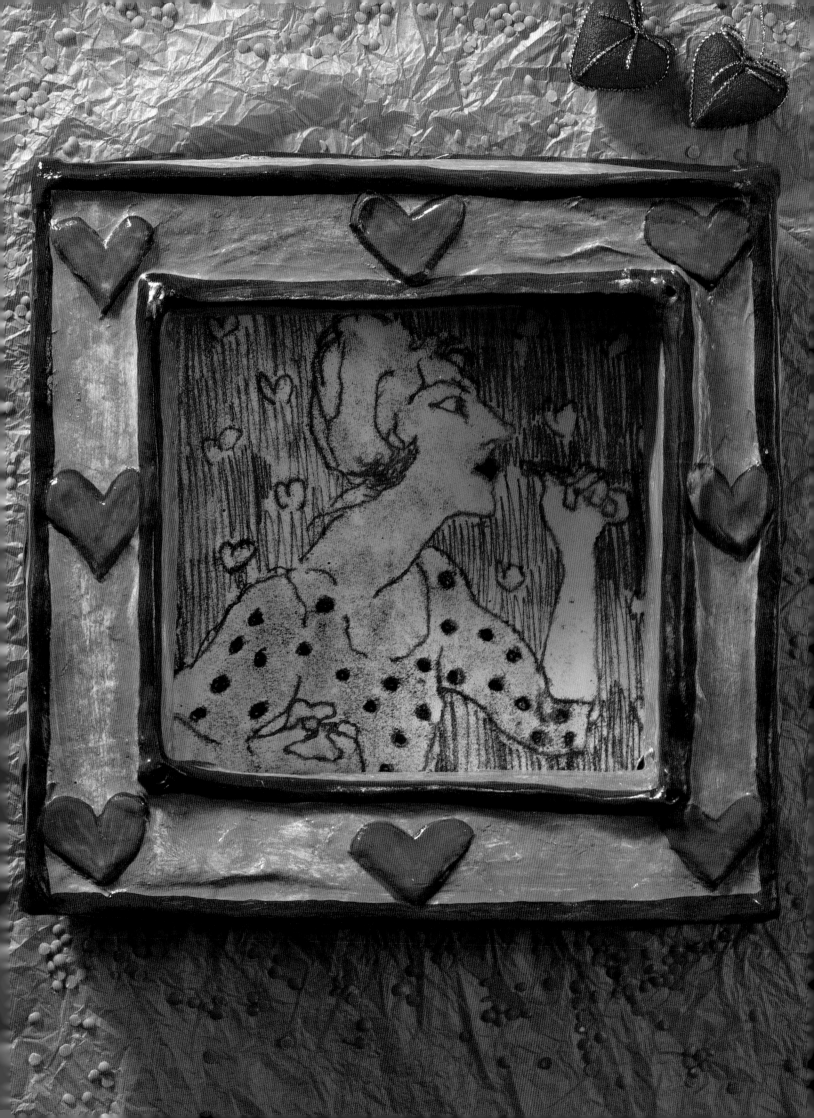

Crackle-Glazed Print

Antique prints are expensive, but with this technique you can create your own thoroughly original design very cheaply. Use a photocopier to enlarge or reduce motifs and practise arranging them until you have a design that appeals.

You Will Need

Materials
selection of black and white
cupid prints
spray adhesive
tea bags and instant coffee
PVA (white) glue
hardboard or card
acrylic medium
clear acrylic gloss varnish
burnt umber acrylic paint

Equipment
scissors
large soft Chinese
paintbrush
household and fine
paintbrushes
paint-mixing container

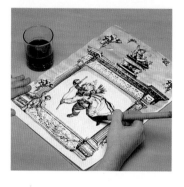

1 Cut out the prints and lightly coat them on the back with spray adhesive. Arrange the prints until you are happy with the result. By using spray adhesive, you can reposition the designs as many times as you like. Photocopy the final result.

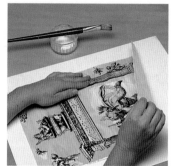

2 Make a "cocktail" of one tea bag and three teaspoons of coffee and let it cool. Apply to the print with a Chinese paintbrush. You can experiment with brews of different strengths and apply the mixture several times, to create depth. Allow to dry.

3 Mix equal parts of PVA (white) glue and water and apply the mixture to the back of the print with a household paintbrush. Smooth the print on to the hardboard or card backing. (You can also apply the print directly to a wall or a piece of furniture.) Brush the PVA (white) mixture on top of the print and backing and allow to dry.

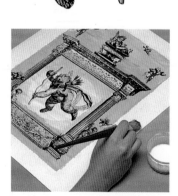
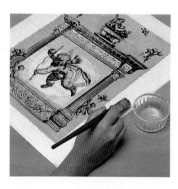
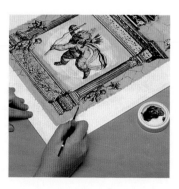

4 Cover the print and backing with acrylic medium in the same way. This may cause the paper to wrinkle, but don't worry: once dry, the wrinkles will vanish.

5 Coat with acrylic varnish, to give a shiny finish and add an antique look.

6 Mix burnt umber acrylic paint into the varnish and paint cracks with a fine paintbrush. Add more shadows and blend them in softly. Finally, apply another coat of acrylic varnish and allow to dry.

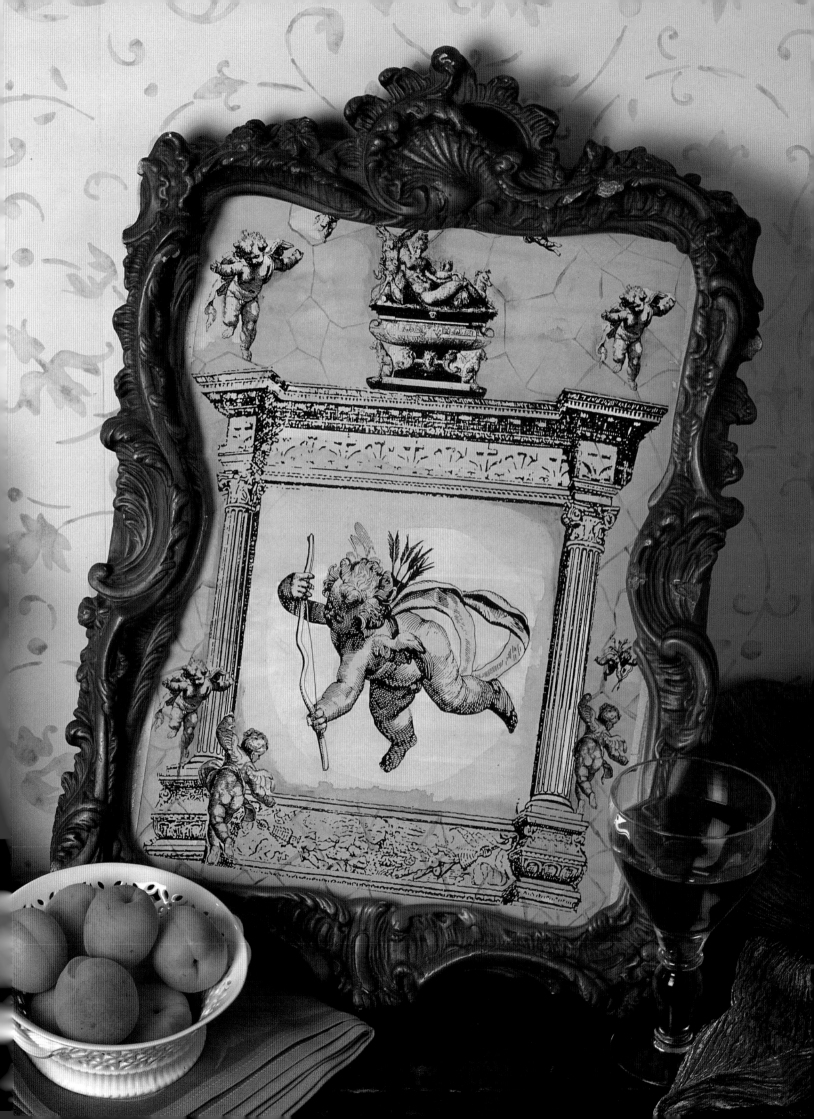

• PAPERCRAFTS AND PAPIER-MACHE •

Water Bearer's Shrine

Aquarius, the water bearer, carries the waters of creation and symbolizes death and renewal. An original tribute to him is this charming wall plaque.

You Will Need

Materials
thin card or paper
corrugated card
masking tape
paper pulp (see Basic Techniques)
newspaper
wallpaper paste
PVA (white) glue
white acrylic primer
gouache paints: pale blue, dark blue, orange and red
gloss varnish
gold enamel paint
epoxy resin glue
mirror-hanging plate

Equipment
pencil
craft knife
cutting mat
bowl
paintbrushes

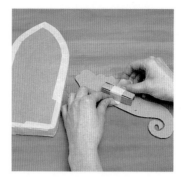

1 Draw templates for the shrine, its sides and figure, and transfer them to corrugated card. Cut them out and assemble them using masking tape. Make a small rectangular "step" from card and fix it to the figure's back.

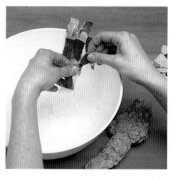

2 Apply paper pulp to the front of the figure to give a rounded shape. When dry, cover the figure and plaque in several layers of newspaper strips soaked in wallpaper paste. Allow to dry.

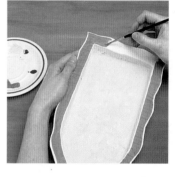

3 Paint on a coat of PVA (white) glue followed, when dry, by a coat of white acrylic primer. Decorate the plaque and figure with gouache paints.

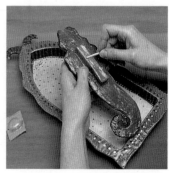

4 Varnish, then, when dry, highlight the details with gold enamel paint. Use epoxy resin glue to secure the figure in place and fix a mirror-hanging plate to the back.

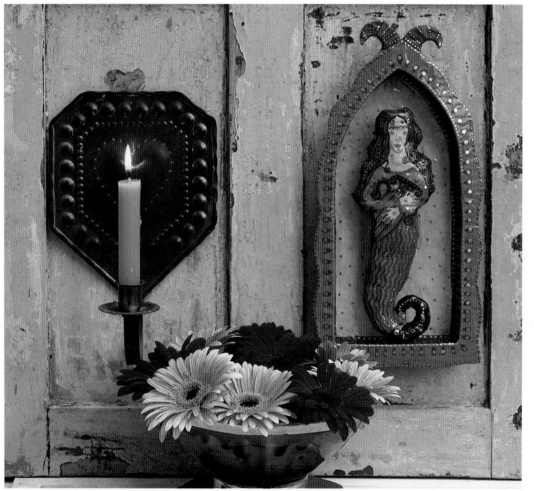

• PAPERCRAFTS AND PAPIER-MACHE •

Gold-rimmed Bowl

This attractive bowl is delicately hand-painted and decorated with gold paint. Its cheerful, sunny design will brighten up any dull corner. Use it purely as decoration, or to hold trinkets, nuts or sweets.

YOU WILL NEED

MATERIALS
*petroleum jelly
newspaper
paper pulp (see Basic Techniques)
PVA (white) glue
white undercoat paint
gold "liquid leaf" paint
acrylic paints: white, yellow, ochre, turquoise and brown
paper tissue
fixative spray
gloss varnish*

EQUIPMENT
*bowl
scissors
large, medium and fine paintbrushes
pair of compasses
pencil
paint-mixing container*

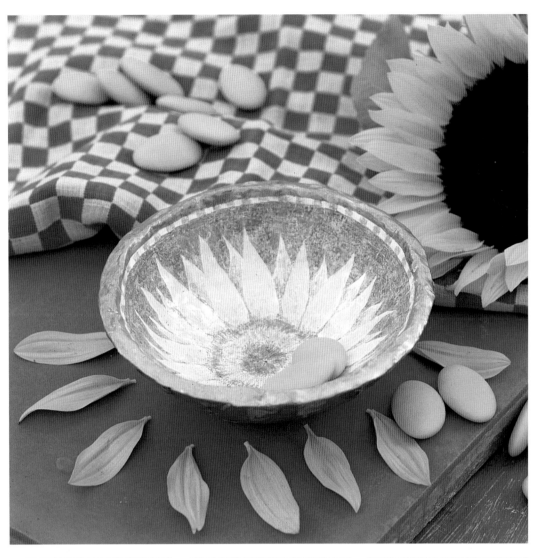

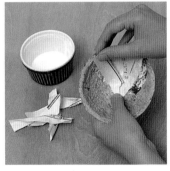
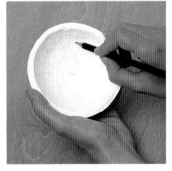
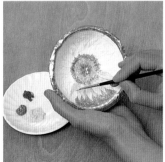

1 Apply a coat of petroleum jelly to the inside of the bowl. Line it with strips of wet newspaper. Put the paper pulp into the bowl in an even layer about 1 cm/½ in deep. Allow to dry in an airing cupboard for about five days. Release the bowl from the mould. Dip strips of newspaper in PVA (white) glue and cover the bowl.

2 Give the bowl two coats of white undercoat. Use a pair of compasses to help you centralize the flower motif. Draw the flower freehand.

3 Paint the rim with gold "liquid leaf". Decorate the bowl with the acrylic paints. Mix white into all the colours to lighten them and, before the paint dries, dab some off with a paper tissue so that the undercoat shows through in places. Allow to dry. Spray with fixative spray, then give the bowl a coat of varnish.

• PAPERCRAFTS AND PAPIER-MACHE •

MIRRORED KEEPSAKE BOX

This box is made from an old poster tube decorated with mirror shards. It is an original idea for storing jewellery.

YOU WILL NEED

MATERIALS
section of poster tube
card
masking tape
PVA (white) glue
newspaper
4 marbles
wallpaper paste
epoxy resin glue
chemical metal filler
(i.e. car-body repair filler)
mirror fragments
white acrylic primer
selection of gouache paints
glossy varnish
gold enamel paint

EQUIPMENT
pencil
scissors
pair of compasses
small and fine paintbrushes
paint-mixing containers

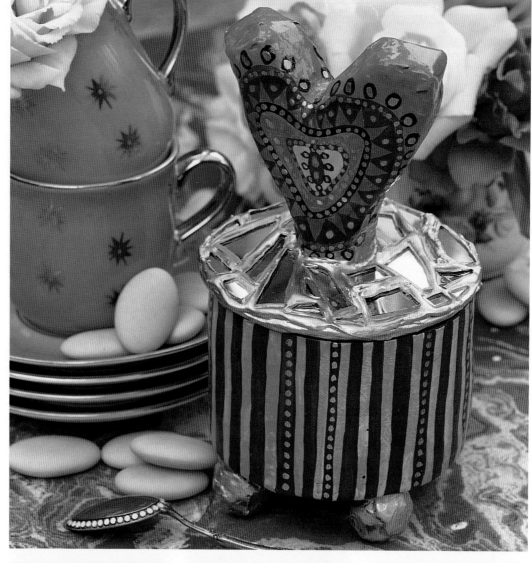

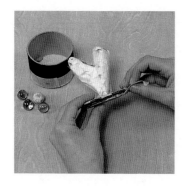

1 Draw around the poster tube end on card, cut it out and tape it to the tube. Cut out a slightly larger lid and another circle 1 cm/½ in less in diameter. Glue together. Bend a roll of newspaper into a heart shape and tape it to the lid. Cover the marbles with masking tape.

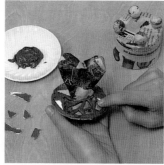

2 Cover the box, lid and marbles with several layers of newspaper strips soaked in wallpaper paste. When dry, glue the marbles to the box base with epoxy resin glue. Mix up the filler, spread it on to the lid, and carefully push in the mirror fragments.

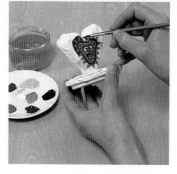

3 Paint the box, excluding the mirror pieces, with PVA (white) glue. When dry, prime the box and paint the design with gouache paints.

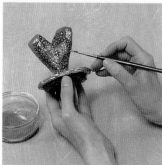

4 Coat the box with several layers of glossy varnish, and allow to dry thoroughly. Add detail in gold enamel.

• PAPERCRAFTS AND PAPIER-MACHE •

Floating Leaves Mobile

Featherlight paper leaves will flutter delicately in the merest whiff of air. Use a variety of textures for the cut-outs — look out for handmade paper incorporating leaves and flower petals.

You Will Need

MATERIALS
*thick silver florist's wire
tracing paper
thin card or paper
selection of coloured and textured papers
matching sewing thread*

EQUIPMENT
*wire-cutters
round-nosed pliers
pencil
scissors
needle*

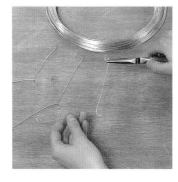

1 Cut two lengths of wire 20 cm/8 in and one length 30 cm/12 in. Twist each piece of wire in the middle to make a loop. Make a small loop, pointing downwards, at each end of each length.

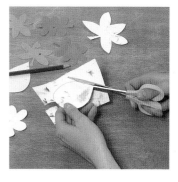

2 Trace the templates from the back of the book, enlarging if necessary. Transfer them to card or paper and cut out. Draw round them on coloured and textured papers, then cut out the shapes.

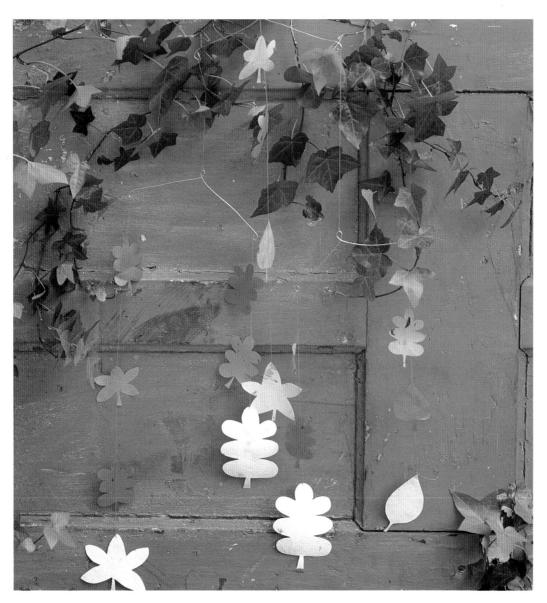

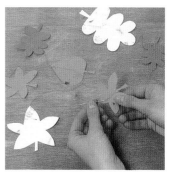

3 Use a needle to attach an assortment of leaves on to a length of thread to hang from each wire loop.

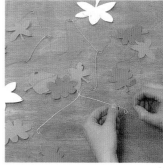

4 Use thread to hang the two shorter wires from the ends of the longer one. Tie the leaves to each wire loop. Fasten a length of thread to the top loop to hang the mobile.

• PAPERCRAFTS AND PAPIER-MACHE •

Decorated Box

This mirror box has a wonderful corrugated texture. The mirror is hidden behind doors, which can be closed when not in use.

YOU WILL NEED

MATERIALS
*corrugated card
PVA (white) glue
newspaper
masking tape
white undercoat paint
gouache paints: red, blue,
orange, yellow and white
gloss varnish
gold "liquid leaf" paint
mirror
epoxy resin glue
2 small brass door hinges*

EQUIPMENT
*craft knife
cutting mat
metal ruler
pencil
fine paintbrushes
paint-mixing container*

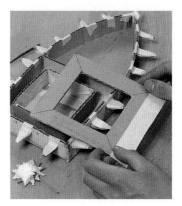

1 Cut out the box pieces from corrugated card. The back is 26 cm/10 in high and 13 cm/5 in wide at the base. The sides are 3.5 cm/1½ in deep. Create a recess 3.5 cm/1½ in deep and 8 cm/3 in square, for the mirror to sit in. Cut a 13 cm/5 in flat square frame for the outside of the recess. Cut a 7 cm/2¾ in square piece of card in half for the doors. Cut out the petals for the sides of the box. Cut out the sunflowers and the stems, bulking out the middles by gluing on scrunched-up newspaper with PVA (white) glue. Assemble the box, using masking tape. Leave off the doors.

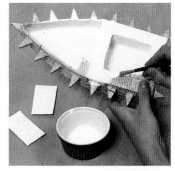

2 Cover the box with layers of newspaper soaked in diluted PVA (white) glue. Allow to dry. Paint with undercoat.

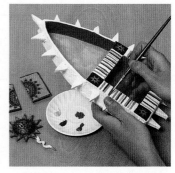

3 Paint all the pieces with gouache paints. When dry, apply several coats of varnish. Add details in gold and glue on the mirror. Pierce three holes in the shelf and glue in the sunflowers with epoxy resin glue. Glue the hinges and doors in position.

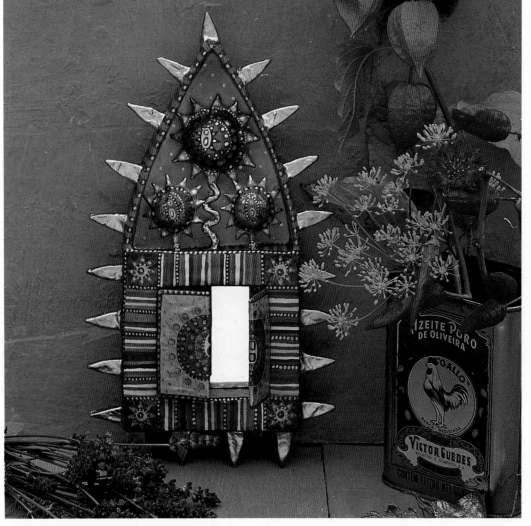

• PAPERCRAFTS AND PAPIER-MACHE •

Love Token Bowl

This delightful container for a Valentine's gift uses a simple but very decorative technique.

You Will Need

Materials
petroleum jelly
newspaper
paper pulp (see Basic Techniques)
PVA (white) glue
white acrylic primer
tracing paper
masking tape
gouache or acrylic paints: blue, white, red, yellow and gold
clear gloss varnish

Equipment
bowl
medium and fine paintbrushes
pencil
scissors
paint-mixing container

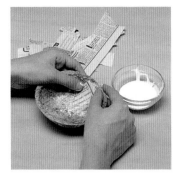

1 Coat the inside of the bowl with a layer of petroleum jelly, followed by strips of newspaper. Press a layer of paper pulp into the bowl. When dry, release from the bowl. Cover the pulp with newspaper strips dipped in PVA (white) glue.

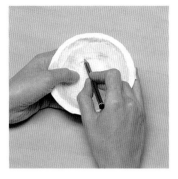

2 When dry, cover with white primer. Trace the template from the back of the book, enlarging if necessary. Snip the edges so the template can be taped flat inside the bowl, and transfer the outline.

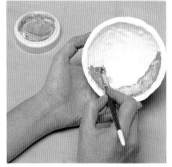

3 Paint the background pale blue, dabbing on lighter shades for a mottled effect.

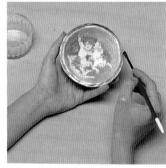

4 Paint the design, mixing the colours to achieve subtle shades. Paint the rim gold. When dry, give the bowl a coat of varnish.

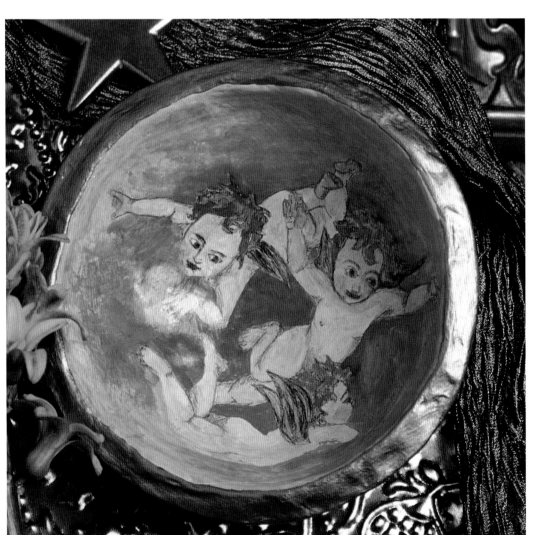

• PAPERCRAFTS AND PAPIER-MACHE •

WALL PLAQUE

Although the heart and farm animal motifs call to mind folk art, the strong pastel colours used to paint this plaque give it a more contemporary feel. It would be at home in a light, modern interior.

YOU WILL NEED

MATERIALS
*galvanized wire, from a coat hanger
card, 13 x 13 in/5 x 5 in
masking tape
newspaper
wallpaper paste
white emulsion (latex) or poster paint
self-hardening clay
acrylic or poster paints: pink, mauve, blue, green and yellow
clear varnish*

EQUIPMENT
*scissors
medium and small paintbrushes
clay-modelling tools
paint-mixing containers*

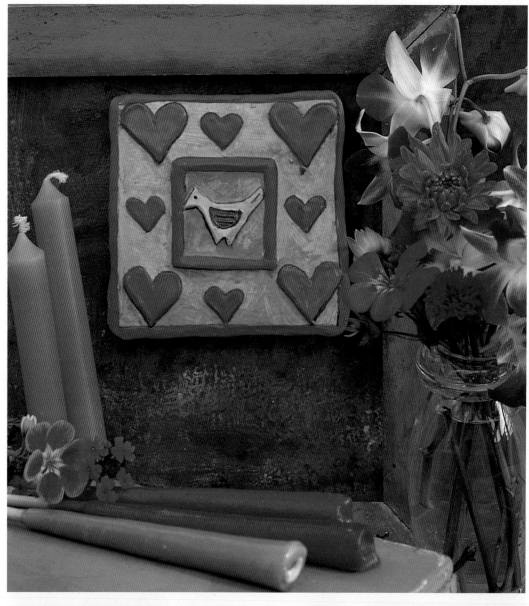

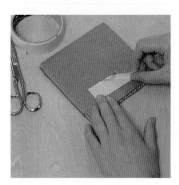

1 Shape a hook from the wire and tape it on to the back of the card with masking tape.

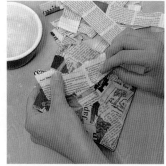

2 Tear the newspaper into small strips. Dip them into the wallpaper paste and cover both sides of the card with a layer of newspaper.

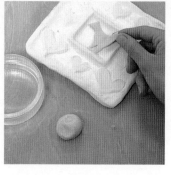

3 Prime both sides of the plaque with white paint and allow to dry. Mould decorative borders, heart shapes and a central chicken motif in the self-hardening clay. Allow to dry thoroughly.

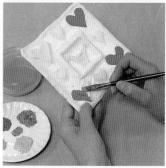

4 Decorate with the paints and allow to dry. Finish with a coat of varnish.

SCHERENSCHNITTE

Intricately cut paper designs existed for many centuries in the Middle and Far East before they became popular in Europe and America. This papercraft technique is also known by the German term "Scherenschnitte" as it was particularly practised in Switzerland and Germany.

YOU WILL NEED

MATERIALS	EQUIPMENT
tracing paper	*pencil*
paper	*craft knife*
thin black paper	*metal ruler*
spray adhesive	*cutting mat*
mounting paper	

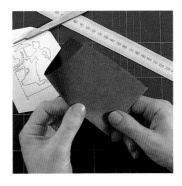

1 Trace the template from the back of the book, enlarging if necessary. Transfer it to paper. Fold the thin black paper in half.

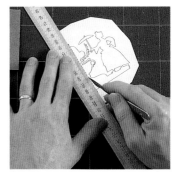

2 Cut along the centre edge of the design using a craft knife and a metal ruler.

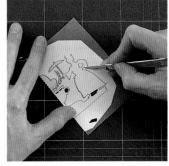

3 Give the reverse side of the tracing a very light coat of spray adhesive and stick it to the back of the black paper. Cut out the shapes using the tip of the craft knife. Move the paper around as you cut, so that you always cut at the easiest angle.

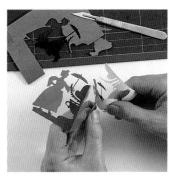

4 Very carefully, separate the black paper from the tracing, making sure that the picture does not tear. Unfold the picture and display it on mounting paper.

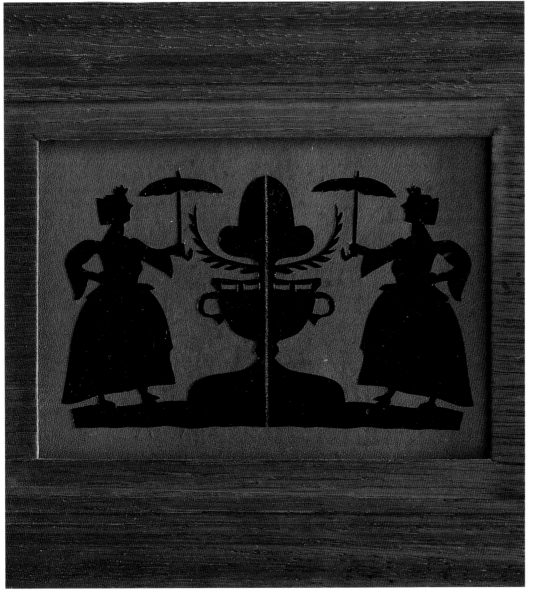

• Papercrafts and Papier-mache •

Cardboard Gift Boxes

It is simple to transform a flat sheet of thin card into an attractive gift box to make an ideal receptacle for that special present. Stamp rows of scampering dogs diagonally on to your box before folding it to add a frivolous touch, or select your own motif for an individualized look. The box can be scaled up or down, depending on the size you require, and the surface can be decorated with different designs to suit the occasion.

You Will Need

MATERIALS
thin coloured card
piece of paper (optional)
stamp pad
double-sided tape

EQUIPMENT
pencil
ruler
craft knife
cutting mat
rubber stamp
set square (optional)
blunt knife

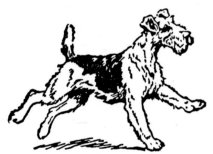

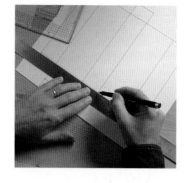

1 Follow the design from the back of the book, scaling it up or down to the required size, but taking care to keep the proportions the same.

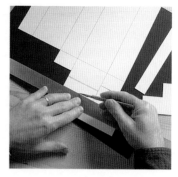

2 Cut out the box from coloured card using a ruler and craft knife to ensure that you make neat and accurate lines for it.

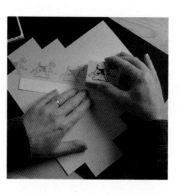

3 Using a straight-edged piece of paper or a ruler as a guide, stamp rows of motifs diagonally across the card.

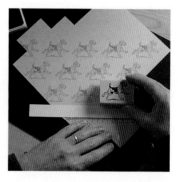

4 Make sure that you extend the pattern over the edges by stamping partial motifs at the ends of each alternate row.

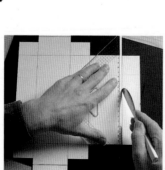

5 On the wrong side of the card, hold a set square or ruler against the fold lines and score along them with a blunt knife. Make sure that you do not break the surface of the card at all.

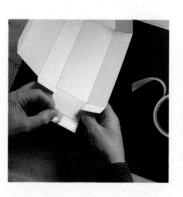

6 Fold along the score lines, making sure that all the corners are square. Apply double-sided tape to the joining edges, then peel off the backing paper and press the sides of the box together.

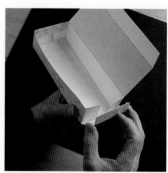

7 Continue folding and sticking the card in this way, ensuring that all the edges fit together neatly. Finally, fold in the end pieces to complete the card box.

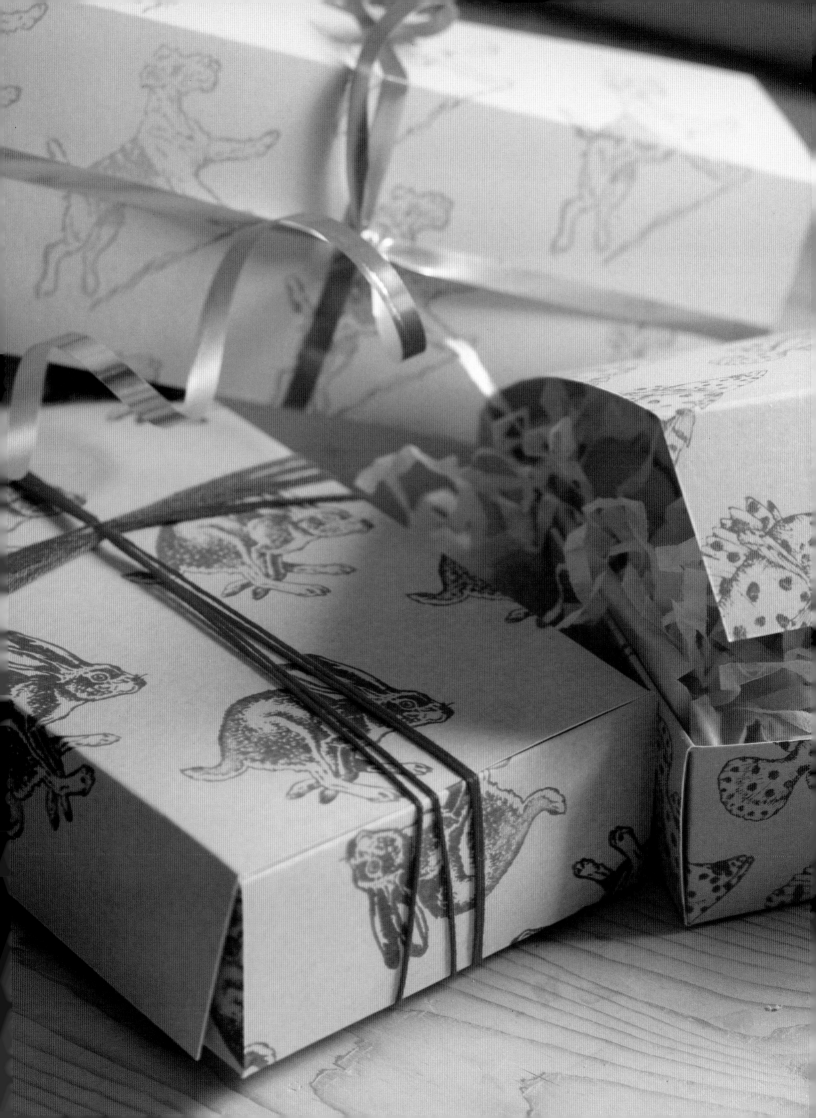

Crepe Paper Bags

These bags can be decorated with any motif – use stickers of cartoon characters, cars, animals or planes to decorate gift bags for children's parties.

You Will Need

Materials
*bright crepe paper
contrasting thread
metallic stick-on stars
gold or silver cord*

Equipment
*pinking shears
sewing machine, with
zigzag attachment*

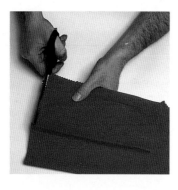

1 Decide on the size of your bag and, using pinking shears, cut out two rectangles from the crepe paper.

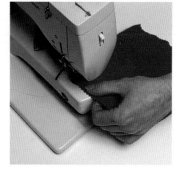

2 Set the sewing machine to a large zigzag stitch. Place the triangles together and sew along the three edges.

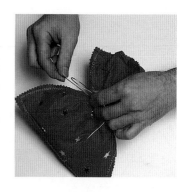

3 Place the stars randomly over the bag, then fill it with your gifts, and tie up the bag with gold or silver cord.

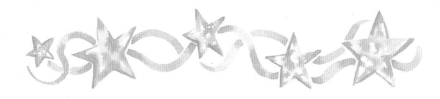

Carrier Bags

It really is great fun making bags, and they can be used for all sorts of objects – buttons, sweets, jewellery and, of course, for presenting gifts.

You Will Need

Materials
*tracing paper
stiff coloured paper
double-sided tape
cord or ribbon*

Equipment
*pencil
blunt knife or scissors
ruler
hole punch*

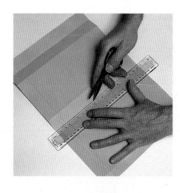

1 Trace the template from the back of the book, enlarging if necessary. Transfer it to stiff paper. The dotted lines indicate mountain folds and the dashed lines are valley folds. Use a blunt knife or scissors and a ruler to score along the fold lines. Cut out the shape.

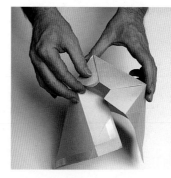

2 Stick the bag together using double-sided tape along the seams. Using the hole punch, carefully make two sets of holes opposite each other on the top seam.

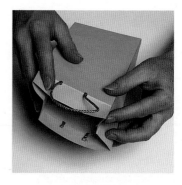

3 Place a square of tape below each hole. Thread the cord or ribbon through the holes, peel off the backing paper and press together to hold the handles in place between the bag and the overlapping seam.

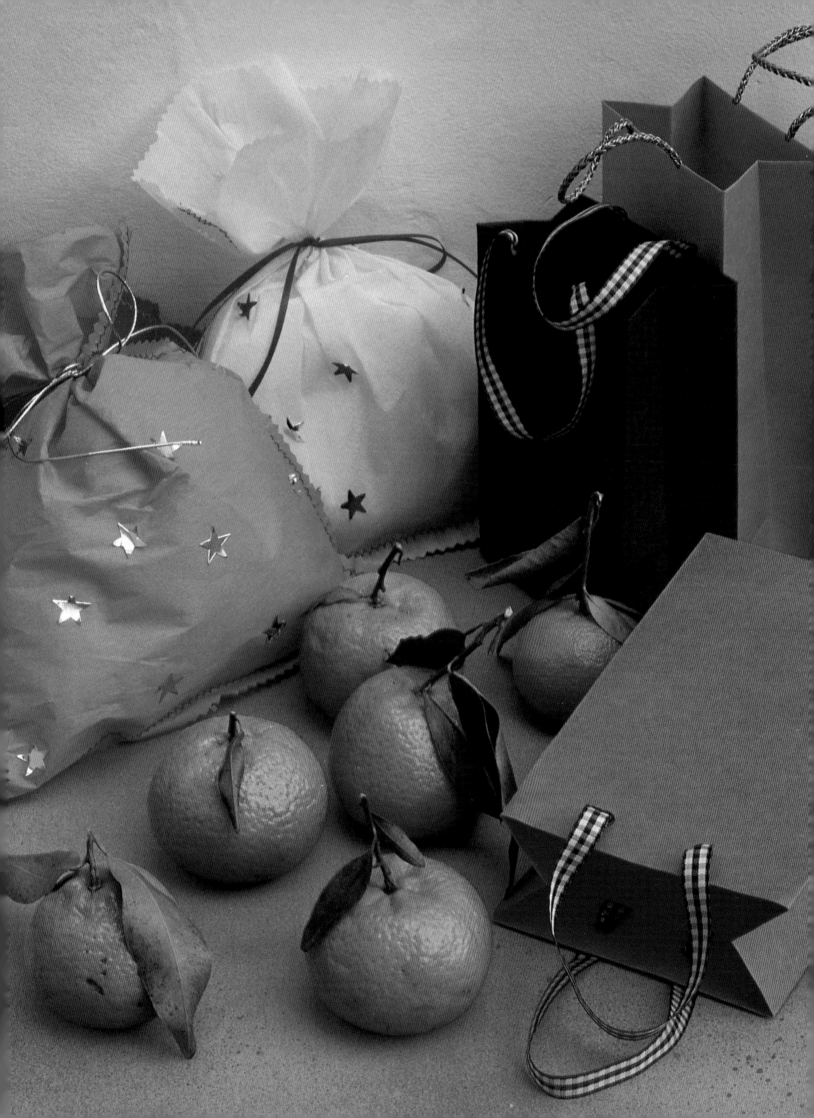

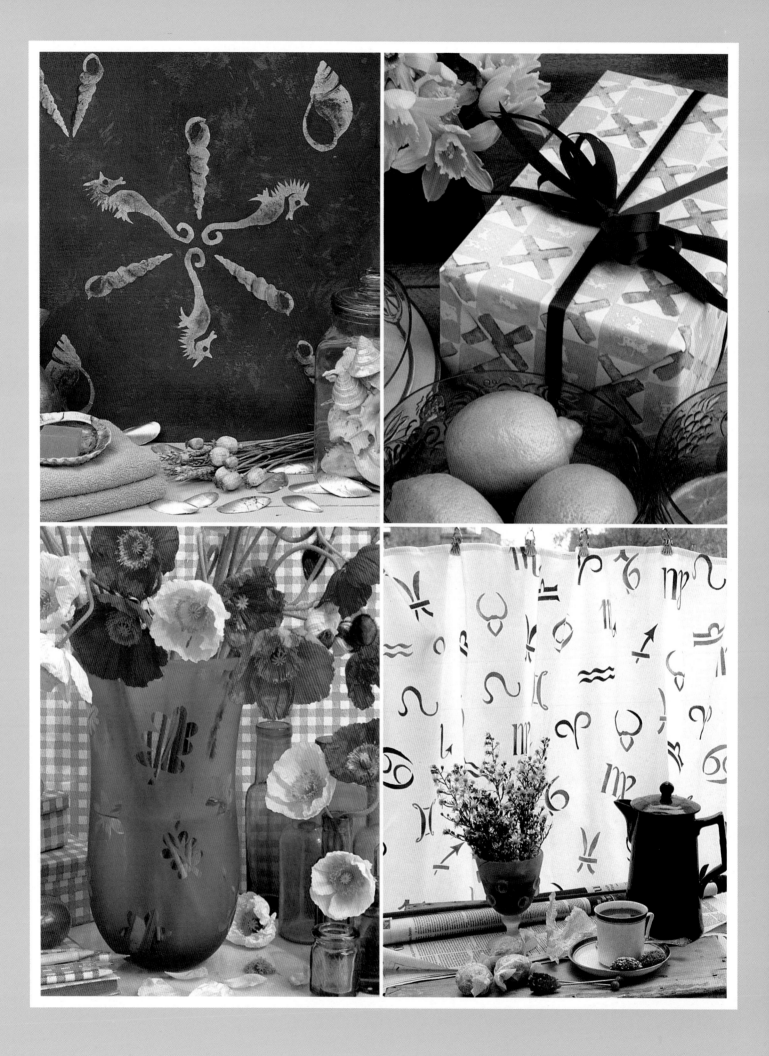

Stencilling, Stamping and Printing

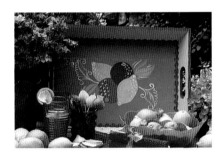

In this section you can find projects which, in their different ways, all involve transferring an image or motif to a surface, which can be anything from paper to plaster, floors to fabric. Stamping – whether using commercial stamps or the home-made kind – is probably the easiest method there is of transforming a plain surface. You can use the techniques to cover large areas, such as the walls of a room, or small, such as notepaper or gift wrapping.

In addition to stamping, there are exciting print projects for linocuts and potato prints, and a great selection of stencilling ideas from cork tiles to curtains. All the projects are easily adaptable to suit your needs and will inspire you to make up your own motifs and patterns!

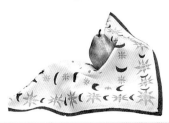

• STENCILLING, STAMPING AND PRINTING •

Basic Stamping Techniques

Stamping is a simple and direct way of making a print. The variations, such as they are, come from the way in which the stamp is inked and the type of surface to which it is applied. It is a good idea to experiment and find a method and effect that you find most pleasing.

RIGHT *Printing is fun as well as decorative. Here is a selection of the materials you may find yourself using.*

FAR RIGHT *You can buy ready-made commercial stamps, or make them yourself from plastic foam, linoleum blocks – and, of course, the humble potato.*

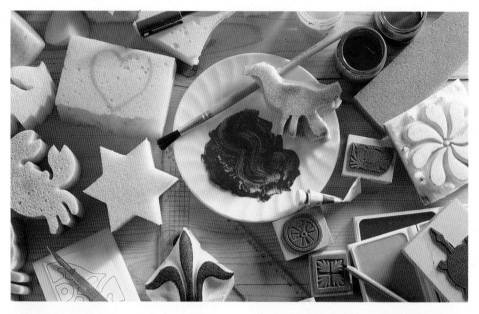

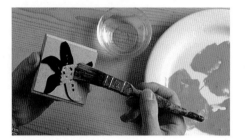

Stamping with a brush
The advantage of this technique is that you can see where the colour has been applied. This method is quite time-consuming, so use it for smaller projects. It is ideal for inking an intricate stamp with more than one colour.

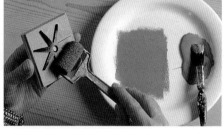

Stamping with a foam roller
This is the very best method for stamping large areas, such as walls. The stamp is evenly inked and you can see where the colour has been applied. Variations in the strength of printing can be achieved by only re-inking the stamp after several printings.

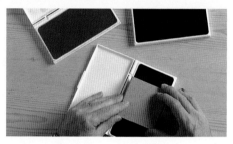

Stamping with a stamp pad
This is the traditional way to ink rubber stamps, which are less porous than foam stamps. The method suits small projects, particularly printing on paper. Stamp pads are more expensive to use than paint, but they are less messy and produce very crisp prints.

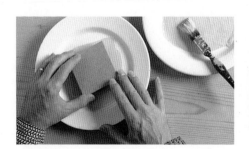

Stamping by dipping in paint
Spread a thin layer of paint on to a plate and dip the stamp into it. This is the quickest way of stamping large decorating projects. As you cannot see how much paint the stamp is picking up, you will need to experiment.

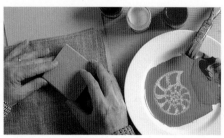

Stamping with fabric paint
Spread a thin layer of fabric paint on to a plate and dip the stamp into it. Fabric paints are quite sticky and any excess paint is likely to be taken up in the fabric rather than to spread around the edges. Fabric paint can also be applied by brush or foam roller, and is available with integral applicators.

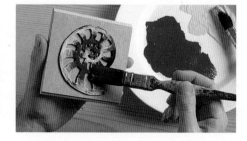

Stamping with several colours
A brush is the preferred option when using more than one colour on a stamp. It allows greater accuracy than a foam roller because you can see exactly where you are putting the colour. Two-colour stamping is very effective for giving a shadow effect or a decorative pattern.

Basic Stamping Techniques

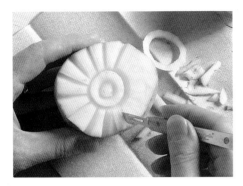

Potato

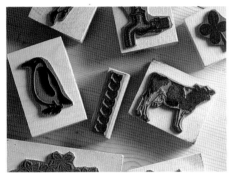

Commercial

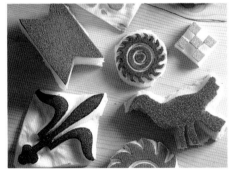

Foam

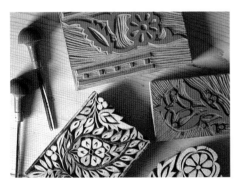

Lino

Surface applications

The surface on to which you stamp or stencil your design will greatly influence the finished effect. This page gives hints and tips for best results.

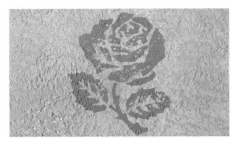

Rough plaster
You can roughen your walls before stamping or stencilling by mixing the filler to a fairly loose consistency and spreading it randomly on the wall. When dry, roughen it with coarse sandpaper, using random strokes.

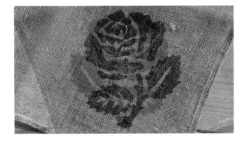

Fabric
As a rule, natural fabrics are the most absorbent, but to judge the painted effect, experiment first on a small sample. Fabric paints come in a range of colours, but to obtain the subtler shades, you may need to combine the primaries with black or white. Card behind the fabric will protect your work surface.

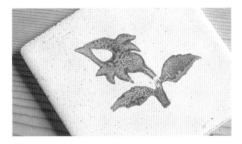

Tiles
Wash tiles in hot water and detergent to remove any dirt or grease, and dry thoroughly. If the tiles are already on the wall, avoid printing in areas which require a lot of cleaning. The paint will only withstand a gentle wipe with a cloth. Loose tiles can be baked to add extra strength and permanence to the paint. Always read the manufacturer's instructions before you do this.

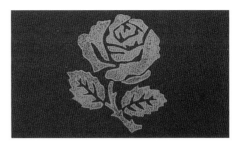

Smooth plaster or lining paper
If you are using a stamp, ink it with a small foam roller to achieve the crispest print. Re-create perfect repeats by re-inking with every print, or give a more hand-printed effect by making several prints between inkings.

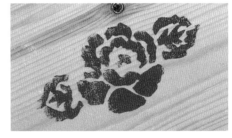

Wood
Rub down the surface of any wood to give the paint a better "key" to adhere to. Some woods are very porous and absorb paint, but you can intensify the colour by over-printing later. If you stamp or stencil on wood lightly, the grain will show through. Seal your design with matt varnish.

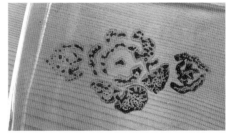

Glass
Wash glass in hot water and detergent to remove any dirt or grease, and dry it thoroughly. It is best to print on glass for non-food uses, such as vases. Practise on a spare sheet of glass first. As glass has a slippery, non-porous surface, you need to apply your print with a direct on/off movement.

• STENCILLING, STAMPING AND PRINTING •

Stencilled Sprig Curtain

This regular repeat pattern is easy to achieve by ironing the curtain fabric to mark a grid before you start to stencil. Alternatively, the leaf motif could be stencilled randomly across the fabric for a more informal look. Wash and iron the fabric before you start work.

You Will Need

Materials
*tracing paper
thin card or paper
cotton voile, to fit window
newspaper
masking tape
spray adhesive
fabric paints: green, blue, brown and pink
matching sewing thread
curtain wire*

Equipment
*pencil
craft knife
cutting mat
iron
thick and thin stencil brushes
paint-mixing container
sewing machine*

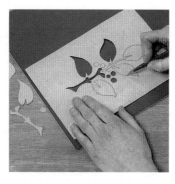

1 Trace the template from the back of the book, enlarging it to 17 cm/6½ in high. Transfer it to thin card and cut it out. Fold the fabric into 20 cm/8 in vertical pleats and 25 cm/10 in horizontal pleats, then iron it lightly to leave a grid pattern. Cover your work surface with newspaper and tape the fabric down so that it is fairly taut.

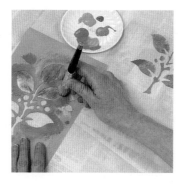

2 Spray the back of the stencil with adhesive and place it in the first rectangle. Mix the paints to achieve subtle shades. Paint the leaves in green, adding blue at the edges for depth. Paint the stem in brown and the berries in a brownish pink. Repeat the design in alternate rectangles.

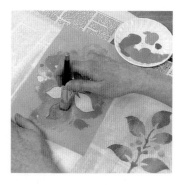

3 Turn the stencil upside-down and paint the top leaf in the centre of the plain rectangles pink. Add a darker shade at the tip and mark the stalk in brown. Fix the paints according to the manufacturer's instructions. Hem the sides and lower edge of the curtain. Make a 2.5 cm/1 in channel at the top and insert the curtain wire.

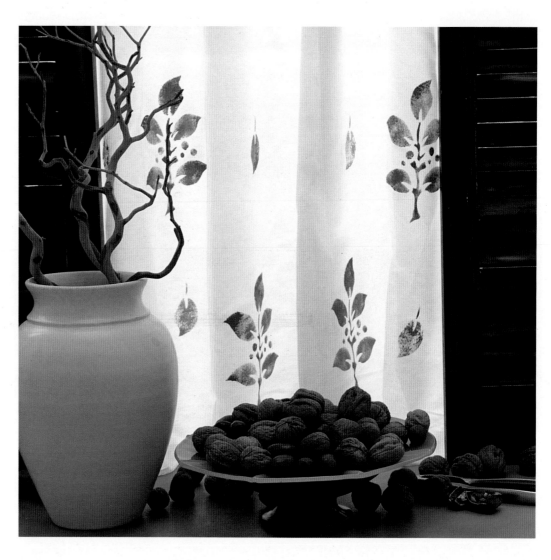

• STENCILLING, STAMPING AND PRINTING •

SUNS AND MOONS NAPKIN

Transform plain napkins by decorating them with golden suns and blue moons. To achieve the best result, cut the stencils carefully and register them accurately, with the help of the cross-points you draw on the napkin.

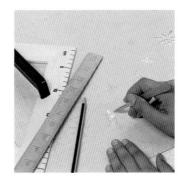

YOU WILL NEED

MATERIALS	EQUIPMENT
tracing paper	pencil
2 sheets of thin card, size of the napkins	ruler
spray adhesive	craft knife
napkins	cutting mat
fabric paints: gold and blue	iron
	fabric marker
	sponge or stencil brush

1 Trace the template from the back of the book, enlarging it if necessary. Rule grids on the card to help you position the motifs. Transfer the motifs on to the thin card; you will need to make one stencil for the suns and one for the moons. Cut out the stencils

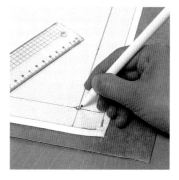

2 Spray adhesive on the sun stencil. Iron a napkin and lay it on the stencil, smoothing it outwards from the centre. With a fabric marker, draw the registration marks on the napkin, parallel to the edges. The lines should cross at the centre of the corner sun motif.

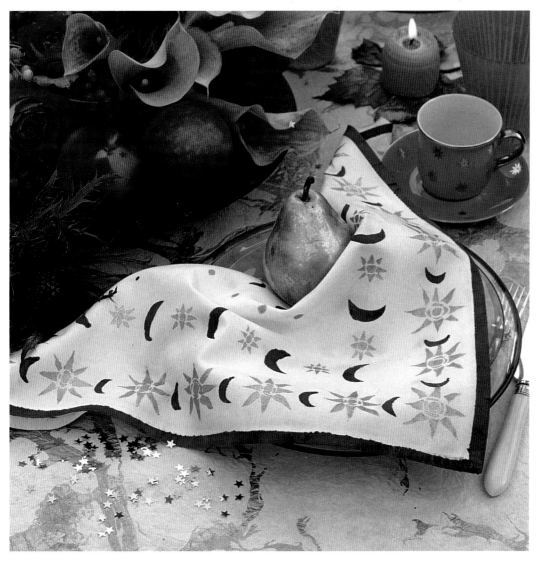

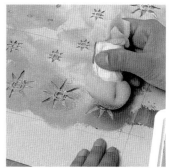

3 Spray adhesive on the reverse of the sun stencil and register the stencil on the cross-points. Using a sponge or stencil brush, apply the gold paint. Remove the stencil, then allow to dry. Repeat with the moon stencil and blue paint, registering the stencil as before. Fix the paints according to the manufacturer's instructions.

• STENCILLING, STAMPING AND PRINTING •

STYLISH LAMPSHADE

*U*nusual *lampshades can be very expensive, so the solution is to take a plain lampshade and apply some surface decoration that will transform it from a utility object into a stylish focal point. The design, which resembles a seedpod, is easy to cut from high-density foam and it makes a bold, sharp-edged print that is highly effective.*

YOU WILL NEED

MATERIALS
tracing paper
card
spray adhesive
high-density foam
thinned emulsion (latex)
paints: cream-yellow and
pale blue
plain lampshade

EQUIPMENT
pencil
craft knife
cutting mat
2 plates
small rubber roller

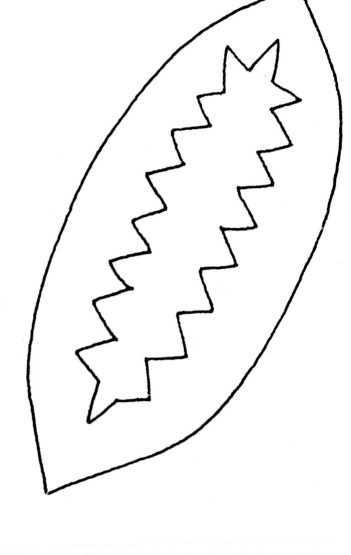

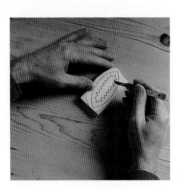

1 Trace the template on this page, enlarging it if necessary. Transfer it to a piece of card and cut it out. Lightly spray the shape with adhesive and place it on the foam. Cut around the outline, going all the way through the foam. Then cut around the centre detail to a depth of about 1 cm/½ in. Undercut and scoop this section away before cutting away the background.

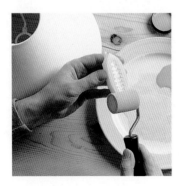

2 Spread some cream-yellow paint on to a plate and coat a small roller evenly. Use it to apply a coat of paint to the foam stamp.

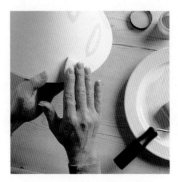

3 Make the first print a partial one, using only the top end of the stamp. Continue to print at random angles, leaving plenty of spaces for the second colour. Wash the stamp to remove all traces of yellow.

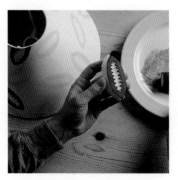

4 Spread some pale blue paint on to a second plate and coat the roller evenly. Use it to apply a coat of paint to the foam stamp.

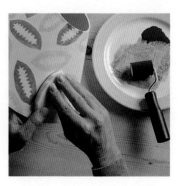

5 Stamp pale blue shapes at random angles in between the cream-yellow ones. Be sure to make some partial prints so that the pattern continues over the edges.

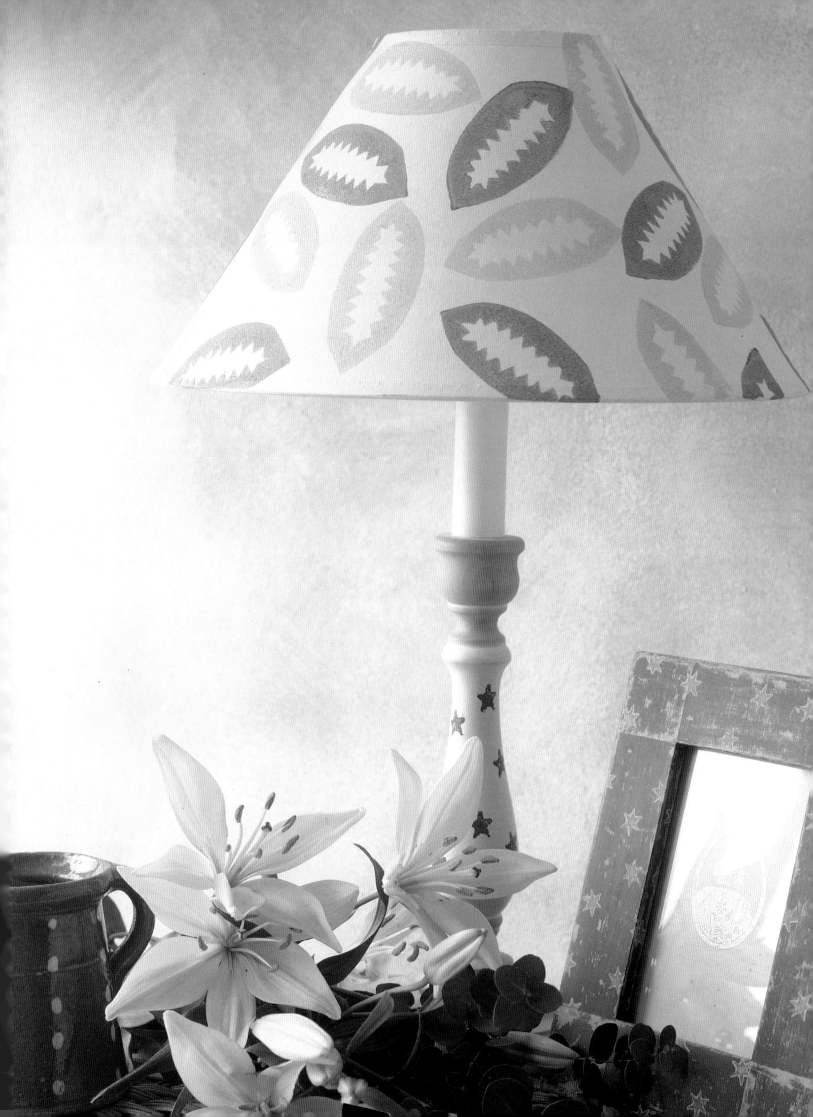

• STENCILLING, STAMPING AND PRINTING •

CREEPY CRAWLY HANDKERCHIEF

A handkerchief full of little bugs sounds alarming, but these prints adapted from nineteenth-century folk art woodcuts are anything but! If the handkerchief has a self-weave pattern, use it as a guide for the prints; if not, scatter them about but make sure they are evenly spaced over the fabric. Practise first on a spare piece of fabric.

YOU WILL NEED

MATERIALS
*lino tile, 15 x 15 cm/6 x 6 in
tracing paper
fabric paints in various colours
fabric paint medium
laundered white handkerchief*

EQUIPMENT
*lino tools
craft knife
pencil
paintbrush*

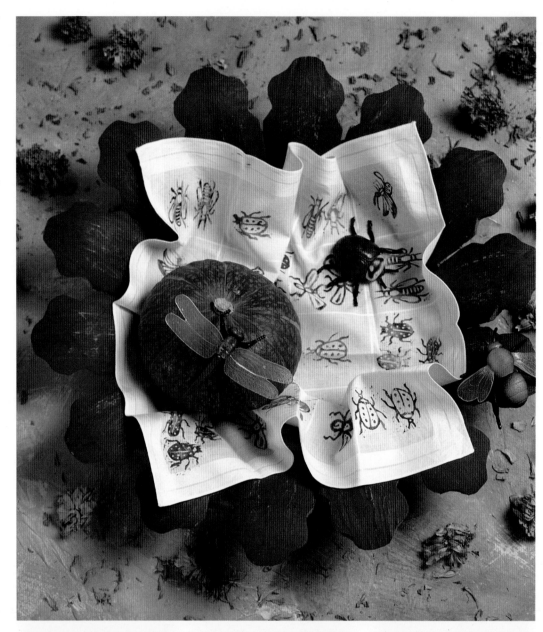

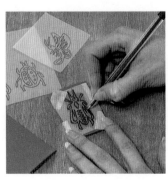
1 Cut the lino tile into six pieces, each measuring 5 x 7.5 cm/2 x 3 in. Trace the templates from the back of the book and transfer them to the lino pieces.

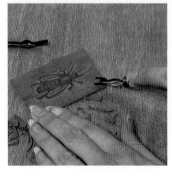
2 Using a V-shaped lino tool, carefully cut around the outlines of the bug templates. Then use a wider lino tool to cut away the remainder of the background.

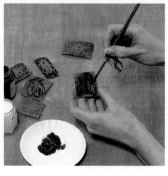
3 Apply fabric paints to the blocks. Using a paintbrush, blend the colours to achieve interesting paint effects. Dilute the paint as necessary with fabric medium.

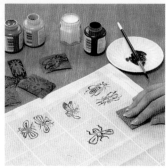
4 Place the block on the fabric, press evenly over the back and lift it up carefully to avoid smudging the print. Fix the paints according to the manufacturer's instructions.

• STENCILLING, STAMPING AND PRINTING •

Seashore Spongeware Set

Imagine the effect of a whole tea-set of this seashore design, set out on shelves or a dresser. Painting your own is an inexpensive way of transforming plain, white china, and the end result is unique.

You Will Need

Materials	Equipment
cellulose kitchen sponge	*ballpoint pen*
all-purpose glue	*scissors*
corrugated card	*plate*
ceramic paints: dark blue	*rag*
and dark green	*fine black magic marker*
paper towels	*stencil brush*
white china	*cosmetic sponge (optional)*
white spirit	

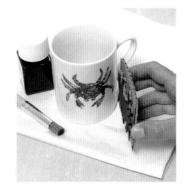

1 Draw your crab shape freehand on the sponge. Cut the crab out and glue it to a small square of corrugated card. Trim the card as close to the crab as possible. Pour a small amount of dark blue ceramic paint on to a plate. Lightly press the sponge into the paint and blot off any excess paint with paper towels. Gently apply even pressure to stamp the crab on to the china. Carefully lift off the sponge, in a single movement. Repeat the pattern as often as necessary for your design. Remove any mistakes with white spirit on a rag. Fix the paint according to the manufacturer's instructions.

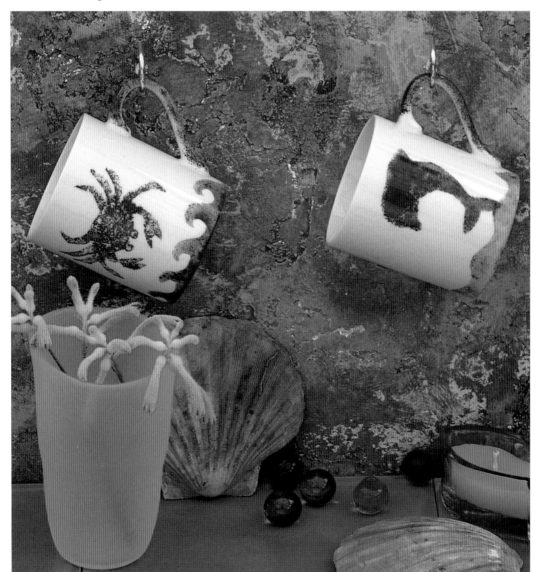

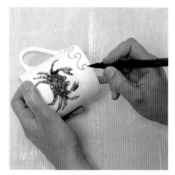

2 With the magic marker, draw the border freehand around the bottom of the mug. Fill in the waves using a stencil brush and fix the paint again.

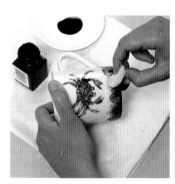

3 Alternatively, use the cosmetic sponge to sponge the border around the mug. Use both the blue and green paints, to give depth to the border. Fix the paint.

• STENCILLING, STAMPING AND PRINTING •

CHECKERBOARD POTATO PRINT

Potato prints are one of the easiest and most satisfying ways of creating a personalized repeat design. Here, one potato half is cut into a square stamp and the other half is given the same treatment with a cross shape added to make a checkerboard design.

YOU WILL NEED

MATERIALS
potato
acrylic paints: cadmium-yellow and cobalt-blue
sheet of white paper
thin blue ribbon
florist's wire (optional)

EQUIPMENT
chopping board
sharp knife or craft knife
2 plates
paper towels
scissors

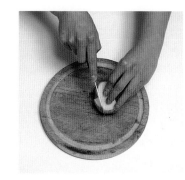

1 On the chopping board, cut the potato in half with one smooth movement. Cut the sides of one half to make a plain square.

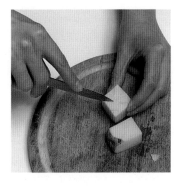

2 Cut the other potato half into a square, then cut out a cross shape by removing triangular sections around the edge and squaring off the corners of the cross.

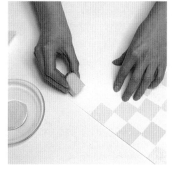

3 Put the paints on separate plates and have some paper towels handy. Print the yellow squares first on a sheet of paper, starting in one corner and working down and across the sheet.

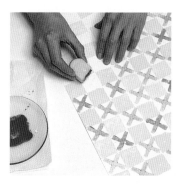

4 Print the blue crosses in the white squares and allow to dry thoroughly.

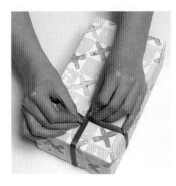

5 Wrap a gift in the paper and use a thin blue ribbon, set off-centre, as a trimming.

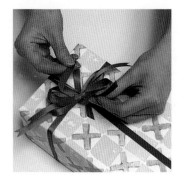

6 If you like, make a separate bow, securing loops of ribbon with some florist's wire.

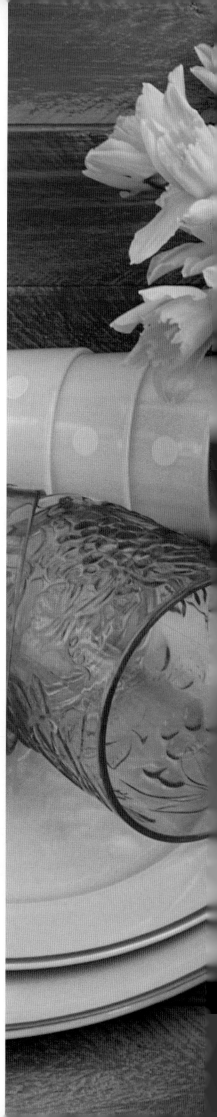

54

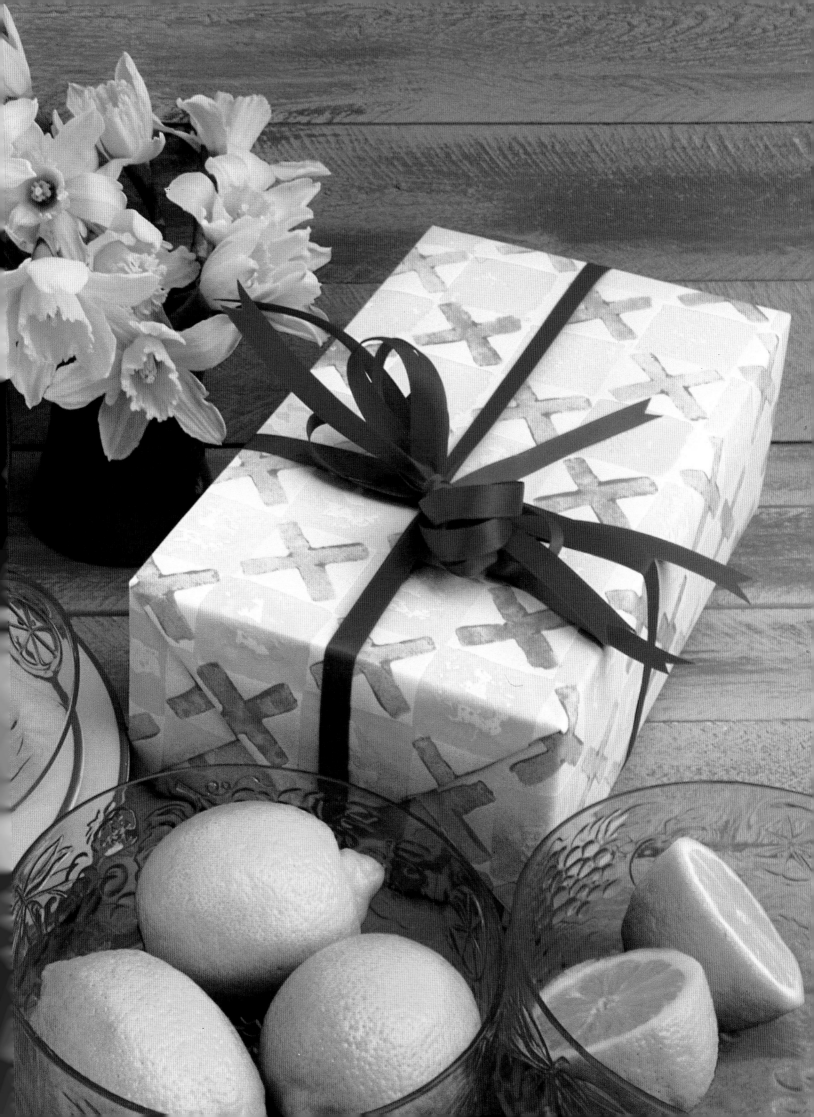

• STENCILLING, STAMPING AND PRINTING •

Zodiac Cafe Curtain

Use gold fabric paints to dramatize a plain muslin (cheesecloth) curtain. Stencil the shapes at random all over the curtain, but try to plan your design so that they all appear fairly regularly. Add variety by blending the two shades of gold on some of the designs that you make.

You Will Need

Materials
tracing paper
thin card or paper
scrap fabric
fabric paints: light and dark gold
paper towels
newspaper
white muslin (cheesecloth), to fit window
masking tape
spray adhesive
matching sewing thread
curtain clips and metal rings

Equipment
pencil
craft knife
cutting mat
2 stencil brushes
iron
needle

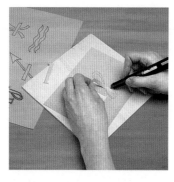

1 Trace the templates from the back of the book, enlarging if necessary. Transfer on to 12 rectangles of thin card or paper and cut out the shapes with a craft knife. Before working on your curtain, practise your stencilling technique on some spare fabric. Don't overload your brush and wipe off any excess paint on paper towels before you begin.

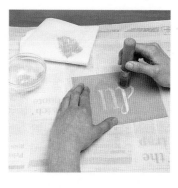

2 Cover your work table with newspaper. Iron the muslin (cheesecloth), then fix one corner to the table with masking tape, keeping it flat. Coat the back of each stencil lightly with spray adhesive before positioning it on the fabric. Start with the light gold, then paint over the edges of the motif with dark gold to give depth. Allow to dry, then gently peel the card off.

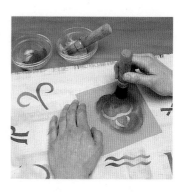

3 Cover the rest of the fabric with the motifs, repositioning it on the work table as necessary and stencilling one section at a time. Fix the paint according to the manufacturer's instructions. Iron, then hem the edges and attach the curtain clips to the upper edge.

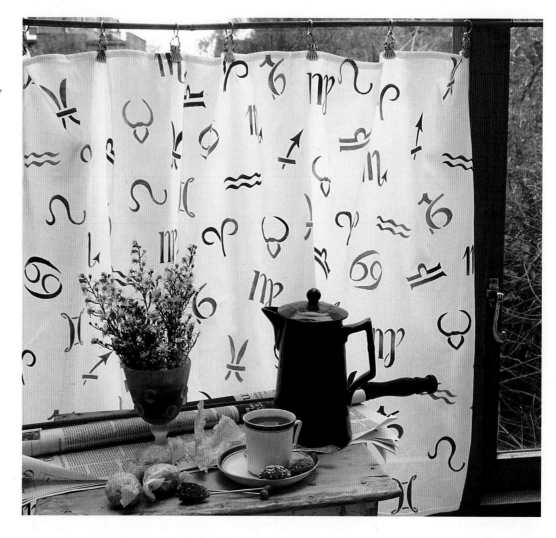

• STENCILLING, STAMPING AND PRINTING •

LEAFY PENCIL POT

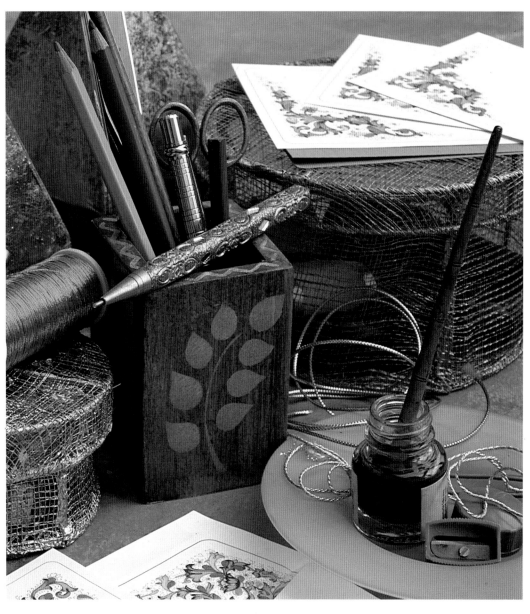

This useful pencil pot is stencilled with a simple leaf motif over a dark green background which is painted with a "dragged" effect.

YOU WILL NEED

MATERIALS
*pine slat, 8 x 45 mm/
⅜ x 1¾ in
pine slat, 8 x 70 mm/
⅜ x 2¾ in
wood glue
masking tape
sandpaper
white undercoat paint
thin card
acrylic paints: green, blue
and yellow
PVA (white) glue*

EQUIPMENT
*ruler
fretsaw
paintbrushes
pencil
craft knife
cutting mat
paint-mixing container*

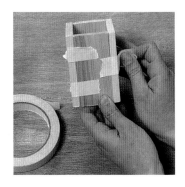

1 Cut two 9 cm/3½ in lengths of each pine slat. Glue with wood glue to form the sides of the pot. Hold with masking tape until the glue is dry.

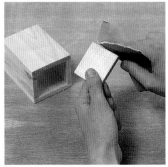

2 Sand all the rough edges. Measure the inside dimensions of the pot and cut a piece of wood to make the base. Glue it in place and allow to dry.

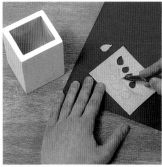

3 Paint with two coats of white undercoat, sanding lightly between coats. Cut a piece of thin card the same size as the broad side of the pot. Draw a leaf design and cut out with a craft knife.

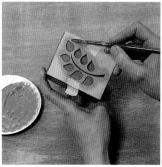

4 Mix the paints to blue-green and yellow-green. Apply blue-green paint with a stiff brush to show the brush strokes. Stencil the leaf pattern in yellow-green. Finish with a coat of diluted white glue.

· STENCILLING, STAMPING AND PRINTING ·

STAMPED BEDLINEN

Matching bedlinen is the last word in luxury. The white pillowcases have an all-round border of horse chestnuts and the top sheet folds back to reveal a matching pattern. Smooth cotton with straight edging is a dream to work with because the stamps can be confidently lined up with the edges and the sheeting absorbs the paint well to give a very crisp print.

YOU WILL NEED

MATERIALS
*fabric paints: dark green and blue
scrap paper
sheet and pillowcase
thin card
scrap fabric*

EQUIPMENT
*rubber stamp
scissors*

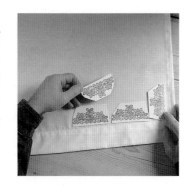

1 To plan your design, stamp out several motifs on scrap paper and cut them out. Arrange these along the sheet edge or the pillowcase border to work out the position and spacing of your pattern.

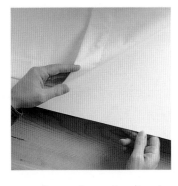

2 Place a sheet of card under the sheet or inside the pillowcase to prevent the paint from soaking through.

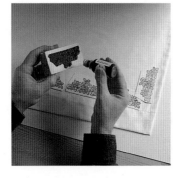

3 Follow the manufacturer's instructions and apply green paint to half of the stamp.

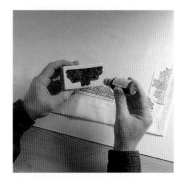

4 Apply blue paint to the other half of the stamp.

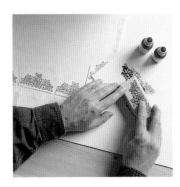

5 Test the distribution of the paint by making a print on a scrap of fabric. Re-apply and test the paint until you feel confident enough to make the first print on the bedlinen.

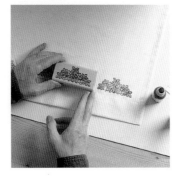

6 Check the arrangement of the paper-stamped motifs, then lift one at a time and stamp the fabric in its place. Press quite firmly to give the fabric time to absorb the paint.

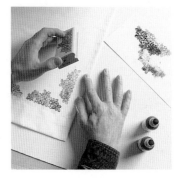

7 Continue to re-coat and test the stamp as you print all the way around the edges to complete a matching bedlinen set. Fix the paint according to the manufacturer's instructions.

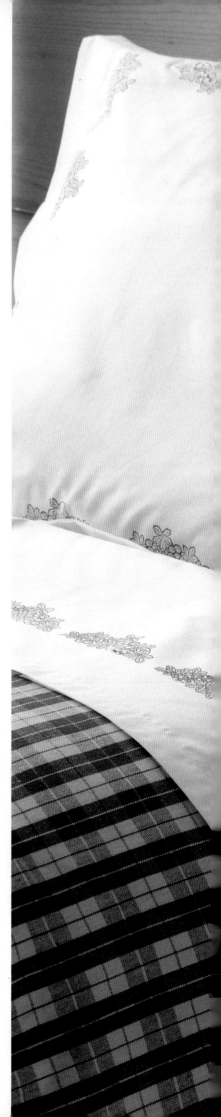

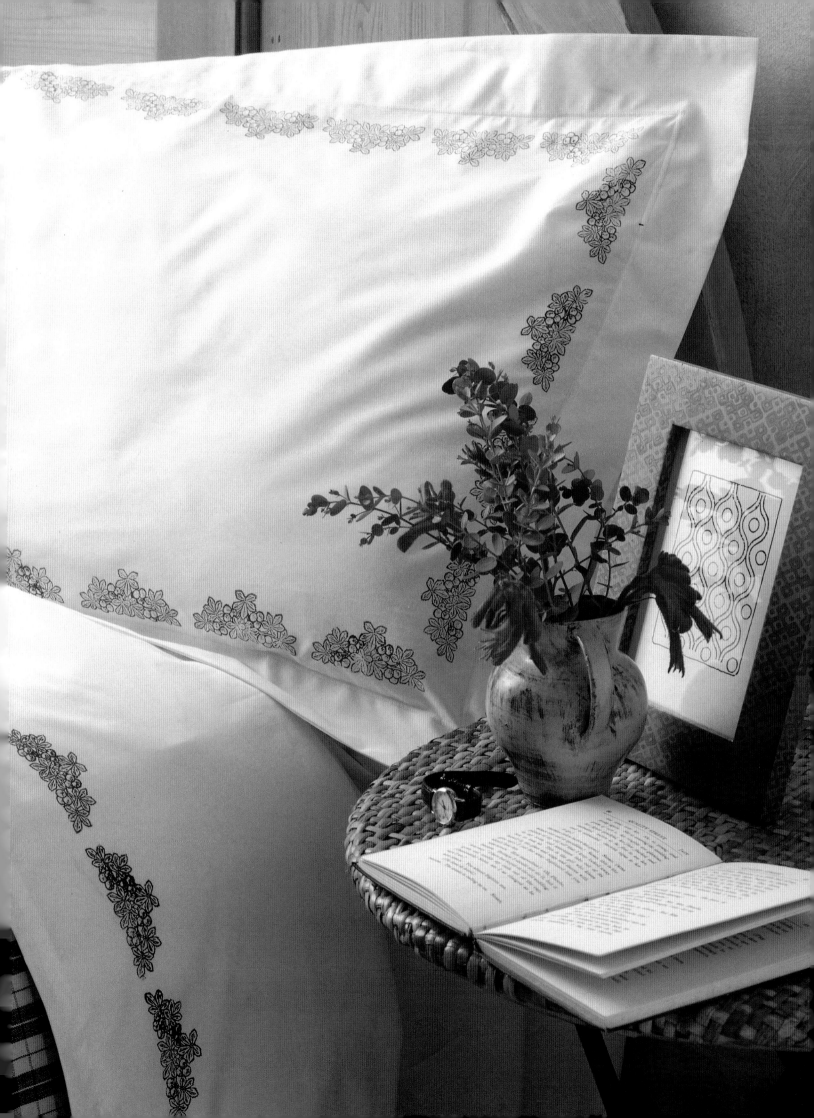

• STENCILLING, STAMPING AND PRINTING •

STENCILLED SEA WALL

*T*his unusual idea for a wall decoration capitalizes on the shininess of ordinary kitchen foil. The effect is shimmering and glittering, with an underwater feel that is ideal for a bathroom wall. It can also be done directly on a wall surface.

YOU WILL NEED

MATERIALS
sheet of hardboard
emulsion (latex) paint
gloss paints: dark blue and
olive-green
tracing paper
thin card
aluminium foil
clear gloss varnish
artist's oil colours: dark
blue and chrome-yellow

EQUIPMENT
decorator's paintbrush
sponge or rag
pencil
scissors
dressmaker's pins
fine paintbrush

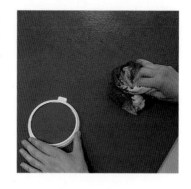

1 Paint the hardboard with an undercoat of emulsion (latex) paint. Paint the surface with dark blue gloss paint. When it is dry, sponge or rag roll the green paint in blotches all over the hardboard surface.

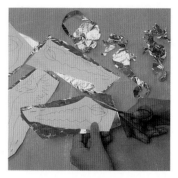

2 Trace the templates from the back of the book, enlarging if necessary. Cut out the templates very roughly on thin card and lay them, face-up, on one or two pieces of foil, slightly larger than the templates. Pin the layers together, then cut out the shapes and separate the layers.

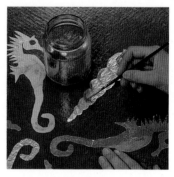

3 Brush some varnish on to the hardboard and apply foil shapes to the surface. Tint some of the varnish with the artist's colours. Add detail and texture with varnish tinted with artist's colours, using a fine paintbrush. When the varnish is dry, give the whole design a further coat of tinted varnish.

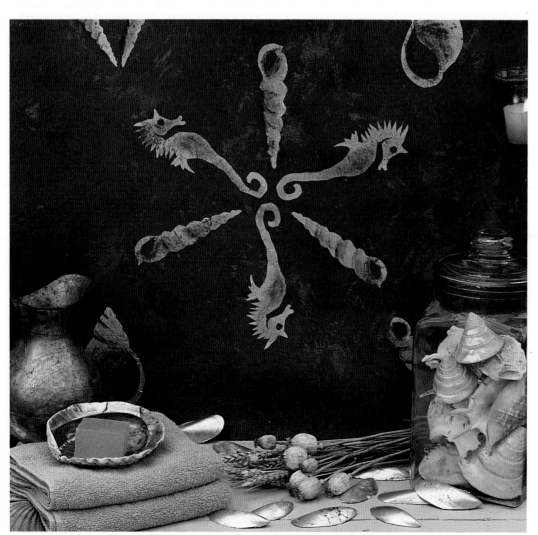

• STENCILLING, STAMPING AND PRINTING •

FLEUR-DE-LYS TILES

This design is based on some original tiles from a medieval flooring. The modern version can quickly be stencilled on to plain tiles using a little imagination and some acrylic paint. Experiment with different colours and sizes to come up with an individual design for your tiles.

YOU WILL NEED

MATERIALS

*tracing paper
thin card
unglazed terracotta tiles,
13 x 13 cm/5 x 5 in
detergent
spray adhesive
cream acrylic paint
clear matt acrylic spray
varnish*

EQUIPMENT

*pencil
craft knife
cutting mat
stencil brush*

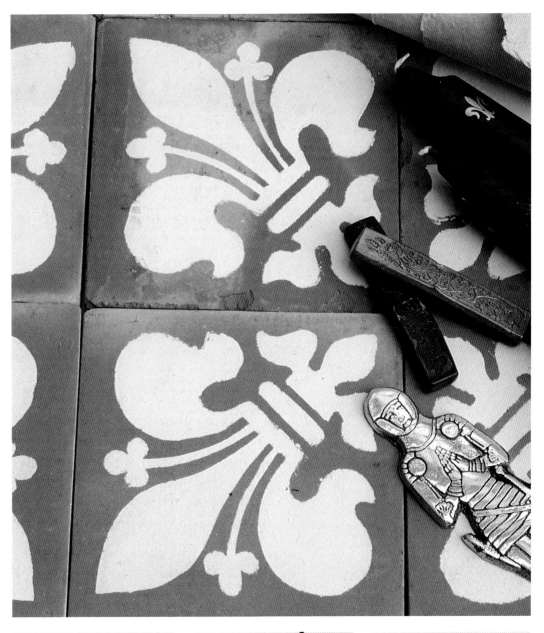

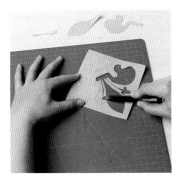

1 Trace the template from the back of the book, enlarging if necessary to fit on to a tile leaving a narrow border. Transfer it to thin card and cut out with a craft knife.

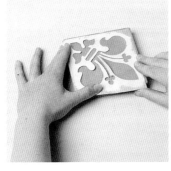

2 Wash the tiles with detergent to remove grease and dust. Allow to dry. Spray the back of the stencil lightly with adhesive and smooth in place on the first tile.

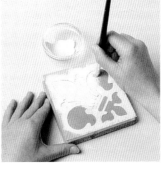

3 Paint in the design with small circular movements of the brush. Be careful not to overload the brush with paint.

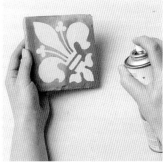

4 Peel off the stencil and leave the paint to dry thoroughly. Then seal with several coats of clear matt acrylic spray varnish.

• STENCILLING, STAMPING AND PRINTING •

LEAFY ESPRESSO CUPS

Browsing around antique stalls, you sometimes come across coffee cups hand-painted with broad brush strokes and lots of little raised dots of paint. It is simple to decorate your own coffee service in this style.

YOU WILL NEED

MATERIALS	EQUIPMENT
white ceramic cup and saucer	*acetone or other grease-dispersing alcohol*
thin card or paper	*cotton buds*
sticky-backed plastic	*pencil*
green acrylic ceramic paint	*scissors*
pewter acrylic paint with nozzle-tipped tube	*paintbrush*
	hair dryer (optional)
	craft knife

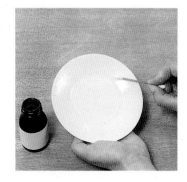

1 Clean any grease from the surface of the china to be painted, using the acetone or alcohol and a cotton bud.

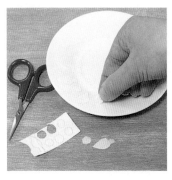

2 Draw leaves and circles freehand on to thin card or paper. Cut them out and draw around them on the backing of the sticky-backed plastic. Cut out. Peel away the backing paper and stick the pieces on the cup and saucer.

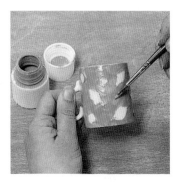

3 Paint around the shapes with the ceramic paint, applying several coats to achieve a solid colour. Leave each coat to air-dry or use a hair dryer for speed.

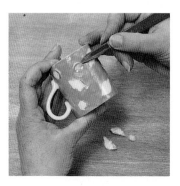

4 To ensure a clean edge, cut around each sticky shape with a craft knife, then peel off.

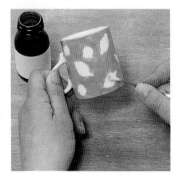

5 Clean up any smudges with a cotton bud dipped in acetone or water.

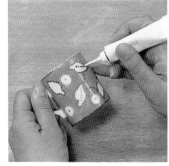

6 Using pewter paint and the nozzle-tipped paint tube, mark the outlines and details of the leaves with rows of small dots. Allow to dry for 36 hours. Fix the paints according to the manufacturer's instructions. The paint should withstand general use and gentle washing up, but not the dishwasher.

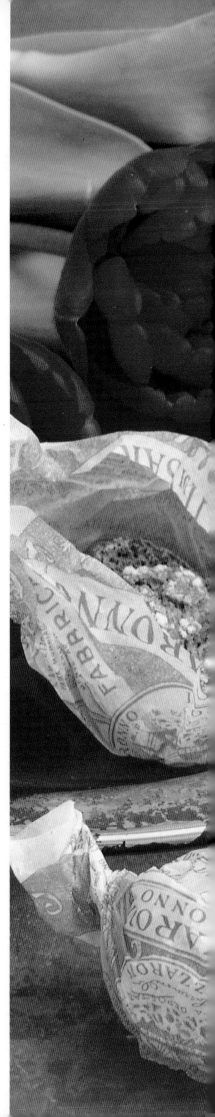

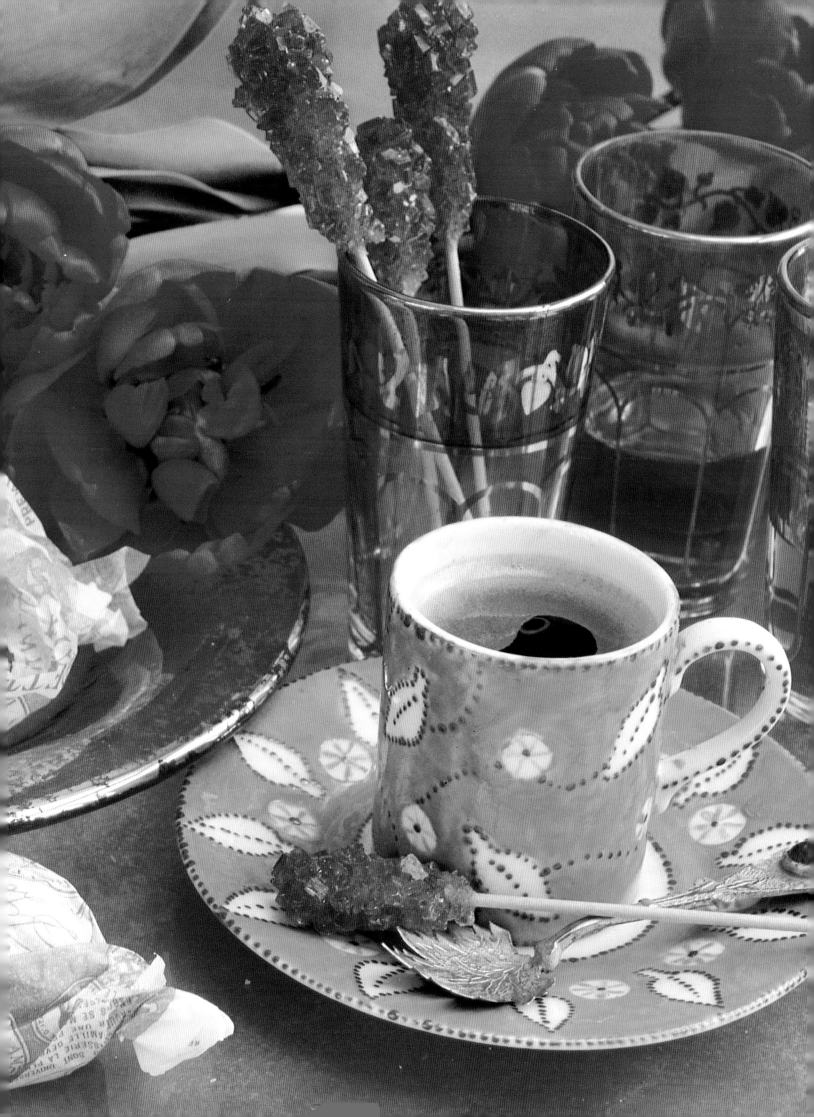

• STENCILLING, STAMPING AND PRINTING •

SGRAFFITO EGGS

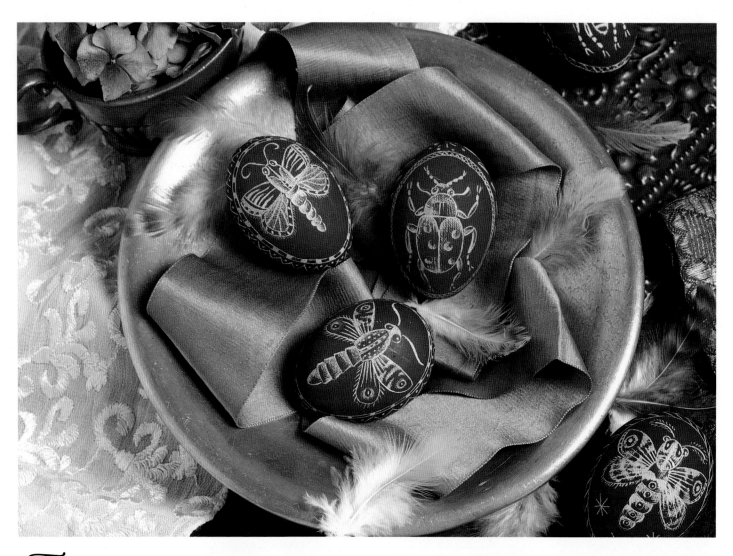

The familiar scraper-board technique has a wonderful new delicacy when it is applied to the fragile surface of a real eggshell.

YOU WILL NEED

MATERIALS
*blown egg
acrylic paints: purple-brown and dark blue*

EQUIPMENT
*pencil
paintbrush
craft knife
white marker pencil*

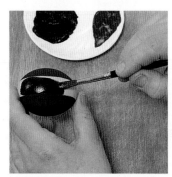

1 Draw a cameo outline on the front and back of the eggshell in pencil. Paint the two oval shapes in purple-brown acrylic paint, allowing one side to dry before you turn the egg over. You may need two coats. Paint the band around the egg in dark blue, again using two coats if required. Allow to dry.

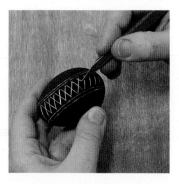

2 Use the point of a craft knife blade to scratch double lines between the purple-brown and blue sections. Make a criss-cross pattern across the blue section and mark a dot in each diamond. Scratch a series of dots between the double lines of the borders.

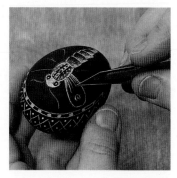

3 Using a white marker pencil, very lightly sketch the outline of an insect in each purple-brown oval. You can copy the moth in the photograph or use a natural history print as a reference. Engrave the design following the white pencil line, adding in more intricate details.

• STENCILLING, STAMPING AND PRINTING •

STENCILLED PICTURE FRAME

The stylish raised leaf patterns around these frames are simple to create using ordinary white interior filler instead of paint to fill in the stencilled shapes.

YOU WILL NEED

MATERIALS
*2 wooden frames
dark green acrylic paint
fine-grade sandpaper
tracing paper
thin card
ready-mixed interior filler*

EQUIPMENT
*paintbrush
pencil
scissors
stencil brush*

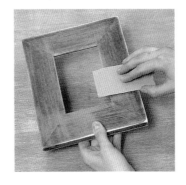

1 Paint the wooden frames dark green. When dry, gently rub them down with sandpaper to create a subtle distressed effect.

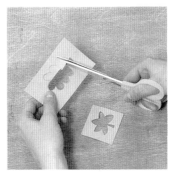

2 Trace the templates from the back of the book, enlarging to fit the frames. Transfer the designs to thin card and cut them out.

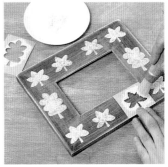

3 Position a stencil on the first frame and stipple ready-mixed filler through the stencil. Reposition the stencil and continue all around the frame. Allow to dry.

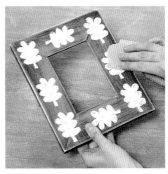

4 Repeat with a different combination of motifs on the second frame. When the filler is completely hard, gently smooth the leaves with fine-grade sandpaper.

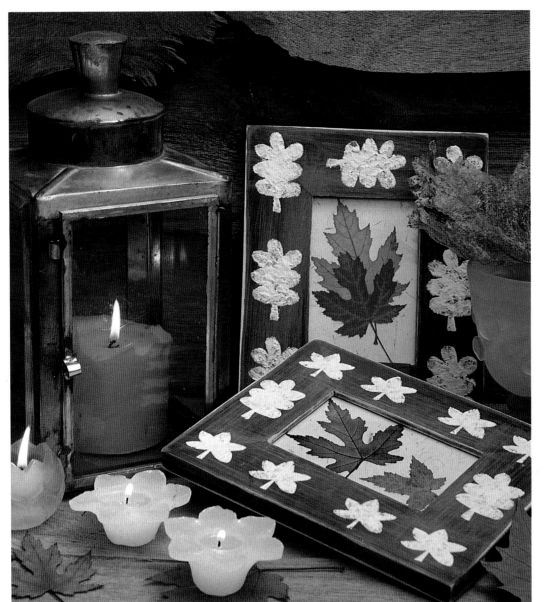

• STENCILLING, STAMPING AND PRINTING •

Mexican Citrus Tray

Breakfast in bed will really wake you up if it is presented on this flamboyant tray. The bold fruit motif, painted in zingy, sunny colours, is full of the energy and simplicity of folk art.

You Will Need

Materials	Equipment
sandpaper	medium and fine
wooden tray	paintbrushes
matt emulsion (latex) paints:	hard and soft pencils
dark emerald, lime-green	
and turquoise	
tracing paper	
acrylic gouache paints	
matt polyurethane varnish	

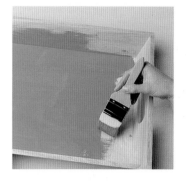

1 Sand the tray to remove any varnish. Paint the whole tray a dark emerald-green colour, then paint the inside of the tray lime-green, and the base turquoise. Allow to dry thoroughly.

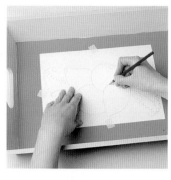

2 Trace the templates from the back of the book, enlarging to fit the base and sides of the tray. Rub over the outlines on the reverse of the tracing with a soft pencil, then transfer the designs to the tray.

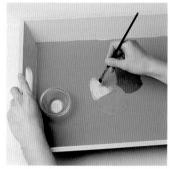

3 Paint the oranges, lemons and leaves on the base of the tray, and the flower motif on the sides, using acrylic gouache. When dry, add the details in white.

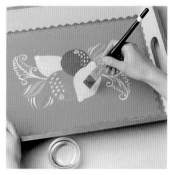

4 Paint a pink wavy border around the edge and the base of the tray. Paint the handle holes in bright orange. When the paint is dry, protect with several coats of varnish.

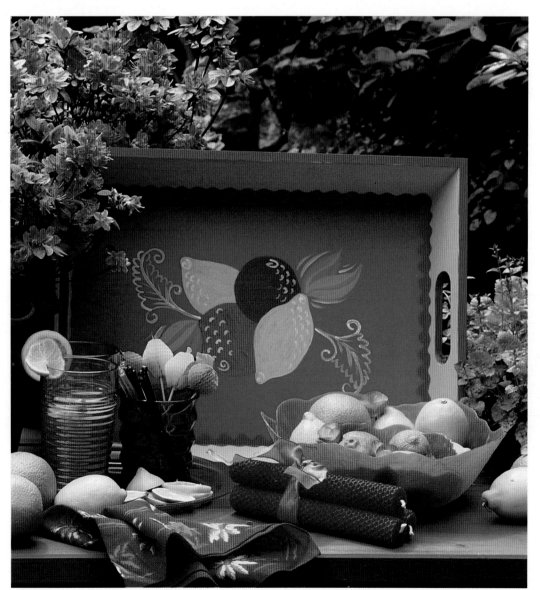

• STENCILLING, STAMPING AND PRINTING •

CUPID LINOCUT

Linocut images have a pleasing graphic simplicity. Here, the marvellous texture and light-enhancing qualities of gold metallic organza are contrasted with the solidity of the image. The beauty of linocuts is that the lino block can be used lots of times, so this idea can be adapted for making, for example, your own greetings cards.

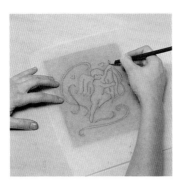 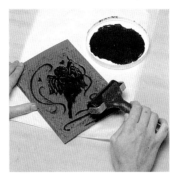 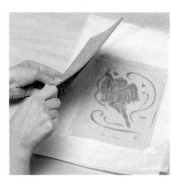

1 Trace the template from the back of the book, enlarging if necessary, and transfer to the lino block. Cut the design with the lino cutting tools: use the scoop to cut out large background areas and the nib for the fine details.

2 Squeeze the printing inks on to a plate and use the roller to mix the colours to get a deep burgundy shade. Coat the roller evenly, then roll over the surface of the linocut.

3 Tape the corners of the metallic organza to scrap paper to ensure the fabric is wrinkle free. Put the linocut over the organza and press evenly to ensure a crisp print. Use the decorative paper to create a mount, then frame.

YOU WILL NEED

MATERIALS
*tracing paper
printing inks: red and blue
masking tape
gold metallic organza
scrap paper
decorative paper
picture frame*

EQUIPMENT
*pencil
lino block
lino cutting tools:
U-shaped scoop and
V-shaped nib
plate
paint roller*

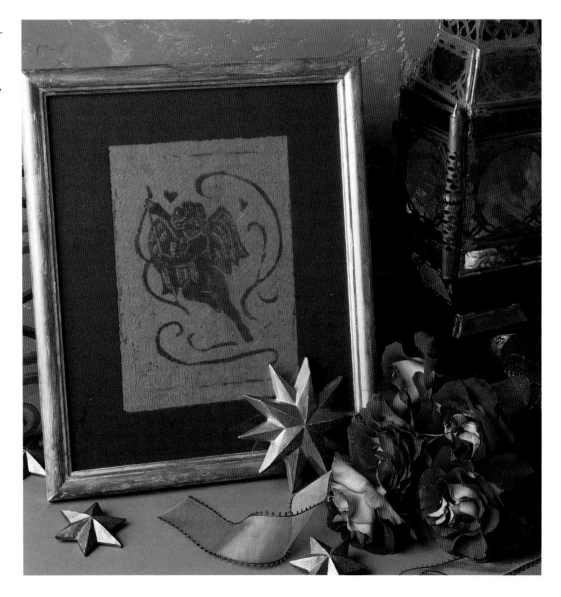

• STENCILLING, STAMPING AND PRINTING •

MEDIEVAL CORK TILES

Transform ordinary unsealed cork tiles to look like medieval terracotta by using a variety of wood stains. They give just the right range of muted shades, and you can mix them together to add further subtlety. Use the template provided for all of your tiles or find other mythical beasts in heraldic books to create a variety of designs.

YOU WILL NEED

MATERIALS	EQUIPMENT
unsealed, unstained cork tiles, 30 x 30 cm/12 x 12 in	pencil
wood stains: pine-yellow, red and brown-mahogany	ruler
tracing paper	brown crayon
thin card or paper	fine and medium paintbrushes
permanent black ink	scissors
waterproof gold ink (optional)	dip pen
matt polyurethane varnish	

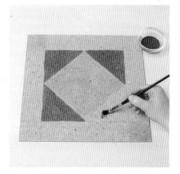
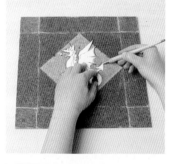
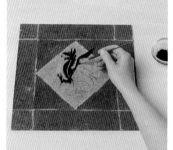
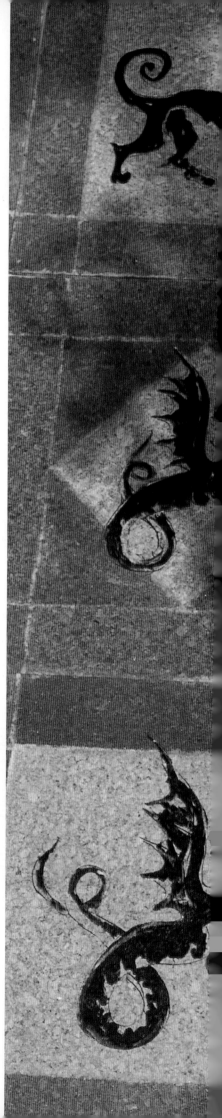

1 Mark the geometric pattern on a tile: use a brown crayon which will merge in with the design. Paint with the various wood stains. They spread on the cork, so don't overload the brush and start in the middle of each area, working outwards. A narrow gap between each colour looks very effective.

2 Scale up the animal template from the back of the book as required, transfer to thin card or paper and cut out. Position it in the centre of the tile and draw around it with permanent black ink, using a dip pen.

3 Use a fine brush to fill in the animal design in black. Highlight the design with gold ink, if you wish, then seal the tile with several coats of polyurethane varnish.

• STENCILLING, STAMPING AND PRINTING •

Gilded Wall Border

This simple version of stencilling produces an extremely effective and eye-catching border. Buy a cheap roll of wallpaper border paper and use the wrong side, then stick the completed design in place. This gets over the problem of stencilling on to a vertical surface.

You Will Need

Materials
tracing paper
paper glue
thin card
aerosol gloss paint
wallpaper border paper
emulsion (latex) paints:
warm-blue and white
masking tape
silver acrylic paint
rub-on gold paint

Equipment
pencil
craft knife
cutting mat
scissors
paintbrush
paint-mixing container
sponges

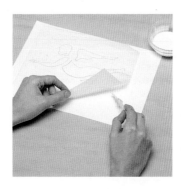

1 Trace the template from the back of the book, enlarging if necessary. Using a few dabs of paper glue, stick the template on to the card for the stencil.

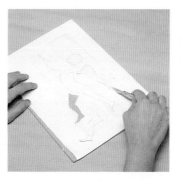

2 Cut out the stencil and remove the template.

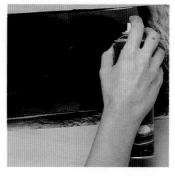

3 Spray both sides of the stencil with gloss paint.

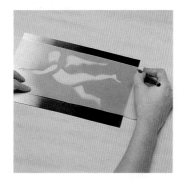

4 In order to line up the design on the border, cut a strip of tracing paper to the width of the border paper. Trace the cupid design on to it, placing it centrally. Place this tracing over the stencil, lining up the cupids. Mark the edges of the stencil at the edges of the tracing paper. Cut notches in the stencil to mark the top and bottom edges of the border. Use these to line up the stencil on the border paper.

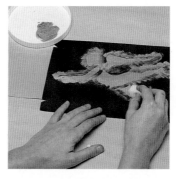

5 Paint a background colour of warm-blue emulsion (latex) on the border paper. Place the stencil over the border, lining up the notches with the top and bottom, and fix it in place with masking tape. Dip a sponge into the silver paint and apply it sparingly over the whole stencil. Allow to dry. Repeat along the length of the border. You can use the stencil several times before it becomes clogged, then you will have to cut a new one.

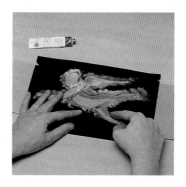

6 Use your finger to apply the gold paint to give depth to the body.

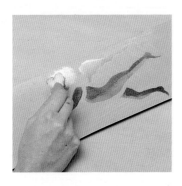

7 Remove the stencil template and sponge hair on to the cupids.

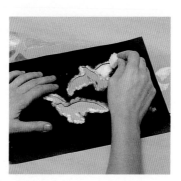

8 Apply the doves randomly between the cupids, using white emulsion (latex) paint and a second sponge.

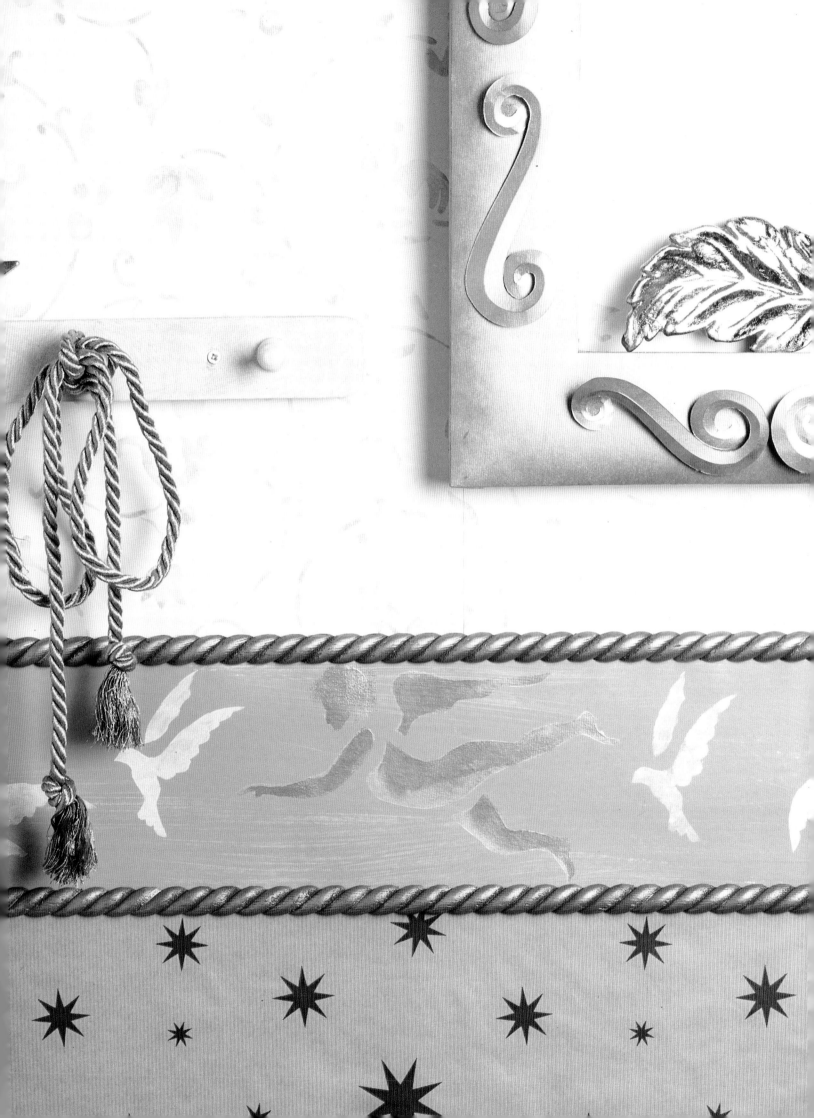

• STENCILLING, STAMPING AND PRINTING •

Art Nouveau Rose Box

*I*nspired by the motifs of early 20th-century art nouveau, this design for a simple wooden box combines sinuous lines, swirling leaf shapes and stained-glass-style roses to dramatic effect.

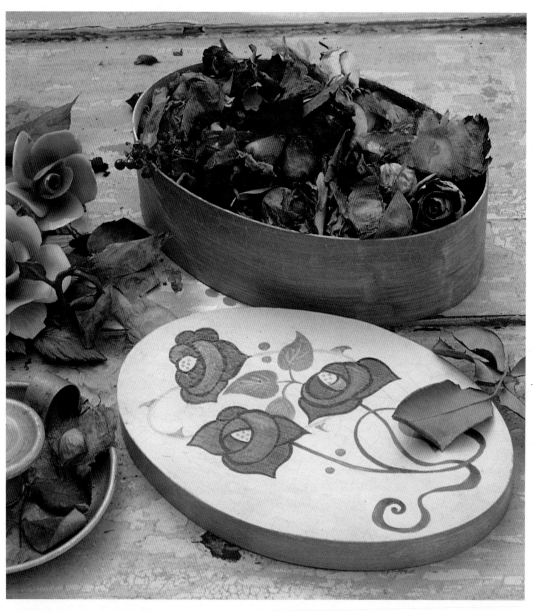

You Will Need

Materials
*fine-grade sandpaper
oval wooden craft box, with lid
white primer paint
tracing paper
acrylic paints: rose-pink, green, yellow, white, black and blue
clear acrylic or crackle varnish*

Equipment
*thick bristle and fine hair paintbrushes
hard and soft pencils
paint-mixing container*

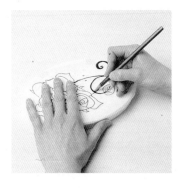

1 Sand the box and lid and give them three layers of primer. Trace the template from the back of the book, enlarging if necessary, to fit the lid of the box. Transfer it to the lid, with a soft pencil and tracing paper.

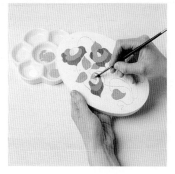

2 Paint the rose petals and the leaves as solid blocks of colour.

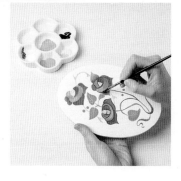

3 Paint the stems and thorn ring; add shade and tone to the flowers. Paint the veins on the leaves. Paint a black outline around the rose petals.

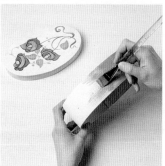

4 Colour-wash the outside rim of the lid with watered-down rose paint. Paint the box blue in the same way. Seal the surface with a coat of varnish (crackle varnish will give an antique effect).

• STENCILLING, STAMPING AND PRINTING •

Frosted Flower Vase

This is a magical way to transform a plain glass vase into something stylish and utterly original. Check the vase all over to make sure that it is evenly frosted before you peel off the leaf shapes: it may be necessary to paint on another coat of etching cream.

You Will Need

Materials	Equipment
coloured glass vase	*pencil*
tracing paper	*scissors*
sticky-backed plastic	*paintbrush*
etching cream	

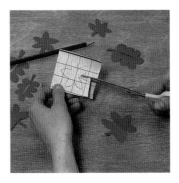

1 Wash and dry the vase. Trace the templates from the back of the book, enlarging if necessary. Cut them out and draw around them on to the backing of the plastic and draw small circles freehand.

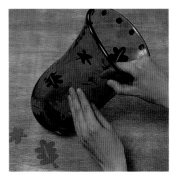

2 Cut out the shapes and peel off the backing paper. Arrange the shapes all over the vase, then smooth them down carefully to avoid any wrinkles.

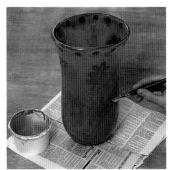

3 Carefully paint the etching cream all over the cleaned vase and leave it in a warm place to dry, following the manufacturer's instructions.

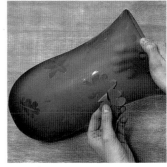

4 Wash the vase in warm water to remove the cream. If the frosting looks smooth, you can remove the shapes. If not, repeat with another coat of etching cream, then wash before removing the shapes.

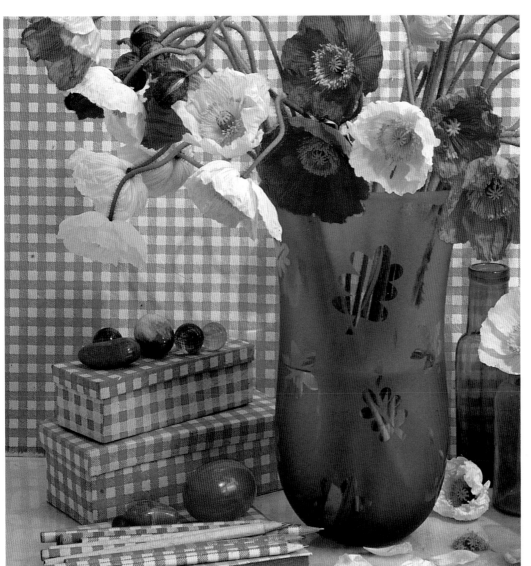

• STENCILLING, STAMPING AND PRINTING •

Country-style Shelf

Simple in shape but conveying a universally understood message, the heart has been used in folk art for centuries. Here, the outline of a heart is drawn in four positions on a foam block, then cut out to make a stamp that resembles a four-leafed clover. The smaller heart is a traditional solid shape that fits neatly along the edges of the shelf supports.

You Will Need

Materials
tracing paper
spray adhesive
high-density foam
country-style shelf
deep-red acrylic or emulsion (latex) paint
scrap paper

Equipment
pencil
craft knife
plate
paintbrush (optional)

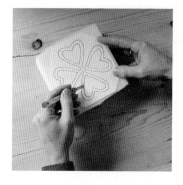

1 Trace the templates from the back of the book, enlarging if necessary. Lightly spray the shapes with adhesive and place them on the foam. Cut around the outline of the shapes with a craft knife.

2 Cut out the single heart shape. First cut out the outline, then part the foam and cut all the way through.

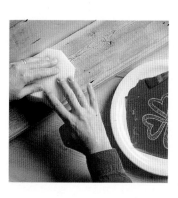 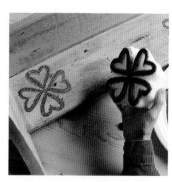 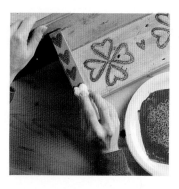

3 Use the foam stamp as a measuring guide to estimate the number of prints to fit along the back of the shelf. Mark the positions with a pencil. Spread some deep-red paint on to a plate.

4 Coat the clover-leaf stamp evenly and make a test print on scrap paper to ensure that it is not overloaded with paint. (You may find it easier to apply the paint to the stamp with a paintbrush.) Using the pencil guidelines, make the first print on the shelf.

5 Continue until you have completed all of the clover-leaf shapes. Try not to get the finish too even; this is a rustic piece of furniture and an uneven effect is more suitable.

6 Finish off the shelf with a row of small hearts along the support edges, then add one heart between each of the larger motifs.

74

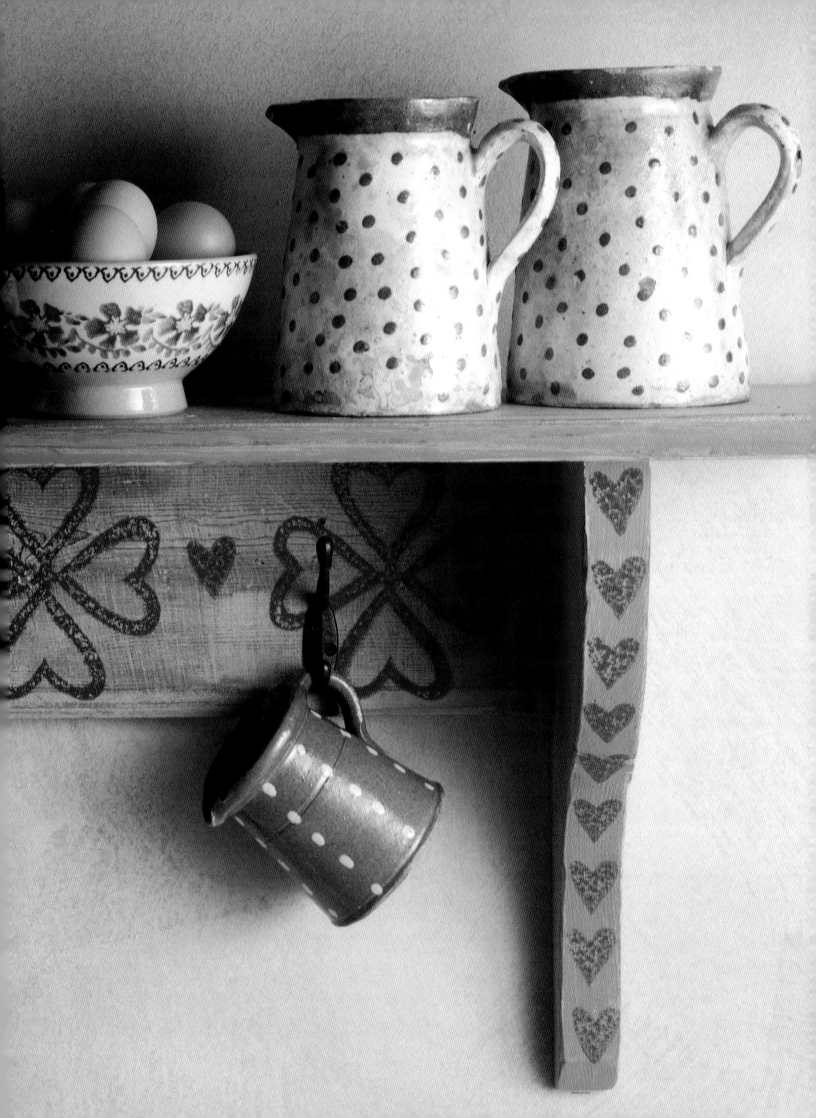

• STENCILLING, STAMPING AND PRINTING •

Foam-block Printing

Printing with cut-out foam blocks must be the easiest possible way to achieve the effect of hand-painted wallpaper. A special feature of this project is the paint used – a combination of wallpaper paste, PVA (white) glue and gouache colour. This is not only cheap, but it also has a wonderful translucent quality all of its own that really does produce a unique finish.

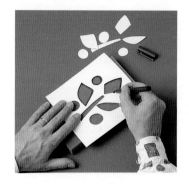 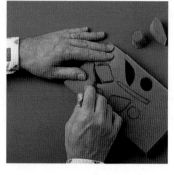

YOU WILL NEED

MATERIALS	EQUIPMENT
tracing paper	pencil
thin card	scissors
high-density foam	felt-tipped pen
paper, 15 x 15 cm/6 x 6 in	craft knife
wallpaper paste	plumb-line
PVA (white) glue	plate
gouache paints: viridian, deep-green and off-white	paintbrush (optional)
clear matt varnish (optional)	

1 Trace the templates on this page, enlarging if necessary. Transfer them to thin card and cut them out. Trace the design on to the foam, outlining it with a felt-tipped pen.

2 Cut out the shapes. First cut around the pattern and then part the foam slightly and carefully cut through the entire thickness.

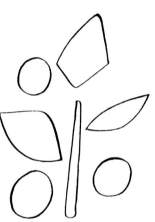

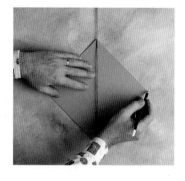

3 Prepare the wall for decorating. Attach the plumb-line to the wall or ceiling in one corner of the room. Turn the paper square on the diagonal and let the plumb-line fall through the centre. Make pencil dots on the wall at each corner of the paper. Move the paper down the plumb-line, marking the corner points each time. Then move the plumb-line along sideways and continue marking dots until the wall is covered in a grid of dots.

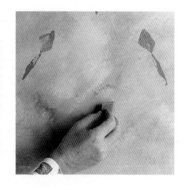 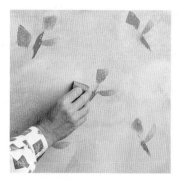 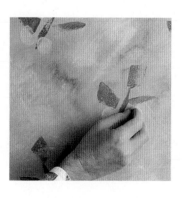

4 Mix the wallpaper paste according to the instructions. Add PVA (white) glue, in the proportion three parts paste-to one part glue. Add a squeeze of viridian and deep-green paint and blend.

5 Put some paint mixture on to a plate and dip the first sponge into it. Wipe off any excess paint and then print on the wall, using a light rolling motion. Use the dots to position the stamp.

6 Use the second sponge to complete the sprig design with leaf shapes, varying the angle slightly to add life.

7 Use the dot-shaped sponge and off-white to complete the design with berries, adding the colour to the PVA (white) mixture as before. If liked, protect the wall with a coat of varnish.

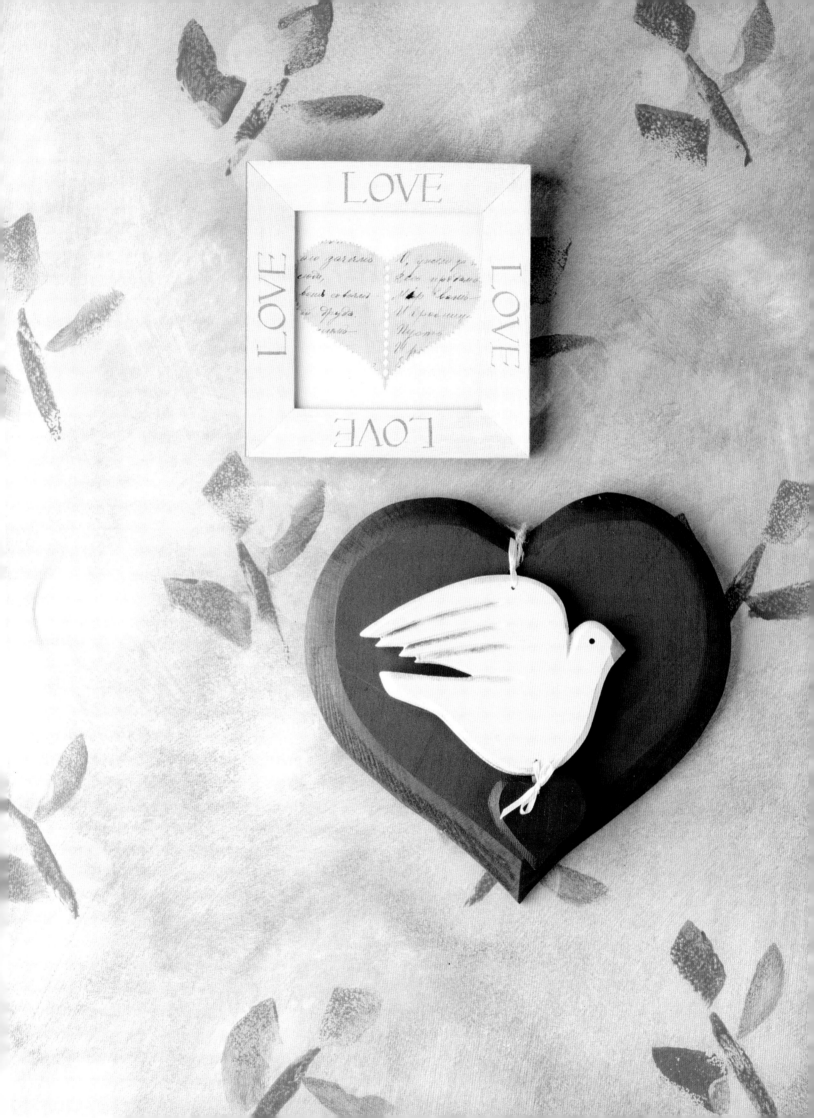

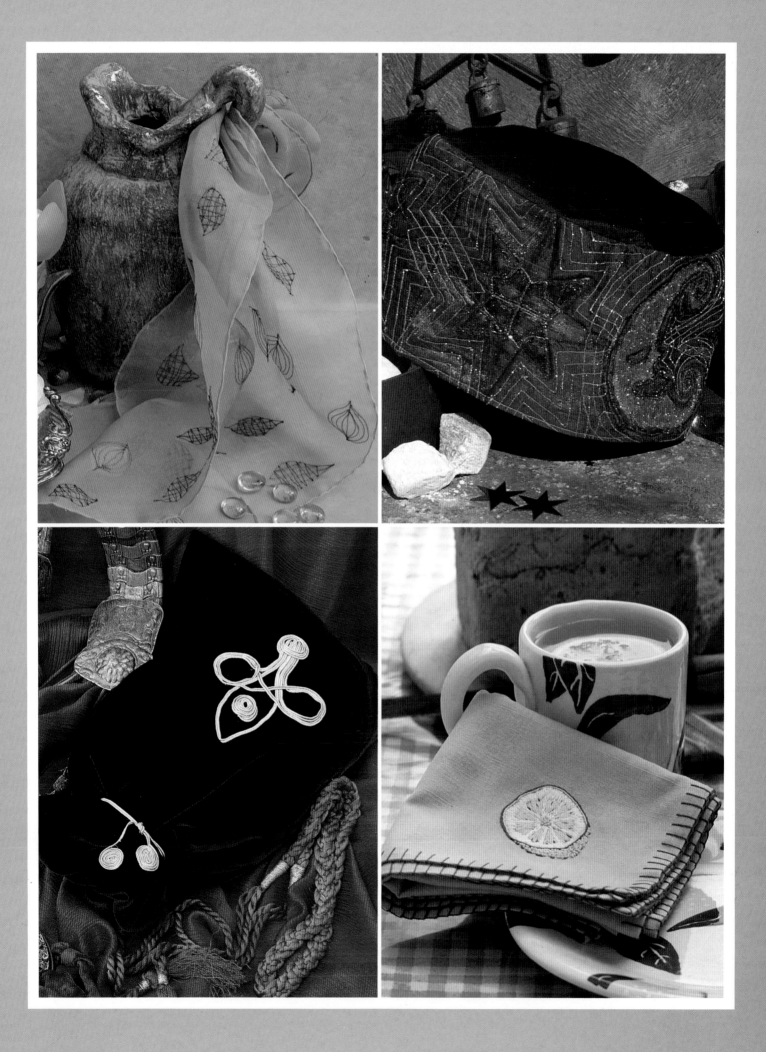

E M B R O I D E R Y

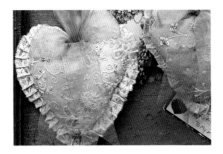

*E*mbroidering detail on to fabric – whether by hand or by machine – is a beautiful method of decoration, and it can be applied to a wide range of materials and objects, including clothes, linens and pictures. The wealth of threads available today means that your embroidery can be bright and vivid or muted and subtle – whatever mood you wish to evoke, there will be a thread available for you. The range of fabrics in varying colours, textures and strengths is quite astounding, and you can choose to work on a small square of fabric to create a purse, or enhance a baby's outfit with fine stitching.

Whatever project you choose to embark on, you will soon find that your embroidery skills increase with practice and experimentation. So, gather needle and thread together and enjoy one of the most rewarding of decorative crafts.

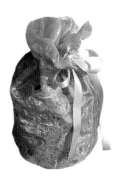

Embroidery

Materials and Equipment

Most of the materials used for embroidery can be purchased from craft suppliers or department stores. The range of fabrics available is immense, so consider how the texture will affect your finished piece when making your fabric choice. Cotton and silk are easy to handle, and felt, plastic and leather produce interesting results. Some key materials and pieces of equipment to help you with your embroidery are given below.

Bobbins are useful to have in a fair quantity so that you don't have to unwind and rewind them with each different thread colour.

Buttons and beads come in a range of shapes and sizes and a variety of materials, such as plastic, glass, wood and bone.

Dressmaker's carbon is used to transfer designs to fabric.

Embroidery hoops A wooden hand embroidery hoop can also be used for machine embroidery if the inner ring is wrapped with strips of cotton to improve tautness. Specialized **machine embroidery hoops** with spring closures are more convenient.

Fabric glue can be used instead of fusible bonding web.

Fabric paints are water-based non-toxic paints that are fixed by ironing.

Feet For most machine embroidery, a foot should be used, although a presser foot will give a cleaner satin stitch. You can work without a foot, but the thread will tend to snap more often.

Fusible bonding web is used to bond appliqué fabrics to the ground fabric temporarily during stitching. Templates can be marked out on the paper backing.

Hand embroidery threads are available in skeins and can be couched or stitched to enhance machine embroidery.

Machine embroidery threads are available in every imaginable colour and in different strengths. They are more lustrous than sewing threads.

Metallic embroidery threads are very popular and are available in many colours as well as shades of gold, silver and bronze. Be careful when stitching at high speeds on a machine, as occasionally the thread will snap.

Scissors Use dressmaker's scissors for cutting fabrics and embroidery scissors for cutting away threads and trimming.

Sewing machine The machine should have a free arm and a detachable bed for ease of movement. Take care of the machine and oil and clean it regularly to prevent stitch problems.

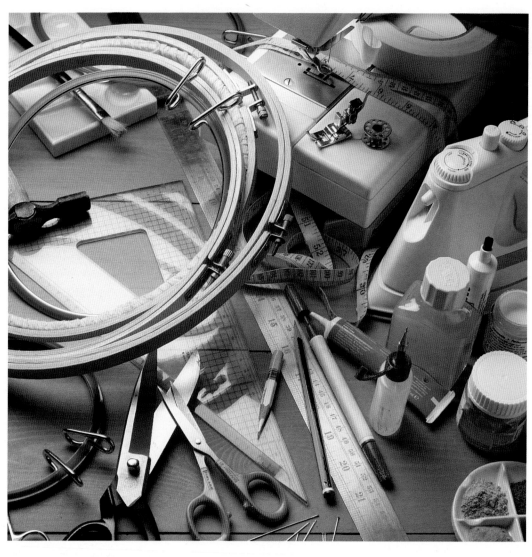

ABOVE *Equipment required for embroidery – whether by hand or by machine – can be easily obtained from crafts suppliers. Each embroidery project in this section tells you exactly what you will need for best results.*

Stabilizers should be used to prevent the fabric from puckering and distortion. Water-soluble polythene will stabilize open-work and sheer fabrics, and is easily dissolved in cold water.

Vanishing fabric markers are available in pink and purple and will fade with exposure to air or water.

• EMBROIDERY •

WORKING WITH DIFFERENT STITCHES

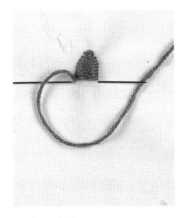 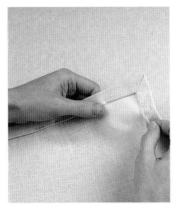 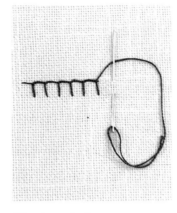 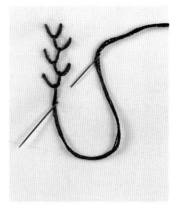

Satin stitch
Satin stitch is used for filling in and outlining. Ensure the fabric is held tautly in a frame to prevent puckering. Carry the thread across the area to be filled, then return it back underneath the fabric as near as possible to the point from which the needle emerged.

Slip stitch
Slip stitch is used to join together two folded edges, and for flat-hemming a turned-in edge. It should be nearly invisible. Pick up two threads of the single fabric and slip the needle through the fold for about 5 mm/¼ in. Draw the thread through to make a tiny stitch.

Blanket stitch
Blanket stitch can be used for finishing hems and, when the stitches are worked closely together, for buttonholes. It is used decoratively for scalloped edging. Working from left to right, bring the needle down vertically and loop the thread under its tip before pulling it through.

Feather stitch
Feather stitch is a looped stitch, traditionally used for smocking and decorating crazy patchwork. It can be worked in straight or curved lines. Bring the thread through the fabric and make slanting stitches, working alternately to the right and left of the line to be covered.

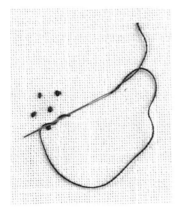  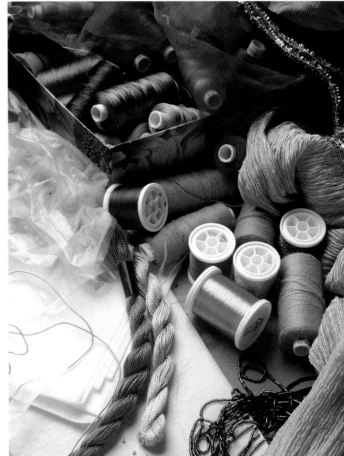

French knot
French knots are used sparingly as accents, or worked more closely together to produce a texture. The stitch should be worked with the fabric in a frame, leaving both hands free. Bring the thread through and hold down. Twist the thread around the needle a few times and tighten. Holding the thread taut, insert the needle back into the fabric with the other hand, at the point from which it emerged. Pull the needle through the thread twists to form the knot.

Tacking
This is a temporary stitch, used to hold seams together before sewing by machine. The stitches should be between 0.5–1 cm/¼–⅜ in long and evenly spaced. Use a contrasting thread to make the stitching easy to unpick.

RIGHT *For machine embroidery projects, keep a number of bobbins ready-wound with threads of different colours.*

Embroidered Insect Display

This pretty design is inspired by old Victorian display cases containing rows of beetles and bugs. It's ecologically sound, however, because these stylish black bugs are embroidered on calico.

You Will Need

Materials
*thick tracing paper
natural calico,
30 x 30 cm/12 x 12 in
embroidery threads: black, ochre, emerald and yellow
thick card, 20 x 20 cm/
8 x 8 in
strong button thread
3 small labels
wooden frame, to fit
20 x 20 cm/8 x 8 in*

Equipment
*transfer pencil
iron
embroidery hoop
embroidery needle
large needle
pen*

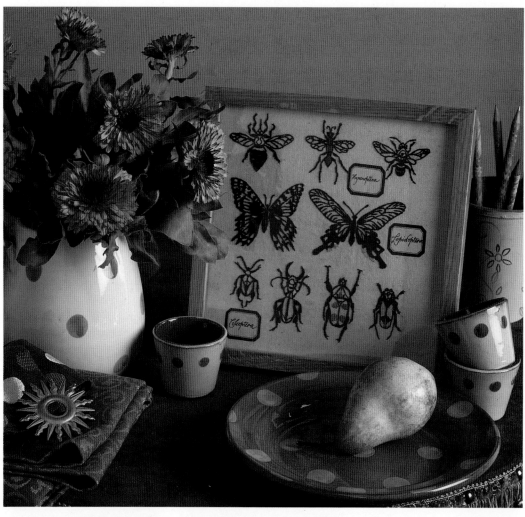

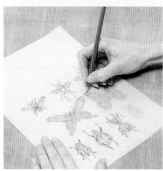

1 Using a transfer pencil, trace the template from the back of the book, enlarging if necessary, on to the calico. Fix the design according to the manufacturer's instructions.

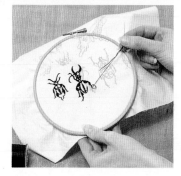

2 Stretch the calico in an embroidery hoop and work over the design outlines using two strands of black embroidery thread in simple straight and satin stitches. Work legs and antennae in small chain stitch and pick out a few details in colour. Iron lightly from the wrong side.

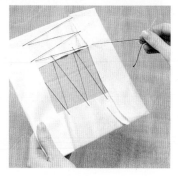

3 To mount the embroidery, place the card centrally on the back of the work and fold two opposite sides over it. Lace together with strong thread, then repeat with the other two sides. Write labels for the three orders of insects: Hymenoptera (bees and wasps), Lepidoptera (butterflies) and Coleoptera (beetles). Fix these to the fabric and insert it in the frame.

• EMBROIDERY •

Embroidered Organza Scarf

Use muted, autumnal colours for this delicate, sheer scarf. The painted and embroidered leaves create an almost abstract pattern.

You Will Need

Materials	Equipment
laundered silk organza or chiffon	*embroidery hoop*
fabric paints: green and blue	*fine paintbrush*
machine embroidery threads: orange and red	*paint-mixing container*
matching sewing thread	*iron*
	sewing machine, with darning foot
	dressmaker's scissors
	needle

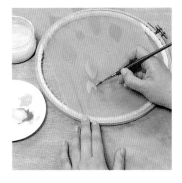

1 Stretch the fabric taut in an embroidery hoop. Paint the leaf shapes freehand in greens and blues, mixing the paints to achieve subtle shades. Allow to dry. Iron the silk to fix the paint, according to the manufacturer's instructions.

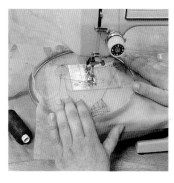

2 Select the darning or free stitch mode on the sewing machine and attach a darning foot. With the fabric in an embroidery hoop, stitch the details on the design in orange and red thread over the painted leaves.

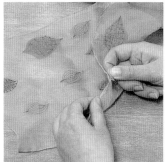

3 Trim and roll the raw edges of the scarf and slip stitch the hems in place.

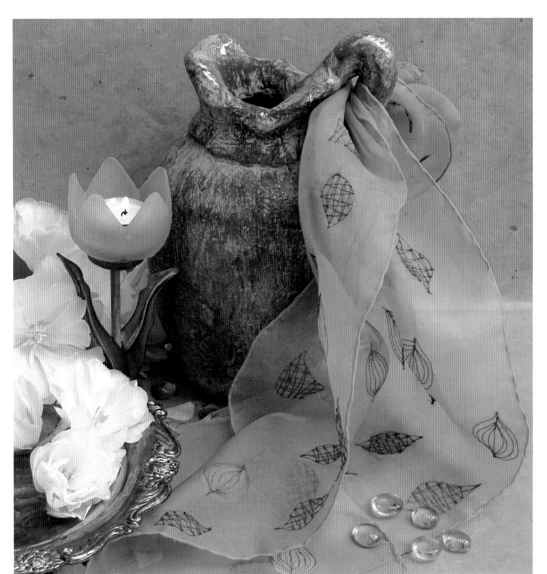

• EMBROIDERY •

Lemon Slice Napkins

These lovely yellow napkins embroidered with cool lemon slices would look delightful on a table set for a summer lunch in the garden.

You Will Need

Materials

tracing paper
large yellow napkin
embroidery threads: dark
and pale yellow, off-white
and dark green

Equipment

soft and hard pencils
dressmaker's pins
embroidery needle
iron

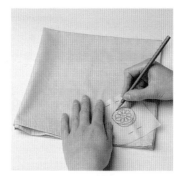

1 Trace the template at the back of the book, enlarging if necessary. Rub over the lemon motif on the reverse of the tracing with a soft pencil. Pin the tracing in the corner of the napkin and transfer the motif on to it.

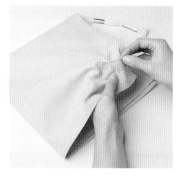

2 Using dark yellow thread, work French knots in the centre of the lemon. Fill the segments in stem stitch using pale yellow. Fill the pith in stem stitch using off-white, and fill the skin area with dark yellow French knots.

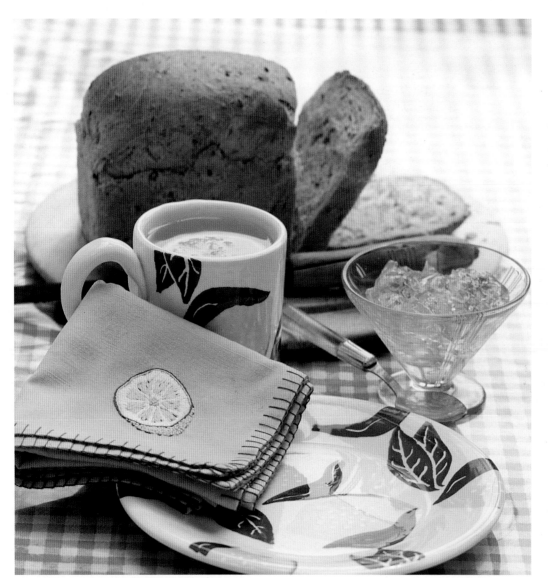

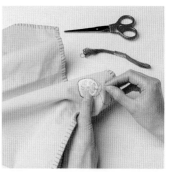

3 Work dark green blanket stitch around the hem of the napkin. The stitches can be worked over the existing machine stitching. Work a row of dark yellow stem stitch around the edge of the lemon pith and another row outside that in green. Work a dark green running stitch around the edge of the French knots and add some small dark green stitches as shading in the segments to complete the design. Iron the embroidery on the reverse side.

• EMBROIDERY •

FLEUR-DE-LYS SHOE BAG

Rich purple velvet and opulent gold braid suit the regal motif on this luxurious bag for your best party shoes. The appliquéd braid technique could easily be adapted to other items such as cushions and throws.

YOU WILL NEED

MATERIALS
cotton velvet fabric,
53 x 38 cm/21 x 15 in
tracing paper
thin card or paper
gold embroidery thread
gold braid
matching sewing thread
black satin ribbon,
4 cm/1½ in wide
elastic, 1 cm/½ in wide

EQUIPMENT
dressmaker's scissors
dressmaker's pins
pencil
needle
sewing machine
safety pin

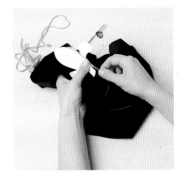

1 Cut the velvet in half across the width and mark the centre of one piece with a pin. Trace the template from the back of the book on to thin card and pin it to the centre of the velvet towards the lower edge. Use gold thread to sew on the gold braid, pinning it around the template as you stitch. Work in a continuous pattern around the outline. Add the swirls.

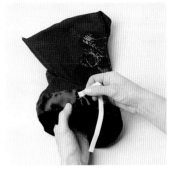

2 Machine stitch the sides and hem, leaving a seam allowance of 1 cm/½ in. Neaten the raw edges. Fold down the top edge, leaving a generous cuff. Cover the raw edge with satin ribbon, stitching along both edges to form a casing. Fold under the ends of the ribbon and butt them together. With a safety pin, thread some elastic through the casing and stitch the ends together.

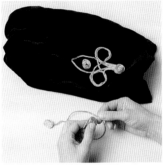

3 Complete the bag by making a tie with another length of braid, coiling and stitching the ends. Attach to one side seam and tie around the neck of the bag.

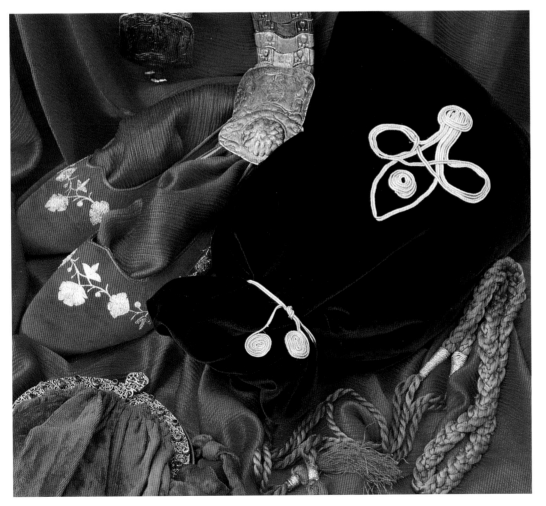

• EMBROIDERY •

BEADED ORANGE PURSE

This luxurious purse is embroidered to look like slices of fruit with tiny beads to echo the texture.

YOU WILL NEED

MATERIALS
*velvet or brocade pieces,
1 orange and 1 yellow,
15 cm/6 in
2 pieces yellow silk,
15 cm/6 in
tracing paper
embroidery threads: white,
crimson, orange, yellow
and lime-green
small glass beads: yellow,
orange and clear
tacking (basting) thread
zip, 12 cm/4¾ in
matching sewing thread*

EQUIPMENT
*dressmaker's scissors
pencil
tailor's chalk
embroidery needle
dressmaker's pins
needle*

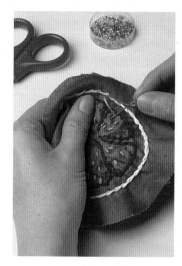

1 Cut circles, 14 cm/5½ in in diameter: one each of orange and yellow velvet and two of silk. Trace the template from the back of the book, enlarging to fit the circle, and transfer it to the velvet with tailor's chalk. Sew chain stitch in white for the pith. On the orange side, sew crimson segments and orange flesh; on the lemon side, sew yellow segments and lemon and lime flesh. Use chain stitch for the segments and back stitch for flesh. Add coloured beads for the skin and clear beads for moisture. With right sides together, pin and tack (baste) the zip, leaving a 1 cm/½ in allowance.

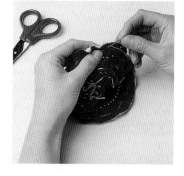

2 Stitch along the zip. Open it and complete the seam around the rest of the circle.

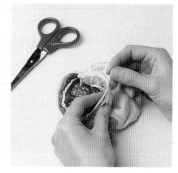

3 With right sides together, sew the two pieces of silk halfway round. Turn to the right side. Put the purse, inside out, inside the lining. Turn in the lining seam allowance and slip stitch it to the zip.

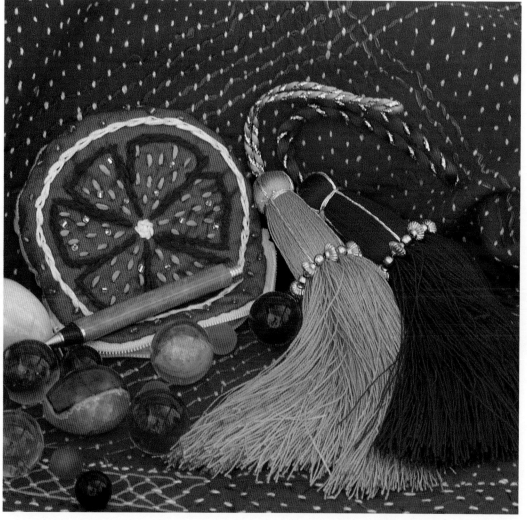

• EMBROIDERY •

HEAVENLY BAG

This delicate and pretty bag is ideal for lingerie.

YOU WILL NEED

MATERIALS
*2 rectangles silver metallic organza, 65 x 28 cm/ 26 x 11 in
2 circles silver metallic organza, 18 cm/ 7 in in diameter
2 rectangles gold metallic organza, 24 x 26 cm/ 7 x 11 in
contrasting metallic machine threads
tacking (basting) thread
tracing paper
ribbon*

EQUIPMENT
*sewing machine, with darning foot
tape measure
needle
dressmaker's scissors
fabric marker*

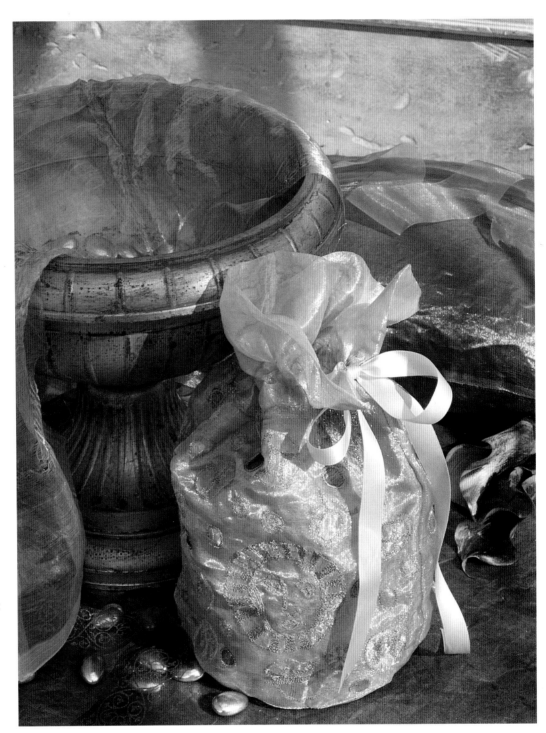

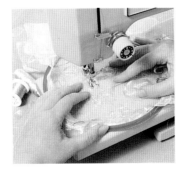

1 Fold the rectangular pieces of fabric in half widthways. Stitch an 8 cm/3 in seam from the folded edge on both side edges. Turn the rectangles right sides out. To make the ribbon casing, stitch two parallel lines 8 and 10 cm/3 and 4 in from the folded edge. Make a grid of tacking (basting) lines to attach a gold rectangle to a silver rectangle, matching the bottom edges.

2 Using a fabric marker, trace the template from the back of the book, enlarging if necessary, and transfer it to the gold side of the two silver and gold pieces. On the sewing machine, set the dial to the darning or free embroidery mode. Work the circles in straight stitch, with contrasting thread in the top and bobbin.

3 Cut away the gold organza inside the stitched line. Work the remaining signs in contrasting colours. Cut away and discard the organza again. Top stitch 1.5 cm/⅝ in from the top edge and pull away the weft threads, to produce a gold fringe. Remove the tacking (basting). Lay the two embroidered sides right sides together.

4 Stitch the sides to make a tube-shaped outer, embroidered bag, with a lining formed by the folded half. Stitch one silver circle to the bottom of the outside tube, and the other to the bottom of the lining. Turn right sides out. Tuck the lining inside the bag and slip stitch the gap. Thread a ribbon through the casing.

87

Sparkling Ivy Garland

Make this beautiful jewelled crown of leaves for a midsummer night's party, or perhaps for a summer wedding.

You Will Need

Materials
water-soluble fabric
paper or thin card
fine green wool or green
embroidery thread
metallic threads: silver and
blended gold and silver
sewing threads: dark and
light green
paper towels
fine silver or brass wire:
0.6 mm for circlet,
0.4 or 0.2 mm for leaves
selection of beads

Equipment
embroidery hoop
fabric marker
large-eyed needle
sewing machine, with
size 11 needle
dressmaker's scissors

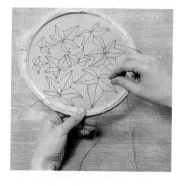

1 Stretch the water-soluble fabric on to the embroidery hoop. Using a fabric marker, trace the template from the back of the book, enlarging if necessary, on to the fabric. For the first style of leaf, hand stitch the central veins in fine green wool or embroidery thread. Use a running stitch and a thicker thread for the larger leaves.

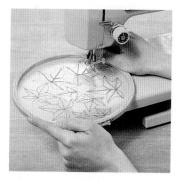

2 For the second style of leaf, work the veins and outlines on the machine with a straight stitch, using silver metallic thread in the bobbin and dark green sewing thread in the needle. Fill in between the veins with the lighter green. For the first style of leaf, fill in with blended gold and silver thread in the bobbin and silver thread in the needle.

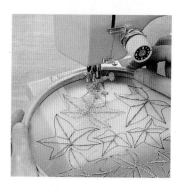

3 Sew randomly across the machined lines within each section of leaf to make the tiny veins. (This also holds the embroidery together.)

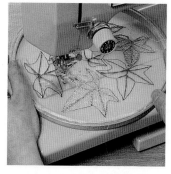

4 Work a zigzag stitch up the central veins and around the outer edge of each leaf to stiffen it.

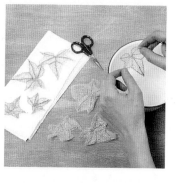

5 Cut the leaves off the hoop and dissolve the fabric of each one in turn in water. Pat dry on paper towels. While still damp, fold each leaf in half and press with your fingers to make a crease along the central vein. Open out and allow to dry.

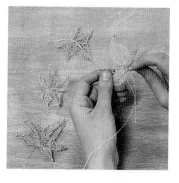

6 Continue to embroider more leaves in both styles to make enough for the whole garland. Sew each leaf on to fine wire.

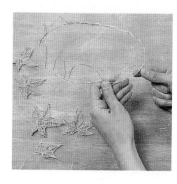

7 Twist a piece of thicker wire into a band to fit your head. Twist on more wire to make loops for attaching the leaves. Make the loops higher at the front of the garland.

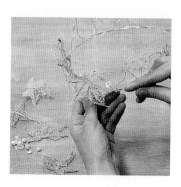

8 Wind the wired leaves on to the loops on the band, using the larger leaves at the front. Add beads threaded with more wire. Bend and arrange the leaves into shape.

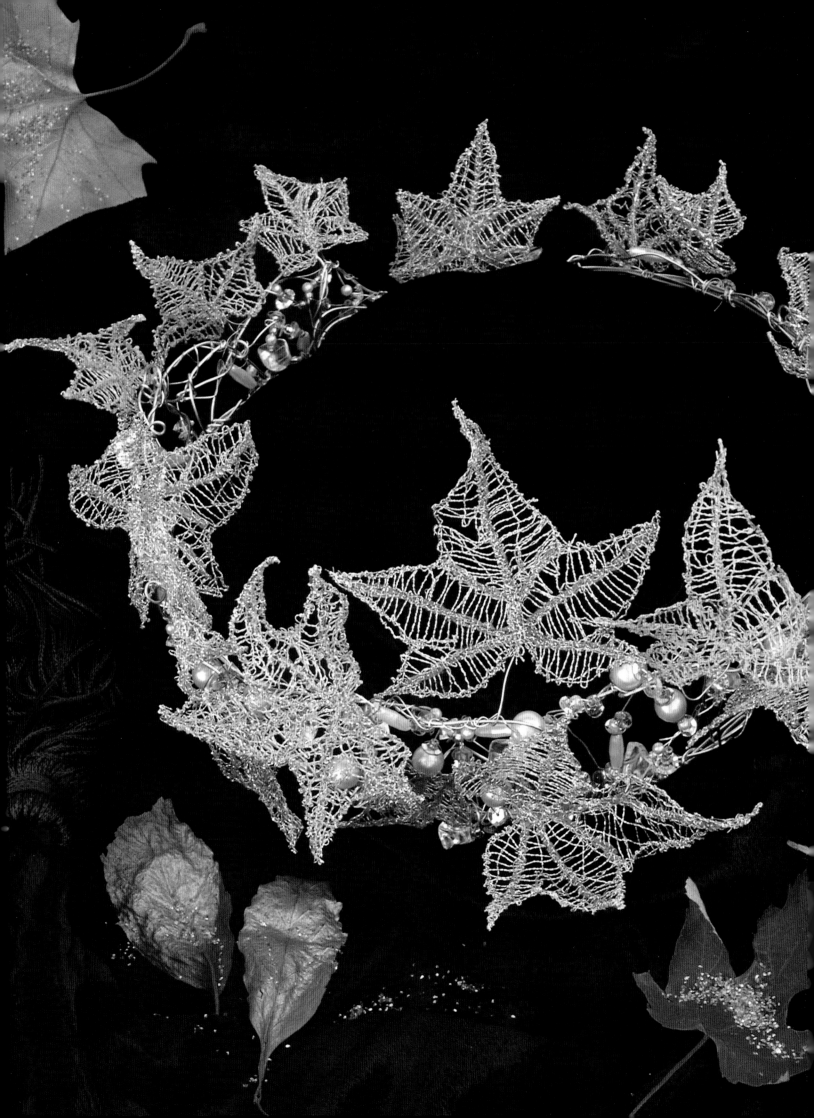

• EMBROIDERY •

TUDOR ROSE BUTTON

These buttons take up the theme of the Tudor Rose, a famous heraldic union of the red rose of Lancaster and the white rose of York.

YOU WILL NEED

MATERIALS
water-soluble fabric
machine embroidery
threads: green, red
and white
fine metallic thread
a few small pearl beads
self-cover buttons,
22 mm/¾ in
piece of metallic fabric
piece of sheer organza
PVA (white) glue

EQUIPMENT
embroidery hoop
fine magic marker
embroidery needle
sewing machine
dressmaker's scissors
fine paintbrush

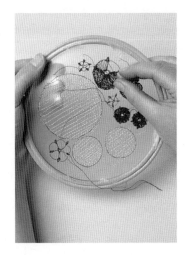

1 Stretch the water-soluble fabric on to the embroidery hoop. Trace the template from the back of the book on to the fabric using a fine magic marker. Hand or machine embroider the leaf detail in green, using straight stitch and sewing back and forth to link the stitches. Cut off the trailing green threads and hand or machine embroider in red or white over the flower, making sure that you interlock the stitches. To make the mesh, thread the machine with metallic thread and sew straight rows, first one way then the other, to make a net. Remove the embroidery from the hoop.

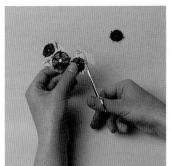

2 Cut around the flowers and mesh and sew them together, adding a few beads, before you dissolve the water-soluble fabric.

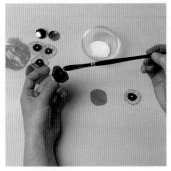

3 Follow the manufacturer's instructions to cover the buttons. Cut circles of metallic and sheer fabrics and dab a little glue in the centre of each button before covering with the layers of fabric.

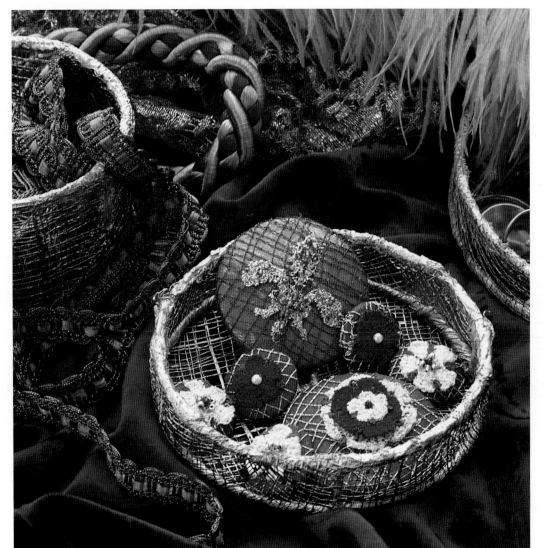

• EMBROIDERY •

Underwater Picture

The effect of the layers of delicate blue and green chiffon is marvellously evocative of an undersea scene. This tranquil picture would be ideal in a bedroom, where its calm, reflective quality is bound to induce plenty of sweet dreams.

You Will Need

Materials
*shot organza in shades of green and blue
white paper
metallic organza
shot velvets
shot silk
shot organza
pearlized lamé
metallic embroidery threads*

Equipment
*dressmaker's scissors
dressmaker's pins
embroidery hoop
sewing machine, with embroidery foot*

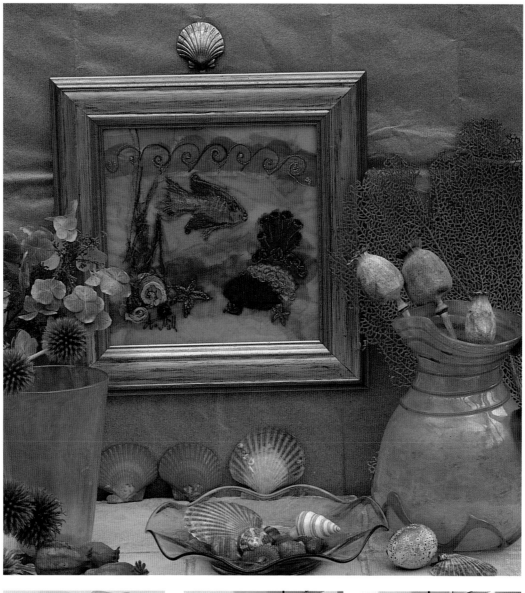

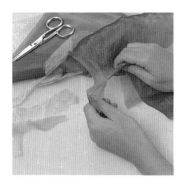

1 Use one sheet of organza as the base of the sea. Tear strips of organza to form the sea background.

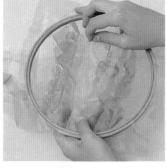

2 Assemble all the strips, pin them together, and fit them into the embroidery hoop. Pin them in place.

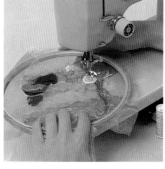

3 Make shell, fish and starfish paper templates. Cut out shells from the metallic organza, fish from the velvets and silk, and starfish from the shot organza and lamé. Pin and machine stitch to the sea base, using metallic threads.

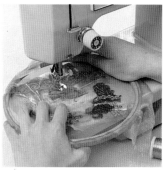

4 Build up the design with texture and colour. Remove the embroidery from the hoop and stretch it back into shape, ready for framing.

• EMBROIDERY •

UNICORN PENNANT

This richly embroidered pennant uses the unicorn as its motif. Cool colours are used to great effect to reflect his elusive nature.

YOU WILL NEED

MATERIALS
*4 toning cotton fabrics,
15 x 21.5 cm/6 x 8½ in
matching sewing thread
tracing paper
fusible bonding web
unbleached calico,
25 x 25 cm/10 x 10 in
gold machine
embroidery thread
1.5 m/1½ yd wire-edged
fleur-de-lys ribbon
tacking (basting) thread
cotton backing fabric,
28 x 40 cm/11 x 16 in
wooden pole, 36 cm/14 in
dark blue craft paint*

EQUIPMENT
*sewing machine
iron
pencil
dressmaker's scissors
needle
dressmaker's pins
paintbrush*

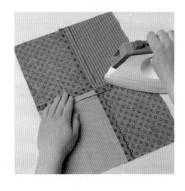

1 Join the fabric rectangles in pairs along the long edges. Iron the seams open, then join the two pairs to form a large rectangle. Iron the seams open.

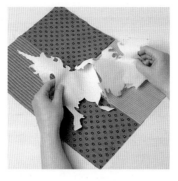

2 Trace the template from the back of the book, enlarging it to 23 cm/9 in across. Transfer it, in reverse, to the backing paper of the fusible bonding web. Iron it on to the calico, then cut it out along the outline. Peel off the backing paper and iron it on to the centre of the patchwork. Draw on the features.

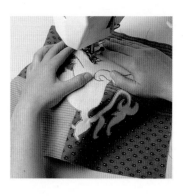

3 Using a narrow satin stitch and gold thread, sew around the outside edge of the motif and over the various details of the design.

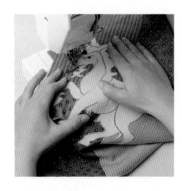

4 Embroider the eye, tongue and nostril by hand or with a machine.

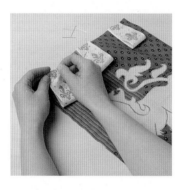

5 Cut three 15 cm/6 in lengths of ribbon, that match the design, and remove the wire from the edges. Fold each piece in half, then pin and tack (baste) in place on the upper edge of the banner so that the loops are facing downwards.

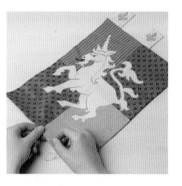

6 With right sides facing, pin the backing fabric to the banner and sew around the edge leaving a 1 cm/½ in seam allowance. Leave a 10 cm/4 in gap at the lower edge for turning. Trim the corners and turn. Iron.

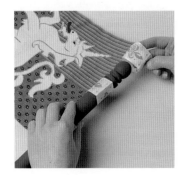

7 Paint the pole and allow to dry, then thread the banner on to the pole.

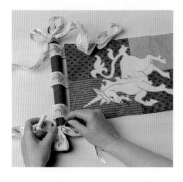

8 Tie each end of the remaining ribbon to the pole in a bow. Secure with a few stitches and pull the wired edges of the loops into shape.

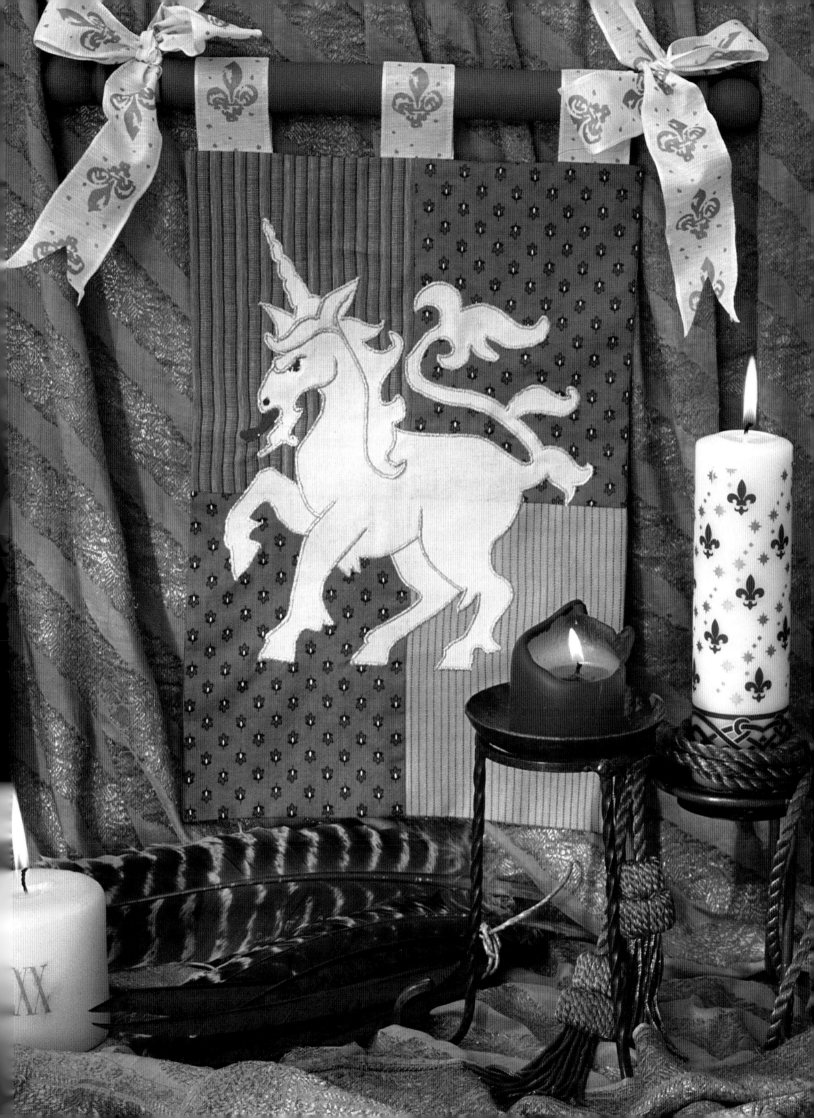

• EMBROIDERY •

WILD ROSE CHIFFON SCARF

Shimmering silk chiffon or organza and glittering silver metallic paint combine here to make a ravishing scarf that would completely transform a plain outfit. You do not have to wear this, though; it is a technique that could equally well be used to make beautiful fabric wall hangings.

YOU WILL NEED

MATERIALS
*silk chiffon or organza,
30 x 50 cm/12 x 20 in
tracing paper
silver metallic fabric paint
metallic paint with nozzle-tipped dispenser*

EQUIPMENT
*iron
wooden frame
drawing pins
pencil
paintbrush
fabric marker
needle*

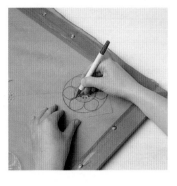

1 Wash, dry and iron the silk. Fold it in half and iron twice. Fold diagonally and iron. Unfold and stretch the fabric taut on the frame using drawing pins. Trace the template on this page, enlarging if necessary, on to the back of the silk at the centre. Trace eight more motifs around it, using the pressed folds as a guide.

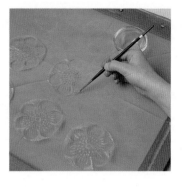

2 Turn the frame over and go over the outlines of the design with silver paint on the front of the fabric. Allow to dry. Unpin the scarf and fix the paint according to the manufacturer's instructions. Stretch the fabric again.

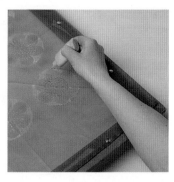

3 Using the nozzle-tipped tube, make dots of metallic paint around the outer edges of each rose and fill in the details. Mark lines of dots 5 cm/2 in from the edges of the scarf, with the marker. To fray the edges, work one side at a time. Use a needle to separate and remove threads from the raw edges, then pull away up to the dotted edges.

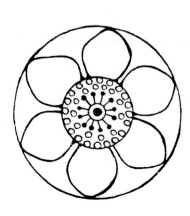

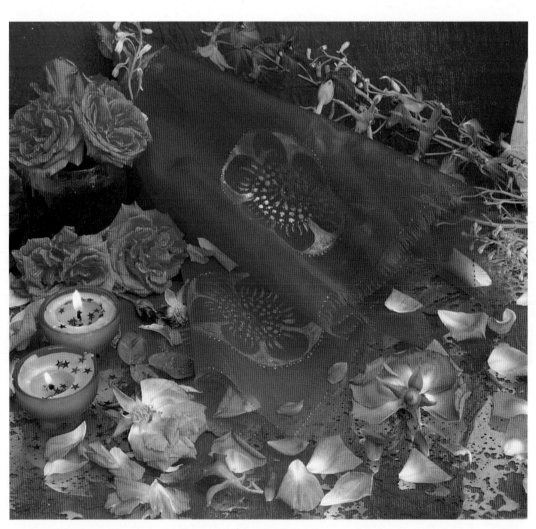

• EMBROIDERY •

HEAVENLY HAT

This richly coloured hat is made from a circle and a rectangle. Measure your head and add a 5 cm/2 in seam and shrinkage allowance. The height of the hat shown is 12 cm/4¾ in plus a 2.5 cm/1 in seam allowance. Cut a circle for the top, according to the size required, and add on a seam allowance of 2.5 cm/1 in.

YOU WILL NEED

MATERIALS
*3 colours of dupion silk
heavy iron-on interfacing
velvet, 10 x 10 cm/4 x 4 in
paper
contrasting cotton threads
contrasting metallic
machine embroidery
threads
metallic fabric paints*

EQUIPMENT
*dressmaker's scissors
tape measure
iron
pencil
dressmaker's pins
sewing machine, with
darning foot
paintbrush*

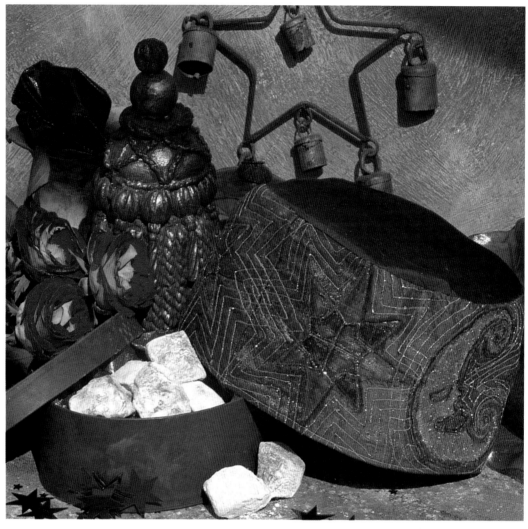

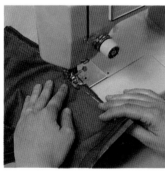

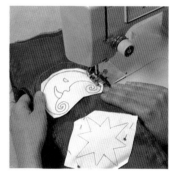

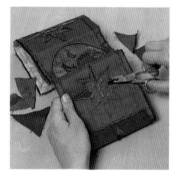

1 Cut three rectangles of silk and one of interfacing to the correct size. Iron the interfacing on to the back of the bottom layer of silk. Stitch around the edge of the rectangles, leaving a gap in one long seam. Insert the square of velvet slightly larger than the moon template through the gap, on top of the top layer of silk.

2 Draw and cut out the sun and moon shapes and pin on to the silk. With the machine in embroidery mode, stitch on top of the moon template, then stitch the features. Stitch the stars and outline stitching in the same way, using different coloured threads. Go over all the stitching twice, then tear away the paper.

3 Next, cut out the fabric layers to reveal your desired colours. Random whip stitch in a loop fashion inside the moon, with metallic thread. Paint areas of the hat with metallic fabric paints. Stitch the crown and top of the hat together and clip into the seam allowances.

• EMBROIDERY •

Dragonflies

These beautiful iridescent creatures look almost ready to fly away! If you've never tried free machine embroidery, look in your sewing machine manual for detailed instructions.

You Will Need

Materials
*water-soluble fabric
tracing paper
opalescent cellophane
(or cellophane sweet wrappers)
small pieces of sheer synthetic organza: brown and green
fine metallic thread
thicker metallic thread
paper towels
piece of card
spray varnish
glitter pipecleaners
fine wire and a few glass beads, for the butterflies*

Equipment
*embroidery hoop
fine magic marker
dressmaker's pins
sewing machine, with fine needle
dressmaker's scissors
needle*

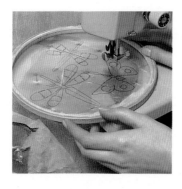

1 Stretch the fabric on to the hoop. Trace the template from the back of the book on to the fabric with the magic marker. Sandwich the cellophane between the sheer fabrics and pin under the hoop. Machine around the wing details in straight stitch with fine thread.

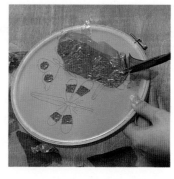

2 Remove the hoop from the machine and trim away the spare fabric and cellophane with scissors.

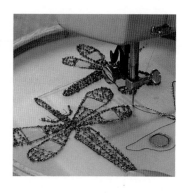

3 With fine metallic thread in the needle and the thicker metallic thread on the bobbin, machine all round the outlines of the insects in ordinary straight stitch.

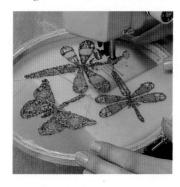

4 Put the fine thread on the bobbin and fill in between the outlines, joining all of the design. To stiffen the edges, go over the outlines in zigzag.

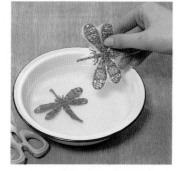

5 Hold the work to the light to check that the outlines are linked. Remove from the hoop and dissolve the fabric in water. Dry on paper towels.

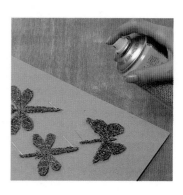

6 Pin the insects out flat on a piece of card and spray with varnish. Allow to dry.

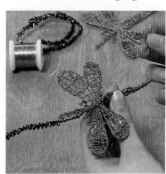

7 Cut a piece of glitter pipecleaner longer than the dragonfly body and sew it to the underside of the body part as far as the head. Trim it.

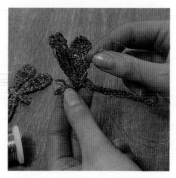

8 Bend the rest of the embroidery under the head and upper body to cover the pipecleaner. Stitch in place. Finally, fold the wings together and secure with a few stitches near the body so that the wings are raised.

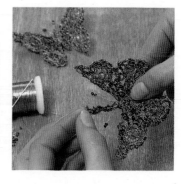

9 Thread some small glass beads on to fine gold wire and twist into two antennae for the butterfly. Thread these on to the head, and then complete it as for the dragonfly.

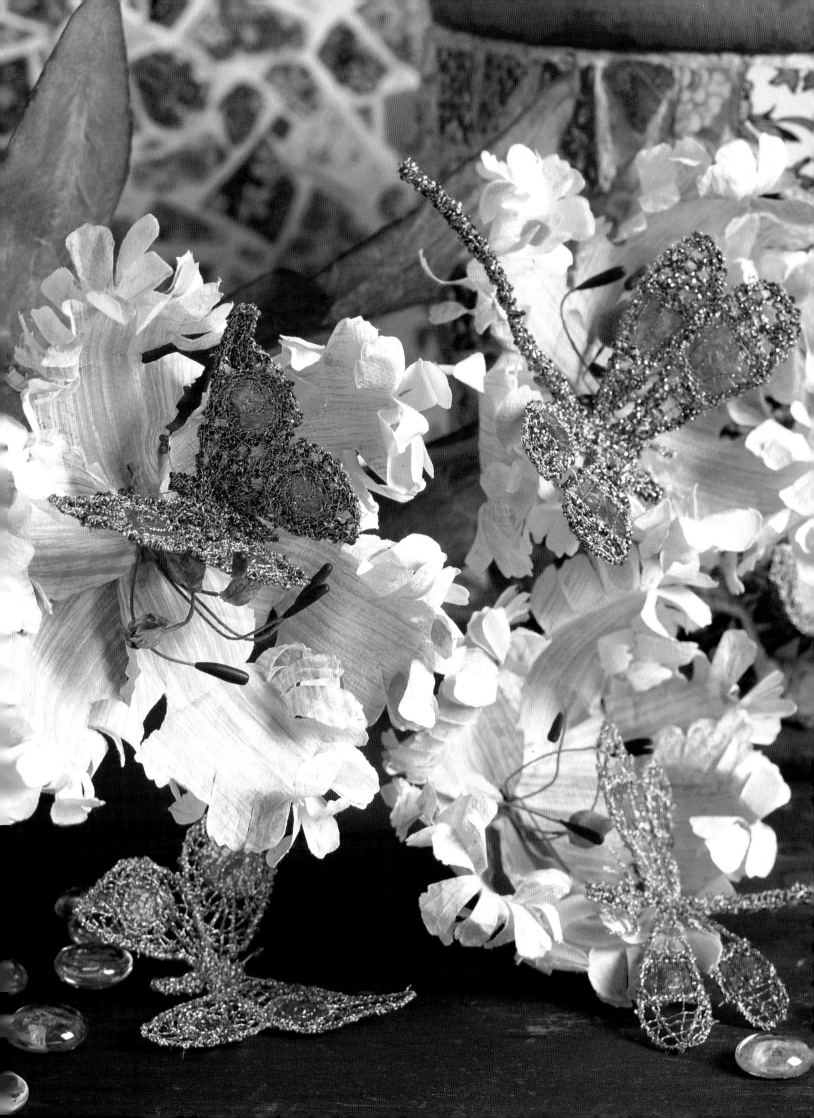

• EMBROIDERY •

CONTEMPORARY TABLEMAT

Here, a very traditional and popular motif is depicted in bright and bold modern colours.

YOU WILL NEED

MATERIALS	EQUIPMENT
light grey Zweigart Annable evenweave fabric, 38 x 56 cm/ 15 x 22 in	*tape measure*
	dressmaker's scissors
matching and black sewing thread	*dressmaker's pins*
	sewing machine
tacking (basting) thread	*iron*
tracing paper	*needle*
Anchor "Marlitt" shades 836, 815, 801 and 1032	*pencil*

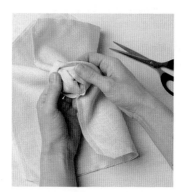

1 Cut two fabric rectangles, 28 x 38 cm/11 x 15 in. Pin them together and stitch around the edges, 1.5 cm/⅝ in from the edge, with matching thread and leaving a gap on one side. Mitre the corners, turn right side out and iron. Top stitch 1 cm/½ in from the edge. Tack (baste) guides around the edge of the mat, 2.5 cm/1 in and 4 cm/1½ in from the edge. Machine zigzag stitch over the top of the guidelines, using black thread. Use the presser foot as a guide to stitch the crossways lines. Stitch in the thread ends on the reverse side.

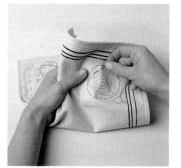

2 Trace the template from the back of the book, enlarging if necessary. Pin in position. Tack (baste) around the lines, then tear the tracing paper away. Machine zigzag along the lines and sew in the ends.

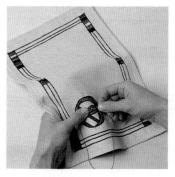

3 Fill in the coloured areas of the border in satin stitch, using two strands of Marlitt. Ease the satin stitches on the rose to fit round the curves, and fill in the centre to complete.

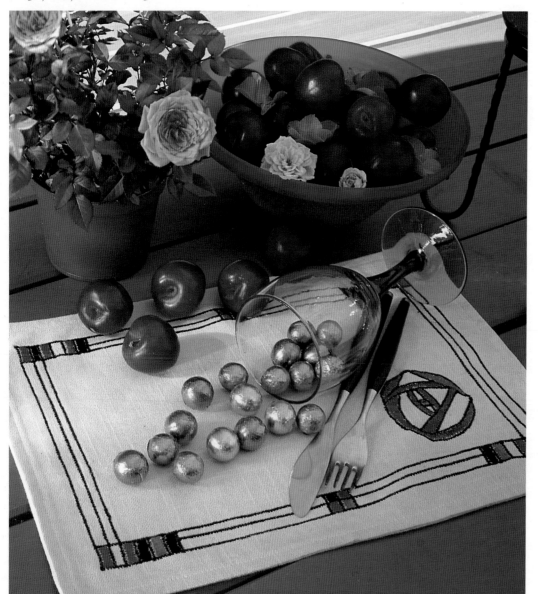

• EMBROIDERY •

Embroidered Dress

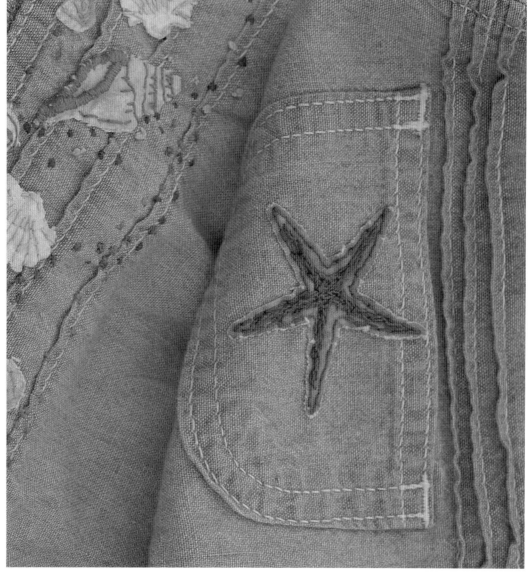

Seashore motifs make for a pleasing decoration on this denim dress. Shown here as a repeat pattern, the shell and starfish shapes are appliquéd, then decorated with embroidery; the embroidered detail helps to unify the design as a whole.

You Will Need

Materials
*ironed white cotton
lining paper or newspaper
selection of fabric paints
tracing paper
dress
fabric glue
embroidery threads*

Equipment
*paintbrush
paint-mixing container
iron
pencil
embroidery scissors
selection of needles
towel*

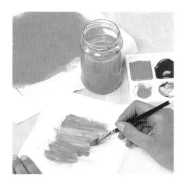
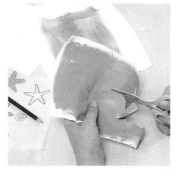
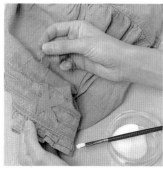
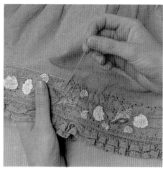

1 Lay the cotton on a larger sheet of paper and paint separate pieces of fabric in different colours. Allow to dry for 24 hours, then fix them, according to the manufacturer's instructions. Draw starfish and shell shapes on tracing paper.

2 Transfer the shapes several times on to the painted fabric. Cut them out, leaving a 5 mm/¼ in border outside the outlines. Lay the shapes on the hem of the dress and work out a pleasing pattern. Glue the shapes down sparingly.

3 Embroider a running stitch, or a continuous double running stitch, around the template outlines.

4 Embroider details to represent sand, stones, etc. Tidy loose threads and iron on the wrong side, over a towel.

• EMBROIDERY •

BABY SUIT

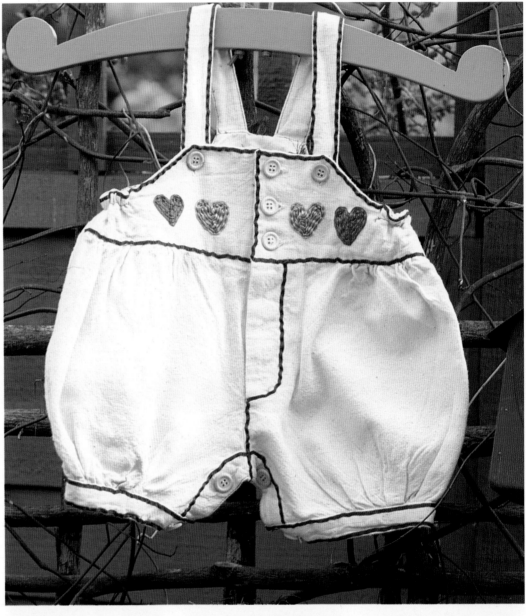

This ribbonwork decoration for a ready-made romper or sunsuit is easy to achieve and it looks really delightful. This type of ribbonwork is simple, because you can follow the existing oversewn garment seams, which act as sewing lines. Choose a plain, not patterned, suit, without any motifs.

YOU WILL NEED

MATERIALS

*chocolate-brown ribbon, 6 m/6 yd
romper or sunsuit
tracing paper
rust ribbon, 3 m/3 yd
sewing threads: orange and chocolate-brown
salmon or peach ribbon, 3 m/3 yd*

EQUIPMENT

*needle
pencil
fabric marker
dressmaker's scissors*

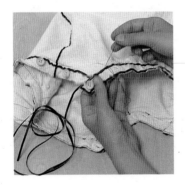

1 Use running stitch to attach chocolate-brown ribbon to the seams of the suit. Turn under, and finish the ends.

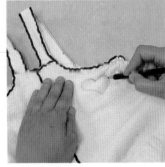

2 Trace the template from the back of the book, enlarging if necessary. Transfer to the suit four times. As an alternative, draw your own motifs with a pencil or marker.

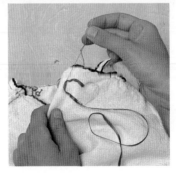

3 Turn under the end of the rust ribbon. Working anti-clockwise from the top of the heart, sew in place with running stitch in orange thread.

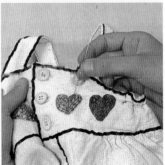

4 Repeat the process with the salmon or peach ribbon, using chocolate-brown or orange thread.

• EMBROIDERY •

MIDNIGHT SKY PICTURE

Glittering metallic threads against shimmering dark blue shot silk create a real feeling of the night sky in this picture, which combines appliqué and machine embroidery techniques.

YOU WILL NEED

MATERIALS
thin card
pearlized chiffon and lamé
dark blue shot silk,
23 x 23 cm/9 x 9 in
embroidery threads:
metallic silver, gold and blue
wadding (batting)
thick card
all-purpose glue

EQUIPMENT
pencil
scissors
fabric marker
embroidery hoop
ruler
dressmaker's pins
sewing machine, with darning foot

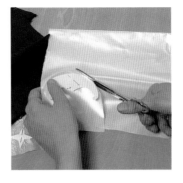

1 Draw the moon and stars freehand on to thin card and cut out to use as templates. Draw round the templates on the pearlized fabrics, using the fabric marker, and cut them out.

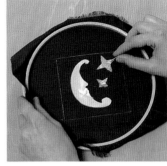

2 Stretch the silk in an embroidery hoop. Mark out a 10 cm/4 in square in the centre, using the fabric marker. Position the pearlized shapes and pin them in place.

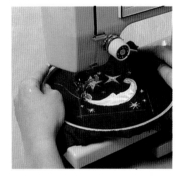

3 Using metallic thread and with the machine on the darning or free embroidery mode, define the shapes with machine embroidery. Continue building up colours and layers. Take the piece out of the hoop. Cut 10 cm/4 in squares of wadding (batting) and thick card. Lay the embroidery face down and place the wadding (batting) and card on top. Glue the edges of the card and then stretch the silk over and press it down firmly. Add a few stitches to hold the silk.

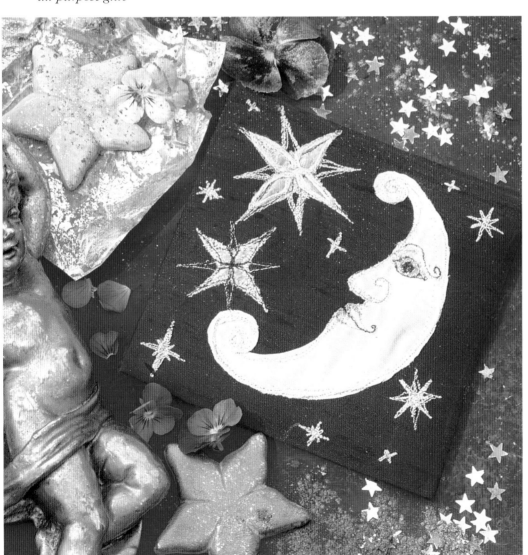

• EMBROIDERY •

VELVET SCARF

This sinuous velvet scarf is encrusted down its full length with the "sigils", or abstract symbols, of the twelve signs of the zodiac. The shiny metallic decorations contrast deliciously with the silky smooth fabric. Choose some darkly glowing colours to wear on a starry evening. Before sewing the seams, make sure that the pile of each piece of velvet is running in the right direction.

YOU WILL NEED

MATERIALS
*velvet in main colour,
1.5 m x 64 cm/60 x 26 in
velvet in toning colour,
36 x 64 cm/14 x 26 in
matching sewing thread
tracing paper
metallic organza
matching embroidery
thread*

EQUIPMENT
*dressmaker's scissors
tape measure
sewing machine
pencil
tailor's chalk
embroidery hoop
needle*

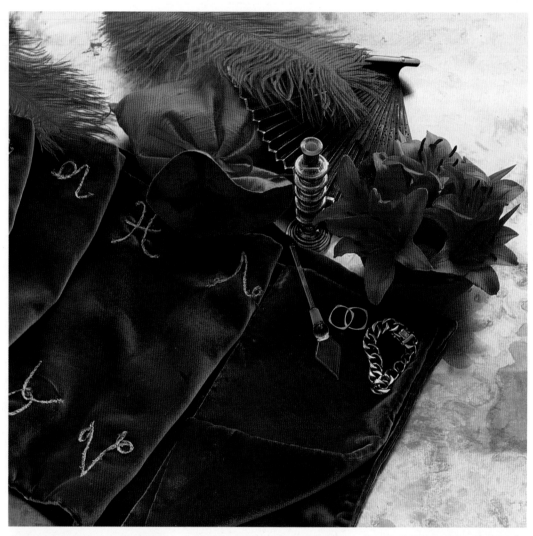

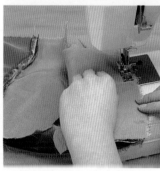

1 Cut two lengths of velvet to 1.5 m x 32 cm/ 60 x 13 in in the main colour, and four pieces 18 x 32 cm/7 x 13 in in the toning velvet. With right sides together and a 1 cm/½ in seam allowance, machine stitch one toning panel to each end of each scarf length.

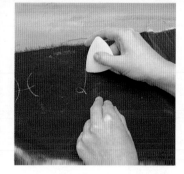

2 Mark out the positions for the astrological signs along the side of the scarf length, placing them 2 cm/¾ in from the seam line and at 13 cm/5 in intervals. Trace the templates from the back of the book, enlarging if necessary. Copy on to the velvet using tailor's chalk.

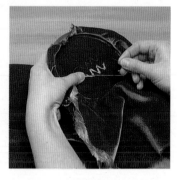

3 Place the velvet in a hoop. Cut 2 cm/¾ in strips of metallic organza. Stitch one end of the organza to the marked line, twist the strip tightly and stitch in place. Work all the designs in the same way. With right sides together, join the two scarf lengths, leaving a small opening. Turn to the right side and slip stitch the opening.

• EMBROIDERY •

Silver Moth Scarf

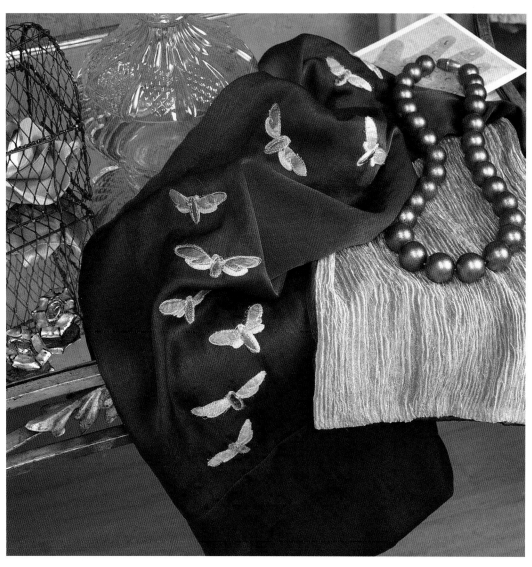

Ethereal silver moths flutter delicately over one side of this lovely silk scarf, their glitter reflected in the pleated organza on the other side. Your sewing machine manual will provide details of how to do free machine embroidery.

You Will Need

Materials
*tracing paper
fusible bonding web
small amounts of contrasting silk, velvet and organza
silk satin, 142 x 30 cm/56 x 12 in
matching fine machine embroidery thread
pleated metallic organza, 142 x 30 cm/56 x 12 in
matching sewing thread*

Equipment
*pencil
iron
dressmaker's scissors
embroidery hoop
sewing machine
dressmaker's pins
needle*

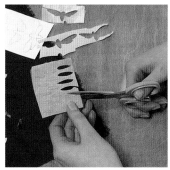
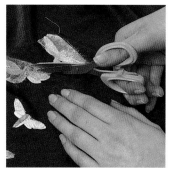
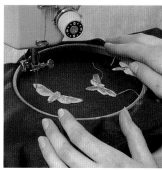

1 Trace the templates from the back of the book, enlarging if necessary. Lay the bonding web over the templates and trace the moths. Iron the bonding to the wrong side of the silk. Trace the same number of body shapes on the bonding and iron to the wrong side of the velvet. Cut out the shapes.

2 Remove the backing paper and iron the shapes to the right side of the silk satin. Place the satin in a hoop. Cut some pieces of organza slightly larger than the moths and machine stitch them to the satin along the wing outlines. Trim the organza close to the line of stitching round each motif.

3 Work two or three lines of stitching around each moth to conceal the raw edges. Pin the pleated organza to the satin with right sides together, and stitch all around the edge, leaving a gap of 10 cm/4 in on one side. Turn the scarf to the right side and slip stitch the gap.

• EMBROIDERY •

FISHY ORNAMENTS

These charming fish are quickly made and would be a rewarding project for children. The symbol of Pisces represents coming and going, past and future, so hang them to swim in different directions!

YOU WILL NEED

MATERIALS
scrap paper
thin card or paper
scraps of woollen fabric
mother-of-pearl buttons
embroidery cotton in
contrasting colours
scraps of polyester wadding
(batting), 5 mm/¼ in thick

EQUIPMENT
pencil
dressmaker's pins
dressmaker's scissors
needle

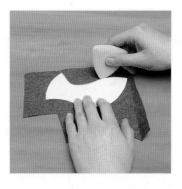

1 Draw a fish motif on to scrap paper and transfer it on to thin card or paper to make a template. Pin it to two layers of the fabric and cut out the fish. (No seam allowance is required for these shapes.)

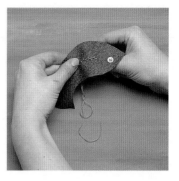

2 Separate the pieces and sew on the buttons to make eyes. Embroider each side of the fish, using three strands of embroidery cotton, in cross stitch, stem stitch and feather stitch as shown in the picture.

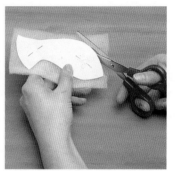

3 Cut a piece of wadding (batting) using the template, then trim it so that it is slightly smaller all round than the fish.

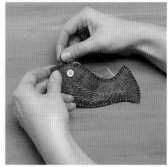

4 Sandwich the wadding (batting) between the two sides and attach a length of thread for the hanger. Blanket stitch round the edge to join the sides together.

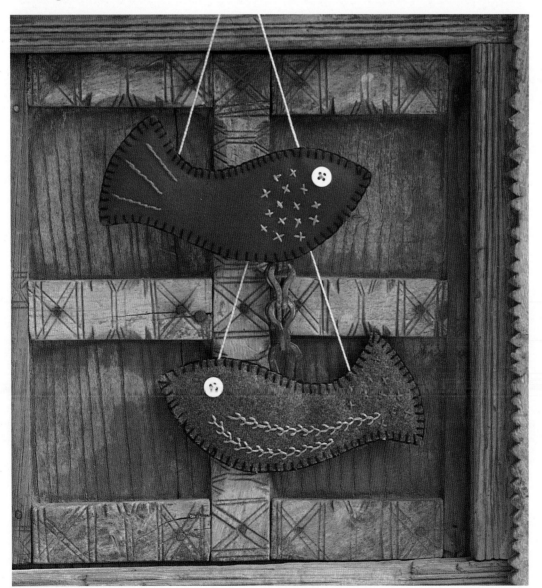

104

• EMBROIDERY •

BRIDAL HEART

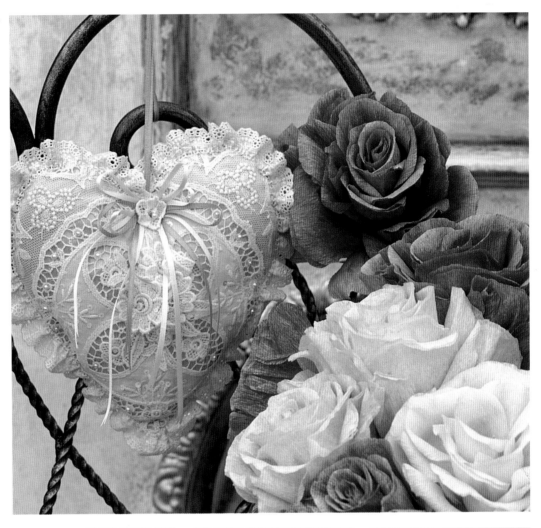

Pink satin and lace are the essence of femininity; this delicate bridal favour would be the perfect loving touch for the wedding day of a daughter, sister or friend. The decoration of sequins, pearls and motifs can be as simple or elaborate as you like, and you can be sure that no two of these will ever be the same.

YOU WILL NEED

MATERIALS

tracing paper
pink satin fabric,
40 x 20 cm/16 x 8 in
lace fabric or mat,
20 x 20 cm/8 x 8 in
contrasting tacking
(basting) thread
ready-made silk flowers
(optional)
matching sewing thread
flat sequins
seed pearls
polyester wadding (batting)
narrow lace edging,
60 cm/24 in
short lengths of matching
satin ribbon

EQUIPMENT

pencil
dressmaker's scissors
dressmaker's pins
very fine needle
sewing machine (optional)

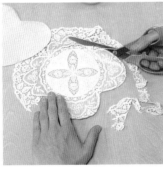

1 Trace the heart template from the back of the book, enlarging if necessary. Cut out two hearts from pink satin. Place one under the lace fabric or mat, and move it about to find the most attractive pattern area. Pin and then tack (baste) through both layers. Cut the lace, carefully following the outline of the satin heart.

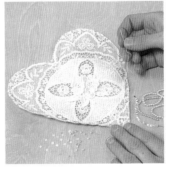

2 From the remaining lace, cut flowers and motifs. Sew to the centre of the lace heart. (Or use silk flowers.) Add sequins and pearls. Pin the hearts together, right sides facing. Stitch 1 cm/½ in in from the edges, leaving a 5 cm/2 in gap. Trim seams and clip curves. Turn right side out. Fill the heart with wadding (batting) and slip stitch the gap.

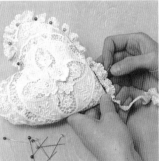

3 Run a gathering thread along the straight edge of the lace edging and pin one end to the top of the heart. Adjusting the gathers evenly, continue to pin the lace around the outside edge and then slip stitch it firmly in place with small, invisible stitches. Remove the gathering thread. Finish with a hanging loop, small ribbon bows and additional beads and sequins.

• EMBROIDERY •

Decorative Pincushion

An essential item on Victorian dressing tables, pincushions are still as useful as they are decorative. There is no more appropriate way to personalize them than with the pins themselves. The symbols used here are Capricorn and Taurus.

You Will Need

Materials
*plain velvet,
28 x 14 cm/11 x 5½ in
brass-headed pins,
1 cm/½ in long
matching sewing thread
polyester wadding (batting)
fine white tissue paper*

Equipment
*dressmaker's scissors
tailor's chalk
sewing machine
needle
pencil
tracing paper
dressmaker's pins*

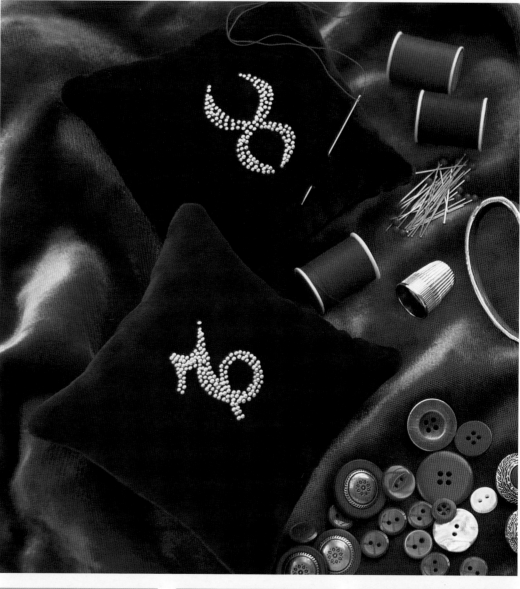

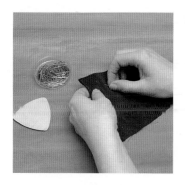

1 Cut the velvet into two 14 cm/5½ in squares and pin them together with right sides facing. Mark a 1 cm/½ in seam allowance with tailor's chalk. Machine around all four sides, leaving a 5 cm/2 in gap in the centre of one side.

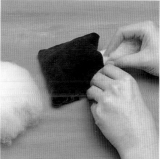

2 Trim the seam allowance at the corners of the cushion and turn it to the right side, easing out the corners with the points of the scissors. Stuff very firmly with polyester wadding (batting). Sew up the opening neatly by hand along the seam.

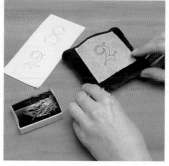

3 Trace the signs you want from the templates in the back of the book, enlarging if necessary, and transfer them to fine white tissue paper. Centre and pin a motif on the pincushion.

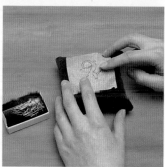

4 Work the motif with the brass-headed pins. When complete, tear away the tissue, gently pulling any bits from between the pins.

• EMBROIDERY •

Cupid Camisole

This beautiful camisole will make you feel like a million dollars. You will need a commercial paper pattern for a camisole, which you can then embellish with machine embroidery. You can embroider over the tissue paper pattern first and then tear away the paper, leaving an outline to be filled in with colour.

You Will Need

Materials
satin fabric, 1 m x 90 cm/
1 x 1 yd
tissue paper
machine embroidery
threads: cream, white,
gold and grey

Equipment
commercial camisole
pattern
dressmaker's scissors
dressmaker's pins
embroidery hoop
sewing machine, with
darning foot

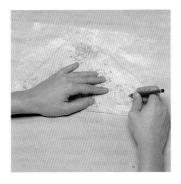

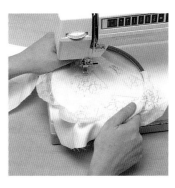

1 Cut out the pattern from the satin, with 1 cm/½ in extra all around to allow for any shrinkage during embroidery. Make a tissue paper duplicate of the front pattern piece. Trace the template from the back of the book, enlarging if necessary, and trace it on to the tissue paper duplicate, rotating it each time and avoiding the darts.

2 Use the tissue paper duplicate for embroidering by pinning it to the satin. Place the satin in the embroidery hoop. Set the machine to darning mode and attach the darning foot. With cream thread, stitch along the outline of the design.

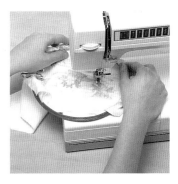

3 Remove the tissue paper and fill in the design. Use white thread for the face, body and hearts, gold for the hair and features and grey for the wings and cloud. Make up the camisole according to the pattern instructions.

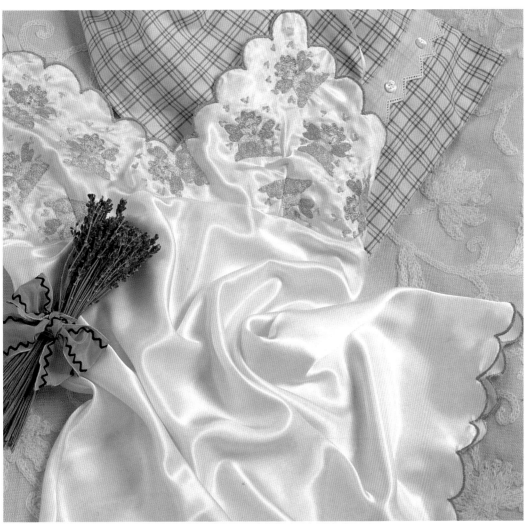

• EMBROIDERY •

NEEDLEPOINT BEETLE

This delightful beetle on its subtly coloured background is easy to work in tent stitch. Measure the frame you have chosen and work enough of the background to ensure that no bare canvas will be visible when the picture is framed.

YOU WILL NEED

MATERIALS
*needlepoint canvas,
25 x 25 cm/10 x 10 in
with 24 holes per 5 cm/
12 holes per 1 in
picture frame
masking tape
tapestry wools: as listed in
key at the back of the book*

EQUIPMENT
*waterproof magic marker
dressmaker's scissors
tapestry needle
iron
damp cloth
dressmaker's pins
(optional)*

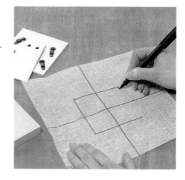

1 To prepare the canvas, mark a vertical line down the centre and a horizontal line across the centre using a magic marker. Mark the edges of the aperture in the frame you intend to use, positioning it centrally over the marked lines.

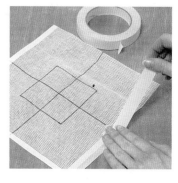

2 Bind the edges of the canvas with masking tape to keep it straight and prevent the yarn catching as you sew.

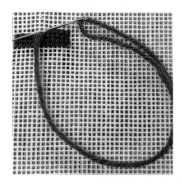

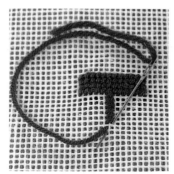

TENT STITCH Begin with a knot on the right side of the canvas, bringing the needle up again about 2.5 cm/1 in away. Work the first few stitches over this thread to secure it; the knot can then be cut away neatly. To work tent stitch, insert the needle one row up and one row to the right, bringing it back up through the hole to the left of your starting point. All the stitches must slant in the same direction – at the end of a row, turn the canvas upside down in order to work the next row.

VERTICAL TENT STITCH Tent stitch is worked horizontally, but it can be worked vertically where necessary. Always keep the stitches on the reverse side longer and more sloping than those on the front to avoid distorting the fabric. Try to keep an even tension and do not pull too tightly.

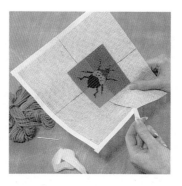

3 Cut a 45 cm/18 in length of tapestry wool and work the design from the chart at the back of the book in tent stitch. Start from the centre and work outwards to help keep the piece from distorting as you sew. When the design is completed and the background is large enough to fill the frame, remove the masking tape.

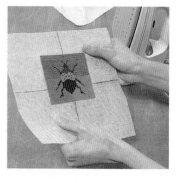

4 Use a hot iron and a damp cloth to steam the work gently, pulling it into shape as you go. If the canvas is very distorted, pin it into shape on the ironing board before steaming it. Dry the canvas thoroughly and quickly.

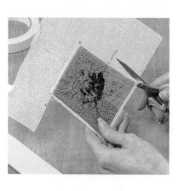

5 Cut away the excess canvas and mount your picture into the frame.

108

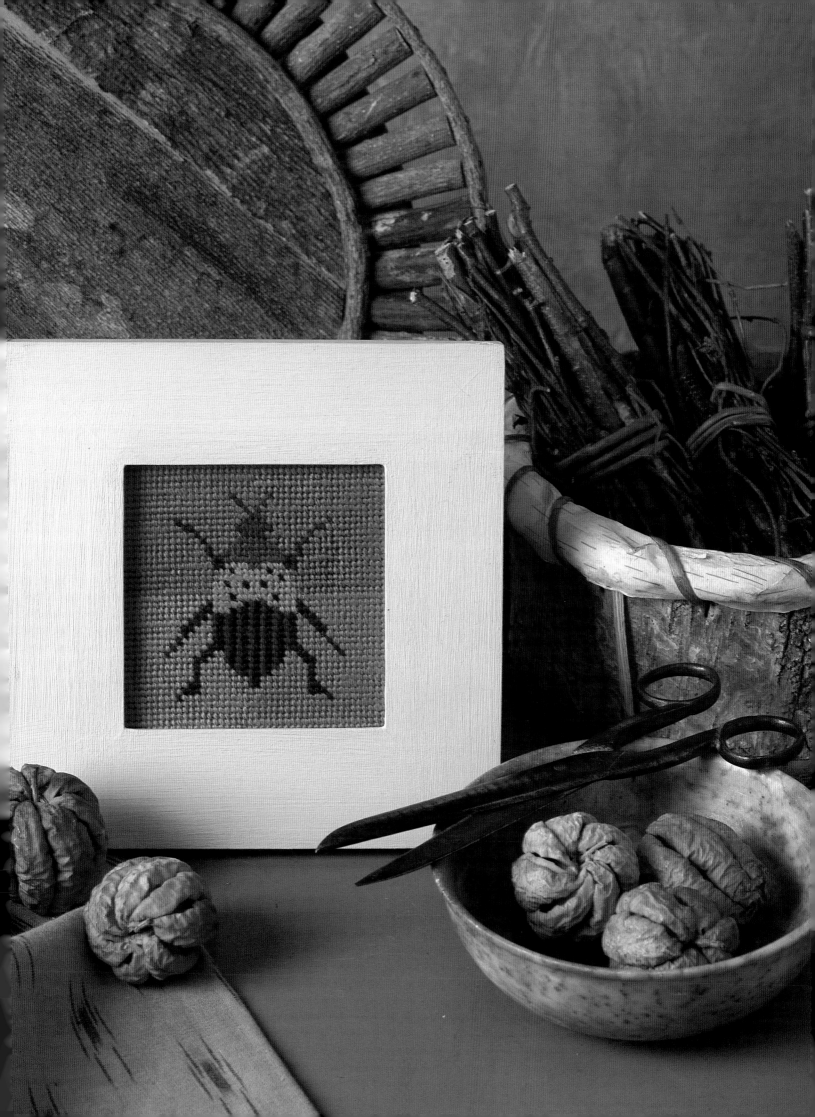

• EMBROIDERY •

SWEET HEARTS

*T*he heart is the ultimate symbol of devotion, so heart-shaped gifts have a special significance, whether they are given to friends and family, or exchanged by lovers. These padded hearts are made from leftovers of old lace fabric, embellished with tiny beads and gauze ribbons. The golden versions are filled with pot-pourri and edged with metallic lace, giving an antique richness.

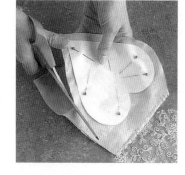

1 Cut out two hearts from the backing fabric and one from lace, leaving a 1 cm/½ in seam allowance all around.

YOU WILL NEED

MATERIALS
silk backing fabric
small pieces of lace fabric
matching sewing thread
polyester wadding (batting)
rocaille embroidery beads
lace, 50 x 2.5 cm/20 x 1 in
gauze ribbon, 1 m x 4 cm/
1 yd x 1½ in

EQUIPMENT
dressmaker's scissors
dressmaker's pins
needle

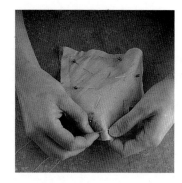

2 Pin the hearts together, sandwiching the lace heart between the two layers of silk. Sew together along one straight edge, leaving a 4 cm/1½ in gap for turning through.

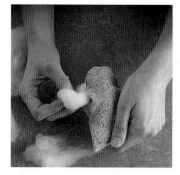

3 Turn the heart the right way out and stuff it firmly, ensuring that the wadding (batting) fills out the point of the heart. Slip stitch the sides, making sure that the fabric lies flat and has no wrinkles.

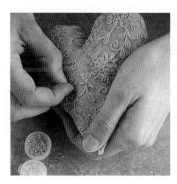

4 Sew the beads on to the lace, picking out and highlighting the various designs within the pattern of lace itself.

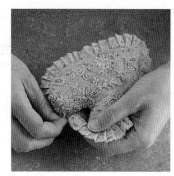

5 Gather the length of lace to fit around the outside edge of the heart, then stitch it in place.

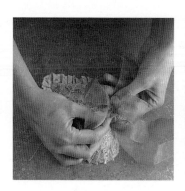

6 Cut a 30 cm/12 in length of gauze ribbon and sew it to the top of the heart to form a hanging loop. Make a bow from the rest of the ribbon and sew it to the base of the loop.

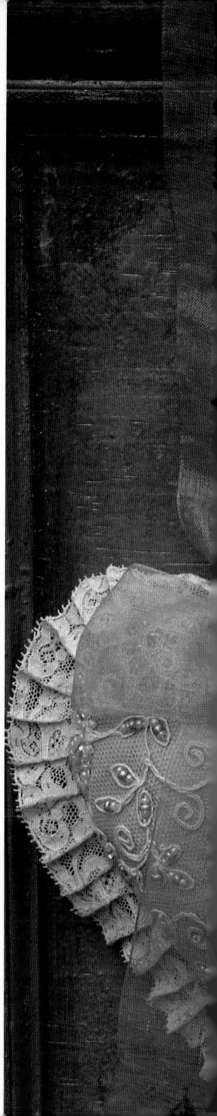

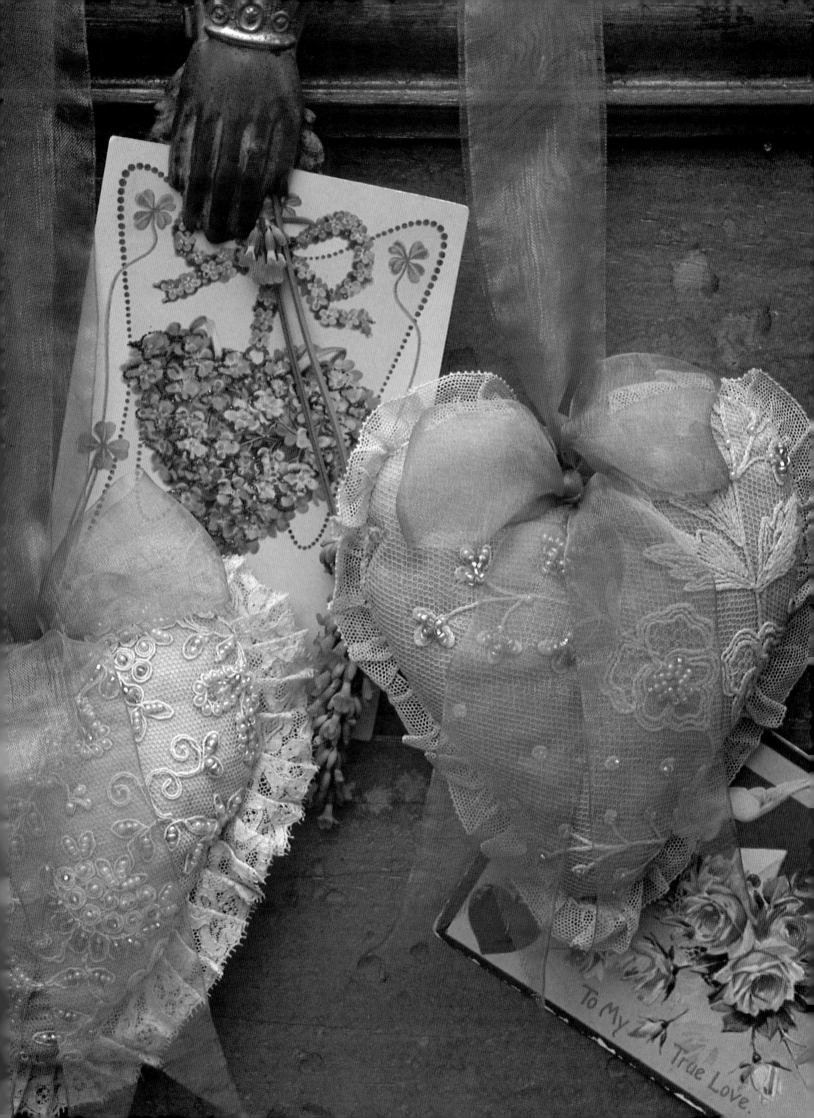

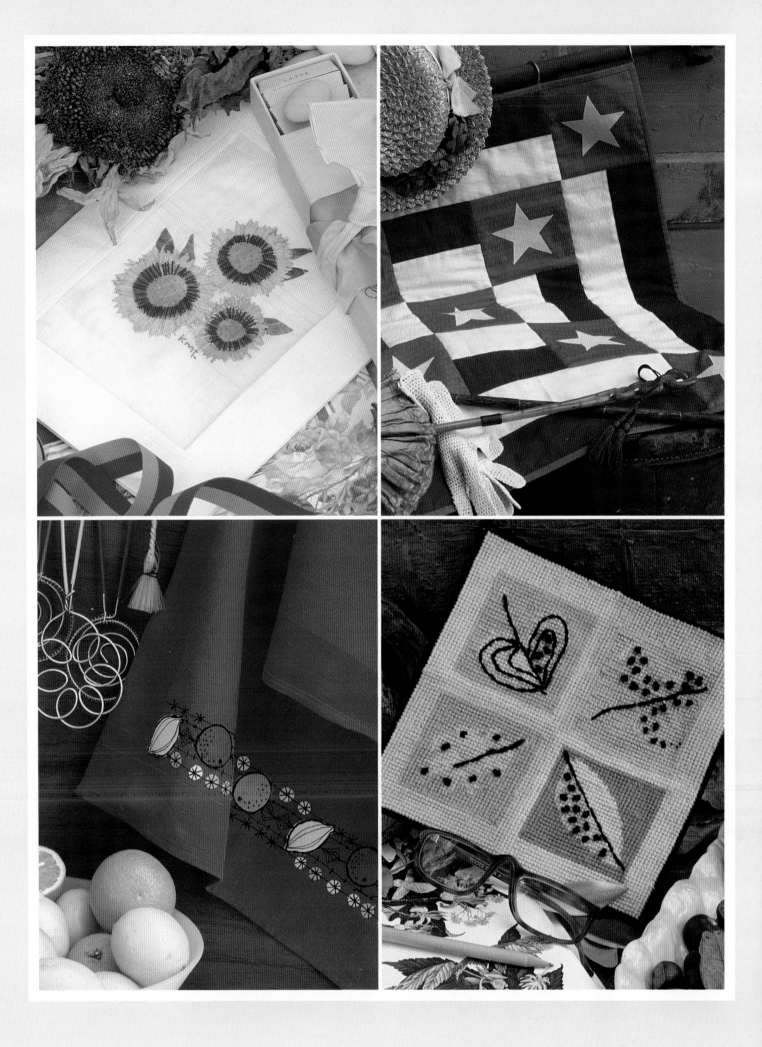

APPLIQUE, PATCHWORK AND CROSS STITCH

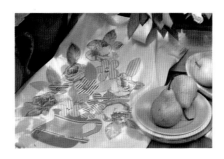

Appliqué and patchwork are crafts requiring only a modicum of skills that nevertheless produce individual and stunning results. The techniques can be used to give an extra sparkle to a whole range of items such as cards, bags, towels and mats as well as bed linen and clothes. The materials needed are all readily available, and most needleworkers will probably already have most of the equipment required. Once you have mastered the techniques, you will be able to experiment fully to create your own designs and projects on fabrics of your choice.

There are few constraints with these needlework techniques, as even the most unassuming scraps of fabric and old clothes can be rejuvenated given a little imagination and some basic know-how. In addition there is a selection of cross-stitch projects for enthusiasts of this most popular of needlecrafts!

• Applique, Patchwork and Cross Stitch •

Basic Techniques

The materials and equipment required for appliqué, patchwork and cross stitch are more or less the same as those for hand and machine embroidery.

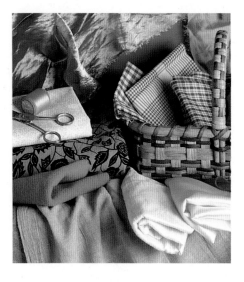

ABOVE *Appliqué and patchwork projects make full use of any fabric remnants.*

Using fusible bonding web

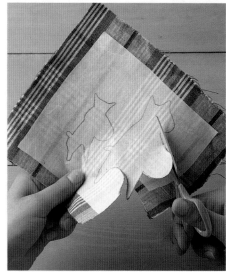

1 Fusible bonding web is useful for stabilizing appliqué pieces, as it binds on to the fabric when pressed with an iron. You can then cut around the shape to be appliquéd, with the bonding web in place to act as a stiffener.

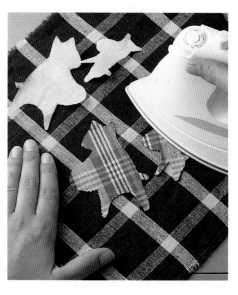

2 Fusible bonding web has a backing paper that can be peeled off. The pieces can then be pressed in place on the ground fabric.

Basic cross stitches

Cross stitch can either be worked as a single stitch or in a row that is completed in two journeys. Irrespective of which method is used, the top stitch should always face in the same direction. If working a border or a detailed piece of cross stitch, it is helpful to put a pin in the work showing the direction that the top stitch should face.

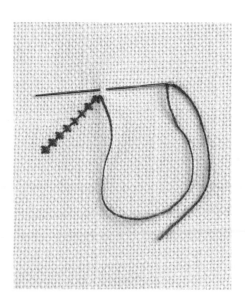

Single cross stitch

This produces a slightly raised cross and should be used for individual stitches and small details. It is also ideal when stitching with tapestry wool.

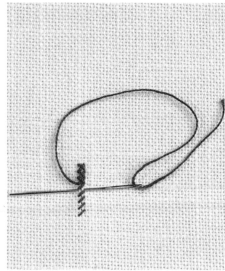

Row of cross stitches

First work a row of cross stitches either diagonally or in a straight line. Complete the cross stitches by stitching the other half on the way back.

Basic Techniques

Simple appliqué

Embroidered appliqué pieces

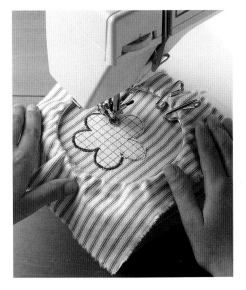

Draw the shape on the fabric with a fabric marker and embroider the pattern over the edges of the outline.

Straight stitch appliqué

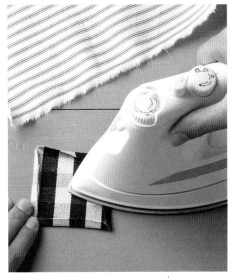

1 Cut out the shape, making sure to leave a 1 cm/½ in allowance all round. Press the allowance to the wrong side, snipping away corners and curves.

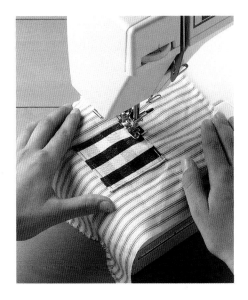

2 Pin the piece to the fabric and work a straight stitch all round.

Zigzag or satin stitch appliqué

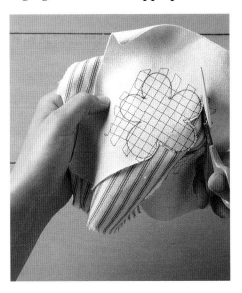

Pin the appliqué piece to the ground fabric and stitch around the outline. Trim away the excess fabric close to the stitched line. Work a zigzag stitch around the outline, covering raw edges. This can be followed by a second line of satin stitch.

Shadow appliqué

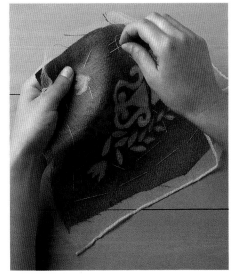

1 Work the appliqué pieces using one of the methods described before, then pin and tack a piece of sheer fabric over the design.

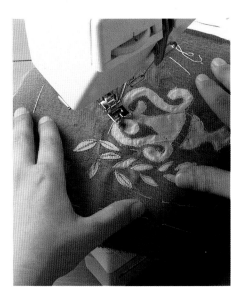

2 Use matching thread to stitch over the sheer fabric, close to the stitches on the appliquéd pieces.

· APPLIQUE, PATCHWORK AND CROSS STITCH ·

OAK LEAF POTHOLDER

Many quilt patterns are inspired by natural images. This oak-leaf pattern is based on a block from an appliqué quilt made in 1850.

YOU WILL NEED

MATERIALS

*thin card or paper
fusible bonding web
green felt,
15 x 15 cm/6 x 6 in
checked cotton fabric,
22 x 30 cm/9 x 12 in
2 polyester wadding
(batting) squares,
22 cm/9 in
thick cotton backing fabric,
18 x 18 cm/7 x 7 in
tacking (basting) thread
matching sewing thread
small eyelet screw
wooden toggle*

EQUIPMENT

*pencil
tape measure
fabric marker
iron
dressmaker's scissors
dressmaker's pins
needle*

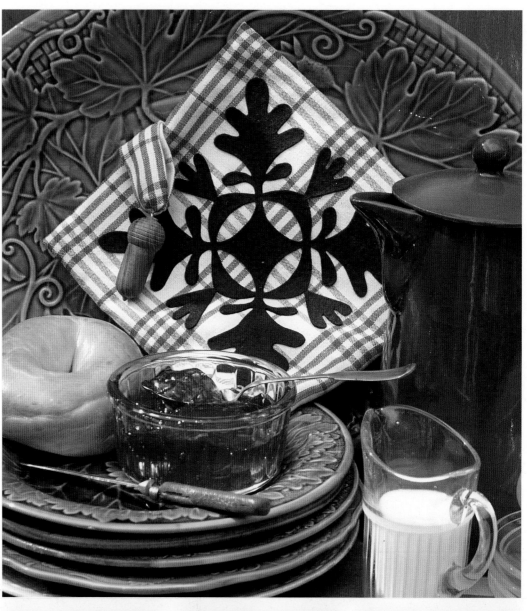

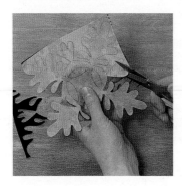

1 Trace the template from the back of the book, enlarging it to 14 cm/5½ in across. Transfer the outline to the bonding web with a fabric marker and iron it on to the green felt. Cut out the shape.

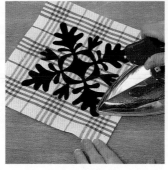

2 Cut a 22 cm/9 in square from the checked cotton fabric. Peel off the backing paper from the felt square and iron it centrally on to the cotton fabric square. Iron under a hem of 1 cm /½ in.

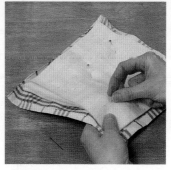

3 Pin the polyester wadding (batting) squares between the backing fabric and the decorated square. Pin, tack (baste) and slip stitch the turned edge over the backing square to conceal the raw edges.

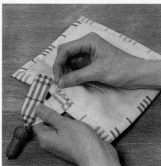

4 For the hanger, sew together the long sides of the remaining checked cotton fabric. Screw the eyelet into the toggle and thread the hanger through. Fold it in half and sew it in place.

· APPLIQUE, PATCHWORK AND CROSS STITCH ·

HERALDIC TABLEMAT

Medieval retainers used to wear circular badges with a distinctive family motif on their clothes to identify them with their feudal overlord: such emblems were much simpler designs than armorial bearings and were often animals or flowers. For this project, you could create your own heraldic design.

YOU WILL NEED

MATERIALS	EQUIPMENT
PVC (vinyl) coated cotton fabric: plain blue, plain red and co-ordinating print	pair of compasses
PVA (white) glue	pencil
tracing paper	scissors
thin card or paper	paintbrush
baize or felt, for backing	sheet of plastic
quilting thread	sewing machine, with leather needle

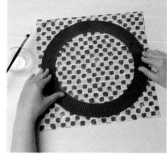

1 Decide on the diameter of your mat, then draw and cut out a rim of plain blue fabric. Glue this to the background print fabric, to secure it while you sew.

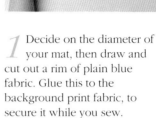

2 Trace an animal template from the back of the book, enlarging if necessary, and transfer it to thin card or paper. Cut it out and draw around it on the reverse of the plain red fabric. Cut it out.

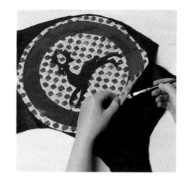

3 Glue the animal in the centre of the mat, and glue a piece of baize or felt to the back. Cover with a sheet of plastic and leave under a weight until it is dry.

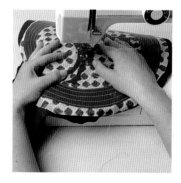

4 Using quilting thread, machine stitch around the edges of the motif and in rows around the border. Use a long, straight stitch. Trim the edge of the mat and wipe off any glue.

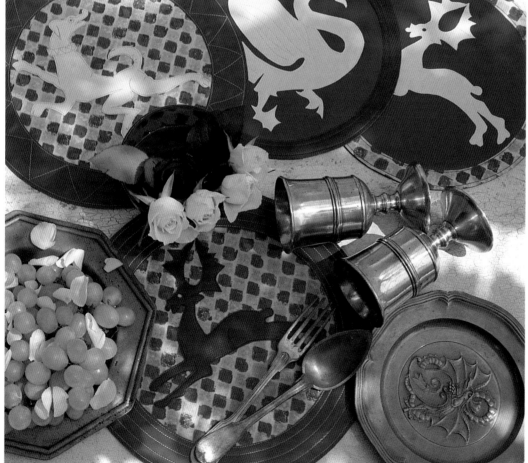

· APPLIQUE, PATCHWORK AND CROSS STITCH ·

Matisse Outfit

The artist Henri Matisse spent his later years creating dynamic and exciting paper collages, characterized by bold colours and strong graphic shapes. They were the inspiration behind this collection of clothes, which shows just how easy it is to customize a ready-made garment and so transform it into something really individual.

You Will Need

MATERIALS
*tracing paper
plain white T-shirt
fusible bonding web
scraps of plain cotton fabric
in bright colours
matching sewing threads
plain white long-sleeved
shirt
coloured buttons
denim jacket*

EQUIPMENT
*pencil
fabric marker
dressmaker's scissors
iron
sewing machine
needle*

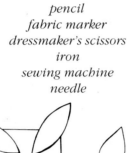

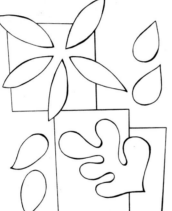

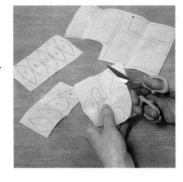

1 Trace the template from the back of the book, enlarging it to fit your T-shirt, and transfer each element of the design, in reverse, on to fusible bonding web with a fabric marker. Cut out roughly.

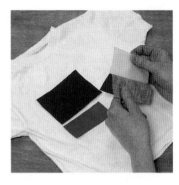

2 Choose three colours for the background shapes and iron one rectangle on to each. Cut out along the outline, peel off the backing paper and iron in place. Stitch around the outside edge with a narrow zigzag stitch in matching thread.

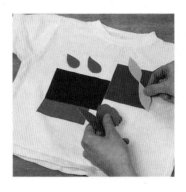

3 Cut out the branched and single leaf shapes in the same way and iron them on to the T-shirt.

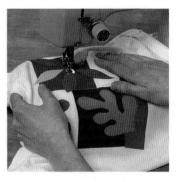

4 Sew each shape in place with zigzag stitch, working accurately around the curves. Iron lightly.

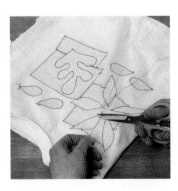

5 Finish off on the reverse of the work, knotting the ends of the threads together and clipping close to the surface.

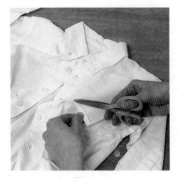

6 Customize a plain white shirt by removing the buttons and pocket. Wash and iron. Sew appliqué motifs to each side of the front, as you did for the T-shirt.

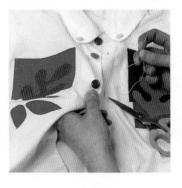

7 Replace the white buttons with brightly coloured ones, chosen to match the appliquéd design.

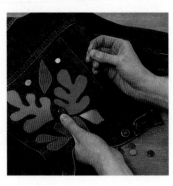

8 Decorate the back of the denim jacket in the same way; again, use coloured buttons to add the final detail.

118

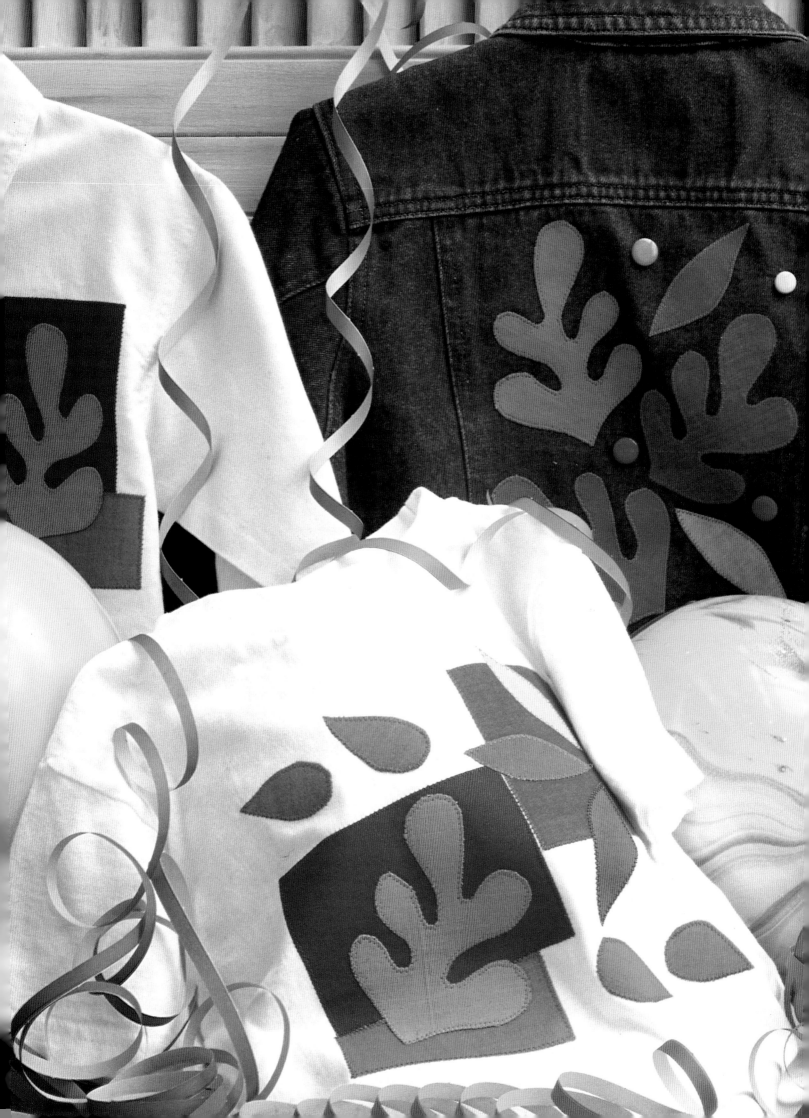

• Applique, Patchwork and Cross Stitch •

Appliqued Sunflower Card

A home-made card is much nicer than a bought one and this cheery sunflower design would be perfect for someone with a high-summer birthday.

You Will Need

MATERIALS
tracing paper
yellow and brown fabric scraps
fabric glue
background fabric
embroidery thread
green paper scraps
blank card and envelope
paper glue

EQUIPMENT
pencil
fabric marker
dressmaker's scissors
needle

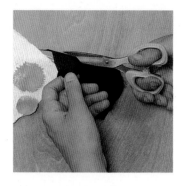

1 Trace the template from the back of the book, enlarging if necessary. Using the fabric marker, transfer the outline to the yellow fabric first and cut it out. Then cut out the smaller centres from brown fabric.

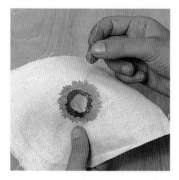

2 Stick the yellow piece on to the background fabric and the brown one on top. Then stick the third piece on top. Sew from the edge of the inner ring, using a running stitch on the centre piece.

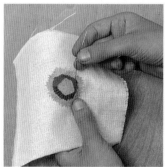

3 On the dark brown ring, sew from the outer to the inner edge in one large stitch, like a very loose, random satin stitch, to give a textured effect. Continue all the way round.

4 On the centre piece, sew running stitches at random, to give the effect of seeds. Sew on green paper leaves. Check for any loose threads on the back and tie them in. Trim the fabric to the correct size for the aperture of the card. Stick the appliqué in position cleanly.

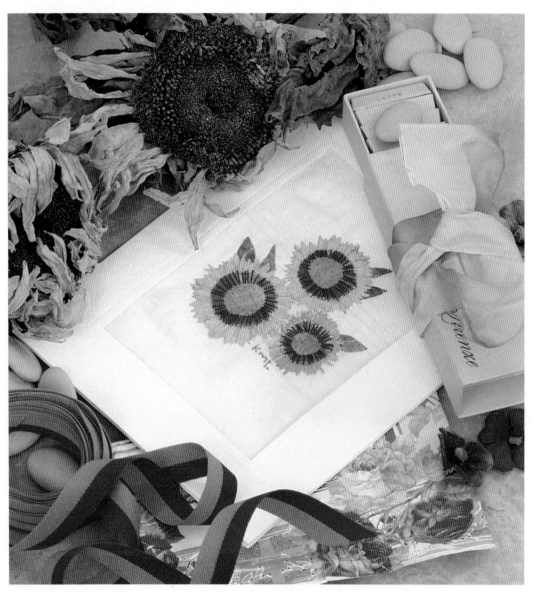

• APPLIQUE, PATCHWORK AND CROSS STITCH •

STAR PATCHWORK SACHET

Patchwork stars made out of diamond shapes appear on many early American quilts; this one is based on the eight-point Lone Star motif. Lining the patches with backing paper is the traditional English way of making patchwork. It keeps the shapes sharp and accurate when joining the points of the star.

YOU WILL NEED

MATERIALS
*tracing paper
thin card
mustard-yellow cotton fabric,
12.5 x 20 cm/5 x 8 in
green and white check cotton fabric,
12.5 x 20 cm/5 x 8 in
dark orange cotton fabric,
20 x 40 cm/8 x 16 in
backing paper
tacking (basting) thread
matching sewing thread
dried herbs or pot-pourri
1 small pearl button*

EQUIPMENT
*pencil
scissors
dressmaker's scissors
ruler
needle
iron
dressmaker's pins*

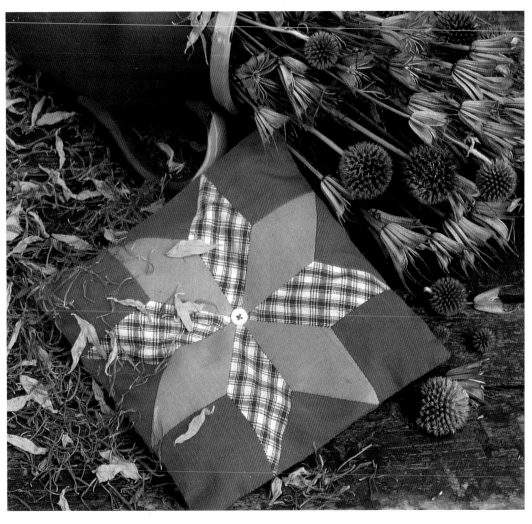

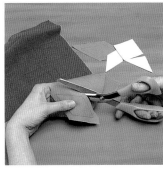

1 Trace the templates from the back of the book, enlarging if necessary. Cut eight diamonds, four squares and four triangles from thin card. Add a 5 mm/¼ in allowance and cut out four yellow and four check diamonds, four orange squares and four orange triangles. Lay the backing paper in the centre of each shape, turn the seam over the paper, folding at the points, and tack (baste) in place.

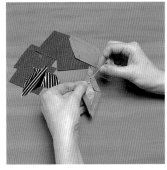

2 Stitch a yellow and a check diamond together along one edge, then sew an orange square into the right angle. Make four of these units, then join together to form a star. Sew the orange triangles into the remaining spaces to complete the square. Iron lightly and remove all the tacking (basting) threads.

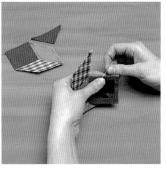

3 Cut a 19 cm/7½ in square from the remaining orange fabric and iron a 5 mm/¼ in seam allowance all round. With wrong sides together, pin this square to the patchwork and overstitch around the outside edge leaving a 7.5 cm/3 in gap on one side. Fill with herbs or pot-pourri and sew up the opening. Sew the button to the centre of the star.

Applique Throw

This appliqué throw recycles an old blanket as its background fabric and is pleasingly quick to put together, using fusible bonding web. Old buttons and bold woollen embroidery stitches add detail and colour.

You Will Need

Materials
cream blanket
matching and contrasting crewel wool
tracing paper
thin card or paper
four pieces of flannel fabric, 25 x 50 cm/10 x 20 in
green, rust and brown felt, 30 x 30 cm/12 x 12 in
fusible bonding web, 1.5 m/1½ yd
assorted shirt buttons (optional)
65 larger brown buttons (optional)

Equipment
dressmaker's scissors
tape measure
tapestry needle
pencil
fabric marker
iron
pressing cloth

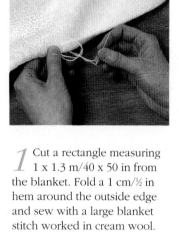

1 Cut a rectangle measuring 1 x 1.3 m/40 x 50 in from the blanket. Fold a 1 cm/½ in hem around the outside edge and sew with a large blanket stitch worked in cream wool.

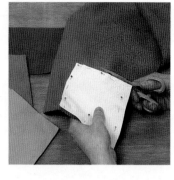

2 Trace the template for the diamond from the back of the book, carefully enlarging it to 20 cm/8 in high. Use this as a guide for cutting 25 diamonds of different colours from the flannel fabric.

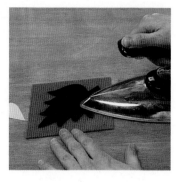

3 Enlarge the leaf templates to fit within the diamonds. For each motif, choose a felt colour that tones with the background fabric. Trace the various leaf outlines, in reverse, on to fusible bonding web with a fabric marker. Cut out roughly and iron on to the felt, then cut out neatly. Peel off the backing paper and iron a leaf to the centre of each diamond.

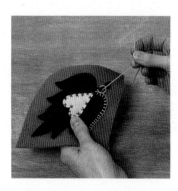

4 Sew the leaves down using a single strand of crewel wool and a running stitch or blanket stitch – follow the picture as a guide. Some of the leaves have an extra appliquéd motif or a cut-out shape; you can make your own variations on these ideas.

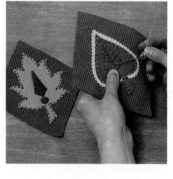

5 Use straight stitch to embroider a vein pattern on some leaves and sew on the extra motifs using a cross or straight stitch.

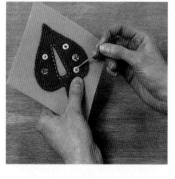

6 Sew on tiny shirt buttons as a finishing touch, or add embroidered stars. (If the throw is for a small child, do not use buttons.) Each leaf can be different, or you could make several in the same colours.

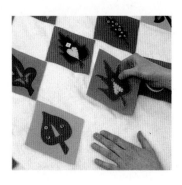

7 Iron fusible bonding web on to the back of each diamond. Peel off the backing paper and arrange them in five rows of five, leaving an even border all around. Iron in place using a pressing cloth.

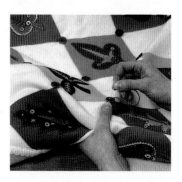

8 If desired, sew a large button over each diamond intersection, using wool in a contrasting colour.

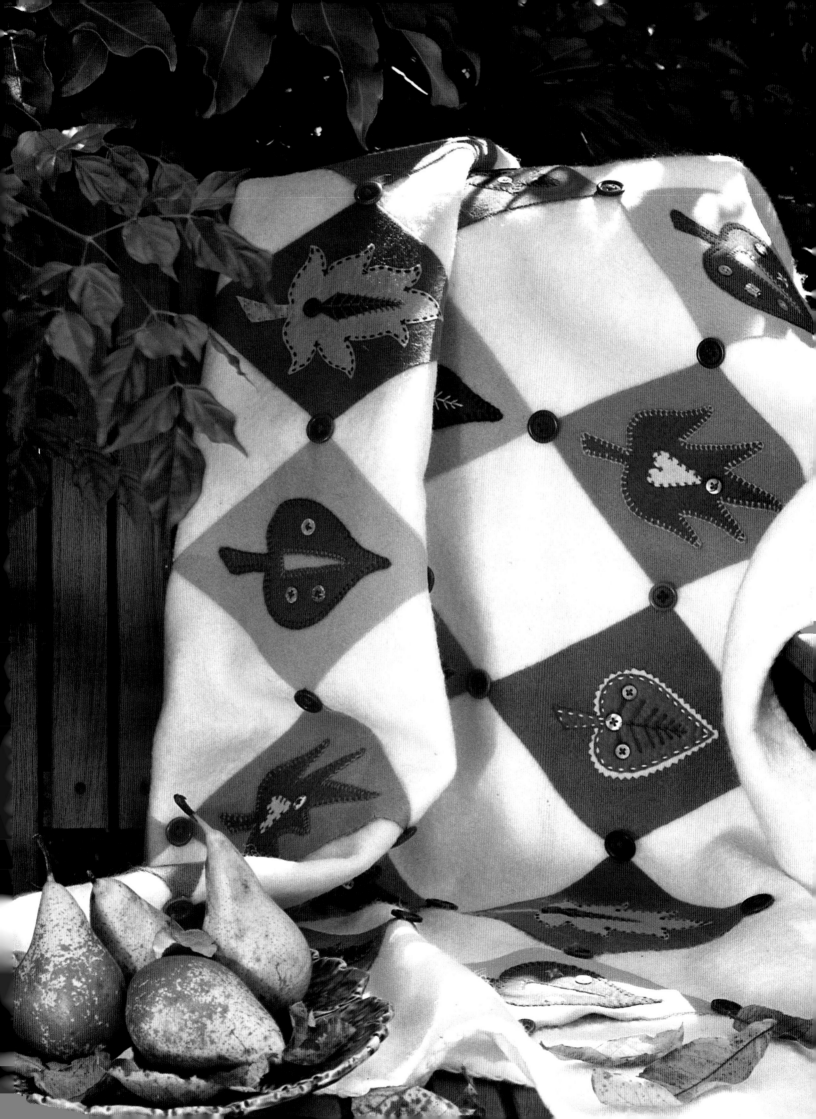

• APPLIQUE, PATCHWORK AND CROSS STITCH •

Rose Applique Bag

This attractive shopping bag recycles old table linen, fabric remnants and buttons. Look for unworn areas of old tablecloths or damask napkins: even the smallest scraps can combine effectively with other kinds of material.

You Will Need

Materials
rose-print furnishing fabric remnant
fusible bonding web
tracing paper
striped or checked table napkins, cloths or remnants
calico, 60 x 83 cm/ 24 x 33 in
matching sewing threads
6 old buttons

Equipment
dressmaker's scissors
iron
pencil
sewing machine
ruler
fabric marker
safety pin
needle

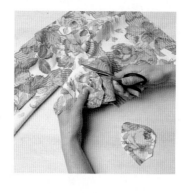

1 Pick out five interesting rose motifs and eight single leaf motifs from the fabric and cut them out roughly.

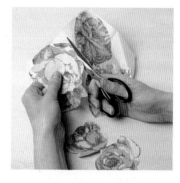

2 Iron the wrong side of the roses and leaves to the bonding web. Cut around the edges, simplifying the outlines to make them easier to sew.

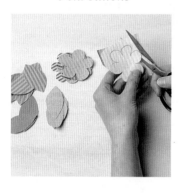

3 Trace the template from the back of the book, enlarging if necessary, and trace six flower shapes on to the paper side of more bonding web. Cut them out roughly and iron them on to the striped or checked fabrics. Cut around the outlines. Make ten leaves in the same way and one large blue and white jug.

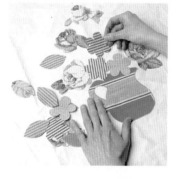

4 Cut a 50 x 83 cm/20 x 33 in calico rectangle and fold it in half widthways. Peel the backing paper from the jug and iron in place on the centre front. Using matching thread and a narrow satin stitch, sew in place. Remove the backing paper from the leaves and flowers and arrange them around the jug. Iron in place.

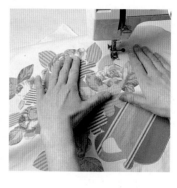

5 Sew the shapes in place with satin stitch, using matching thread and working over the outside edges of the fabric. Finish off all the threads on the wrong side.

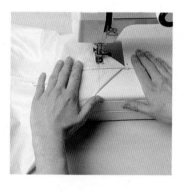

6 Join the bottom and side edges with French seams, for strength. Turn inside out and flatten one corner, to make a right-angled point at the end of the bottom seam. Measure 5 cm/2 in down from the end and mark a line across the corner. Sew across this line. Repeat for the other corner, to make a flat base for the bag.

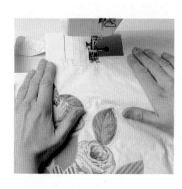

7 Turn under, press and stitch a double hem of 2.5 cm/1 in around the top of the bag. Cut the remaining calico into two equal strips and fold each in half lengthways. Join 1 cm/½ in from the outside edge and, using a safety pin, turn inside out. Top stitch both sides and sew one handle to each side of the bag.

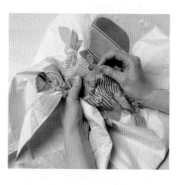

8 Sew a button to the centre of each plain flower, as a finishing touch.

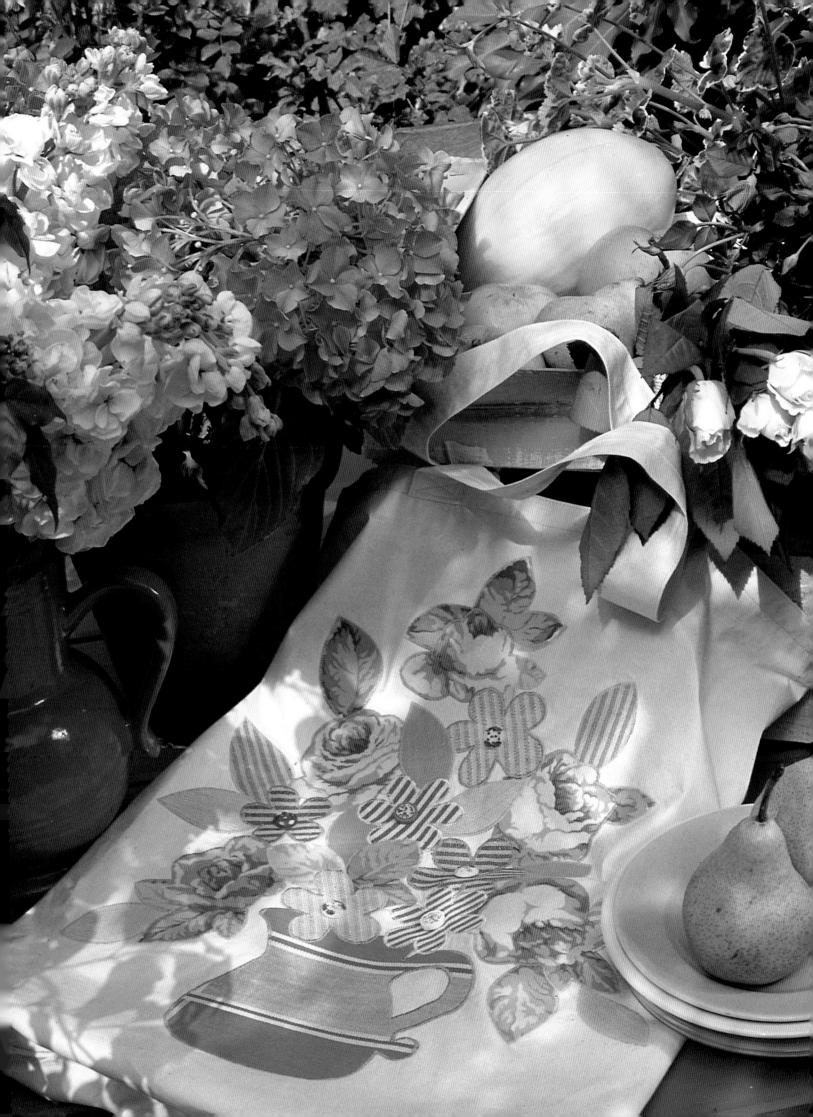

• APPLIQUE, PATCHWORK AND CROSS STITCH •

FLEUR-DE-LYS TIEBACK

Make this smart tieback with a beautifully stylized lily to add restrained elegance to a plain or striped curtain.

YOU WILL NEED

MATERIALS	EQUIPMENT
tracing paper	pencil
white cotton poplin, 20 x 90 cm/ 8 x 36 in	dressmaker's scissors
navy cotton poplin, 30 x 90 cm/ 12 x 36 in	dressmaker's pins
navy-white striped poplin, 50 x 90 cm/20 x 36 in	fabric marker
polyester wadding (batting),	iron
thin card or paper	needle
fusible bonding web, 20 x 90 cm/ 8 x 36 in	sewing machine
tacking (basting) thread	
matching sewing thread	
two white "D" rings	

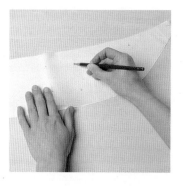

1 Trace the tieback template from the back of the book, enlarging it to fit the width needed for your curtain. Cut out the shape in each of the fabrics and the wadding (batting). Mark the positions of the motifs on the white fabric.

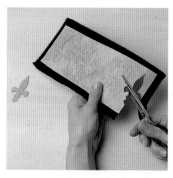

2 Trace the fleur-de-lys motif and cut it out on card or paper. Draw around it seven times on the backing paper of the bonding web and iron on to the remaining navy fabric. Cut out the shapes carefully.

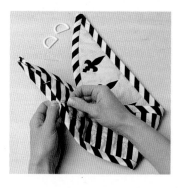

3 Iron the motifs on to the white fabric. Layer the wadding (batting) between the striped and navy fabrics, lay the white fabric on top and tack (baste). Quilt around the motifs. Cut two 6 cm/2¼ in bias strips from the striped fabric. Pin one piece along the top edge and stitch, leaving a 1.5 cm/⅝ in allowance. Fold the binding to the back, turn in the raw edge, pin and hem. Stitch the second strip along the bottom edge. Loop each end of the binding through a "D" ring, turn in the raw edge neatly and stitch.

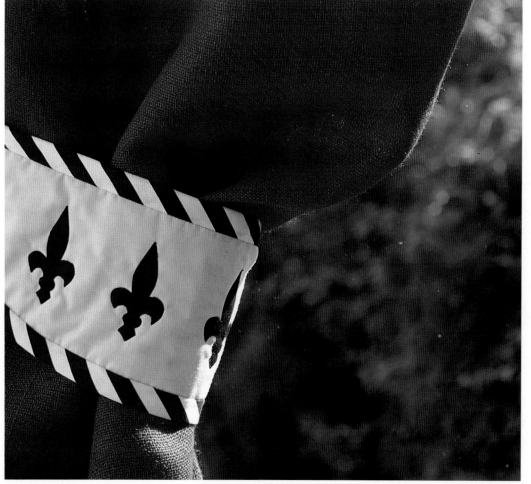

• APPLIQUE, PATCHWORK AND CROSS STITCH •

ORANGE SAMPLER

The fruit basket, piled high with oranges and lemons, was a popular cross-stitch motif in the nineteenth century. You can use the colours suggested here, or experiment with your own shades of embroidery threads to make a more personalized design.

YOU WILL NEED

MATERIALS
*tacking (basting) thread
white cross stitch fabric,
15 x 20 cm/6 x 8 in
stranded embroidery
threads: orange, light
orange, yellow, ochre, dark
olive, light olive and
chocolate-brown
mount board
plain wooden frame, with
9 x 14 cm/3½ x 5½ in
opening*

EQUIPMENT
*needle
tapestry needle
embroidery scissors
iron
craft knife
cutting mat*

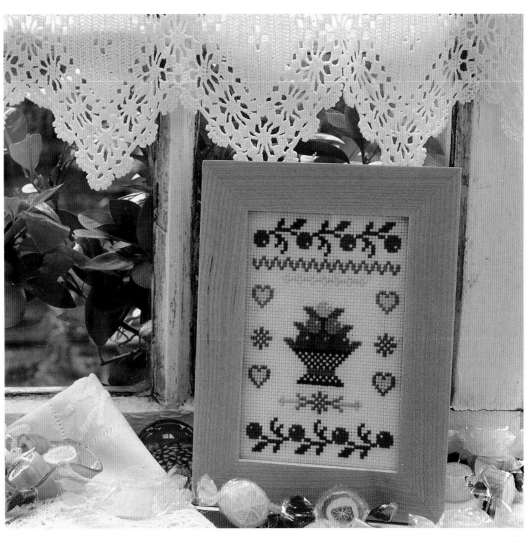

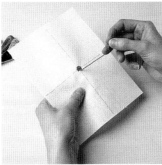
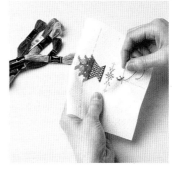
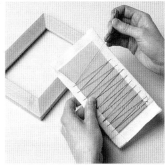

1 Using tacking (basting) thread, mark guidelines vertically and horizontally across the centre of the fabric. Follow the chart at the back of the book; the sampler is worked with three strands of embroidery thread throughout, and one square of the chart represents one cross stitch. Using orange thread, work the centre orange of the bottom row of fruit.

2 Stitch the other oranges, then work the leaves around them and the basket. Use the guidelines to establish the position of the other motifs and count the squares between them carefully. When the design is complete, unpick the tacking (basting) threads and iron lightly from the back of the work.

3 Cut a piece of mount board to fit the finished piece, using the lining paper from the frame as a guide. Place the board centrally on the back of the work and lace the two long sides together using long stitches. Repeat the process with the two short sides, then insert in the frame.

• APPLIQUE, PATCHWORK AND CROSS STITCH •

CRADLE QUILT

With its contrasting patchwork squares and heart motifs reminiscent of American folk art, this embroidered quilt will look really special in a cradle or crib.

YOU WILL NEED

MATERIALS
*blue cotton chambray,
140 x 90 cm/54 x 36 in
white cotton fabric,
15 x 60 cm/6 x 24 in
graph paper,
20 x 20 cm/8 x 8 in
tracing paper
dressmaker's carbon paper
stranded embroidery
threads: white, red
and blue
fusible bonding web,
25 x 37 cm/10 x 15 in
5 scraps of checked or
striped cotton shirting
matching sewing thread
iron-on wadding (batting),
60 x 60 cm/24 x 24 in
tacking (basting) thread
strips of chambray,
5 x 65 cm/2 x 26 in*

EQUIPMENT
*iron
dressmaker's scissors
pen or hard pencil
dressmaker's pins
sewing machine
needle*

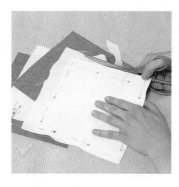
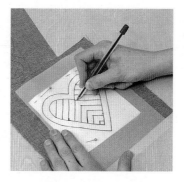
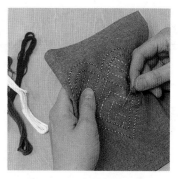

1 Iron the fabric. Using the graph paper as a template, cut four squares of blue chambray and five of white cotton. Make sure that you cut all the squares exactly in line with the grain of the fabric.

2 Trace the heart template from the back of the book, enlarging if necessary. Using dressmaker's carbon paper, transfer it on to the centre of one blue square, using a pen or hard pencil and pressing firmly to achieve a strong line.

3 Using three strands of white thread, work over the lines in a small, regular running stitch. Work a red whipstitch over the inner and outer heart outlines. Work a blue whipstitch over the parallel lines inside the heart. Repeat the process with the three remaining blue squares.

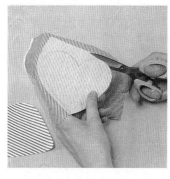
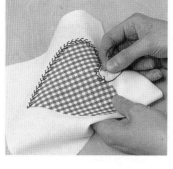
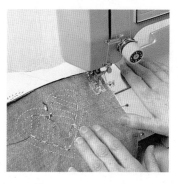

4 Trace just the outline of the heart template on to the paper side of the bonding web. Cut out roughly around the edge and then iron the heart on to a piece of shirting, following the manufacturer's instructions. Make sure that the centre line matches the stripes or checks. Cut out carefully around the outline. Repeat with the remaining fabric scraps.

5 Remove the backing paper and iron the heart on to the centre of a white square. With three strands of embroidery thread, work a row of feather stitching around the outside of the heart, to conceal the raw edges. Repeat with the remaining four pieces of shirting and white squares.

6 Lay the nine squares in three rows of three, with alternating colours. Machine stitch along each row, with right sides facing, and allowances of 1 cm/½ in. Iron with the allowances lying on the blue squares. Pin the rows together, matching the joins. Sew along the long edges with 1 cm/½ in allowances. Clip the seams where the squares meet. Iron the seams towards blue squares.

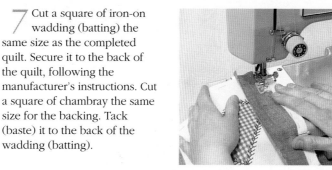

7 Cut a square of iron-on wadding (batting) the same size as the completed quilt. Secure it to the back of the quilt, following the manufacturer's instructions. Cut a square of chambray the same size for the backing. Tack (baste) it to the back of the wadding (batting).

8 Fold the cambray strips in half lengthways and iron the folds. Iron 5 mm/¼ in under each long edge. Pin in the first strip with the raw edge lying 1 cm/½ in from the quilt edge. Sew 2 cm/¾ in from the edge. Fold the facing over, turn in the hem and slip stitch. Repeat for each side. Neaten each corner and remove the tacking (basting).

128

• APPLIQUE, PATCHWORK AND CROSS STITCH •

SEASHELL BEACH BAG

Crisp cream and navy give this smart beach bag a nautical feel. The charm of the project lies in combining colours to give a three-dimensional feel.

YOU WILL NEED

MATERIALS
cream cotton drill or denim,
55 x 75 cm/21½ x 30 in
tracing paper
stencil card
spray adhesive
2 lengths blue cotton drill or denim, 15 x 38 cm/6 x 15 in
dry fabric stencil paints: dark yellow, dark red and navy blue
sewing threads: white, dark orange and blue
cream cord, 2 m/2 yd
masking tape

EQUIPMENT
dressmaker's scissors
craft knife
cutting mat
3 stencil brushes
iron
sewing machine
dressmaker's pins
ruler or tape measure

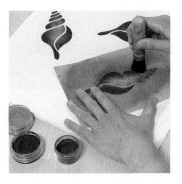

1 Cut the cream cotton drill in two lengthways. Trace the template from the back of the book, enlarging if necessary. Transfer it to stencil card and cut out. Spray the back lightly with adhesive and stencil five shells on to each piece of fabric, using two or three colours. When thoroughly dry, fix the paint according to the manufacturer's instructions.

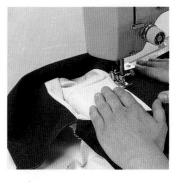

2 With right sides together, sew a blue strip to the top edge of each cream piece, leaving a 1 cm/½ in seam allowance. Press the seam upwards. Pin rectangles right sides together and stitch around the main bag. Press under the seam allowances on the open sides of the blue fabric and top stitch in orange. Fold in half lengthways. Machine stitch parallel to the top stitch.

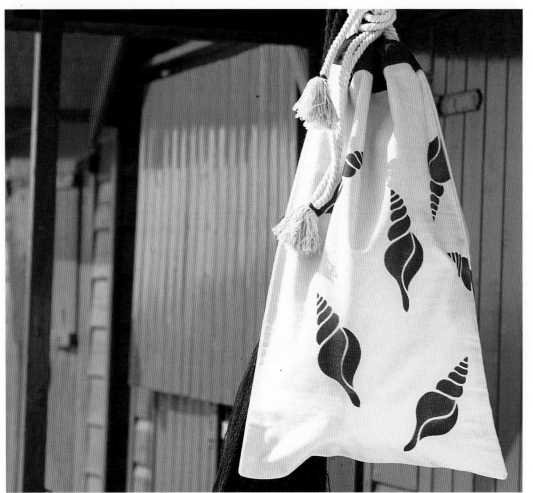

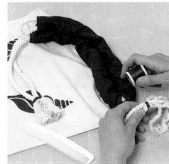

3 Cut the cord in half and bind the ends with masking tape. Thread both pieces through the bag. Remove the tape and bind the ends with blue thread, 5 cm/2 in from the ends. Fringe and comb the cord to make tassels. Trim neatly.

• APPLIQUE, PATCHWORK AND CROSS STITCH •

Star-spangled Scarf

A lavish scattering of gold appliqué and beads on dark velvet creates a luxurious scarf for winter evenings.

You Will Need

Materials
burgundy velvet,
23 x 63 cm/9 x 25 in
gold velvet,
23 x 63 cm/9 x 25 in
tracing paper
fusible bonding web,
23 x 30 cm/9 x 12 in
gold machine
embroidery thread
translucent gold
rocaille beads
matching sewing thread
black velvet,
32 x 122 cm/12½ x 48 in
black glazed cotton,
56 x 89 cm/22 x 34½ in

Equipment
dressmaker's scissors
pencil
iron
pressing cloth
sewing machine
needle
dressmaker's pins

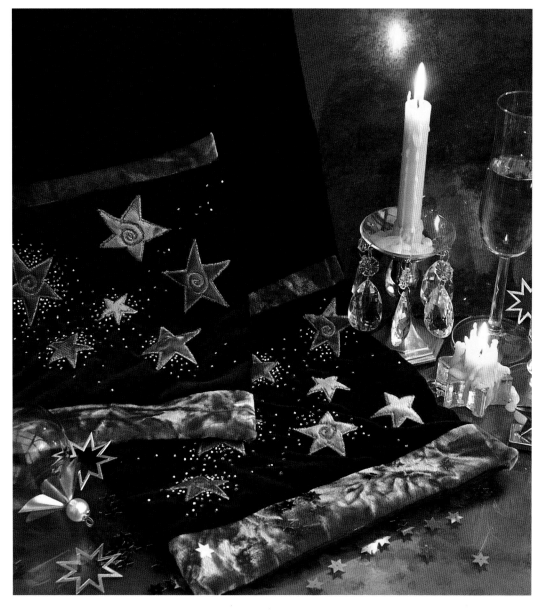

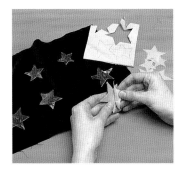

1 Cut the burgundy velvet into two rectangles 23 x 32 cm/9 x 12½ in. From the gold velvet cut two 4 x 32 cm/ 1½ x 12½ in strips and two 6 x 32 cm/2½ x 12½ in strips.

Trace the templates from the back of the book, enlarging if necessary. Draw and cut out each star twice on the fusible bonding. Iron on to the wrong side of the remaining gold velvet. Cut out each star neatly along the outline. Peel off the backing paper and arrange eight stars on each burgundy rectangle. Iron in place using a pressing cloth. Using gold thread, machine around the edge of each appliqué star and work a spiral over the centres of the three largest shapes. Sew a thick sprinkling of beads to the background with double thread.

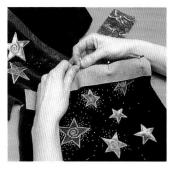

2 Join one wide and one narrow gold velvet strip to the long sides of each burgundy panel, using a 1 cm/½ in seam allowance. Attach a panel to each end of the black velvet, joining the narrow gold strip to the main scarf. Iron all seams open lightly, using a cloth. Cut the lining fabric in half lengthways and join to form one long strip. Press the seam open, then pin the cotton lining to the scarf along the long edges with right sides facing. Stitch, leaving a 12.5 cm/5 in opening in the centre of one seam. Remove the pins and adjust the ends so that an equal amount of velvet lies on each side of the lining. Pin, then stitch across the ends. Clip the corners and turn the scarf to the right side. Press lightly and slip stitch the opening.

• APPLIQUE, PATCHWORK AND CROSS STITCH •

Star-spangled Banner

Make a bold statement with this cheerful wall hanging, based on an American bed quilt from 1876.

You Will Need

Materials
*tracing paper
fusible bonding web,
76 x 142 cm/30 x 56 in
white cotton fabric,
30 x 40 cm/12 x 16 in
blue cotton fabric,
76 x 40 cm/30 x 16 in
matching sewing thread
dark red cotton fabric,
76 x 38 cm/30 x 15 in
medium weight wadding
(batting), 66 x 66 cm/
26 x 26 in
6 curtain rings, 2.5 cm/1 in
curtain pole with decorative
finials, 86 cm/34 in
acrylic paints: dark red
and cream
red cord, 130 cm/50 in*

Equipment
*pencil
dressmaker's scissors
iron
dressmaker's pins
sewing machine
needle
tacking (basting) thread or
safety pins
paintbrush*

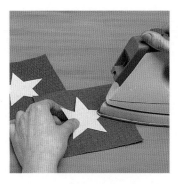

1 Trace the star template from the back of the book, enlarging if necessary. Transfer it to fusible bonding nine times and cut out. Iron them on to white fabric, then cut out and peel off the backing paper. Cut nine 14 cm/5½ in blue cotton squares and fuse a star to the centre of each.

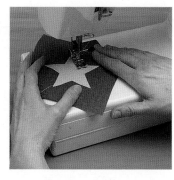

2 Neaten the edges of the stars by stitching over them with a narrow satin stitch in white thread. Cut out four red and four white rectangles, each 7.5 x 14 cm/3 x 5½ in. Press all seams flat and join the red and white pieces in pairs along the longer sides.

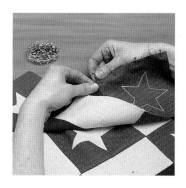

3 Lay the squares alternating with the blue star squares as a border around the central star. Pin and sew together in three rows of three, then join the rows to form a square. Cut out four red and four white rectangles, each 7.5 x 40 cm/3 x 15½ in, and join in pairs along the longer sides.

4 With right sides together, stitch a blue square to each end of two of the rectangles. Stitch the remaining pieces to opposite sides of the central panel, with the white sides on the inner edge, then stitch the longer strips to the other two sides.

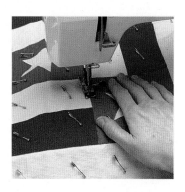

5 Cut 66 cm/26 in squares of wadding (batting) and blue cotton and tack (baste) to the patchwork with tacking (basting) thread or safety pins. Machine or hand quilt along the seam lines, then stitch all round the outside, 3 mm/⅛ in from the edge. Trim.

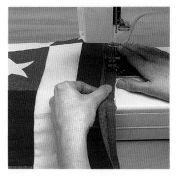

6 From the remaining blue cotton, cut four strips, each 3 x 66 cm/1¼ x 26 in for the binding. Iron in half lengthways, then press under 5 mm/¼ in along one edge. Pin each strip along one side of the quilted square, raw edges even, and stitch. Turn the folded edge to the back and slip stitch in place. Neaten the corners.

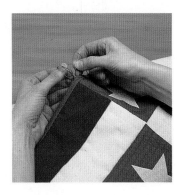

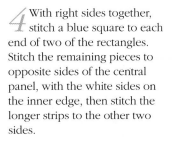

7 Sew the curtain rings to the top of the banner, spacing them evenly.

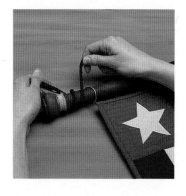

8 Remove the finials from the curtain pole and paint dark red, using a dry brush for a dragged effect. Paint cream stripes or details on the turned ends. Thread the pole through the rings and replace the finials. Attach the cord to one end of the pole and wrap it round, securing with matching cotton. Do the same with the other end, then make a loop in the centre.

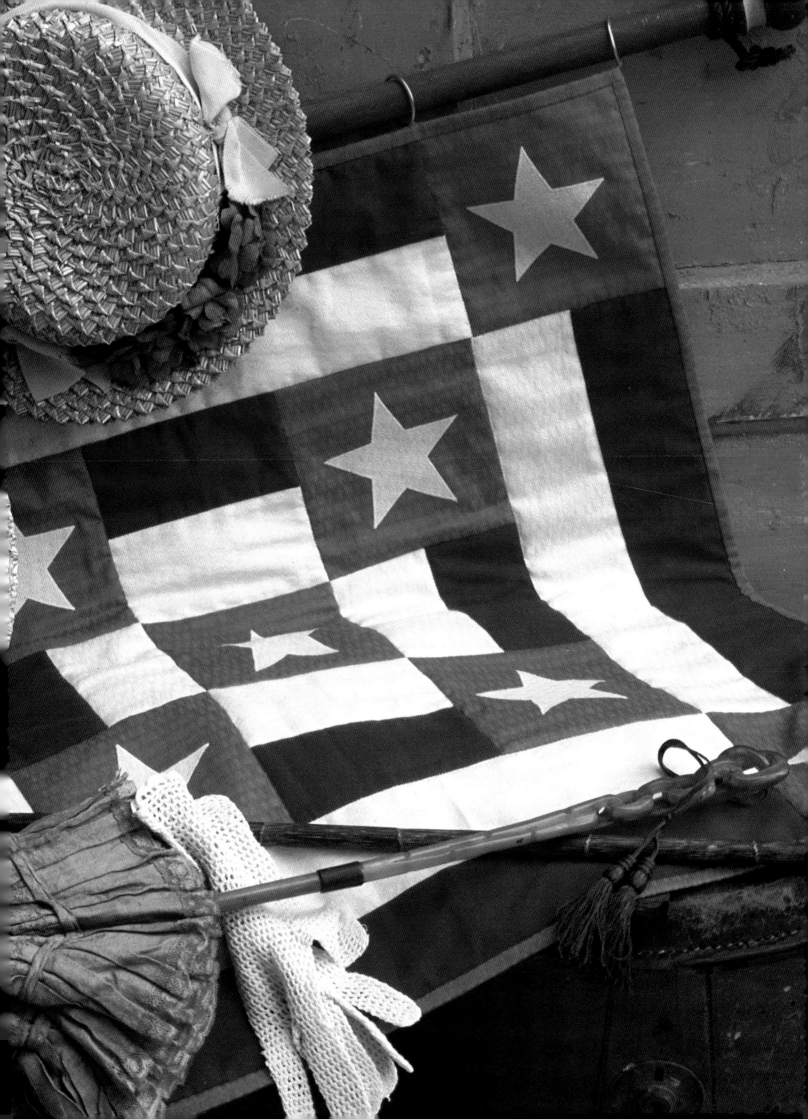

· Applique, Patchwork and Cross Stitch ·

Spice-scented Pot Stand

The lovely homespun look of this pot stand is achieved by tinting all the fabrics with tea. Placing a hot pot on the mat releases a rich, spicy scent of cloves.

You Will Need

Materials
calico, 18 x 18 cm/7 x 7 in
red gingham,
22 x 44 cm/9 x 18 in
blue ticking,
6 x 22 cm/2½ x 9 in
small blue check cotton,
6 x 22 cm/2½ x 9 in
tea bags
tracing paper
stencil card
masking tape
yellow-ochre stencil crayon
paper towels
stranded embroidery
threads: yellow-ochre and
beige
4 buttons
matching sewing thread
whole cloves

Equipment
bowl
iron
pencil
craft knife
cutting mat
metal ruler
masking tape
stencil brush
dressmaker's pins
needle
sewing machine

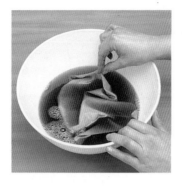

1 Wash all the fabrics to remove any dressing. Brew some strong tea and soak the fabrics until you are satisfied with the colour. It is best to do this in stages, re-dipping if you need to make them darker. Allow to dry and press well.

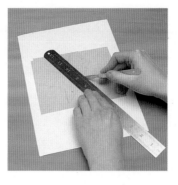

2 Trace the star template from the back of the book, enlarging if necessary. Transfer it to stencil card. Cut out the star using a craft knife and a ruler.

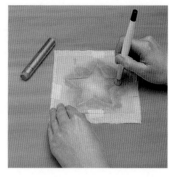

3 Tape the stencil in the centre of the calico. Work around the card with the stencil crayon, scribbling the paint near the edges of the shape, avoiding getting any on the fabric. Work the stencil brush into the crayon and gently ease the paint from the stencil on to the fabric with a light scrubbing action. Add more paint if necessary. Do not try to get an even coverage as this adds to the "antique" effect.

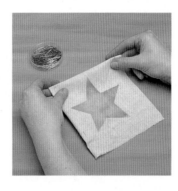

4 Iron the calico on the wrong side between sheets of paper towels to fix the motif and blot excess paint. Fold under the edges of the calico fabric until it measures 11.5 x 12 cm/4½ x 4¾ in. Press.

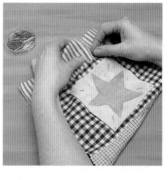

5 Pin the calico in the centre of one gingham square. With your fingers, gently fray one long edge of the ticking and check strips and pin them to opposite sides of the gingham, with the frayed edges pointing inwards.

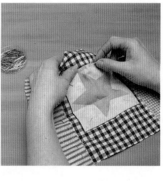

6 Using three strands of yellow thread, stitch the strips to the gingham with a running stitch near the frayed edges. Using beige thread and running stitch, attach the calico square and sew a button in each corner. With wrong sides together, machine stitch the second gingham square to the decorated square, leaving an opening in one side.

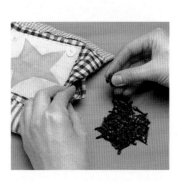

7 Turn the holder to the right side and fill it with cloves. Do not overfill or the pot will be unsteady when resting on the mat. Neatly sew up the opening by hand.

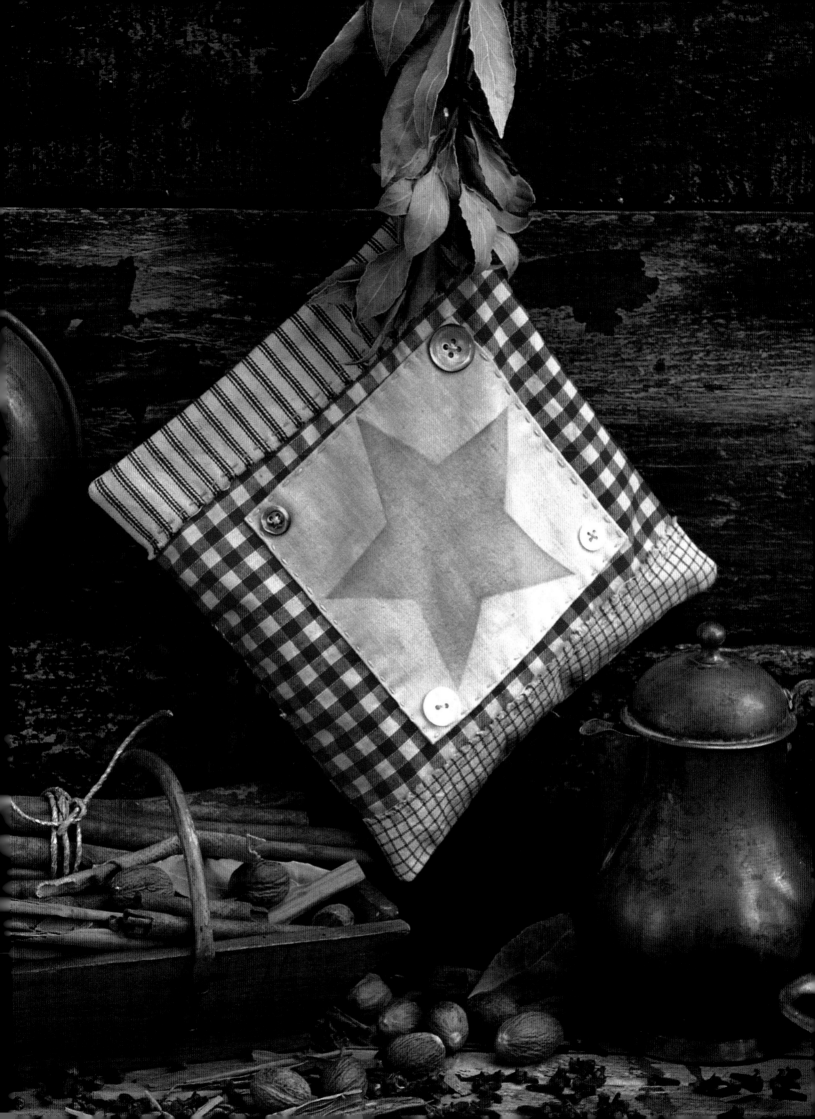

• APPLIQUE, PATCHWORK AND CROSS STITCH •

Oranges Tea Towel

Appliquéd shapes and machine embroidery make a hard-wearing decoration for bright tea towels. Choose a strong base shade to match your own kitchen colour scheme, or use these motifs on a set of towels in different colours.

You Will Need

MATERIALS
*tracing paper
thin card or paper
fusible bonding web
scraps of yellow, orange
and green cotton fabric
tea towel
black machine embroidery
thread*

EQUIPMENT
*pencil
scissors
iron
tailor's chalk
embroidery hoop
sewing machine, with
darning foot
needle*

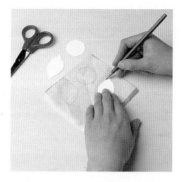

1 Trace the template from the back of the book, enlarging if necessary. Transfer it to thin card or paper and cut out the orange and lemon motifs. Draw around each motif several times on the paper backing of fusible bonding web. Cut out roughly. Iron the web on to the wrong side of the fabric scraps and cut neatly around the outlines.

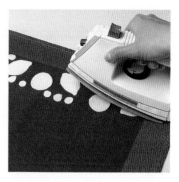

2 Arrange the shapes along the bottom of both ends of the tea towel until you are happy with your design. Remove the paper backing from the fusible bonding web and iron the motifs on to the towel.

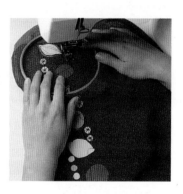

3 Use tailor's chalk to join up the motifs with a series of parallel lines. Put the work in an embroidery hoop. Select the darning or free embroidery mode on the sewing machine and work several lines of black stitching around each fruit. Work down the chalk lines with a series of small embroidered motifs. Hand sew French knots on the oranges.

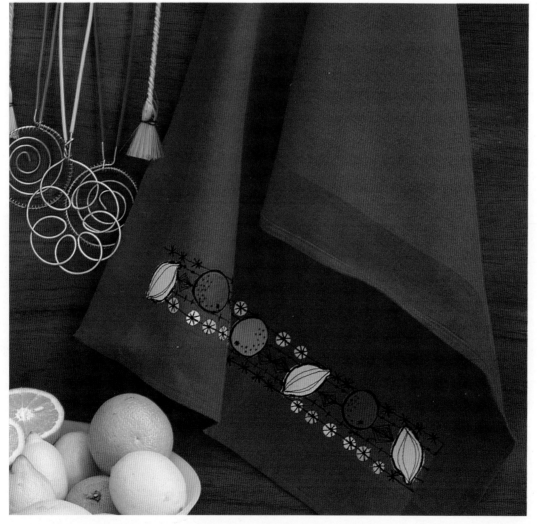

• APPLIQUE, PATCHWORK AND CROSS STITCH •

Shaker Towel

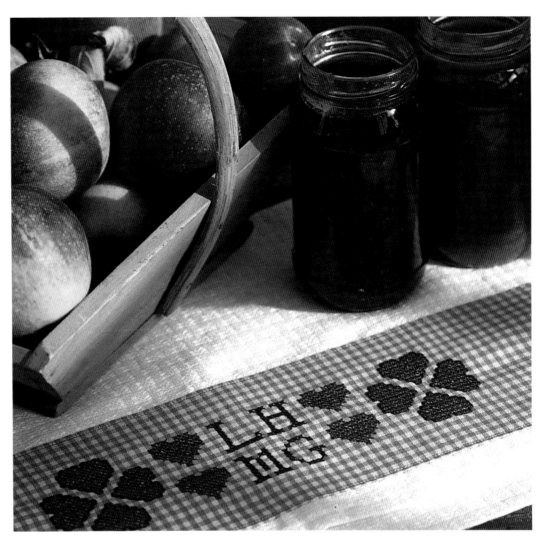

Cross-stitched hearts and initials conjure up the art of the Shakers, for whom the heart was a well-loved decorative image. Hearts denoted not the traditions of romantic love, but the spiritual devotion of the movement's followers, summed up in the saying "Hands to work, hearts to God."

YOU WILL NEED

MATERIALS
*homespun cotton gingham, 20 x 90 cm/8 x 36 in
cotton seersucker towel
tacking (basting) thread
stranded embroidery threads: dark and light crimson and dark turquoise
matching sewing thread*

EQUIPMENT
*dressmaker's scissors
tape measure
needle
embroidery hoop
iron
dressmaker's pins
sewing machine (optional)*

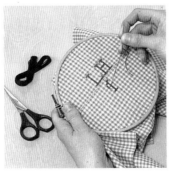 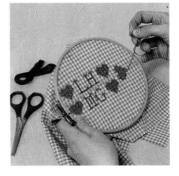 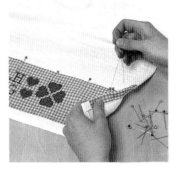

1 Wash the gingham and towel. Cut the gingham 5 cm/2 in wider than the towel. Mark the centre with two intersecting lines of tacking (basting) thread. Stretch the fabric in a hoop. Using the charts at the back of the book, embroider four initials in three strands of dark crimson thread. Work the second diagonal in the same direction each time.

2 Again, following the charts, embroider the four dark turquoise hearts in cross stitch on each side of the monogram. Then work the light crimson hearts. These are given extra definition with an outline of running stitch, worked in dark crimson thread. Press the embroidery lightly.

3 Trim the long edges so that there is 3.5 cm/1½ in of fabric on each side of the embroidery and press under 1 cm/½ in along each side. Fold the towel in half to find the centre point and pin the gingham along the bottom edge. Turn the sides of the gingham to the back of the towel and tack (baste) in place. Then stitch with matching thread.

• APPLIQUE, PATCHWORK AND CROSS STITCH •

Needlepoint Mat

In the 1950s, leaves were a great inspiration to designers, who turned them into almost abstract shapes. The muted colours of this needlepoint are also expressive of the period.

You Will Need

Materials
tacking (basting) thread
needlepoint canvas square
tapestry wools: 3 shades of
cream, 2 shades of green,
yellow, gold and black
card
black velvet, for backing
PVA (white) glue

Equipment
needle
fabric marker
tapestry needle
scissors
metal ruler
craft knife
cutting mat

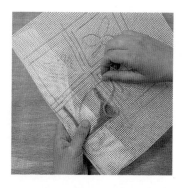

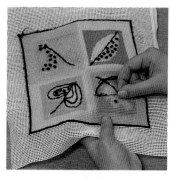

1 Tack (baste) vertically and horizontally across the canvas to mark the centre. Mark the design on to the canvas, following the chart at the back of the book; each square represents a stitch. Work the pattern in half cross stitch.

2 When the half cross stitch is complete, use black wool to embroider the details. Work the straight lines in back stitch and use French knots for the dots.

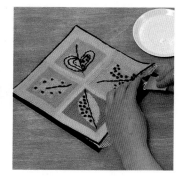

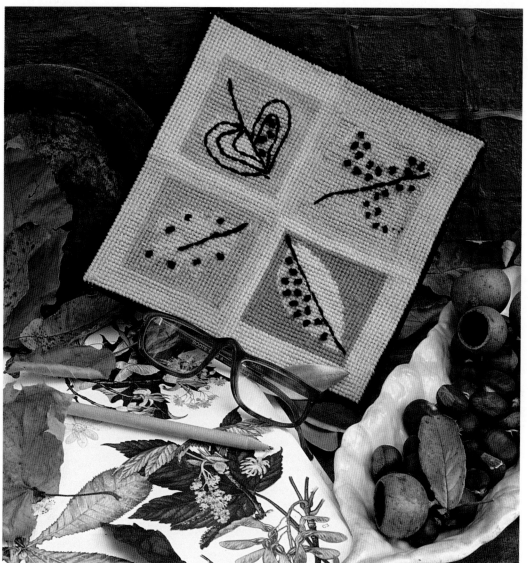

3 Measure the needlepoint and cut out a piece of card to the same size. Cut out a piece of velvet to this size plus a 2 cm/¾ in turning allowance all round. Spread glue on the card and stick it centrally on to the back of the velvet. Clip the corners, fold over the turning allowance and glue in place. Trim the canvas and clip the corners; turn the allowance to the wrong side. Spread glue on the wrong side of the card and press the needlepoint in place.

• APPLIQUE, PATCHWORK AND CROSS STITCH •

Applique Star Card

A beautiful birthday card to treasure, in which the traditional craft of tin-punching is combined with appliqué and embroidery.

YOU WILL NEED

MATERIALS

*light blue check cotton,
16 x 12 cm/6 x 4¾ in
medium blue check cotton,
10 x 12 cm/4 x 4¾ in
blue stranded embroidery thread
dark blue check cotton,
4 x 16 cm/1½ x 6 in
tacking (basting) thread
silver embroidery thread
plain, unridged tin can,
14 x 24 cm/5½ x 9½ in
tracing paper
small piece of wood
all-purpose glue
silver card, folded in half*

EQUIPMENT

*dressmaker's scissors
dressmaker's pins
needle
can opener
tin snips
pencil
hammer
bradawl or large nail*

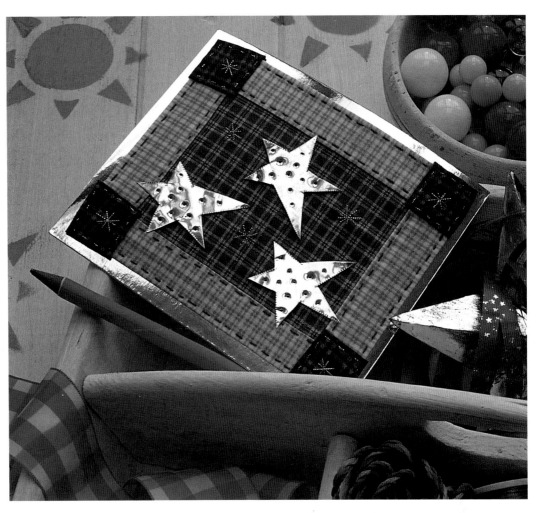

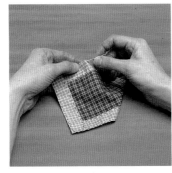

1 Cut the light blue fabric into four 4 cm/1½ in strips. Fold under the raw edge along the long side of each strip and pin it to the medium blue fabric. Using blue embroidery thread, sew small running stitches close to the fold line on both edges.

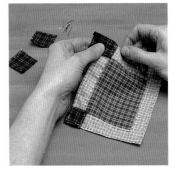

2 Cut out four 4 cm/1½ in squares of dark blue fabric. Turn under the edges of each square and pin in each corner of the panel. Turn under the remaining edges and tack (baste). Sew small running stitches in silver thread around the edges of the corner squares and embroider a simple star in the centre.

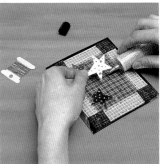

3 Remove the top and bottom of the tin can, cut down the back seam with tin snips and flatten. Trace the template from the back of the book, enlarging if necessary. Cut three tin stars and hammer the points flat. Lay the stars right side up on the wood and punch a star shape using the hammer and bradawl. Embroider three stars in silver thread. Glue the panel to the front of the card. Glue the tin stars in position.

• APPLIQUE, PATCHWORK AND CROSS STITCH •

Applique Notebook

Stitch a delicate appliquéd cover for a special diary, address book or birthday book. This design is appropriate for a gardening or cookery notebook.

You Will Need

Materials	Equipment
scraps of plain cream, green check and orange patterned cotton fabrics	*dressmaker's scissors*
hardback notebook	*pencil*
tracing paper	*iron*
fusible bonding web	*embroidery needle*
stranded embroidery threads: green, orange and cream	*needle*
green cotton fabric	*sewing machine*
tacking (basting) thread	
matching sewing thread	
orange, yellow and green buttons	

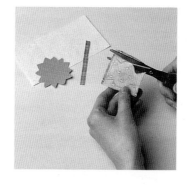

1 Cut a rectangle of cream fabric slightly smaller than the front of your notebook. Trace the template from the back of the book, enlarging it to fit the notebook. Trace the shapes on to the backing paper of the fusible bonding web and cut out roughly. Iron the pieces on to their respective fabrics, then cut out.

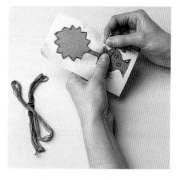

2 Peel off the backing paper and iron on to the cream fabric. Chain stitch around the leaves in green. Work the urn handles in orange, and chain stitch around it. Cut the green fabric for the cover: the width is four times that of the book and the depth 2.5 cm/1 in more. Press under a 2.5cm/1 in fold at each short edge.

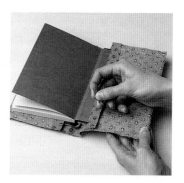

3 Fold in half, wrong sides together, and wrap around the book. Tuck the loose fabric under the front cover and stitch the embroidered panel on the centre front. Fold all the flaps underneath the book covers and loosely tack (baste) the raw edges together at top and bottom. Slip the cover off and machine stitch along the tacked lines. Turn the cover right side out and press. Sew the buttons on to the tree.

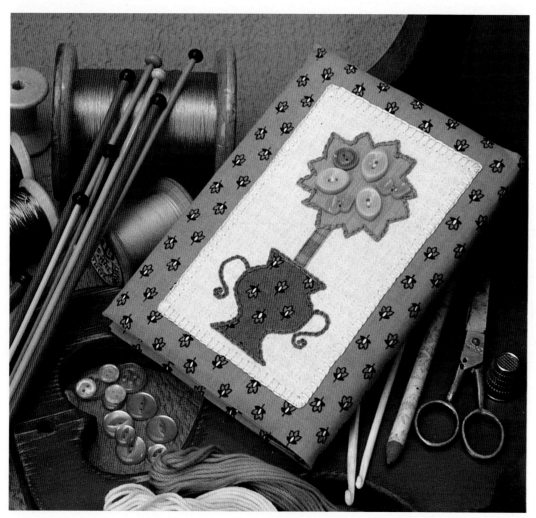

• APPLIQUE, PATCHWORK AND CROSS STITCH •

Hand Towel and Washcloth

Transform a plain white hand towel and washcloth into an individual gift set, by adding appliquéd pansies in velvet and cotton prints.

You Will Need

Materials
tracing paper
velvet, 20 x 15 cm/8 x 6 in
medium-weight iron-on interfacing
3 different cotton floral print fabrics
tacking (basting) thread
matching embroidery thread
white cotton tea towel and washcloth
machine embroidery threads: matching and white

Equipment
pencil
iron
fabric marker
dressmaker's scissors
dressmaker's pins
needle
sewing machine

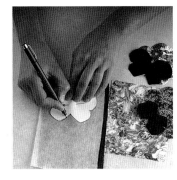

1 Trace the templates from the back of the book, enlarging if necessary. Back the velvet with interfacing. Transfer the pansy to the interfacing and cut out three large and one small petal shape from the backed velvet. Cut one large flower shape from each of the three floral prints and one small flower from one of them.

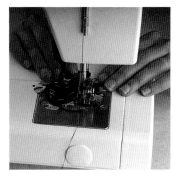

2 Pin and tack (baste) the shapes to the flowers. With matching thread and satin stitch, stitch around the edge of the inner petals. Embroider details on to the flowers. Fill in the centre of each pansy with satin stitch and sew the petal markings with two lines of stem or back stitch. Iron the interfacing on to the back of each flower.

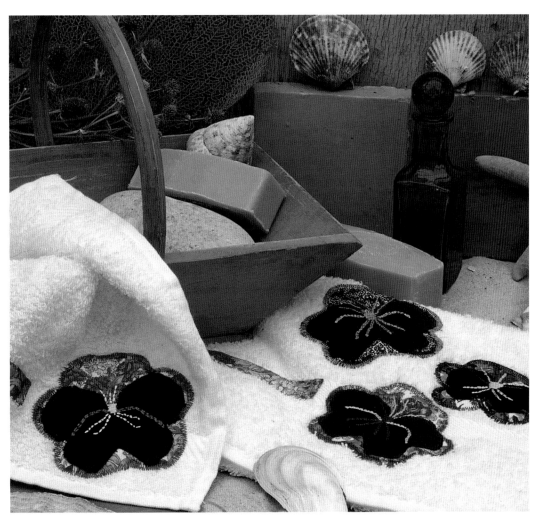

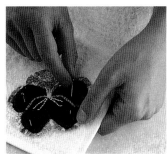

3 Tack (baste) flowers on the towel and cloth. Using matching thread on top and a white spool, appliqué in place.

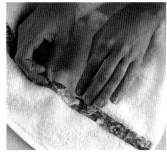

4 Cover the towel borders with strips of floral fabric. Cut a piece 4 cm/1½ in wide to fit from the edge to the pansies with an allowance of 1 cm/½ in at each end. Press, pin and tack (baste) in place. Zigzag to finish.

• APPLIQUE, PATCHWORK AND CROSS STITCH •

Appliqued Sheet and Pillowcase

This bold design gives bedlinen a unique appeal. The shapes can be cut from either patterned or checked fabrics, according to your personal taste.

You Will Need

Materials	Equipment
tracing paper	*pencil*
graph paper	*dressmaker's scissors*
fusible bonding web	*tape measure*
coloured or patterned fabrics	*iron*
sheet and pillowcase	*dressmaker's pins*
matching machine embroidery thread	*sewing machine*

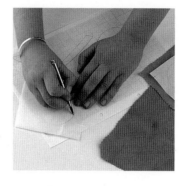

1 Trace selected fabric patterns (or use the template from this book), enlarging as necessary for your design. Cut a piece of bonding web 25 x 25 cm/ 10 x 10 in. Lay it over the designs, and, with paper side facing, trace along the outlines.

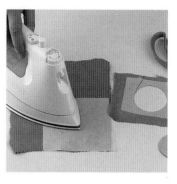

2 Cut four or five pieces of the fabric to squares, each about 20 x 20 cm/8 x 8 in. Iron the bonding web on to the wrong side of the fabric and cut the shapes out.

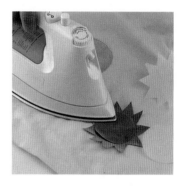

3 Peel away the backing paper and arrange the cutouts on the sheet and pillowcase, parallel to the fabric edge. Pin in place, then iron over the pieces, removing the pins as you go.

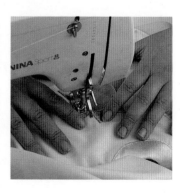

4 Work a zigzag machine stitch all around the fused edges to complete the design.

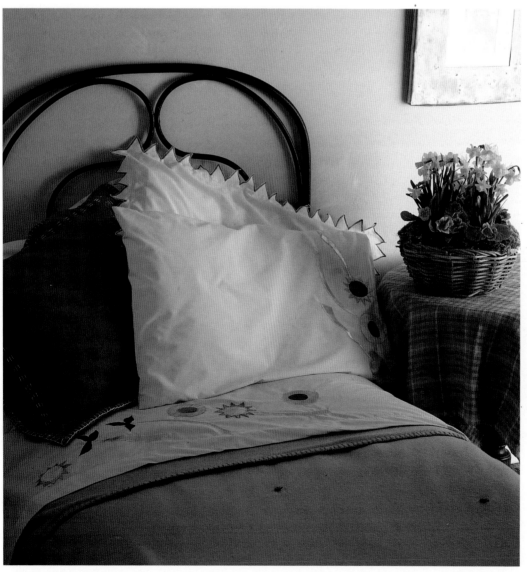

• APPLIQUE, PATCHWORK AND CROSS STITCH •

Child's T-shirt

An ordinary T-shirt is transformed, with appliquéd fabric scraps, machine embroidery and beads, into something really special. There's no reason why the same idea couldn't be used for an adult-size T-shirt.

YOU WILL NEED

MATERIALS
*tracing paper
unbleached cotton T-shirt
fusible bonding web,
30 x 30 cm/12 x 12 in
yellow, orange and brown
cotton fabric scraps
machine embroidery
threads: light orange and
brown
small orange beads*

EQUIPMENT
*pencil
dressmaker's scissors
iron
pressing cloth
sewing machine*

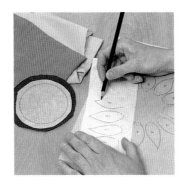

1 Trace the template from the back of the book, enlarging it to fit the T-shirt. Number the petals consecutively 1–12. Trace the even-numbered petals on to the paper side of the bonding and cut out. Iron the bonding to the yellow cotton. Repeat with the other petals in orange, and with brown for the centre.

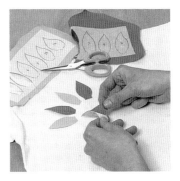

2 Cut out all the shapes around the outlines and remove the backing paper. Place the petals in a circle on the front of the T-shirt, using the template as a guide. Iron them in place, using a cool iron and a pressing cloth.

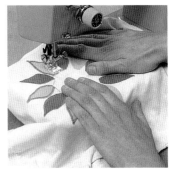

3 Thread the sewing machine with orange thread and set it to a closely spaced medium-size zigzag. Stitch around the edges of all the petals to conceal the raw edges. Iron the flower centre in position and sew around its circumference with brown thread. Using brown thread, sew the beads on to the flower centre, making sure they are evenly scattered.

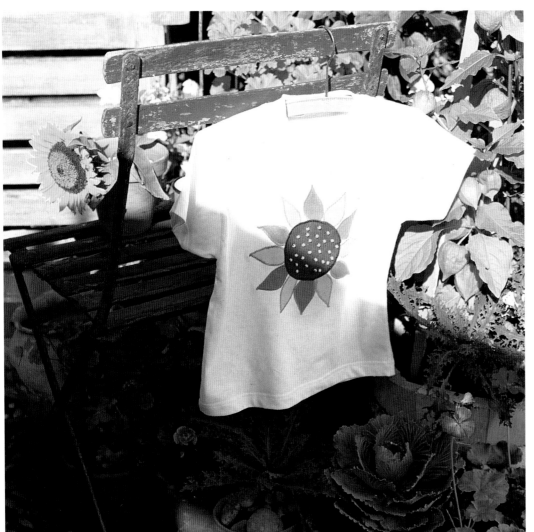

• APPLIQUE, PATCHWORK AND CROSS STITCH •

INITIAL CUSHION

Adapt this design by using the initials of a special person or a couple as the centrepiece. It would make an ideal wedding gift, and a larger version could even include the couple's full names and the date and location of their wedding.

YOU WILL NEED

MATERIALS
stranded embroidery threads
cream cross stitch fabric,
15 x 15 cm, 8 holes per cm/
6 x 6 in, 18 holes per in
cream silk backing fabric
thread
polyester wadding (batting)
cream cotton lace,
1 m x 6 cm/1 yd x 2½ in
4 mother-of-pearl buttons

EQUIPMENT
needle
dressmaker's scissors
dressmaker's pins
tape measure

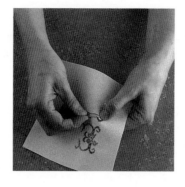

1 Following the chart at the back of the book, or using an alphabet of your own, embroider the initials on to the cross stitch fabric. Work in cross stitch, using two strands of thread. Make sure that the four letters are squared up.

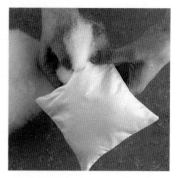

2 Cut the backing fabric to the same size as the front piece of the cushion. Pin with right sides together. Allowing a seam of 1 cm/½ in, stitch together, leaving a 5 cm/2 in gap at one edge. Trim the seam allowance and clip the corners. Turn inside out and stuff firmly. Slip stitch the opening.

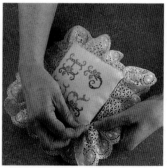

3 Join the ends of the lace together and run a neat gathering thread along the straight edge. Gather the thread to fit around the outside of the cushion and pin it in place, allowing for extra fullness at the corners. Oversew the lace on to the cushion with matching thread, using small, neat stitches. Finish off by sewing a button to each corner.

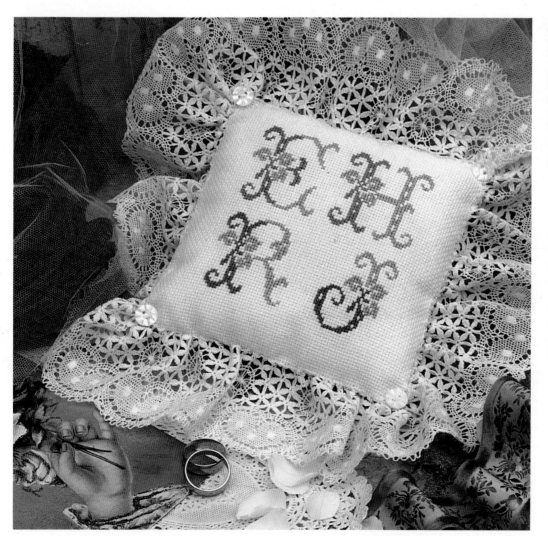

• APPLIQUE, PATCHWORK AND CROSS STITCH •

Country-style Pillowcase

Customize some plain bedlinen and give it a country appeal with this charming heart design. Emphasize the hearts and raise the design with a halo of multi-coloured running stitches.

You Will Need

Materials
*iron-on interfacing,
25 x 25 cm/10 x 10 in
brightly coloured fabric scraps
tacking (basting) thread
pillowcase
matching and contrasting threads*

Equipment
*pencil or fabric marker
dressmaker's scissors
iron
needle
dressmaker's pins
crewel needle*

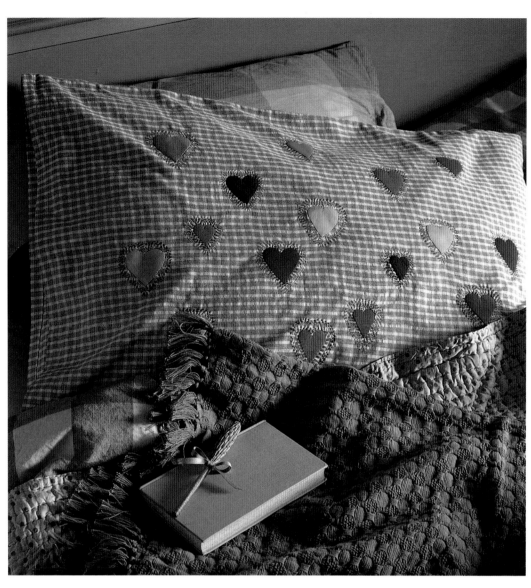

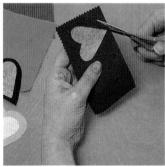

1 Draw 17 hearts on to the interfacing and cut them out. Iron the interfacing to the fabric scraps and cut out the shapes, leaving a 5 mm/¼ in seam allowance.

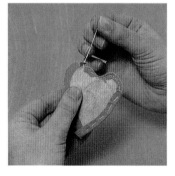

2 Clip the seam allowance around the curves, fold over and tack (baste) in place.

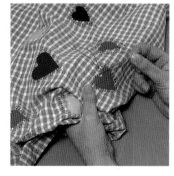

3 Arrange the hearts randomly over the pillowcase. Pin, tack (baste) and then slip stitch them in place. Using an assortment of coloured threads in one strand, work lines of tiny stitches around each heart in halos. Iron to finish the design.

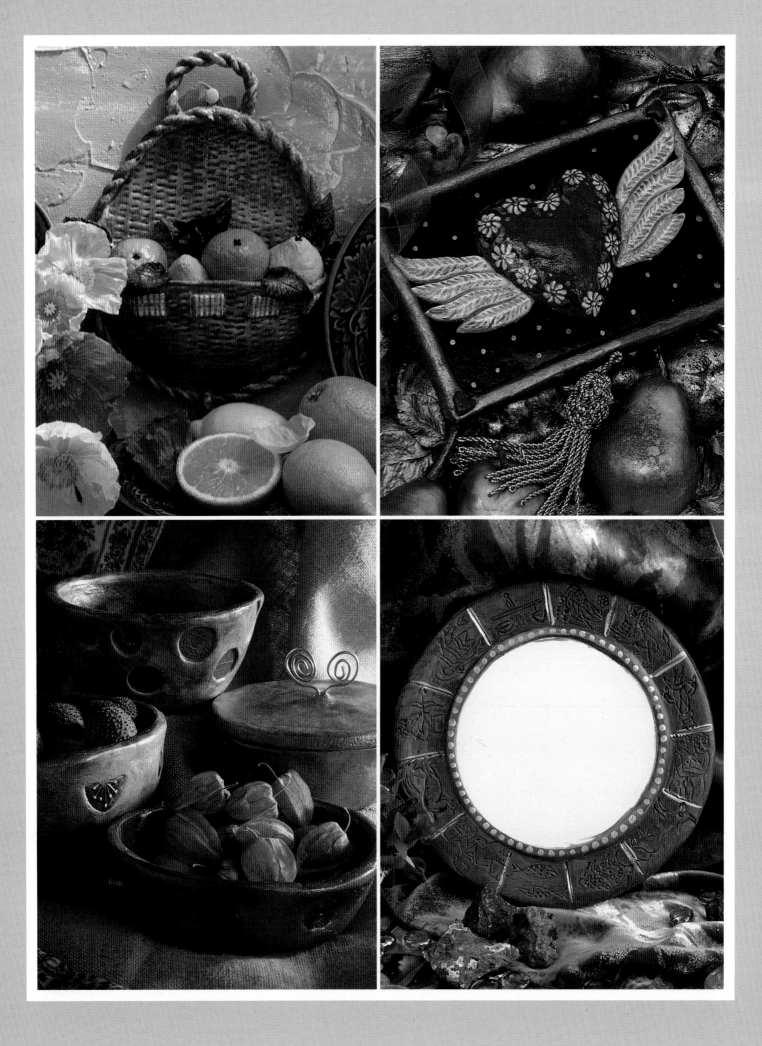

Modelling and Salt Dough

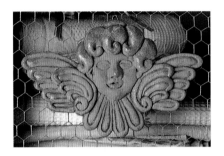

Modelling is a craft particularly suitable for children of any age, as it is soft, safe and a lot of fun to do. The modelling projects in this section use polymer clay, self-hardening clay and salt dough. Working with salt dough has the added attraction that children can take an active part in preparing and baking the dough, as well as shaping it as they wish. When buying commercial modelling materials for use by children, look particularly for non-toxic varieties.

Children and adults alike will find plenty of inspiration within these next pages. There are projects to suit all abilities, ranging from simple and effective motifs that can be stamped on to clay or salt dough using pastry cutters, to more technically challenging three-dimensional creations.

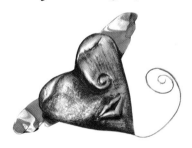

• MODELLING AND SALT DOUGH •

MATERIALS AND EQUIPMENT

Modelling with self-hardening clay or salt dough requires very little in the way of materials and equipment, and you will probably already have the basic items at home. You should work on a clean, smooth, flat surface, and take care to keep sharp implements, glues, paints and varnish well out of the reach of children. Polymer clay (see picture) is a highly adaptable modelling medium that comes in a dazzling array of colours.

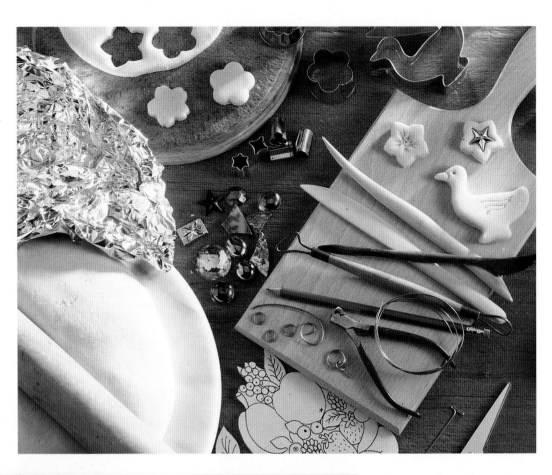

RIGHT *Salt dough is economical to make and easy to use - yet produces wonderfully decorative results. Here you can see a selection of special pastry cutters from the wide range now available.*

Tinting dough and clay

Food colouring is ideal for use on salt dough, and it is available in liquid and paste form. The paste is easier to use and more than one colour can be added to the dough to produce the shade required. Self-hardening clay can be bought from craft suppliers in a variety of colours, or you can colour it with paints and varnishes. Salt dough, too, can be decorated with paints and varnishes.

LEFT *Polymer clay is a versatile, easy-to-handle medium that can be used to make objects as diverse as picture frames and jewellery. Once shaped, it can be baked hard at low temperature in a domestic oven.*

Salt Dough Recipe

Salt dough recipe

Simply follow the method below, adjusting the quantities to make the amount of salt dough you need. The quantities given here are sufficient to make a bowl with a diameter of about 23 cm/9 in.

The addition of 15 ml/1 tbsp vegetable oil to the recipe adds suppleness, while 10 ml/1 tbsp wallpaper paste gives the dough elasticity.

INGREDIENTS

230 g/8 oz/2 cups plain flour
200 g/7 oz/1 cup salt
250 ml/8 fl oz/1 cup water

Raw dough

Once the dough has been kneaded, it is pliable and easily manipulated, suitable for even intricate details.

Remember that salt dough is susceptible to steam and damp, so always keep your creations in a dry atmosphere to prevent deterioration.

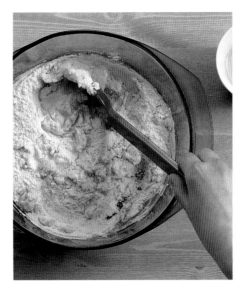

1 Mix together the flour, salt and half the water in a mixing bowl. Knead the mixture, gradually adding more water until the dough has a smooth, firm consistency. Be careful not to add too much water or the dough will sag and become sticky.

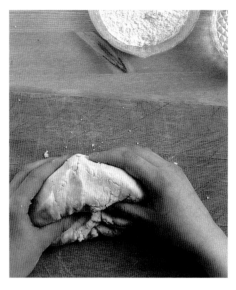

2 Remove the dough from the bowl and continue to knead for 10 minutes. The dough can be modelled immediately, but is best left to rest for 30 minutes in an airtight container. Bake the salt dough in an oven at 120°C/250°F/Gas 1/2 until the dough is completely hardened all over.

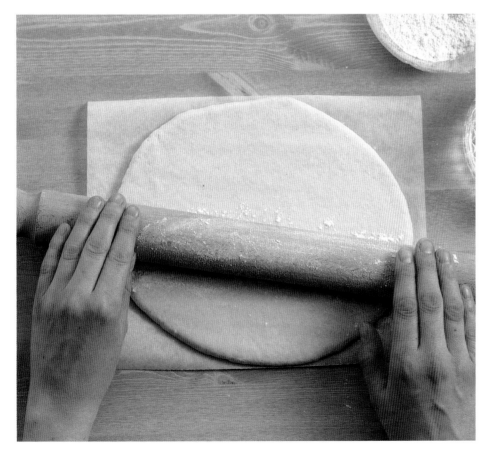

Working with salt dough and clay

Dough and clay can be rolled out flat with a rolling pin. Work directly on baking parchment if you are using salt dough, otherwise work on a clean, flat surface. A small, craft knife or clay modelling tool is indispensable for cutting dough and clay and indenting details. A cocktail stick, knitting needle or thick sewing needle is also useful, and can be used to pierce holes for hanging or decorating models. Make any holes about 3 mm/1/8 in wider than needed to allow for any distortion during painting and varnishing

Various bowls, plates and dishes make suitable moulds for modelling (if the dough is to be baked, then the mould must be heat-resistant). Also, there is an exciting range of beautiful pastry moulds, biscuit cutters and icing cutters that can all be used to great effect.

LEFT *Rolling out salt dough on baking parchment.*

· MODELLING AND SALT DOUGH ·

WHEATSHEAF

The wonderful golden colour of baked salt dough lends itself beautifully to the theme of a sheaf of wheat. This makes an ideal decoration for a kitchen wall, but keep it away from steam.

YOU WILL NEED

MATERIALS

*tracing paper
salt dough (see Salt Dough Recipe)
baking parchment
polyurethane satin varnish*

EQUIPMENT

*pencil
rolling pin
craft knife
clay modelling tool (optional)
baking tray
paintbrush*

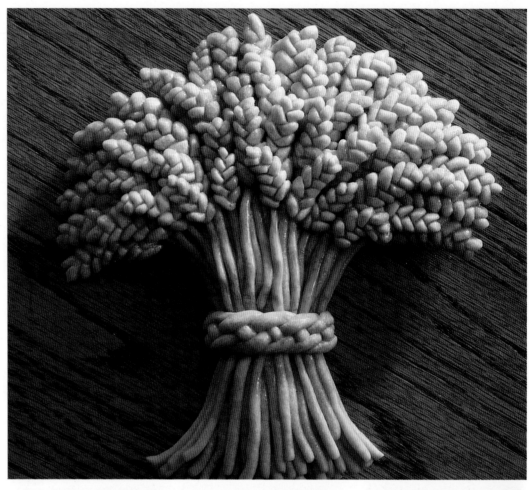

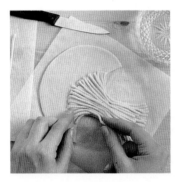 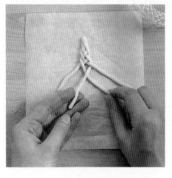 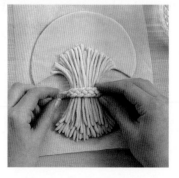 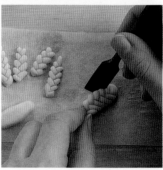

1 Trace the template from the back of the book, enlarging if necessary. Roll out the dough flat on baking parchment to a thickness of 1 cm/½ in. Use the template to cut the wheatsheaf shape. To make the stalks, roll out thin spaghetti-like strands of dough to a length of about 12 cm/5 in and build them up into a bundle as shown. Moisten the strands with a little water to prevent them from drying out.

2 To make the tie for the bundle, roll four strands of dough to a length of 12 cm/5 in. Join the ends together with a little water and gently separate out the strands. Lay the first strand over the second, and the third over the fourth. Then lay what is now the third strand back over the second strand. Repeat these two steps until the plait (braid) is complete. Pinch the bottom ends together, using a little water to moisten and stick in place.

3 Moisten one side of the plait (braid) and place it over the stalks at the narrowest point. Tuck the ends of the plait (braid) neatly under to conceal them. Reserve sufficient salt dough to make the "ears" of the wheatsheaf.

4 Roll sausages from the salt dough, measuring 3 x 1 cm/ 1¼ x ⅜ in. Taper the rolls at one end and flatten them slightly. Use a knife or modelling tool to mark separate grains, curving the edges of each one. Moisten and apply the ears of wheat in overlapping layers. Place the wheatsheaf, on the baking parchment, on a tray and bake at 120°C/250°F/ Gas ½, for 10 hours. Allow to cool. Apply five layers of the satin varnish.

150

• MODELLING AND SALT DOUGH •

GINGERBREAD HEARTS

The designs of these Germanic hearts are based on edible gingerbread and fondant cakes. They are formed from a salt dough base with painted motifs applied in contrasting and complementary patterns.

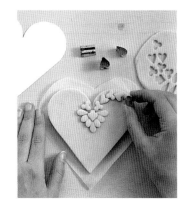

YOU WILL NEED

MATERIALS
*tracing paper
paper or thin card
salt dough (see Salt Dough Recipe)
baking parchment
metal eyelet loop
acrylic gesso or matt emulsion (latex) paint
acrylic or craft paints
polyurethane matt varnish
paper ribbon*

EQUIPMENT
*pencil
scissors
rolling pin
craft knife
aspic cutters
baking tray
paintbrushes*

1 Trace the gingerbread heart template from the back of the book, enlarging if necessary. Transfer it to paper or thin card and cut out. Roll an orange-size ball of salt dough out flat on baking parchment to 1 cm/½ in thick. Place the template on the dough and cut around the edge. Pat the raw edges to round them. Roll some more dough to 5 mm/¼ in thick and cut out shapes with aspic cutters. Moisten the border of the main heart shape and apply the small shapes. Fix the eyelet loop to the top of the heart. Place the model, on the baking parchment, on a tray and bake at 120°C/250°F/Gas ½, for nine hours. Allow to cool.

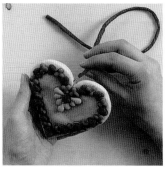

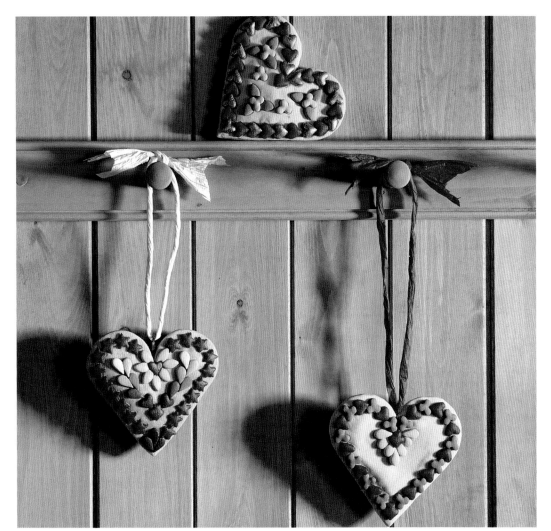

2 Paint on an undercoat of acrylic gesso or matt emulsion (latex) and allow to dry. Pick out the applied decoration with bright acrylic or craft paints, using a fine paintbrush to avoid getting paint on the base heart. When dry, apply five layers of matt varnish, allowing each coat to dry between layers. Cut a 40 cm/16 in length of paper ribbon, thread it through the eyelet and tie in a reef knot about 10 cm/4 in from the heart. Unravel the ribbon and cut out a chevron shape from each end.

Hanging Shapes

Abstract astrological symbols are combined to create an original mobile, decorated with glass panels and beads that will catch the light as the pieces swing in the breeze.

You Will Need

Materials
tracing paper
thin card or paper
1.5 kg/3 lb modelling clay
5 glass circles, 5 mm/¼ in thick, 5 cm/2 in in diameter
1 glass circle, 5 mm/¼ in thick, 3 cm/1¼ in in diameter
0.8 mm copper wire
glass beads in a mixture of colours and sizes
sandpaper
10 cm/4 in thin wire, 2 m/2 yd
2 mm galvanized wire

Equipment
pencil
scissors
rolling pin
clay modelling tools
polythene bag
wire-cutters
jewellery pliers
needle

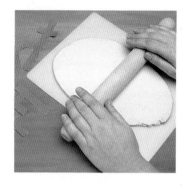

1 Trace the templates from the back of the book, enlarging if necessary. Transfer to thin card or paper and cut out. Roll out the modelling clay to a flat sheet 5 mm/¼ in thick.

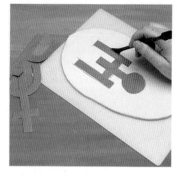

2 Place one shape on to the clay sheet and cut around it with a modelling tool. Return any excess clay to a polythene bag to keep moist. With wet fingers, smooth all the surfaces and edges of the shape.

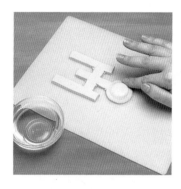

3 Lift up the circular part of the clay shape and hold it gently while positioning a circle of glass centrally underneath. (Use the damp mark left by the clay on the work surface as a guide.) Press the clay around the glass circle with wet fingers.

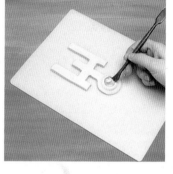

4 Cut out a circle of clay to reveal the glass, leaving a 3 mm/⅛ in border.

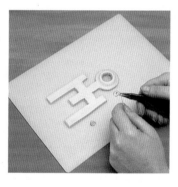

5 Cut the copper wire in half and twist it into two small spirals using pliers. Press gently into the surface of the clay.

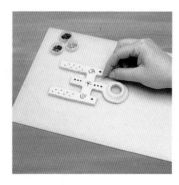

6 Use a needle to help you lift and position the coloured glass beads and press them into the clay.

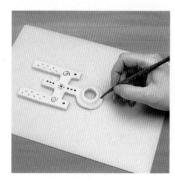

7 Pierce a small hole in the top and bottom of the piece and allow to dry thoroughly. Repeat the process with the other shapes.

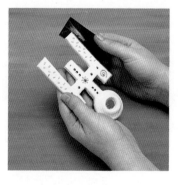

8 Once the pieces have fully dried and hardened, sand down all the edges.

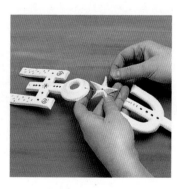

9 Use thin wire to join all the shapes together and then hang them from a galvanized wire hanger.

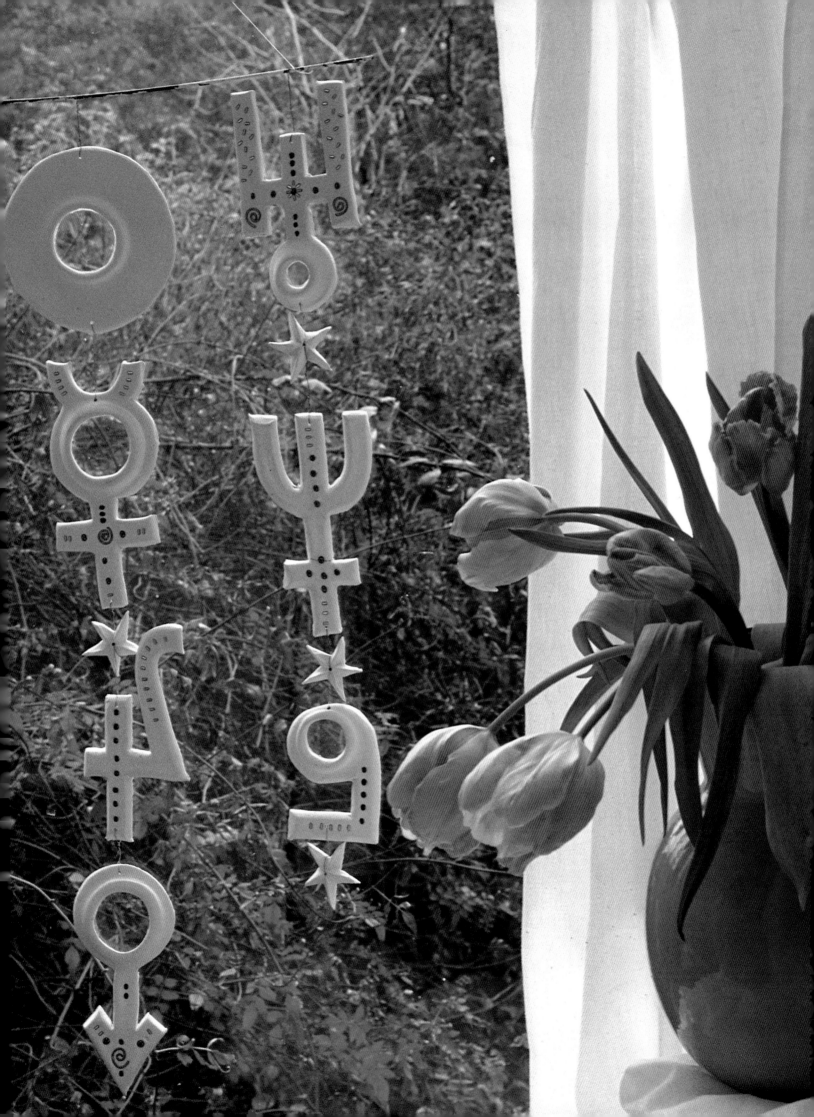

• MODELLING AND SALT DOUGH •

Spider Buttons

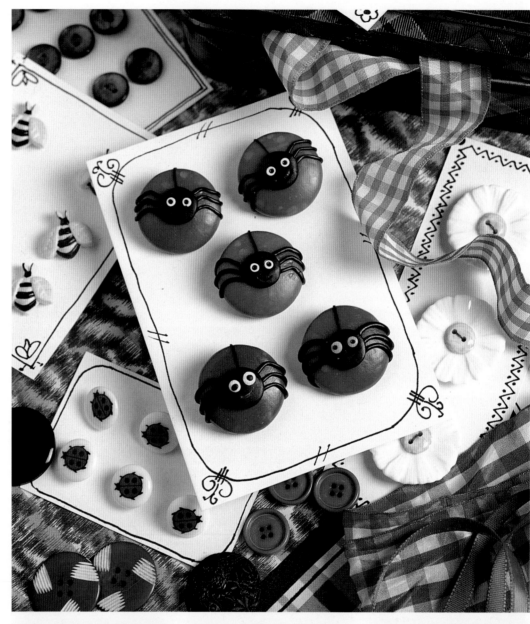

Brighten up a child's coat (or your own!) with these friendly spiders. Use the metal buttons that are sold for covering in fabric and match the size to your buttonholes. Snap the fronts on to the button backs before you start to decorate them. You can coat the baked buttons with a gloss varnish, if you wish.

You Will Need

Materials
*polymer clay: bright green, black and white
set of metal buttons
clear gloss varnish (optional)*

Equipment
*rolling pin
craft knife
cutting mat
paintbrush (optional)*

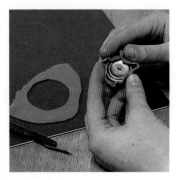

1 Roll the green clay out thinly and cut a circle large enough to cover the button. Mould the clay over the button.

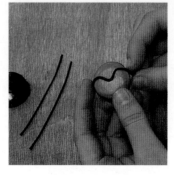

2 Using black clay, roll very thin strands for the legs and press them on to the button. Roll a finer strand for the spider's thread.

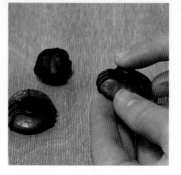

3 Roll a pea-size ball of black clay and press it into the centre of the button for the spider's body.

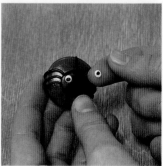

4 Roll two small balls of white clay and press in position to make the eyes. Make the pupils from tiny black balls. Bake in a low oven, following the manufacturer's instructions.

• MODELLING AND SALT DOUGH •

STAR FRAME

A plain frame can be transformed by decorating it with brightly painted cut-out shapes. The result is guaranteed to cheer up any wall.

YOU WILL NEED

MATERIALS
tracing paper
salt dough (see Salt Dough Recipe)
baking parchment
fine-grade sandpaper
acrylic gesso
emulsion (latex) paints
PVA (white) glue
wooden frame
polyurethane satin varnish

EQUIPMENT
pencil
rolling pin
craft knife
baking tray
paintbrushes

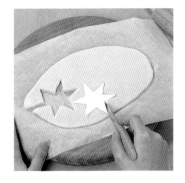

1 Trace the template from the back of the book, enlarging if necessary. Roll out the dough and cut out the star shapes. Place the stars, on baking parchment, on a tray and bake at 120°C/250°F/Gas ½, for five hours. Allow to cool.

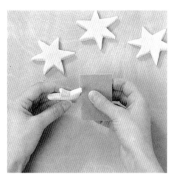

2 Sand all of the baked stars with fine-grade sandpaper.

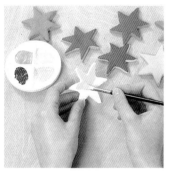

3 Paint each star with gesso and allow to dry. Decorate the stars with a coat of emulsion (latex) paint as a base colour. Allow to dry thoroughly.

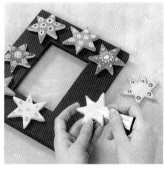

4 Paint patterns in other colours on the stars. Glue the stars to the frame. Finish with a coat of satin varnish.

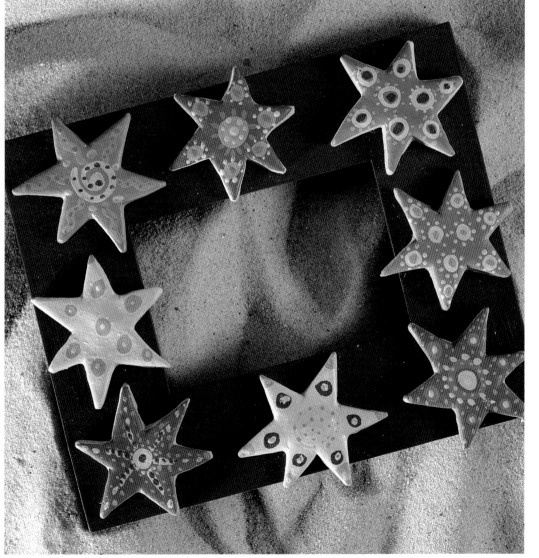

• MODELLING AND SALT DOUGH •

Engraved Mirror Frame

*T*he zodiac stands for the wheeling of the seasons as the sun appears to circle the earth, and astrologers draw it as a circle, with each of the twelve sections presided over by its familiar sign. Here, the ancient calendar is the inspiration for a stunning engraved frame. Secure the hook firmly to the back of the frame to support the weight of the mirror.

You Will Need

Materials
pencil
thin card or paper
1 kg/2¼ lb modelling clay
3 mm/⅛ in thick circular mirror, cut to
15 cm/6 in in diameter
acrylic paints: deep turquoise, white, lemon-yellow and purple
matt varnish
hook
epoxy resin glue

Equipment
plate
rolling pin
clay modelling tools
paint-mixing container
paintbrushes

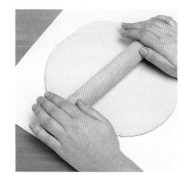

1 Draw around a plate on to thin card or paper to make a template. Roll out the clay to a large flat sheet 5 mm/¼ in thick. Cut two circles of clay.

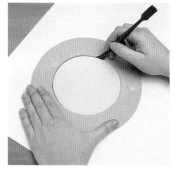

2 Place the mirror on one of the circles and cut around it. Fit the mirror between the two frames, stretching the clay over the edge of the mirror.

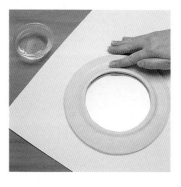

3 Bond the frame by pressing down through both layers with wet fingers at intervals around the outer edge, then smooth the inner and outer edges to leave a neat finish.

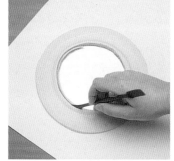

4 Trim the inner edge of the frame to leave an overlap of 5 mm/¼ in around the mirror. Neaten with a modelling tool.

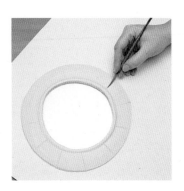

5 Wet and smooth the surface, then divide it into 12 equal sections by engraving straight lines with a wet modelling tool, working from the raised inner border to the edge of the frame.

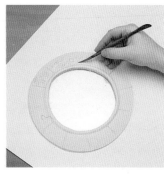

6 Engrave an astrological sign in each section of the frame, following the correct order as shown in the photograph. Allow to harden.

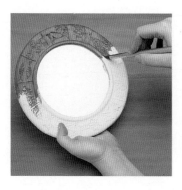

7 Mix turquoise, white and lemon paint, adding water to get a creamy consistency, and paint the frame in two thin coats, allowing the brush strokes to show through. Allow the first coat to dry before applying the second.

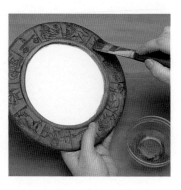

8 Mix purple and white paint, this time to a thicker texture, and apply with a wide dry brush so that the engraved figures and raised inner edge remain green. When dry, coat with a layer of clear varnish and attach the hook to the back with epoxy resin glue.

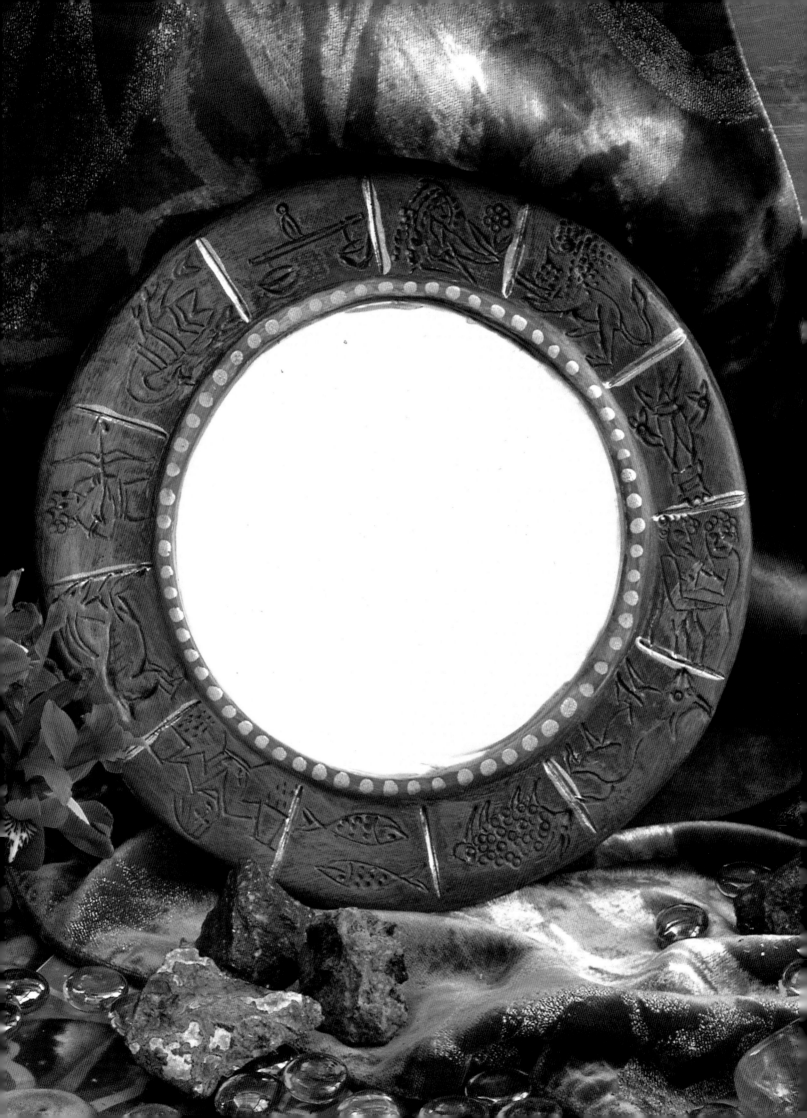

• MODELLING AND SALT DOUGH •

MODELLED MIRROR

A magical frame that uses up little odds and ends you have lying about the house. Use old buttons, beads, shells and even keys.

YOU WILL NEED

MATERIALS
*copper wire
strong glue
odds and ends to decorate,
such as shells, glass and
plastic nuggets
modelling clay
card template, outer
diameter 18 cm/7 in, inner
diameter 20 cm/4½ in
mirror, 9 cm/3½ in
in diameter
2 pieces of aluminium
tubing, 1 cm/½ in in
diameter, 20 cm/8 in long
small plastic drinks bottle
plaster of Paris
acrylic paints*

EQUIPMENT
*wire-cutters
round-nosed pliers
rolling pin
acetate sheet
clay modelling tool
craft knife
paintbrushes*

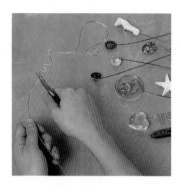

1 Cut the wire into lengths and curl into shapes. Glue odds and ends on one end of each wire. Bend the other ends to make a hook.

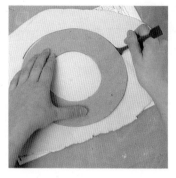

2 Roll out pieces of clay on the acetate sheet. Use the template to cut two circles, 18 cm/7 in in diameter. Cut a 11.5 cm/4½ in circle from one centre.

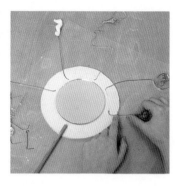

3 Place the mirror in the middle of the circle and arrange the wires around the edge, with the decorated ends outwards. Push the hooked ends into the clay. Put one aluminium tube in the position which you want to become the bottom of the mirror frame.

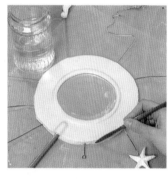

4 Place the clay ring on top and smooth off the overlap around the mirror and the tube with your finger and a little water. Smooth off the sides with the modelling tool. Decorate the front of the frame with small circles of clay. Allow to dry for several days.

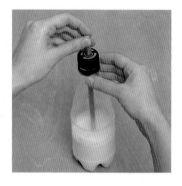

5 Cut the bottle in half and make four 5 cm/2 in cuts around the top half of the bottle. Make a hole in the lid. Mix enough plaster of Paris to half-fill the bottle base and pour it in. Push the top of the bottle part-way into the base and push the second aluminium tube through the hole in the bottle lid down into the plaster.

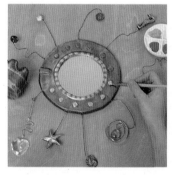

6 When dry, remove the plastic from the plaster. Remove the tube and fit the real tube and mirror into the plaster base. Paint the base, stand and frame with acrylic paints.

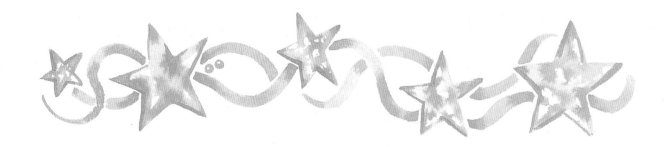

158

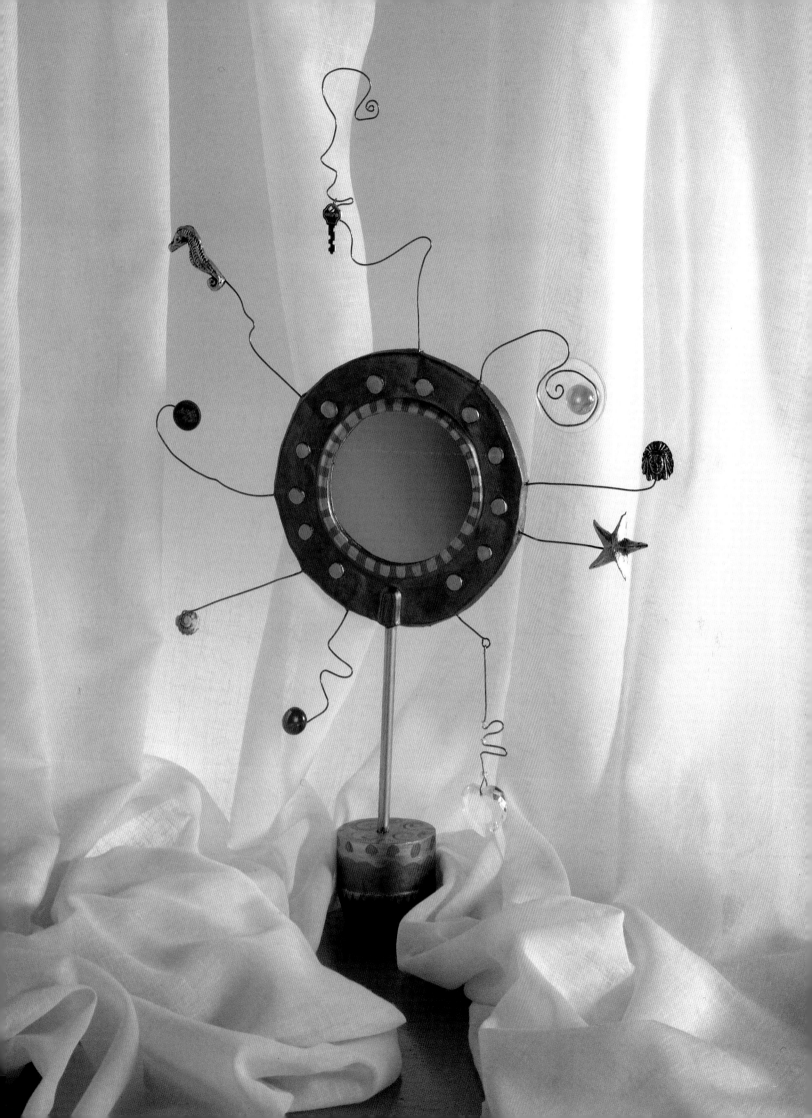

• MODELLING AND SALT DOUGH •

ANTIQUE WALL TILE

The subtle look of this charming tile is achieved very simply by staining it with tea; wiping the design with colour accentuates the relief and you can repeat it as many times as you like until you get the shade you desire.

YOU WILL NEED

MATERIALS	EQUIPMENT
tracing paper	pencil
450 g/1 lb modelling clay	rolling pin
tea bag	clay modelling tools
matt varnish	paintbrush

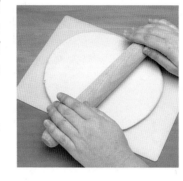

1 Trace the template from the back of the book, enlarging if necessary. Roll out the clay to a flat sheet 1 cm/½ in thick.

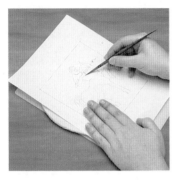

2 Place the tracing on top of the clay and mark all the lines using a modelling tool.

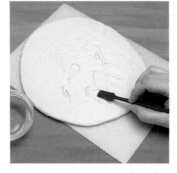

3 Wet the clay surface thoroughly to make it easier to manipulate. Indent the lines of the design, moulding the figure's body to raise it above the background area.

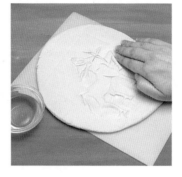

4 Smooth the surface with wet fingers as you work to keep the clay moist.

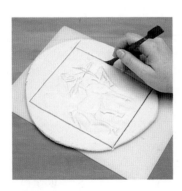

5 Cut out the tile shape and engrave a double border around the edge to frame the central motif.

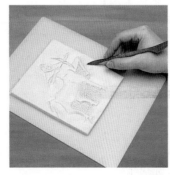

6 Stipple the background with the point of a wet modelling tool to create texture. Then leave the tile to harden completely before staining.

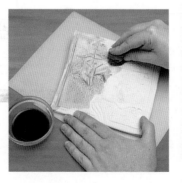

7 Brew a strong cup of tea with a tea bag and use it to stain the clay, wiping over the design with the tea bag. When you are satisfied with the colour, allow to dry, then protect the tile with a coat of matt varnish.

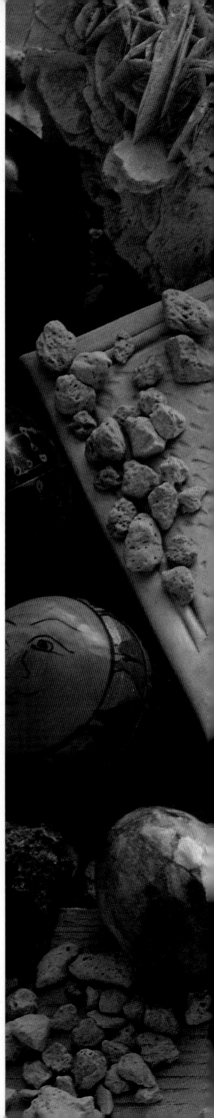

160

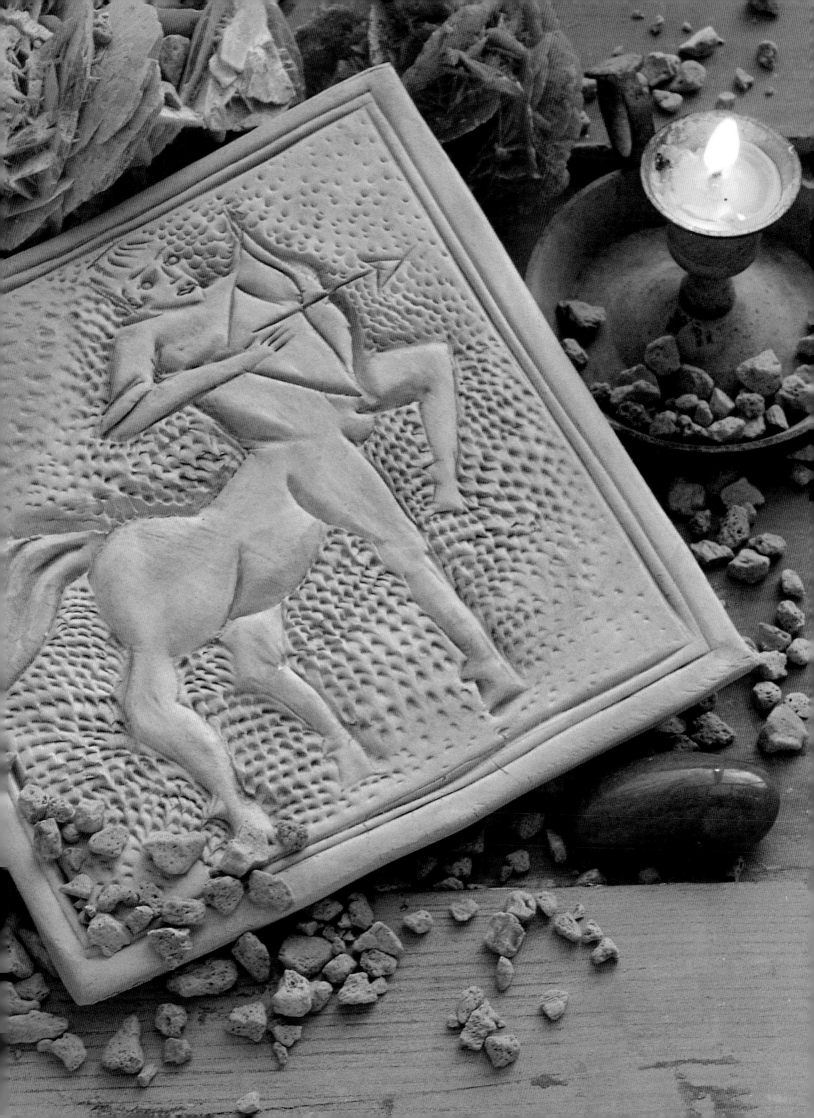

· MODELLING AND SALT DOUGH ·

DISPLAY CASE

This purpose-made unit suits the scale of shells and echoes their sinewy curves in its shape. It is the perfect way of displaying beautiful shells, as the aquamarine colour sets off the tints of the shells and is a reminder of the water that is their natural setting. The gold decoration, like sunlight on water, is the perfect finishing touch.

YOU WILL NEED

MATERIALS
tracing paper
thin card or paper
modelling clay
acrylic paints: turquoise,
white and lemon-yellow
gold powder
clear matt varnish
selection of seashells
epoxy resin glue

EQUIPMENT
pencil
rolling pin
polythene sheet (optional)
clay modelling tools
paint-mixing container
small flat-bristled and fine
paintbrushes

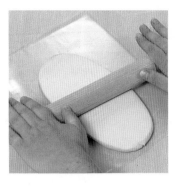

1 Trace the template from the back of the book, enlarging if necessary, and transfer to thin card or paper. Roll out the clay in an approximation of the swirl shape, to 8 mm/⅓ in thick. You may find it helpful to work on a sheet of polythene.

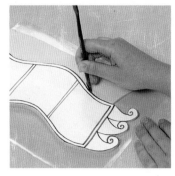

2 Lay the template on the clay and, with a wet modelling tool, cut out the shape for the back of the unit.

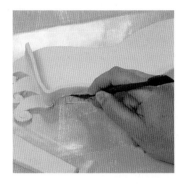

3 Roll out long clay snakes and cut them into rectangles about 2.5 cm/1 in wide, with perfectly straight edges, to make the side walls. Attach the walls to the back, moulding, smoothing the join with a wet modelling tool. Make a hole for hanging in the middle "wave" at the top.

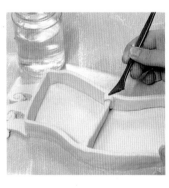

4 Roll out and cut shorter rectangles, for the shelves, and attach them to the back and the walls. Use a small piece of clay, smoothed over the joins, to strengthen them. Allow to dry for several days.

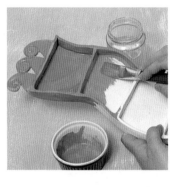

5 Mix the acrylic paints to make a sea-green colour. To achieve a slight verdigris effect, do not mix the colours too thoroughly. Paint the inside and outside of the display unit and allow to dry.

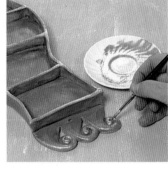

6 Mix the gold powder with varnish, varying the amount of varnish depending on the consistency you wish to achieve. Paint the edges of the display case and the waves gold, using a fine paintbrush.

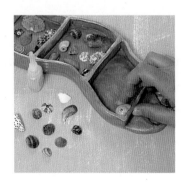

7 Working from the top down, arrange the shells in the compartments and glue them in position.

162

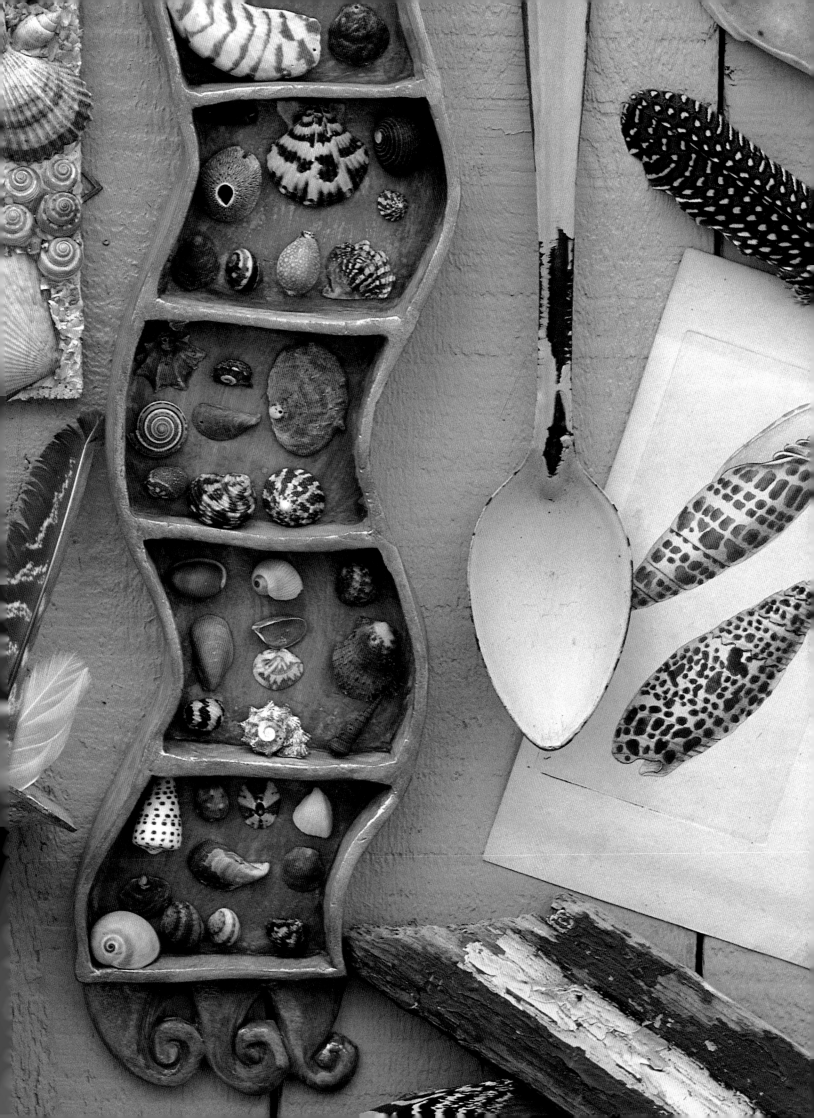

Salt Dough Basket

Make this delightful wall decoration from simple ingredients you are bound to have in your kitchen already. Salt dough is quite durable once it is varnished, but remember not to hang it anywhere damp or steamy as this may make it crumble slightly.

You Will Need

Materials

salt dough (see Salt Dough Recipe)
paper bowl
paperclip
aluminium foil
4 cloves
baking parchment
acrylic paints: green, white, yellow, orange, burnt sienna and black
polyurethane satin varnish

Equipment

rolling pin
craft knife
fork
scissors
cheese grater
heart-shaped pastry cutter
baking tray
paintbrushes

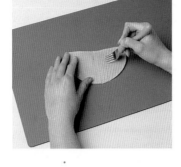

1 Roll out some salt dough to a thickness of 5 mm/¼ in. Cut out a large oval and a half oval. Mark a basket pattern on the dough with a fork.

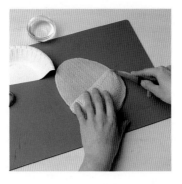

2 Cut the paper bowl in half and trim to fit the large oval. Place the half dough oval on top of the bowl, moisten the edges and stick to the large oval. Cut 2 cm/¾ in slits along the rim for the ribbon.

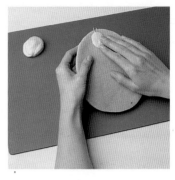

3 Use a thinly rolled piece of dough to attach a paperclip to the top of the basket on the reverse side.

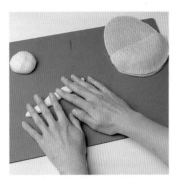

4 Roll out two long thin sausages of dough to fit down the side of the basket. Twist them together, moisten the surfaces and stick them to the edge. Make another twist for the other side. Trim and join invisibly at the top and overlap in a "knot" at the bottom of the basket. Make a smaller twisted length for the handle at the top.

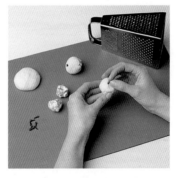

5 Roll four walnut-size balls of aluminium foil. Mould some dough over the foil and make two lemon shapes and two oranges. Roll the fruit over a fine grater to simulate the texture of the skin, and insert a clove at the top. Arrange the fruit inside the basket.

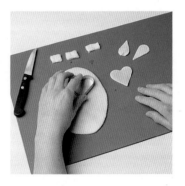

6 Roll out some more dough thinly. Cut small rectangles to fit between the slits to look like ribbon. Cut out four heart shapes, then cut them in half and trim to make leaves. Mark the veins with the point of the knife and shape them. Moisten and arrange around the fruit. Place the basket, on baking parchment, on a tray and bake at 120°C/250°F/Gas ½, for eight hours, or until the basket is hardened. Allow to cool.

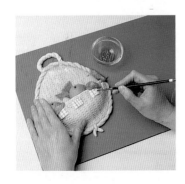

7 Paint the fruit with acrylic paints. Thin the green paint slightly and paint the leaves. Brush off some of the paint with a stiff, dry brush to add highlights. Paint the ribbon white, then allow to dry thoroughly. Paint in a gingham pattern with yellow, orange and green stripes.

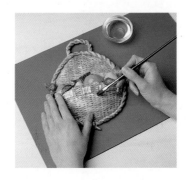

8 Paint the basket with a thin wash of burnt sienna mixed with a little black paint. Brush off the excess with a dry brush. Paint the completed basket with at least two coats of polyurethane satin varnish.

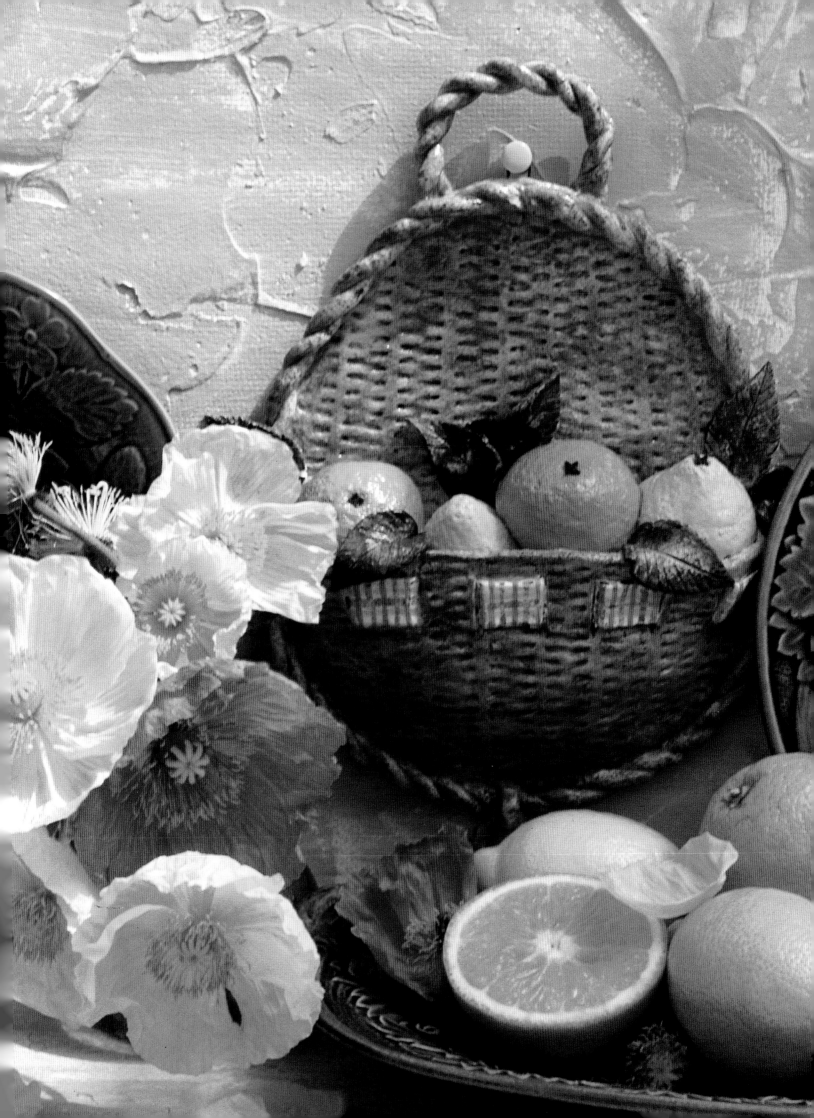

Folk Angel

This plaque-style angel is a perfect model to create from salt dough. On flat pieces of dough, the baking process takes place evenly through the sheet of dough, thus avoiding any hardening inconsistencies.

You Will Need

Materials	Equipment
tracing paper	pencil
salt dough (see Salt Dough Recipe)	scissors
baking parchment	rolling pin
watercolour paints	craft knife
polyurethane matt varnish	dressmaker's pin
coloured string or fine ribbon	wire-cutters
	paperclip
	baking tray
	paintbrushes

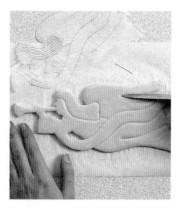

1. Trace the template from the back of the book, enlarging if necessary, and cut out. Roll out the salt dough on baking parchment to 1 cm/½ in thick. Place the template on the dough and cut out the shape. Remove the template and pat the cut edges with a moistened finger to neaten them. Replace the template and transfer the details of the design by pricking along the lines with a pin, working on one layer at a time. Lightly moisten the pricked line, then draw along it with the tip of the knife, leaning the blade towards you then away from you to make an inverted division. Prick and indent all the lines.

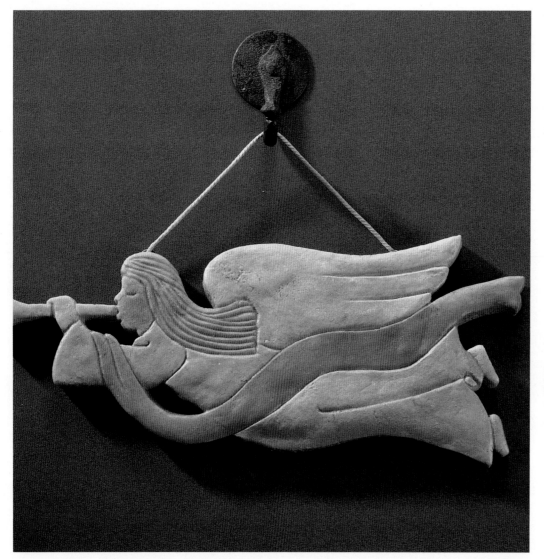

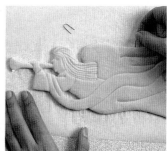

2. Cut a paperclip in half and insert the two outer halves into the edges at the crosses, leaving the loops visible. Bake at 120°C/250°F/Gas ½, for ten hours. Allow to cool.

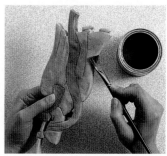

3. Apply the paint thinly to the model, lightening the colours with white. Leave the flesh areas unpainted, but highlight the cheek in pink. Allow to dry. Apply five coats of varnish. Hang up the angel.

• MODELLING AND SALT DOUGH •

Shaker Hand

The unpainted salt dough of this open, friendly hand gives it an amazingly lifelike appearance. The bordered heart motif is typical of the influential Shaker style founded in 18th-century America.

You Will Need

Materials
salt dough (see Salt Dough Recipe)
baking parchment
eyelet loop
polyurethane matt varnish

Equipment
rolling pin
knitting needle
craft knife
heart-shaped cutter (optional)
clay modelling tool
baking tray
paintbrush

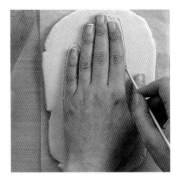 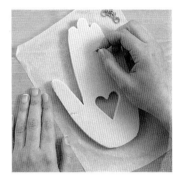

1 Roll out the salt dough on to baking parchment to a thickness of 1.5 cm/⅝ in. Lay your hand flat on to the dough with your fingers together. Use a knitting needle to trace around the edge and mark your fingers, then cut out the outline with a craft knife. Pat the cut edges with a moistened finger to round them.

2 Cut out a heart shape from the palm, either cutting freehand or using a pastry cutter. Turn the hand over and insert an eyelet loop for hanging it up. Bake at 120°C/250°F/Gas ½, for ten hours. Allow to dry, then apply five coats of varnish.

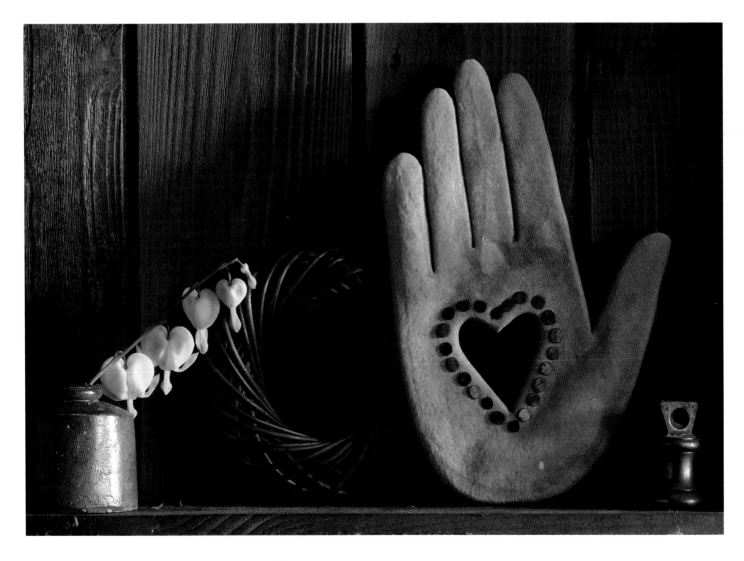

• MODELLING AND SALT DOUGH •

SALT AND PEPPER POTS

A request to pass the salt will be the starting signal for these eager mobile ladybirds to wheel their way down the table to you. They're based on toy trucks with a friction drive, and are sure to be a big hit at family mealtimes.

YOU WILL NEED

MATERIALS	EQUIPMENT
pair of matching toy trucks	screwdriver
stiff card	pencil
matching salt and pepper pots	scissors
polymer clay: black, red and white	rolling pin
coloured paperclips	craft knife
epoxy resin glue	pliers
clear gloss varnish	paintbrushes
enamel paints: red and black	

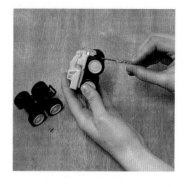

1 Undo the fixing screws and remove the body from each toy truck.

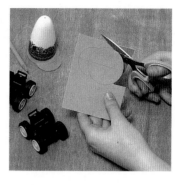

2 Mark out two matching templates on card which will fit over the truck chassis and around the bases of the salt and pepper pots, leaving a rim of about 5 mm/¼ in. Cut them out.

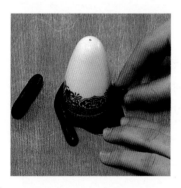

3 Roll a piece of black clay thinly to cover the template. Cut to shape. Stand the salt cellar in position on the base and mould a sausage of clay around it.

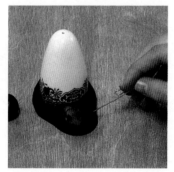

4 Press a ball of clay on to the front of the template and mould it into shape for the head of the ladybird. Make two holes for the feelers with the end of a paperclip. Remove the pot and template carefully. Make a matching base for the pepper pot in the same way.

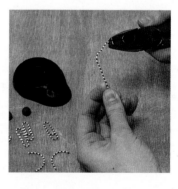

5 Straighten out the paperclips and trim to length to make the feelers. Roll out four small balls of red clay and make a hole in each one with a paperclip. Mould two pairs of eyes from white and black clay.

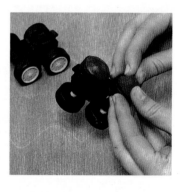

6 Roll a ball of red clay for each truck wheel and press it on, moulding it into a dome shape. Remove carefully.

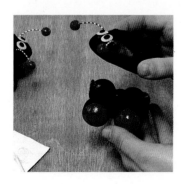

7 Bake the clay elements in a low oven, following the manufacturer's instructions. Fix everything in place with epoxy resin glue, avoiding the drive mechanism in the truck chassis. Varnish the wheel hubs and allow to dry.

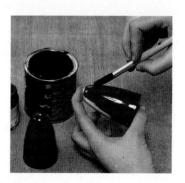

8 Paint the salt and pepper pots in bright red. Allow to dry, then add ladybird spots in black. Allow to dry.

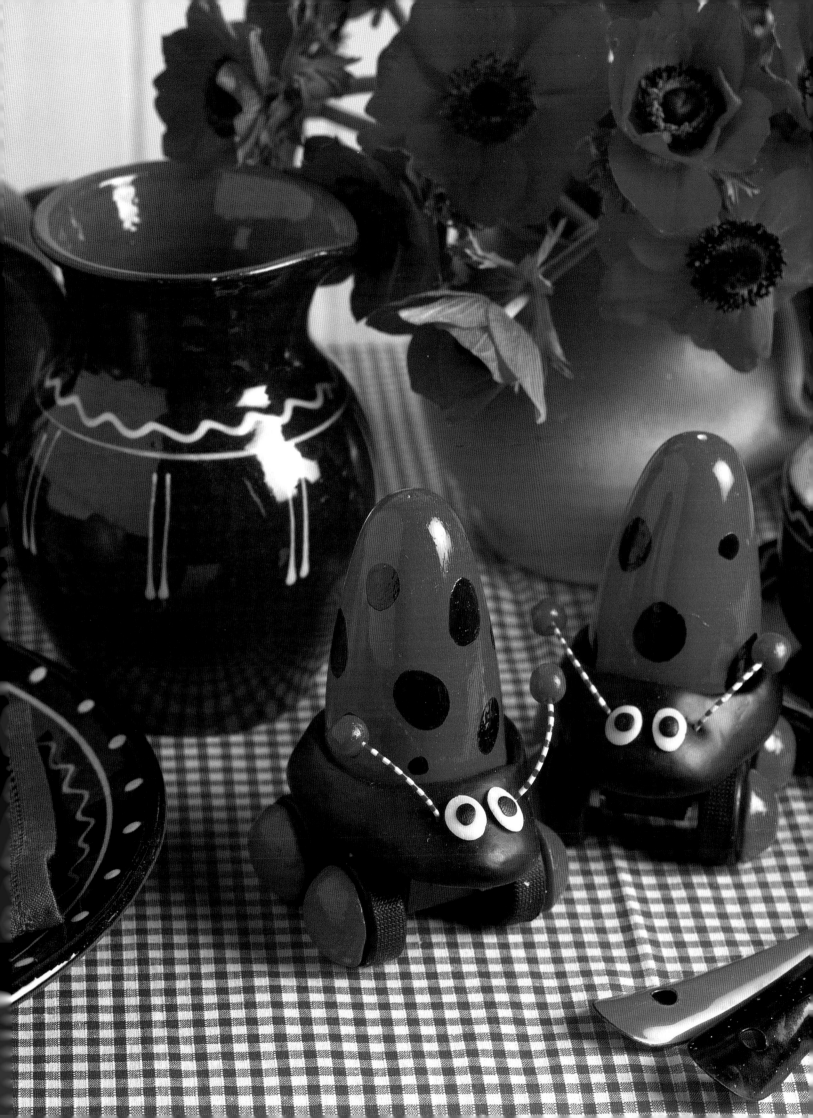

MODELLING AND SALT DOUGH

WINGED HEART

This salt dough wall decoration is a charming way to tell someone absent that you are thinking of them – with a heart that has, literally, taken wing.

YOU WILL NEED

MATERIALS	EQUIPMENT
salt dough (see Salt Dough Recipe)	*pencil*
baking parchment	*scissors*
aluminium foil	*rolling pin*
2 screw eyes	*craft knife*
acrylic paints: red, white, black, green, blue and gold	*clay modelling tools*
clear varnish	*sponge*
length of cord	*paint mixing container*
	small and fine paintbrushes

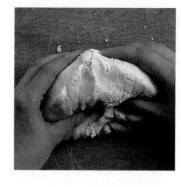

1 Follow the instructions to make the salt dough (see Salt Dough Recipe). Trace the template from the back of the book, enlarging if necessary, on to baking parchment and cut it out.

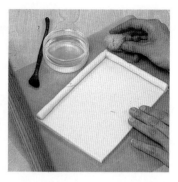

2 Roll about two-thirds of the dough on to a sheet of baking parchment so that it is about 5 mm/¼ in thick. Put the template on the dough and cut around it with a craft knife. Make a thin roll of dough to fit each side of the background. Moisten the edges and put the rolls in place. Smooth the joints with a modelling tool and finish by moulding a small dough heart for each corner.

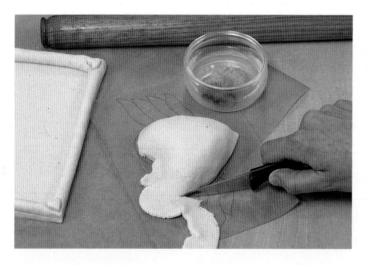

3 Using the template as a guide, mould a solid heart shape from foil. Roll out some dough to 5 mm/¼ in thick and place it over the foil heart. Trim the edges and place the heart in the centre of the background. Smooth with a damp sponge. Roll out some more dough to 5 mm/¼ in thick. Cut out the wing templates from the baking parchment and place them on the dough. Cut around the edges with a modelling tool and make the feather divisions. Moisten the backs and then put them on to the background and smooth the edges.

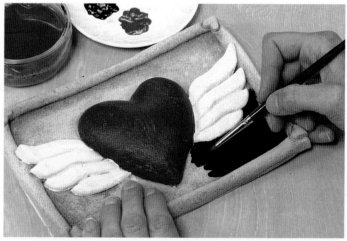

4 Bake the clay heart at 120°C/250°F/Gas ½, for two hours and then remove it and carefully insert the screw eyes on the back, one at each side. Return to the oven for at least six hours, or until it is completely hard. Allow to cool. Paint the heart red, the wings white and background black. Following the template and picture, decorate the heart with a painted daisy chain and add feathery markings to the wings. Highlight with gold paint and then finish with at least two coats of varnish, to protect the dough. When dry, thread the cord through the screw eyes, so you can hang it on the wall.

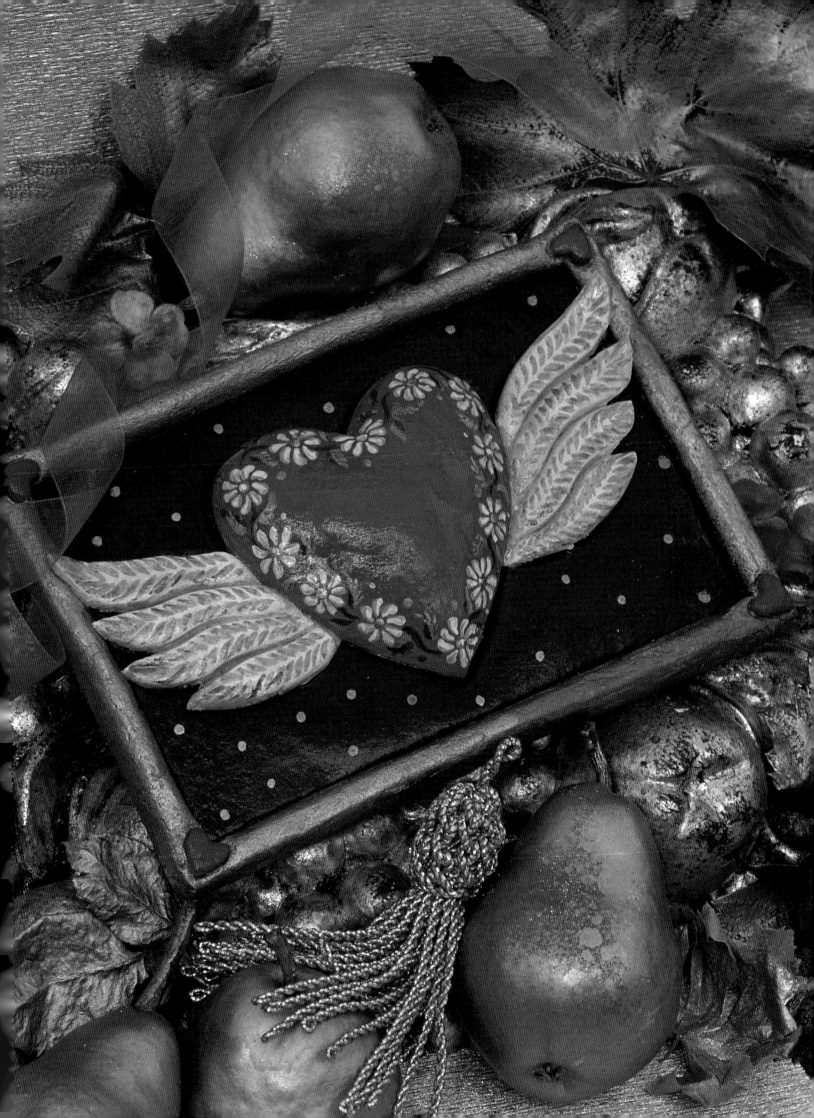

• MODELLING AND SALT DOUGH •

LOVE BUG

A most lovable insect, with a heart-shaped body – this is perfect for giving a friend as a token of your affection.

YOU WILL NEED

MATERIALS

copper wire
tracing paper
thin copper sheet
modelling clay
red acrylic paint
clear varnish
gold powder

EQUIPMENT

round-nosed pliers
pencil
tin snips
rolling pin
acetate sheet
clay modelling tools
small paintbrushes

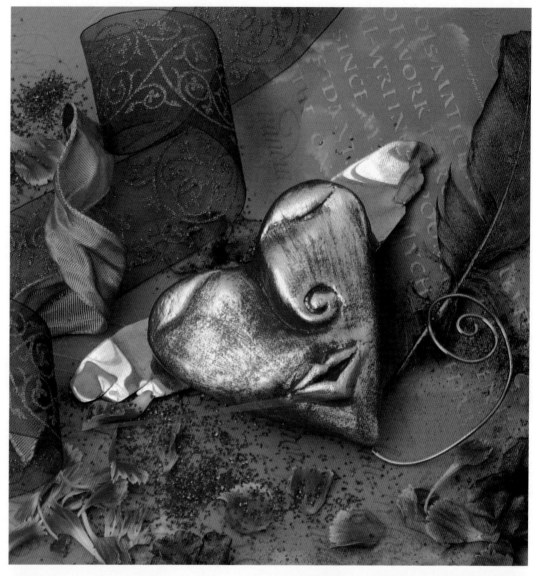

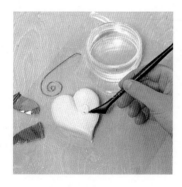

1 Curl the wire. Trace the templates from the back of the book, enlarging if necessary. Trace two wings on to the copper sheet and cut out with tin snips. Roll out the clay on the sheet. Cut out a heart with a wet modelling tool and model the face.

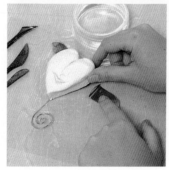

2 Stick the wings and wire curl into the clay and allow to dry for several days.

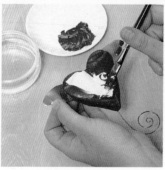

3 Paint the love bug red and allow to dry. Then give it a coat of varnish.

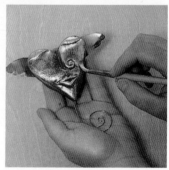

4 With a dry brush, apply gold powder mixed with a little varnish, to finish.

Wall Decoration

Salt dough is a great medium for making architectural-style reliefs. This charming "bronze" wall plaque can easily be incorporated into an interior scheme – or simply used for decoration.

You Will Need

Materials
baking parchment
salt dough (see Salt Dough Recipe)
paperclip
white acrylic primer
acrylic paints: verdigris and bronze

Equipment
pencil
clay modelling tools
flat pliers
scissors
medium and fine paintbrushes
small sponge

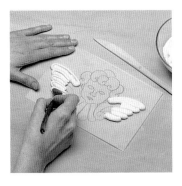

1 Trace the template from the back of the book, enlarging if necessary, on to baking parchment. For the outer wings, make ten thin rolls of salt dough. Moisten the edges and press them gently together on the template. Use a flat-edged modelling tool to make some "feathers".

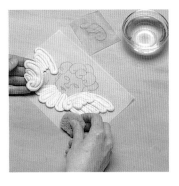

2 Shape the inner wing to fit the parchment outline. Moisten the back of the wing and press it gently in place. Make the face and hair in the same way, shaping the pieces separately and pressing them in place. Cut the paperclip in half with the pliers. Press one piece into the top of the cupid's head for hanging.

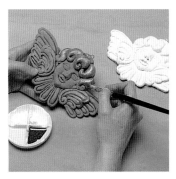

3 Bake the decoration at 120°C/250°F/Gas ½, for at least eight hours. Trim the baking parchment and allow to cool. Leaving to dry between each stage, paint with white acrylic primer, then with the verdigris paint. To complete, burnish the raised details with bronze paint.

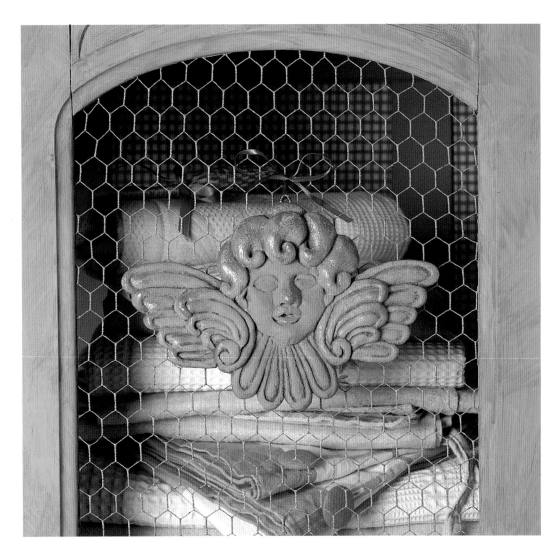

· MODELLING AND SALT DOUGH ·

Cornucopia

A wealth of dusky painted fruit seems to burst from the natural dough base. This harvest cornucopia follows the traditional salt dough theme of natural objects used to decorate the home.

You Will Need

Materials	Equipment
tracing paper	*pencil*
salt dough (see Salt Dough Recipe)	*scissors*
baking parchment	*rolling pin*
2 cloves	*craft knife*
eyelet loop	*dressmaker's pin*
watercolour inks	*clay modelling tools*
polyurethane matt varnish	*knitting needle*
	baking tray
	paintbrushes

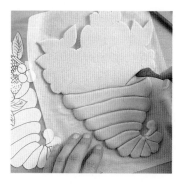

1 Trace the template from the back of the book, enlarging if necessary. Roll the dough out on baking parchment to a thickness of 8 mm/⅜ in. Place the template on the dough and cut around it. Prick out the design with a pin.

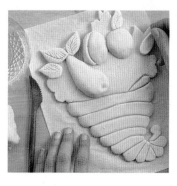

2 Shape a pear, plum and apple from dough, following the template. Moisten with water and press into place. Shape the leaves, with veins, moisten them with water and press into position.

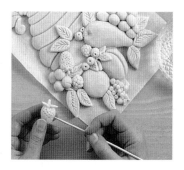

3 Mould grapes, blackberries, cherries, nuts, redcurrants and strawberries. Use a knitting needle to add detail. Moisten each shape and press in place. Make stalks as shown and insert a clove into the bases of the apple and pear.

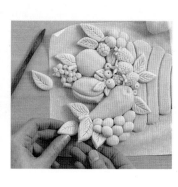

4 Attach four leaves to the underside of the cornucopia. Press an eyelet loop into the back and bake at 120°C/250°F/Gas ½, for 20 hours. Cool, then paint. When dry, apply five coats of varnish.

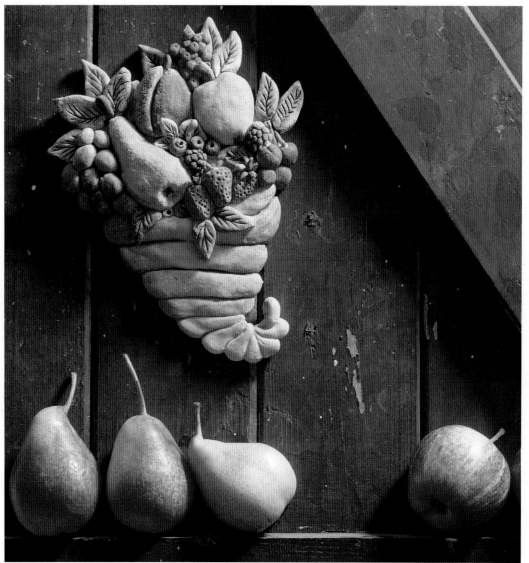

174

• MODELLING AND SALT DOUGH •

Checkered Heart

This heart takes its inspiration from traditional Scandinavian folk art. Although seeming to be separate pieces, the salt dough "squares" are actually formed by deep indentations.

You Will Need

Materials

tracing paper
salt dough (see Salt Dough Recipe)
baking parchment
gold paperclips
acrylic gesso or matt emulsion (latex) paint
cherry-red acrylic or craft paint
polyurethane matt varnish
coloured raffia

Equipment

pencil
rolling pin
dressmaker's pin
craft knife
wire-cutters
baking tray
paintbrushes

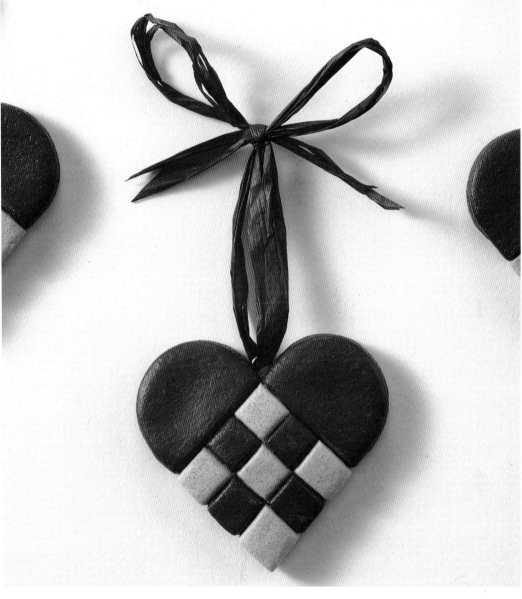

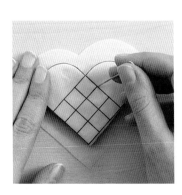

1 Trace the template from the back of the book, enlarging if necessary, and cut out. Roll the dough out on baking parchment to 1 cm/½ in thick. Cover with the template and mark the squares with a pin.

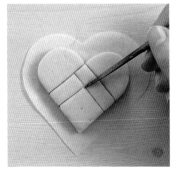

2 Neaten the cut edge by patting it with a moistened finger to round and smooth it. Indent lines on the heart, following the pricked marks, leaning the knife first towards you and then away.

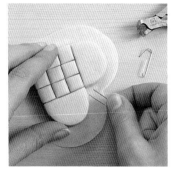

3 Cut a paperclip in half and insert it into the top of the heart. Make two or three more hearts in the same way. Bake on the parchment paper on a tray at 120°C/250°F/ Gas ½, for nine hours.

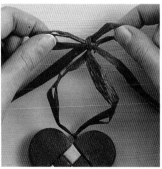

4 Paint with acrylic gesso or emulsion (latex), then paint in cherry-red, leaving alternate squares plain. Allow to dry. Apply five coats of varnish. Thread some raffia through each loop and tie in a bow.

· MODELLING AND SALT DOUGH ·

Gingerbread Cupids

W*hat better token of your affection than a gift of these gilded cherubs? They taste as delicious as they look, and they make excellent decorations.*

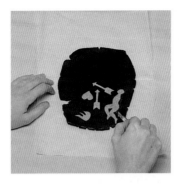 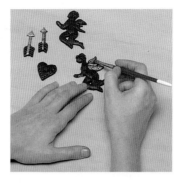 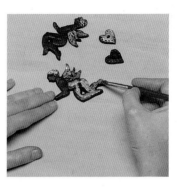

You Will Need

Materials

350 g/12 oz/3 cups plain white flour
15 ml/1 tbsp ground ginger
7.5 ml/½ tbsp ground cinnamon
2.5 ml/½ tsp grated nutmeg
75 g/3 oz/6 tbsp butter, cut into small pieces
50 g/2 oz/4 tbsp soft brown sugar
225 g/8 oz/1 cup black treacle
baking parchment
powdered food colouring: silver and gold

Equipment

mixing bowl
wooden spoon
rolling pin
pencil
scissors
craft knife
baking tray
saucer
spoon
fine paintbrush

1 Place the dough between two sheets of parchment and roll out very thinly. Trace the templates from the back of the book on to baking parchment, cut out and place on the dough, then cut out. Join the sections and mark on details. Place on baking parchment on a baking tray. Bake at 180°C/350°F/Gas 4 for 10–15 minutes. Leave to cool.

2 Mix each food colouring with water, to make a paste. The easiest way is to tip some on to a saucer, add a drop of water and grind into a paste with the bowl of a spoon. Paint the wings and the centre of the arrows silver.

3 Paint the body, the hearts and the flights of the arrows with gold paste. Allow to dry thoroughly.

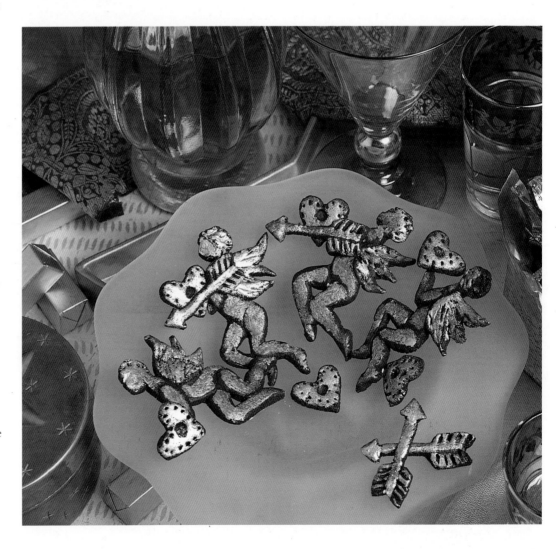

To make the dough

Sieve the flour and spices into a mixing bowl. Add the butter and rub it in with your fingers, until the mixture looks like fine breadcrumbs. Stir in the sugar. Make a well in the centre and pour in the treacle. Mix well and beat until the mixture comes away from the sides of the bowl. Knead until smooth.

• MODELLING AND SALT DOUGH •

COOKIE HEARTS

Delicious to eat – or you can double-bake them to use as decorations.

YOU WILL NEED

MATERIALS
dough (see Gingerbread Cupids)
baking parchment
white royal icing
garden twine
homespun cotton
checked fabric
clear glue or glue gun
cotton gingham fabric
buttons
ribbons
picture-hanging hook
card (optional)

EQUIPMENT
rolling pin
selection of heart-shaped cookie cutters
baking tray
piping bag, with fine icing nozzle
bradawl or skewer
scissors

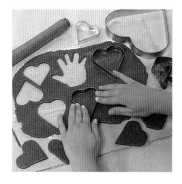

1 Make the dough as for Gingerbread Cupids. Roll out the dough thinly and evenly on a floured board. Cut out the shapes and place on baking parchment on a baking tray. Bake at 180°C/350°F/Gas 4 for 10–15 minutes. Make a hole for hanging while warm, then allow to cool completely.

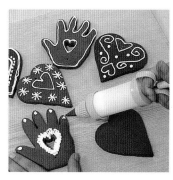

2 For edible cookies, decorate them with white royal icing, using a piping bag and a fine icing nozzle.

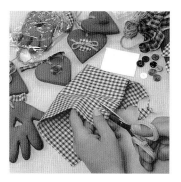

3 If the cookies are not to be eaten, put them back in a low oven for a couple of hours to dry them out. String some together with garden twine. Make bows for tying from checked fabric for some; cut out heart motifs and glue them on others. Do the same with the gingham. Decorate the ties with buttons and ribbons. Use the bradawl to decorate the cookies with a pattern of holes (or do this with a skewer before baking). If the cookie breaks, repair the damage with glue. To make a cookie for hanging on the wall, glue a picture-hanging hook on the back. Large cookies need careful handling and you can glue pieces of card on to the backs, to reinforce them.

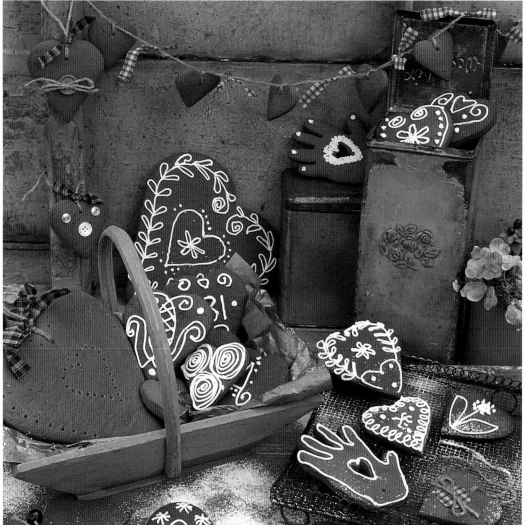

• MODELLING AND SALT DOUGH •

Metal Embedded Bowl

These rustic bowls have the appearance of weather-worn stone. The heat-resistant qualities of metal provide an exciting source of decorative materials to use with salt dough – here, coins, bronze decorations, jewellery, wire and copper motifs are all embedded in the dough.

You Will Need

Materials
cooking fat or vegetable oil
salt dough (see Salt Dough Recipe)
baking parchment
fine copper sheet
metal for embedding, such as jewellery accessories, coins and bonsai wire
paper
watercolour paints
metallic craft paints
polyurethane satin varnish
PVA (white) glue
jewellery stones

Equipment
2 ovenproof bowls
rolling pin
craft knife
old pair of scissors
baking tray
pair of compasses
pencil
ruler
paintbrushes
paint-mixing container
natural sponge

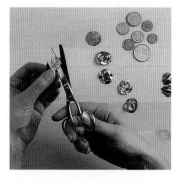

1 Smear the upturned bowls with cooking fat or oil. Roll two pieces of dough on baking parchment to 1 cm/½ in thick. Lift each piece of dough over a bowl and smooth it down. Cut the edges level. To make spirals, cut rough circles from a sheet of copper, then cut into spirals. Press your chosen metal pieces into the dough. Bake at 120°C/250°F/Gas ½, for nine hours, removing the bowls once the dough has dried completely.

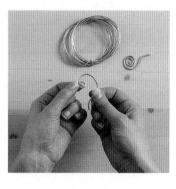

2 To make a flat lid, draw a circle on paper, 2 cm/¾ in larger than the dough bowl. Cut out the circle to use as a template. Roll some more dough out to 1 cm/½ in thick and cut a circle with the template. Roll a ball of dough, moisten it and press to the centre. Smooth the edges and join it to the lid. Coil two lengths of bonsai wire and bend the ends downwards to form two halves of a heart for the handle.

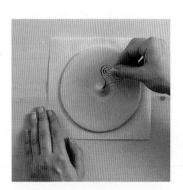

3 Insert the metal handle ends into the centre of the lid. Transfer the lid, on the parchment paper, to a tray and bake as before for five hours, until it is almost hardened. Measure across the dough bowl between the inner edges. Draw a circle on paper with a diameter 1 cm/½ in less than that of the measurement. Cut out and use as a template to cut a circle from dough.

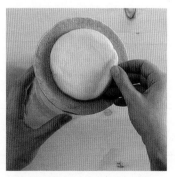

4 Upturn the baked lid and support it on the ovenproof bowl. Moisten the back of the lid and place the smaller circle on top. Return to the oven for five hours until completely hardened.

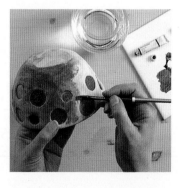

5 Paint the bowls and lid, blending your chosen colours with black or white to dull the colours. Lightly dab the bowls with metallic paints, using a sponge. Allow to dry, then apply five coats of varnish. Glue jewellery stones to the metal decorations.

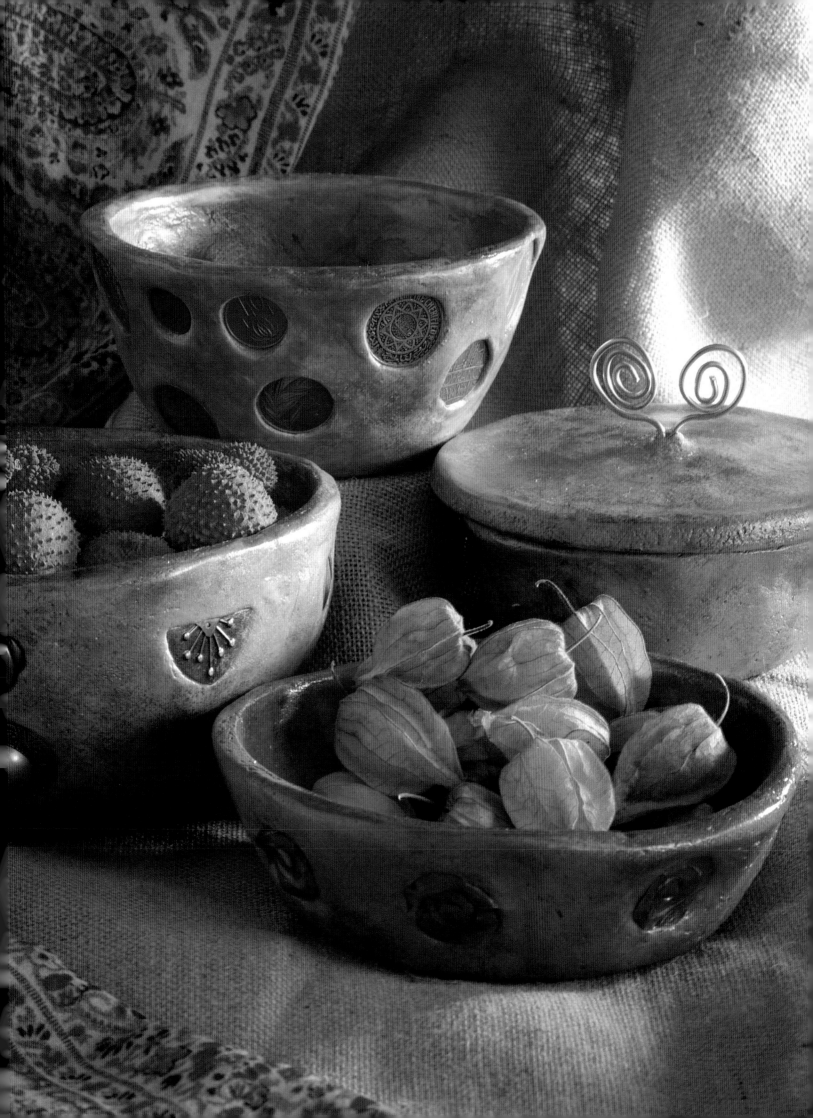

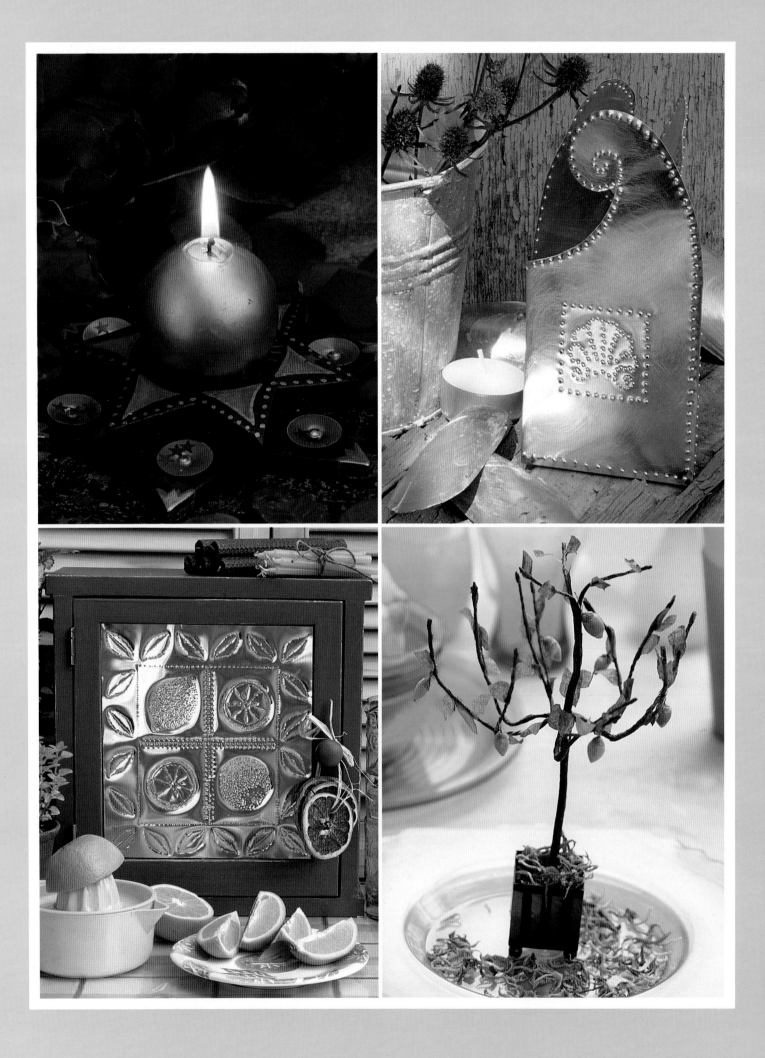

Wood, Wire and Tinwork

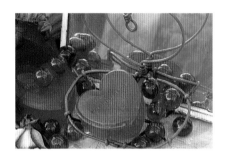

Wood, wire and tin are all everyday materials that can be obtained quite readily. With the recent revival of interest in folk art, wood and tin particularly have had a remarkable resurgence of popularity, and many artefacts, particularly those made from recycled materials, are now being produced in craft workshops throughout the country. Wood, wire and tin can all be formed into products either following a traditional or a contemporary style, and their versatility makes them a popular medium for many craftspeople.

The nature of the materials means that some of the projects require you to wear protective clothing, and some solvents can be very strong, so always work in a well-ventilated area and ensure that children do not get too close.

The projects in this section provide comprehensive instructions if you are a newcomer, but they also aim to inspire the more experienced to experiment and develop the true potential of these exciting craft forms.

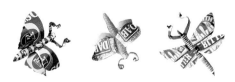

Materials and Equipment

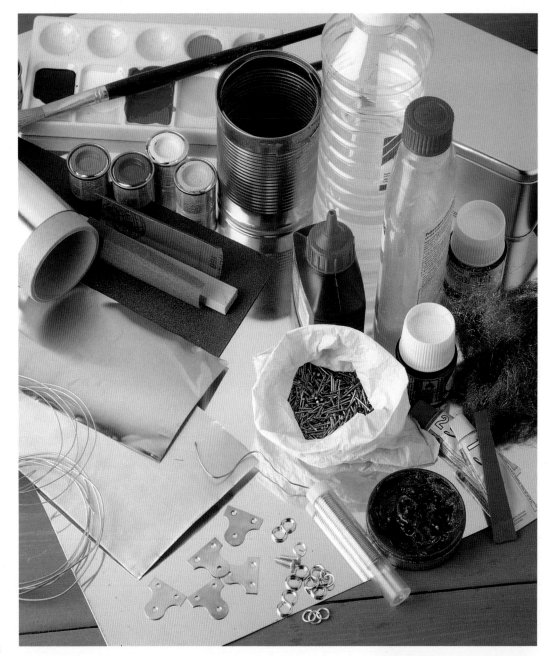

To complete the projects in this book, you can obtain most of the materials and equipment from craft suppliers and hardware shops. For tin plate, metal foils and sheet metals, you will need to visit a metal supplier or, if you wish to opt for recycled materials, a metal merchant or scrap yard dealer. Sheet metal, whether cut or uncut, is extremely sharp and should only be handled when protective leather gloves and a work shirt are worn. The following lists some of the materials you will need for working with wood, tin and wire.

Epoxy resin glue comes in two parts. Only mix up as much glue as you need at one time as it dries very quickly and is wasted otherwise. Once the glue has set firm, which takes about 24 hours, the join is very strong.

Fine wire is used to join pieces of metal together and as a decoration.

A flux is used during soldering to make the area to be soldered chemically clean. As the flux is heated, it runs along the metal, thus preparing the surface so the solder runs smoothly and adheres properly.

Hammers come in a variety of sizes, so always choose the appropriate hammer to suit the project.

Metal foils are thin sheet metals that usually come on rolls in 15 cm/6 in and 30 cm/12 in wide strips. Metal foil is so thin that it can be cut with a pair of household scissors.

Pliers are useful for holding wire and tin when you are cutting them and also for turning over edges.

Protective clothing such as leather gloves and a work shirt should be worn when cutting metals and wire and sawing wood. A mask and goggles are also needed for soldering. Children should be kept away from this work.

Saws are vital for cutting wood. The most useful varieties are a fretsaw, a coping saw and a jigsaw.

Solder is an alloy, or mixture, of metals. Solder is used to join two pieces of metal together by providing a filler of liquid metal between the surfaces. Always follow the manufacturer's instructions carefully when using solder. Solder is applied with a **soldering iron.**

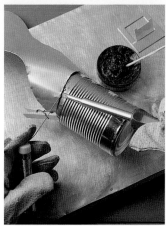

• Wood, Wire and Tinwork •

Materials and Equipment

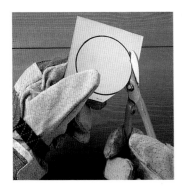

Tin plate is generally used in place of pure tin sheet, which is very expensive. Tin plate is mild sheet steel that has been coated with tin. The tin plating is very bright and will not tarnish in the open air or in humid conditions. Sheet metals come in different thicknesses, or gauges. The higher the gauge, the thinner the metal.

Tin snips and **shears** are needed to cut sheet metal. Try to find a pair with a spring mechanism to open and close the blades.

White spirit is useful for removing excess flux after soldering.

Wire cutters are invaluable for cutting lengths of wire to size.

Wood glue is very strong PVA (white) glue. It is white but becomes clear once it has dried.

OPPOSITE AND BELOW *You'll need quite a few specialist tools for wire and tinwork. But whatever the medium, each project gives clear guidance on the equipment required.*

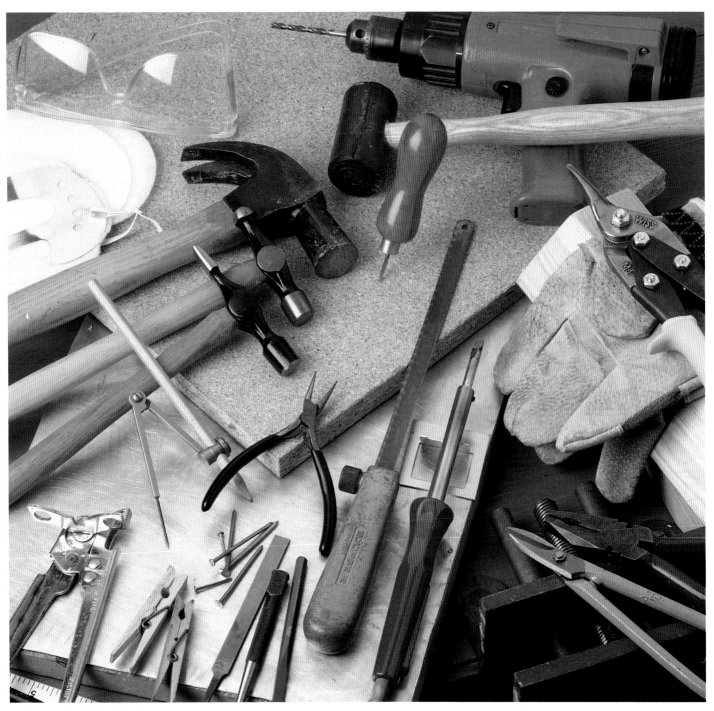

· Wood, Wire and Tinwork ·

Amish Sewing Box

This simply painted box, plain and practical, catches the spirit of Amish crafts.

You Will Need

Materials
*plain wood box
emulsion (latex) paints: duck-egg blue, brick-red and beige
clear water-based varnish
acrylic paints: raw sienna and burnt umber
white knob*

Equipment
*paintbrushes
cloth
screwdriver*

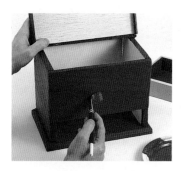

1 Paint the inside of the box with two coats of duck-egg blue. Paint a base coat of red on the outside of the box and beige on the front drawer.

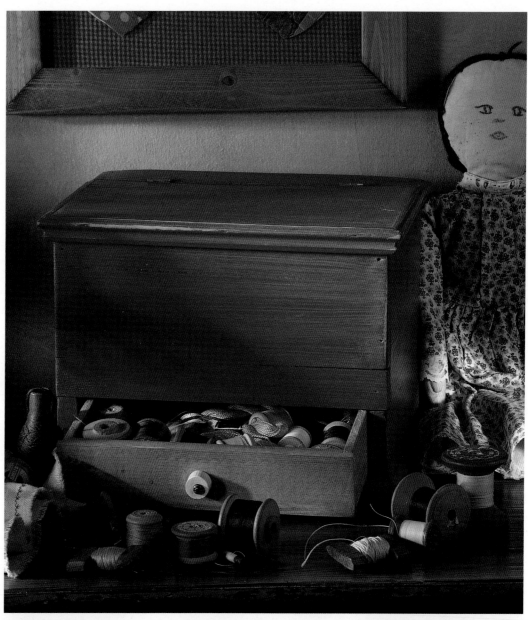

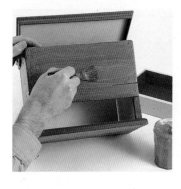

2 Tint the varnish with a small squeeze of raw sienna and burnt umber and paint the outside of the box. Apply it with a thick-bristled brush, using pressure to leave strokes visible.

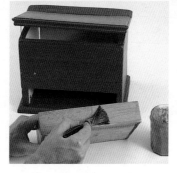

3 Apply the same varnish over the beige base coat on the drawer and while it is still wet, use a dry thick-bristled brush to lift some of the glaze to imitate woodgrain.

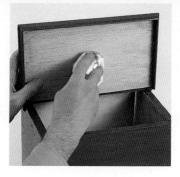

4 Apply a coat of tinted varnish to the inside, and while it is still wet, wipe off patches of it with a damp cloth to imitate wear and tear. Varnish over the whole box.

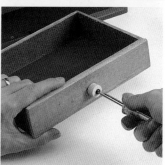

5 Screw on the white knob. If you have bought a new one, try making it look a bit scruffy by scratching on the surface and rubbing it with some burnt umber to age it.

• Wood, Wire and Tinwork •

Punched Tin Panel

Tin-punching is a satisfying and stylish way to transform a panelled door. The graphic outline of the citrus slices and the pitted texture of the peel make the fruits appropriate motifs for this treatment.

You Will Need

Materials	Equipment
tracing paper	pencil
small cupboard with	scissors
panelled door	hammer
3 mm/⅛ in tin sheet, to fit	steel punch
inside door panel	
sheet of card	
masking tape	
strong clear glue	

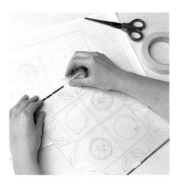

1 Trace the template from the back of the book, enlarging to fit your door panel. Lay the tin sheet on some card and attach the traced design using masking tape.

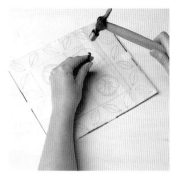

2 Starting with the square boxes around the fruit, hammer the steel punch every 2 mm/¹⁄₁₆ in to make a small dent. Hammer the larger dents to either side of the centre lines. Hammer small dents along all the fruit and leaf outlines.

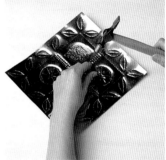

3 Remove the tracing paper and fill in the whole fruit shapes with dents. Fill in the outer rims of the lemon slices with small dents.

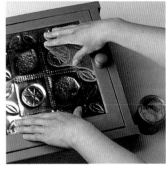

4 Spread strong glue over the back of the tin and on the cupboard panel. Leave until tacky, then glue in position.

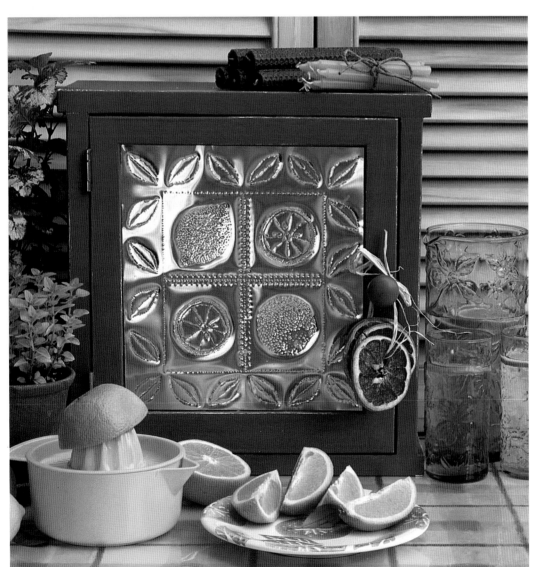

• Wood, Wire and Tinwork •

Ornamental Tree

This tiny ornamental tree will perfume your room with the invigorating aroma of lemon oil.

You Will Need

Materials
florist's medium stub wires
brown florist's tape
modelling clay
yellow acrylic paint
fine brass wire
green crepe paper
tracing paper
thin card
PVA (white) glue
4 small wooden beads
dark green gloss paint
sand or gravel
cotton wool
pure lemon oil
orange and lemon peel

Equipment
wire-cutters or old scissors
paintbrushes
pencil
scissors

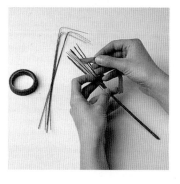

1 Trim 15 pieces of stub wire to a length of 23 cm/9 in. Bind them all together with brown florist's tape for the first 12 cm/4¾ in, then bind each projecting end in turn. Divide the wires into pairs, and bind each pair part way up. Bend them out from the trunk, then inwards to shape the tree.

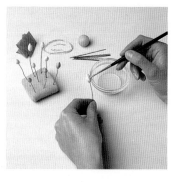

2 Make tiny lemons from clay, spike them on to wire and paint yellow. When dry, replace the wire supports with a loop of fine brass wire, covering the join with green crepe paper.

3 Trace the template from the back of the book, enlarging if necessary, and transfer to card. Make up the box by folding along the lines. Glue, then glue a bead to each corner. Paint dark green. Make a card tube to fit the trunk and glue into the centre of the box. Fill the box with sand or gravel and top with cotton wool.

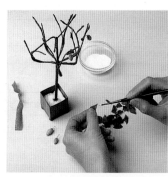

4 Cut the leaves out of green crepe paper. Attach the lemons and leaves to the branches. Drip lemon oil on to the cotton wool and cover with orange and lemon peel.

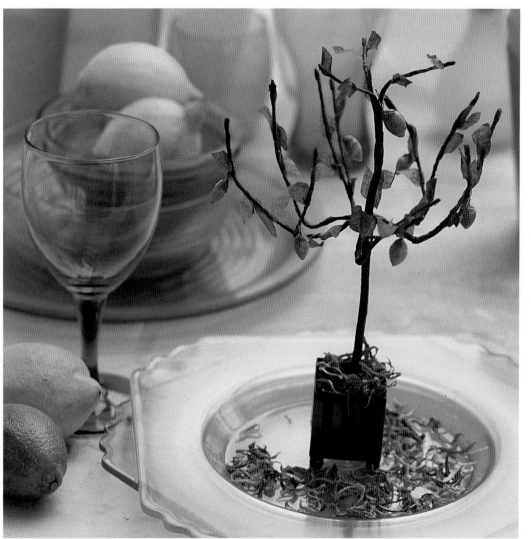

· Wood, Wire and Tinwork ·

Wooden Sheep Sign

*P*ainted signs were a common sight outside shops and taverns in eighteenth-century towns. Here, you can create your own distinct sign.

You Will Need

Materials	Equipment
tracing paper	pencil
5 mm/¼ in plywood,	coping saw or jigsaw
90 x 60 cm/36 x 24 in	paintbrushes
off-white emulsion (latex) paint	stencil brush
acrylic paints: burnt umber,	
deep grass-green and black	
coarse-grade sandpaper	
clear matt water-based	
varnish	
artist's acrylic paints: raw	
umber and raw sienna	

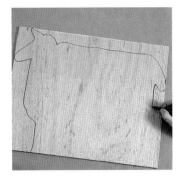

1 Trace the template from the back of the book, enlarging to fit your piece of wood. Cut it out with a coping saw or an electric jigsaw.

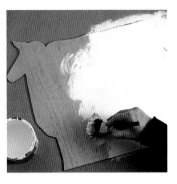

2 Paint the sheep off-white, using random brushstrokes in all directions.

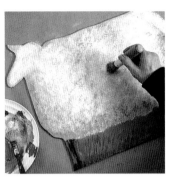

3 Mix some burnt umber into the off-white to obtain two shades of beige, then apply these with the stencil brush. Paint the grass and the black legs, adding highlights to the legs in dark beige.

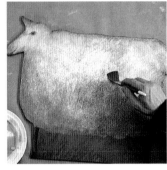

4 Use the darker beige to create the texture of fleece, applying the undiluted paint with a brush. Sand back the paint to reveal a patchy background. Paint an eye and a happy mouth. Apply a coat of varnish tinted with raw umber and raw sienna, and then a coat of clear varnish to finish.

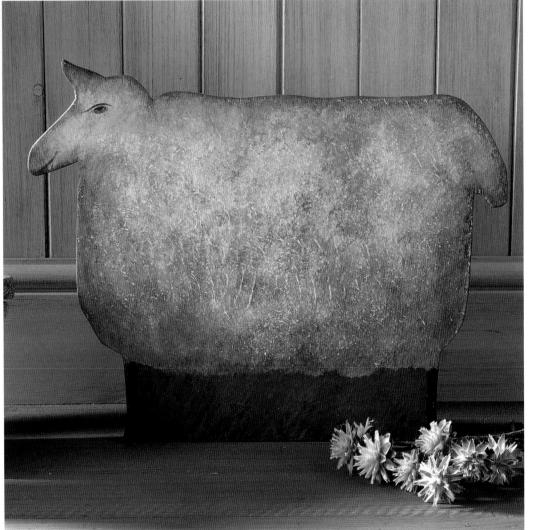

· Wood, Wire and Tinwork ·

Exotic Table Decorations

Make a selection of whole fruit in this design, as well as an ornamental tree in a tub. These table decorations will look lovely underneath a glass bowl or hanging from drinks glasses.

You Will Need

Materials	Equipment
tracing paper	pencil
PVA (white) glue	dried-out ballpoint pen
aluminium foil	old scissors
coloured varnish, or clear	fine paintbrush
varnish tinted with artist's	
oil colours	
fine wire	

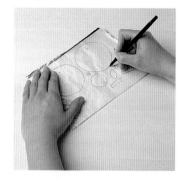

1 Trace the templates from the back of the book, enlarging if necessary. Glue two sheets of foil together, shiny sides outwards. Lay the tracing over the foil and use a pen to draw round the outlines.

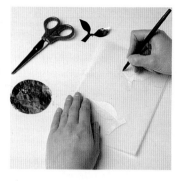

2 Cut out the foil shapes using old scissors, then cover with another sheet of tracing paper to protect the foil. Indent the details on the fruit and leaves with the dried-out ballpoint pen.

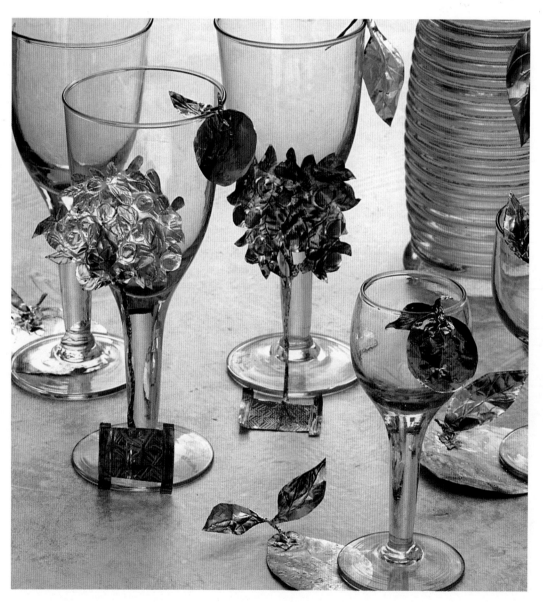

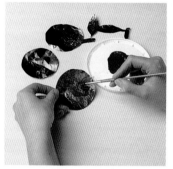

3 Using a fine paintbrush, paint the foil shapes with coloured varnish. Allow to dry.

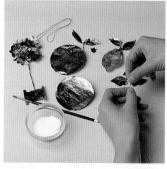

4 Crease the leaves along their central veins and wind the stems around a length of fine wire. Glue them to the fruit. Wire the trunk of the tree.

• WOOD, WIRE AND TINWORK •

LOVE AND KISSES SOAP DISH

A novel idea to brighten up the bathroom – a soap dish made of ordinary gardening wire, spelling out the message with a heart and crosses (kisses). This couldn't be simpler to do, and it will even keep the soap from making a mess into the bargain! If you wish, the soap dish can be attached to the wall by inserting a screw through the pencil-size hoop.

YOU WILL NEED

MATERIALS
thick, plastic-coated gardening wire

EQUIPMENT
*wire-cutters
pencil
pliers*

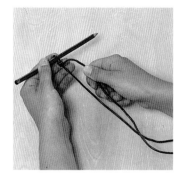

1 Cut an 88 cm/35 in length of wire and wrap it, at the halfway point, around the pencil. Make a coil, by twisting the pencil a couple of times.

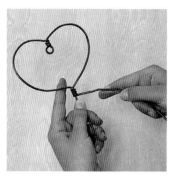

2 Using about 16 cm/6¼ in of wire on each side of the coil, make a heart shape, and then finish off by twisting the wire into a coil again.

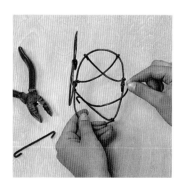

3 Using the wire ends left, hook them together and join the ends by crimping them with pliers. Make this loop into an even oval, which will form the rim of the soap dish.

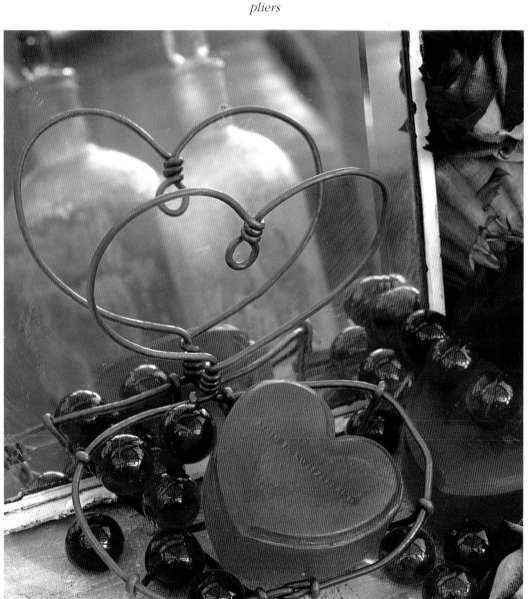

4 Cut four 14 cm/5½ in lengths of wire. Hook over the outside of the oval, making two crosses. Attach a shorter length across the centre.

• WOOD, WIRE AND TINWORK •

Woodburning

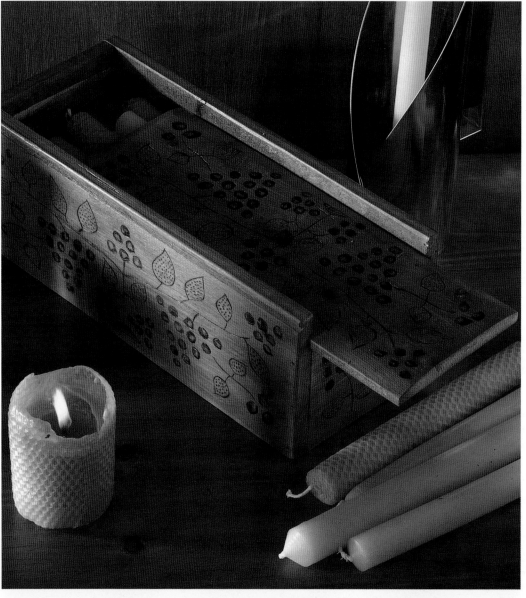

Patterns burnt into wood were a traditional feature of Scandinavian folk art. Nowadays, the specialist tool for the technique is very easily manipulated and gives plenty of scope for creating a pattern to suit every taste.

YOU WILL NEED

MATERIALS
*tracing paper
chalky-based transfer paper
masking tape
woodburning kit, with chisel- and flat-ended tools
clear satin water-based varnish
burnt sienna artist's acrylic paint*

EQUIPMENT
*hard and soft pencils
paintbrush*

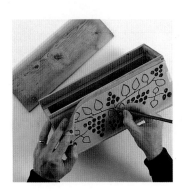

1 Trace the template from the back of the book, enlarging to fit your box. Place the transfer paper between the tracing and the box, tape in place and transfer the design, using a soft pencil.

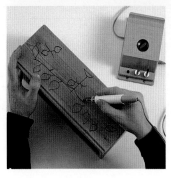

2 Set the woodburner at medium, and follow the lines for the stems and leaf outlines. Use the chisel-ended tool and keep it moving or lift it off the surface as it will burn a deeper hole if held static.

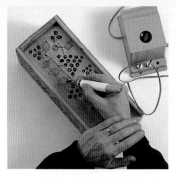

3 Outline the fruit with the flat tool. Fill in the leaf outlines with a pattern of dots using the chisel-ended tool with a prodding movement.

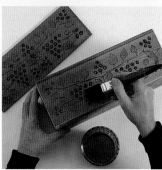

4 Apply two coats of water-based satin varnish tinted with a squeeze of burnt sienna paint, followed by one coat of clear varnish.

• WOOD, WIRE AND TINWORK •

GALVANIZED TRIVET

A practical accessory that is made from galvanized wire, and so will coordinate with and complement your stainless steel kitchen utensils and your pots and pans.

YOU WILL NEED

MATERIALS
2 mm/0.078 in galvanized wire

EQUIPMENT
*pliers
broom handle*

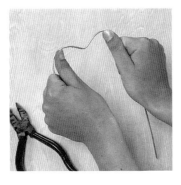

1 Take a 50 cm/20 in length of wire. Using pliers, make a heart shape by bending the wire in the centre, to form the dip in the top of the heart. At the ends, make hooks to join the wires together.

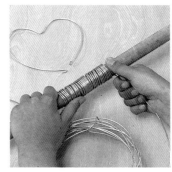

2 Make a coil by tightly and evenly wrapping more wire around a broom handle, about 50 times. Make hooks in the ends in the same way as you did before.

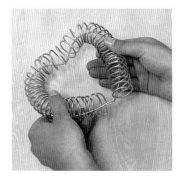

3 Thread the coil over the heart. Connect the ends of the heart by crimping the hooked ends together with pliers. You will need to manipulate the coil to make it sit evenly around the heart shape, before joining and crimping the ends together with pliers.

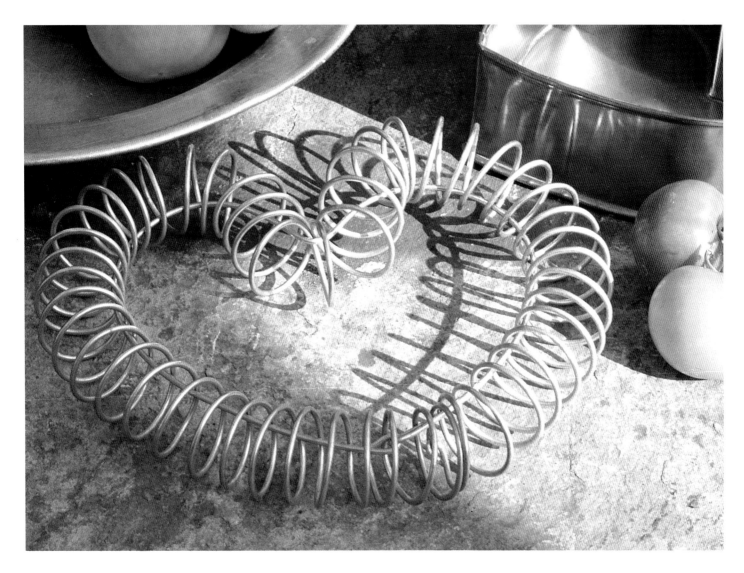

Tin Candleholder

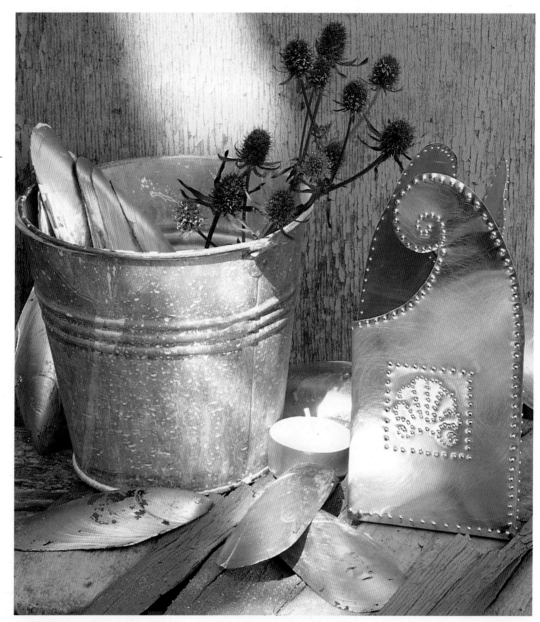

Tin-punching is an ideal technique to use for creating beautiful candleholders, such as this one. The effect is graphic and yet delicately detailed, and the metallic effect will reflect the warm glow of the candlelight. Take care not to leave burning candles unattended.

You Will Need

Materials
*tracing paper
aluminium or tin sheet
magazine or newspaper
epoxy resin glue
candle*

Equipment
*pencil
magic marker
protective gloves
tin snips or sharp scissors
magazine or newspaper
large, strong needle
tack hammer
metal ruler
wire brush*

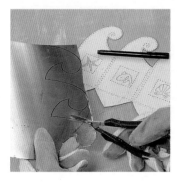

1 Trace the template from the back of the book, enlarging if necessary, and transfer the outline to the metal. Wearing gloves, cut it out, using tin snips or sharp scissors.

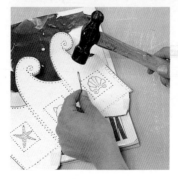

2 Lay the template on a magazine or newspaper to protect the work surface. Using a large, strong needle and a hammer, punch the pattern into the metal sheet.

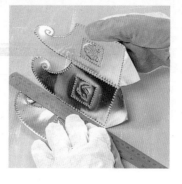

3 Fold the two outer metal panels inwards along the dotted lines, using a metal ruler to crease the sheet cleanly. Do the same with the triangular flaps at the bottom.

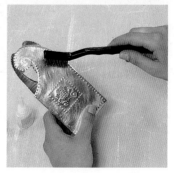

4 Overlap the extra lip to secure the triangular shape, and glue it in place. Scratch the surface all over with the wire brush. Put the candle in the bottom of the container.

Tin Can Insects

There's more than one way to recycle empty cans: these light-hearted designs turn cans into insects to crawl up your garden walls. Use beer or lager cans that have the same logos on the front and back so that your insects look symmetrical. Take care not to cut yourself on the sharp edges of the cans.

You Will Need

Materials
tracing paper
large steel drinks (soda) can, top and bottom removed
masking tape

Equipment
pencil
scissors with small points
large paintbrush with a tapered handle
small long-nosed pliers

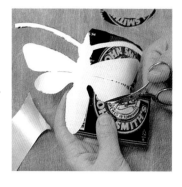

1 Trace the template on this page, enlarging if necessary. Cut up the side of the can opposite the bar code and open out flat. Place the template in position and secure with tape. Cut round the template carefully with sharp scissors.

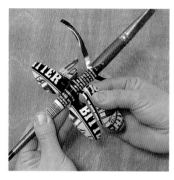

2 Place the body of the insect over the tapered handle of a paintbrush, with the fattest part nearest the head. Shape the body by bending it around the handle. Fold the lower wings very slightly under the body and bend the upper wings forward, folding them slightly over the top part of the body.

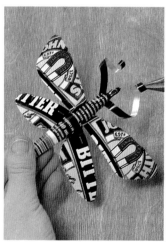

3 Using some long-nosed pliers, twist the antennae back on themselves and curl the ends to complete.

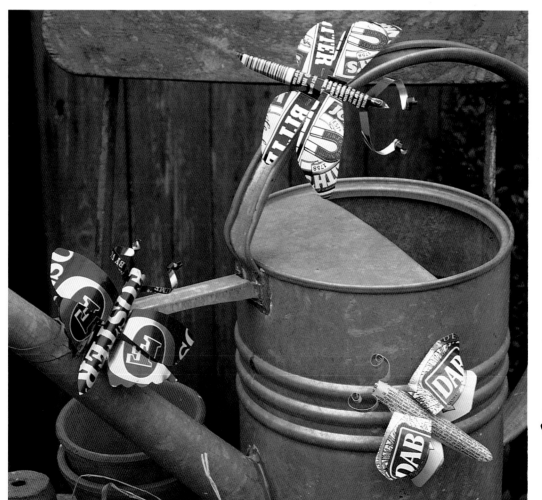

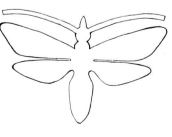

• Wood, Wire and Tinwork •

Pierced Tin Shelf

Tin-piercing is a wonderfully cheap and effective form of decoration. Here, it is combined with a traditional quilting pattern to make a small shelf from a recycled cake tin.

You Will Need

Materials	Equipment
sheet of paper, to fit tin base	scissors
old baking tin	magic marker
scrap wood	tin snips
	pliers
	tack hammer
	fine, sharp nails

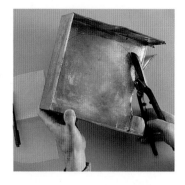

1 Make a pattern for the arch by folding the paper in half and cutting a curve from one half. Select one of the tin's sides and draw the arch above it, using the paper as a guide.

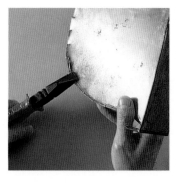

2 Snip 5 mm/¼ in into the raw edges at 2.5 cm/1 in intervals and use pliers to fold it firmly and crimp it until no sharp edges remain exposed.

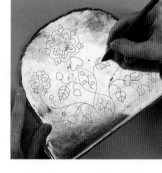

3 Draw your pattern on to the arch. The pattern used here is an old quilting pattern, but a folk-style embroidery pattern would be just as suitable.

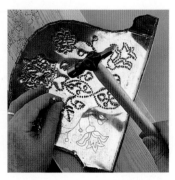

4 Place the tin on a flat piece of scrap wood and use the hammer to tap the nails through the tin and along the dotted lines. The perforations should be quite close to each other without causing the holes to join.

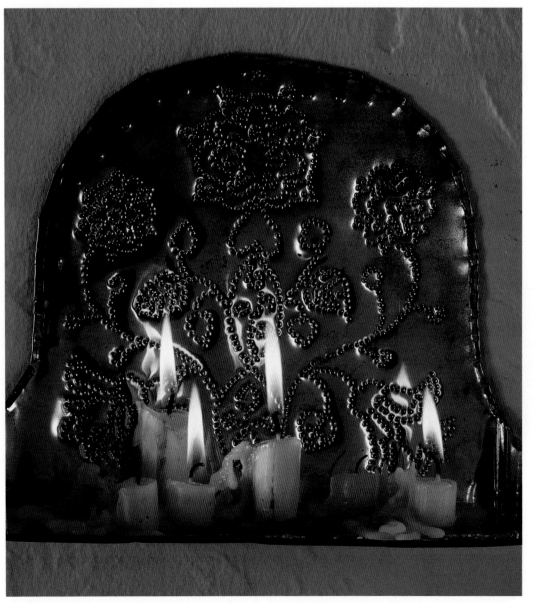

194

• WOOD, WIRE AND TINWORK •

Candle Collars

This is a clever way of making candles look extremely decorative and original.

YOU WILL NEED

MATERIALS
*tracing paper
thin card
masking tape
40 gauge/0.003 in copper foil
wooden block
fine jeweller's wire
glass beads*

EQUIPMENT
*soft and sharp pencil
scissors
bradawl
ballpoint pen*

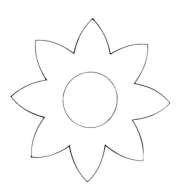

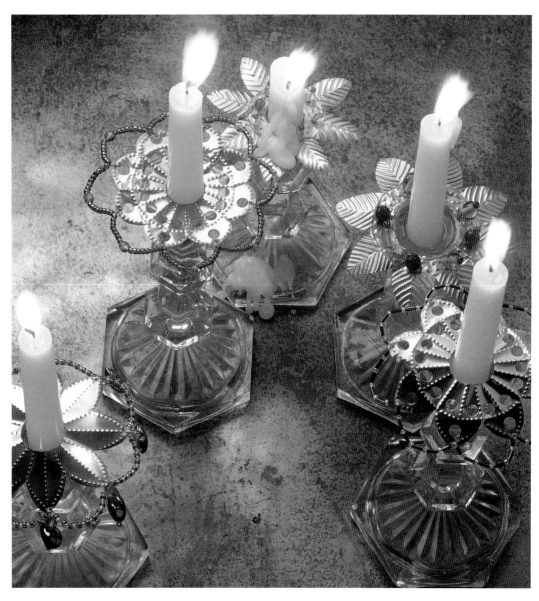

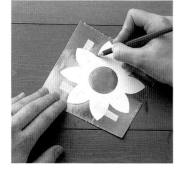
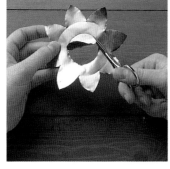
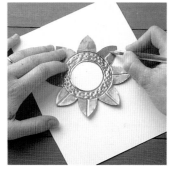
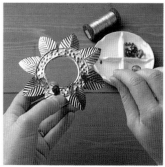

1 Trace the template on this page, enlarging if necessary. Transfer to thin card and cut out. Tape the template to some copper foil. Draw around the template using a sharp pencil to transfer the design.

2 Remove the template and cut around the outside of the collar. Pierce the centre of the collar using a bradawl. Insert the scissors through the hole and carefully cut out the centre of the collar.

3 Place the collar, face down, on a sheet of thin card. Redraw over the lines of the outer and inner circles with a ballpoint pen. Press dots randomly into the surface of the foil between the two rings. Draw veins on each petal.

4 Place the collar, face up, on some wood. Pierce a hole below the centre of each petal. Thread wire through the first hole in the collar, bending the end back to secure. Thread beads on, twisting the wire at the end to hold in place.

· WOOD, WIRE AND TINWORK ·

PAINTED CHEST

*T*he chest used in this project is a mixture of Old and New World influences. The shape is English, but the painted decoration was inspired by an old American dowry chest. You can use this pattern to decorate any chest you like.

YOU WILL NEED

MATERIALS
blanket chest
shellac (optional)
emulsion (latex) paints:
dusky-blue and
regency-cream
tracing paper
antique pine acrylic
varnish

EQUIPMENT
paintbrushes
pencil
pair of compasses
ruler
graining comb
cloth

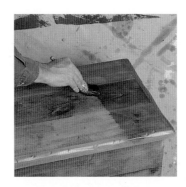

1 If you are starting with bare wood, apply a coat of shellac to seal the surface.

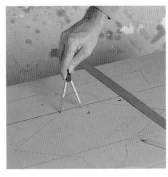

2 Paint the chest with dusky-blue. Trace the templates from the back of the book, enlarging them to fit your box. Use the templates as a guide to position the panels. Draw the panels with a pair of compasses and a ruler.

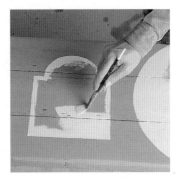

3 Paint all the panel pieces with cream emulsion (latex) paint.

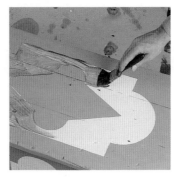

4 Apply a thick coat of varnish to one panel only.

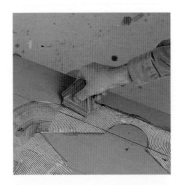

5 Quickly comb the varnish in a pattern, following the shape of the panel. Make one smooth combing movement into the wet varnish, then wipe off the comb to prevent any build-up of varnish. Complete one panel before repeating steps 4 and 5 for the other panels.

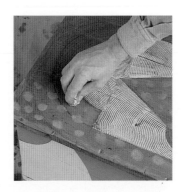

6 Apply a coat of varnish to the whole chest. Immediately, take a just-damp cloth, screw it into a ball and use it to dab off random spots of the varnish.

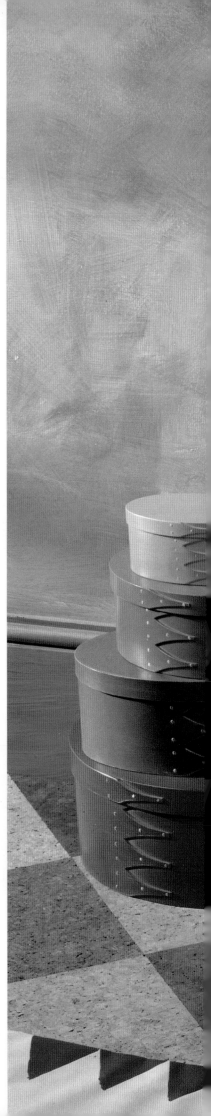

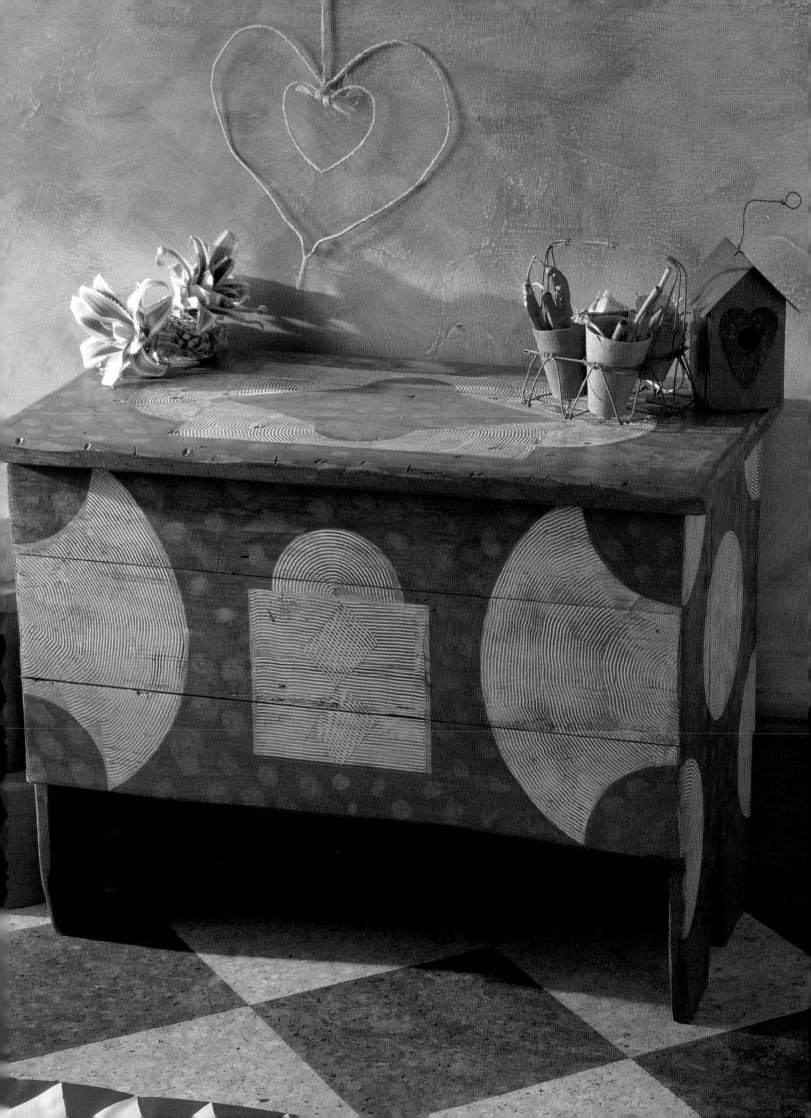

· Wood, Wire and Tinwork ·

Storage Canister

Transform canisters by spraying them with paint and painting cheerful sunflowers all over them.

You Will Need

Materials
*plain metal storage canister
matt blue spray paint
acrylic paints: yellow, orange, brown and cream
acrylic sealer spray*

Equipment
*medium and fine paintbrushes
paint-mixing container*

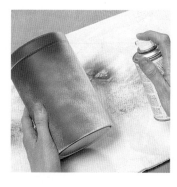
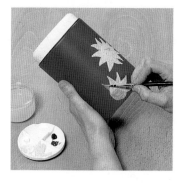
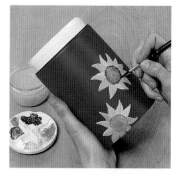

1 Wash the canister to remove any grease and dry thoroughly. Spray the can and lid with the blue paint, building the colour up with several fine layers and allowing each one to dry before applying the next, to prevent the paint from running.

2 Using the acrylic paints, paint in the sunflowers. For each one, paint a yellow circle about 3 cm/1¼ in in diameter and then evenly space the petals around the edge. Repeat the motif, placing it evenly around the canister, until the whole surface is covered. Allow to dry and then apply another layer of paint.

3 Add more colour to the petals, to give a feeling of depth. Paint the centres brown. Paint in the seeds with circles of brown, highlighting with cream. When the paint is dry, spray the canister and lid with an acrylic sealer, to protect the surface. The canister will withstand gentle cleaning, but not the dishwasher.

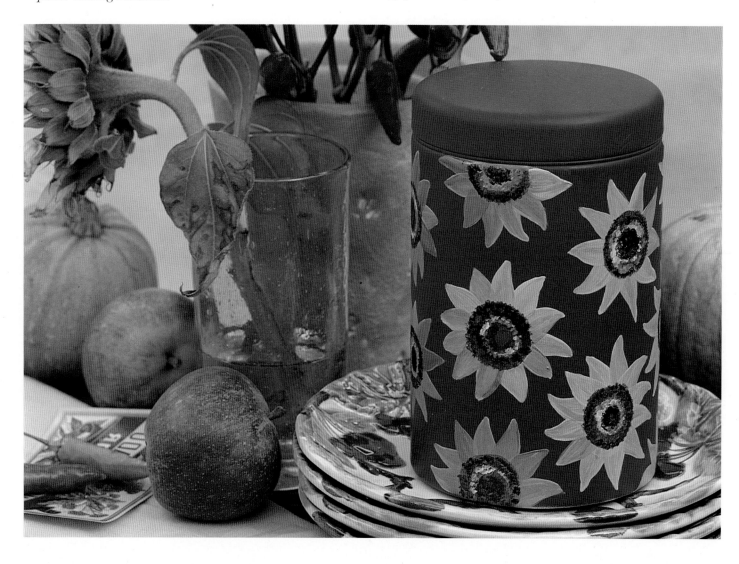

• WOOD, WIRE AND TINWORK •

Wall Sconce

These fashionable room accessories were once essential to every household, and nowadays they restore a bit of the romance that electricity has taken out of life.

You Will Need

Materials
old piece of wood, such as driftwood
brass and black upholstery nails
wood glue
fine nails

Equipment
saw
hammer

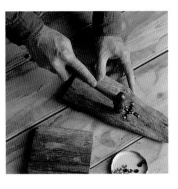

1 Saw through the wood, making two sections to be joined at right angles. Begin the pattern by hammering the upholstery nails in a central line; the pattern can then radiate from it.

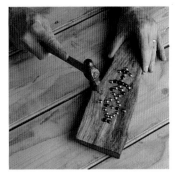

2 Form a pattern of arrows, crosses and diamonds, using the contrast between the brass and black nails to enhance the design.

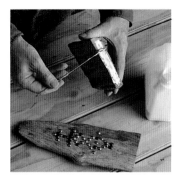

3 Apply a coat of wood glue to the sawn edge of the base. Hammer fine nails through the back into the base.

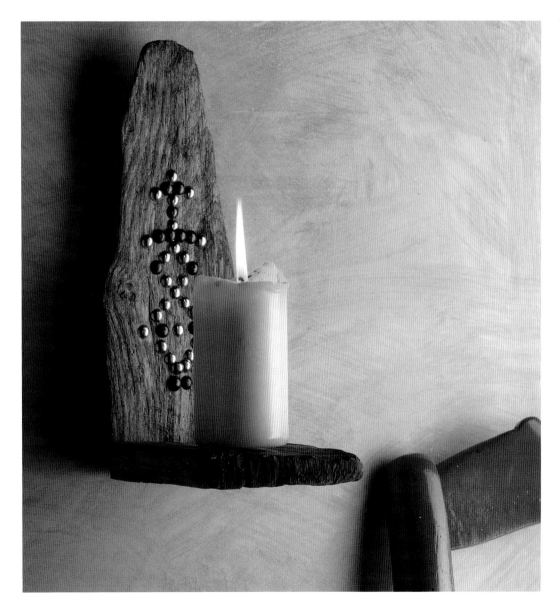

· Wood, Wire and Tinwork ·

Copper Frame

This frame combines two metal foils to create a stunning effect. The embossed shapes and simple nail patterns look very striking indeed.

You Will Need

Materials
sheet of thin copper foil,
1 cm/½ in wider than frame
softwood frame, with sides
at least 7 cm/2¾ in deep
brass escutcheon pins,
1.5 cm/¾ in and 1 cm/½ in
sheet of thin aluminium foil
metal polish

Equipment
large, soft cloth
ballpoint pen
scissors
bradawl
tack hammer
white china marker
soft cloth

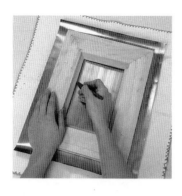

1 Spread out the cloth and put the copper foil on top. Lay the frame upside down on the foil and draw around the outer and inner edges with a ballpoint pen.

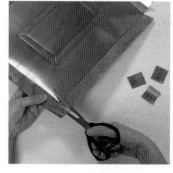

2 Mark on an inner frame 1.5 cm/¾ in deep, to allow for turning around the rebate of the frame. Cut out the outer corners and the middle of the foil with scissors.

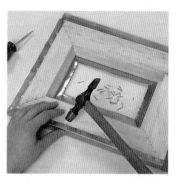

3 Fold the foil around the outer edges of the frame and make holes with a bradawl. Hammer the longer pins through the holes. Fold the foil around the rebate, mark and pin it with the short pins.

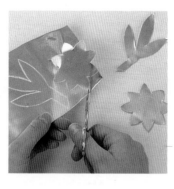

4 Draw simple flower and leaf shapes on the back of the aluminium foil with the china marker. Cut out the shapes with scissors.

5 Place the shapes on the soft cloth and draw decorative patterns on the back of them with a ballpoint pen.

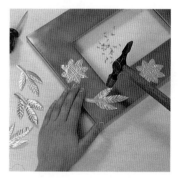

6 Place the flowers and leaves around the frame and prick through both the metals and the wood using a bradawl. Using the long pins, nail the shapes on to the frame through the pricked holes.

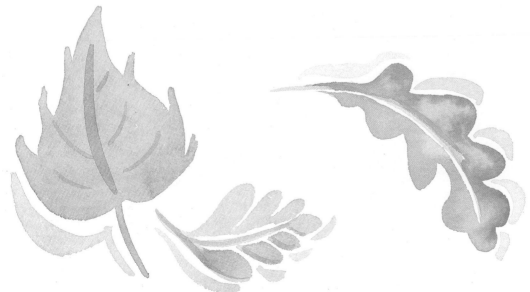

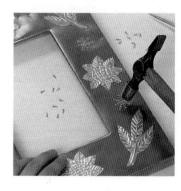

7 Further decorate the frame with more long pins hammered in to form star shapes. Finish off by gently rubbing the whole frame with a soft cloth and metal polish.

200

• Wood, Wire and Tinwork •

Christmas Decorations

These twinkly Christmas decorations were inspired by Eastern European architecture and folk art. Stamped and die-cut artefacts were very popular in many European countries throughout the nineteenth century, when there would have been a tin-worker in every village.

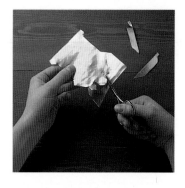

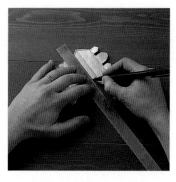

You Will Need

Materials	Equipment
tracing paper	*soft and sharp pencils*
thin card	*scissors*
36 gauge/0.005 in	*embroidery scissors*
aluminium foil	*magic marker*
fine wire	*ruler*
	dressmaker's wheel
	ballpoint pen
	wooden block
	bradawl

1 Trace the templates from the back of the book, transfer to thin card and cut out. Cut a small piece of foil and place the template on it. Draw around the outline with a sharp pencil. Using embroidery scissors, cut out the foil shape. Cut it carefully to ensure that there are no rough edges.

2 Using the picture as a guide, mark the basic lines of the design on the back of the decoration using a magic marker and ruler. Place the decoration face down on card. Trace over the lines with a dressmaker's wheel to emboss a row of raised dots at the front. Trace a second line of dots inside the first, in the decoration's centre.

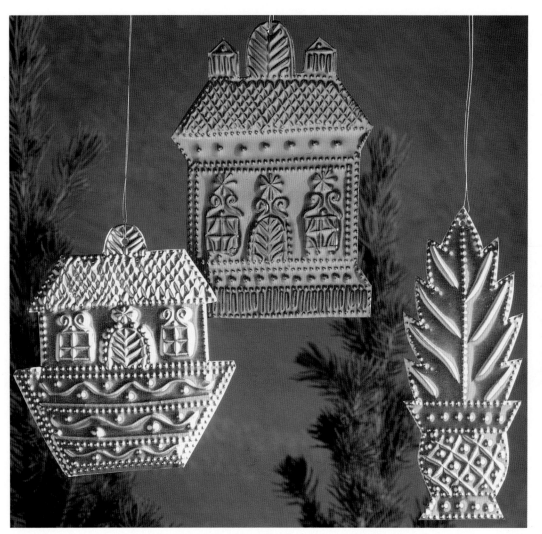

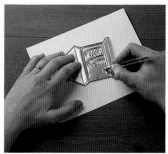

3 Using the picture as a guide, draw the details of the house on the back of the decoration with a pen.

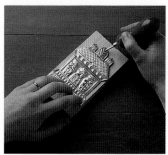

4 Place the decoration face up on a small block of wood. Using a bradawl, make a hole in the top of the decoration, then tie a length of fine wire through the hole to make a hanger.

• WOOD, WIRE AND TINWORK •

SUNFLOWER MAGNET

This sunflower fridge magnet will brighten up the kitchen on the darkest of mornings. In winter, you could consider making a whole row of them, as a reminder of the pleasures of the summer garden.

YOU WILL NEED

MATERIALS
5 mm/¼ in thick birch-faced plywood sheet
medium- and fine-grade sandpaper
wood glue
white undercoat paint
acrylic paints: yellow, red, green, chocolate-brown and gold
gloss varnish
small magnet
epoxy resin glue

EQUIPMENT
pair of compasses
pencil
coping saw or fretsaw
medium and fine paintbrushes
paint-mixing container

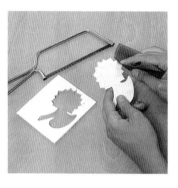

1 With a pair of compasses, draw a circle on the plywood for the centre of the flower. Draw in the petals, leaf and stem freehand. Draw another circle the same size on the plywood and cut the shapes out.

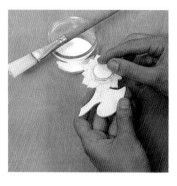

2 Sand any rough edges off the flower shape. Sand the circle's edge to a curve. Then glue the circle to the centre of the flower with wood glue.

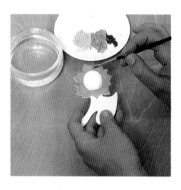

3 Paint with undercoat. Allow to dry and then sand lightly. Paint in the flower details with acrylic paints. Mix a golden-yellow and paint the petals. Paint the stem and leaves green. Paint the centre brown. When dry, add darker detail on the petals, veining on the leaves and gold dots on the centre. When dry, apply a coat of varnish. When the varnish is dry, stick the magnet on the back of the flower.

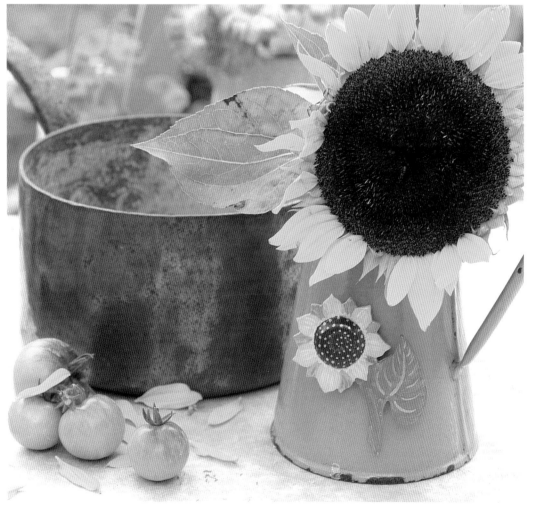

· Wood, Wire and Tinwork ·

Gilded Candlestick

Candlelight gives a magical glow to a room, and this shimmering candlestick will really heighten the atmosphere. Both silver and gold are used here, to dramatic effect. The sunflower motif is a relief design built up with layers of gesso, and the depth of the relief enhances the light and shade effect.

You Will Need

Materials
turned-wood candlestick
red oxide primer
3-hour oil size
aluminium leaf transfer book
acrylic gesso
Dutch gold leaf transfer book
black watercolour paint
methylated spirit-based varnish

Equipment
medium and fine paintbrushes
large stencil brush
paint-mixing container
rag

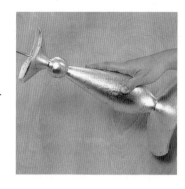

1 Prime the candlestick all over with red oxide and allow to dry. Then paint it with size and allow to dry for three hours. When the size is "squeaky", it is ready for gilding. Begin gilding the candlestick with aluminium leaf, rubbing it with a dry stencil brush, so it adheres to the size. Repeat until covered.

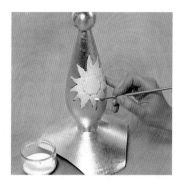

2 Paint a fine layer of acrylic gesso, freehand, in a sunflower shape. Allow to dry. Build up the relief with three or four layers of gesso.

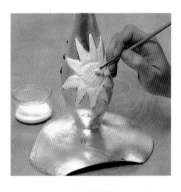

3 Paint lines of gesso in the centre, to make a lattice pattern. Allow to dry.

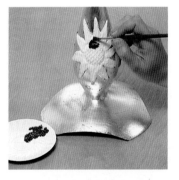

4 Paint the sunflower with red oxide primer, to seal the surface and to act as a base for the gilding. Allow to dry.

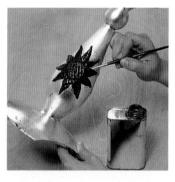

5 Paint the sunflower with size and allow to dry.

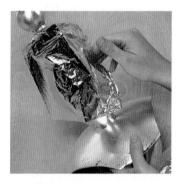

6 Once the size is "squeaky", lay a sheet of Dutch gold leaf on the flower.

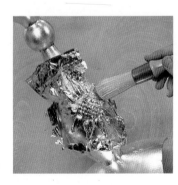

7 Rub it with the stencil brush, using the bristles to push the metal into the grooves, so it adheres.

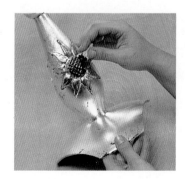

8 Put some black paint on to a rag and rub it into the lattice to darken it, giving it an effect of greater depth. Finally, give the whole candlestick a coat of varnish.

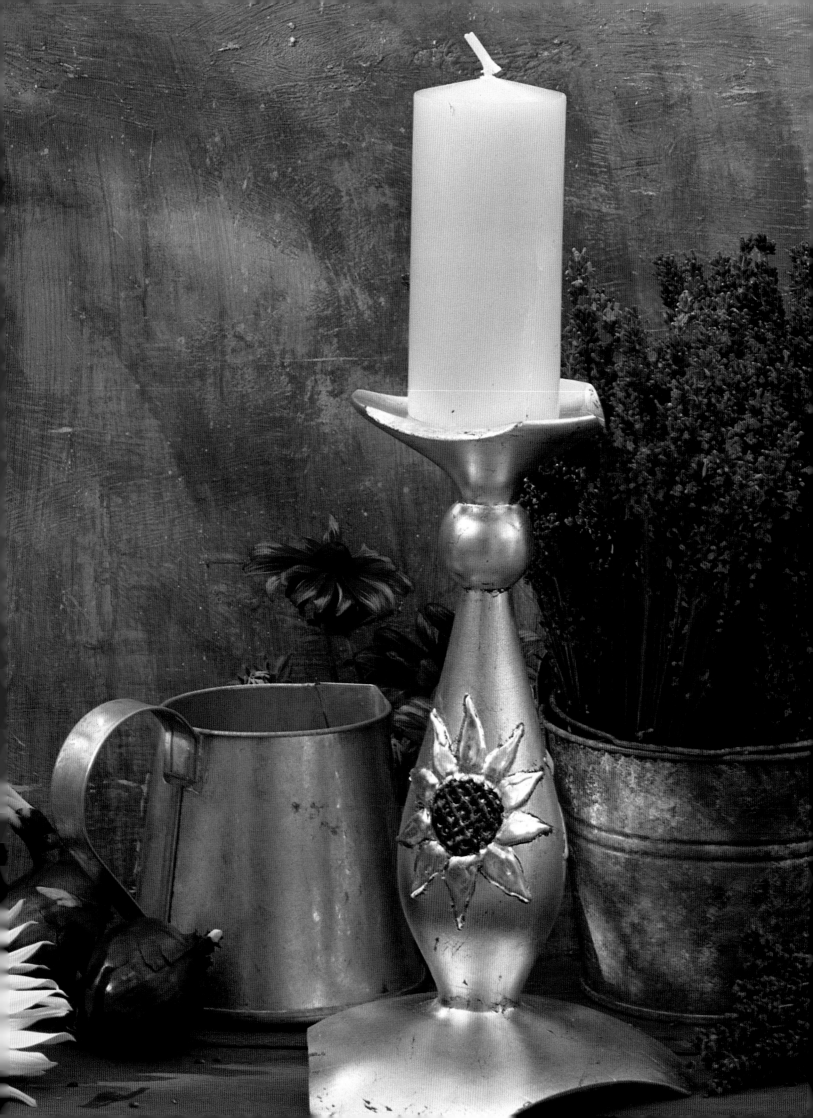

• Wood, Wire and Tinwork •

Grasshopper on a Stick

*P*lant this bold, bright grasshopper in your garden or conservatory, and let it add a splash of colour among the foliage.

You Will Need

MATERIALS
*tracing paper
9 mm/³⁄₈ in pine slat,
5.5 x 23 cm/2¼ x 9 in
2 pieces of 5 mm/¼ in
birch plywood, each
10 x 24 cm/4 x 9½ in
sandpaper
wood glue
5 mm/¼ in dowel,
48 cm/19 in long
white undercoat paint
enamel paints*

EQUIPMENT
*pencil
fretsaw
double-sided tape
craft knife
5 mm/¼ in drill
medium and fine
paintbrushes
empty wine bottle*

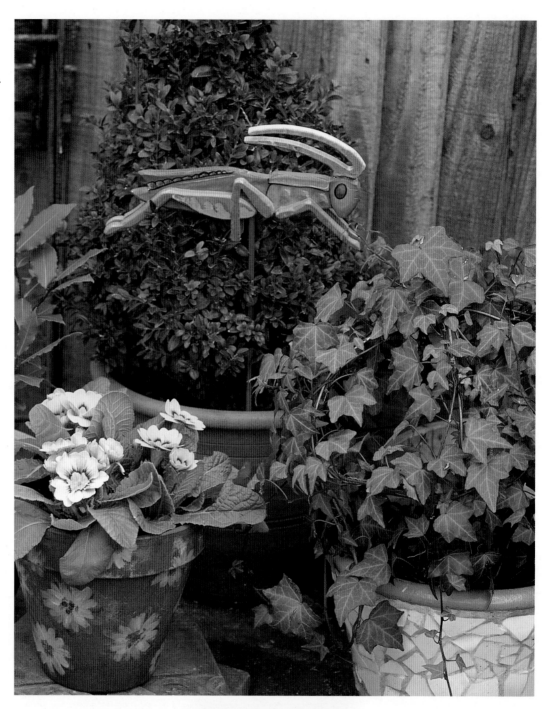

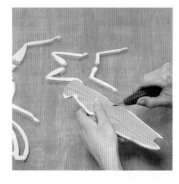

1 Trace the templates from the back of the book, enlarging if necessary. Draw the body on the slat and cut out. Stick the plywood pieces together with tape and cut out the legs, sawing through both pieces at once. Cut out the antennae from plywood. Use a craft knife to whittle the edges. Sand all the rough edges.

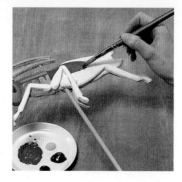

2 Drill a hole in the underside of the body. Glue the legs and antennae in position on the body and stick the dowel in the hole. Paint with white undercoat and allow to dry, standing in an empty wine bottle. Colour the grasshopper with paints.

206

Gilded Candleholder

The gentle glow of candles has an obvious affinity with starlight, and this twelve-pointed star is gilded and studded with copper to reflect the light. Painted in warm, festive colours, it would make a lovely addition to a traditional Christmas table.

You Will Need

Materials
5 mm/¼ in birch plywood sheet
1 cm/½ in pine sheet
sandpaper
wood glue
white undercoat paint
acrylic paints: dark green, red and gold
matt varnish
6 copper disc rivets, 2 cm/¾ in

Equipment
pair of compasses
pencil
ruler
fretsaw
paintbrushes
spike
wire-cutters

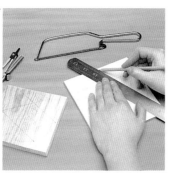

1 Using a pair of compasses, draw a large circle on the plywood. With the same radius, mark the six points of the star around the circle and join with a ruler. Draw a smaller circle on the pine and mark out the second star in the same way. Draw a circle in the centre to fit your chosen candle size.

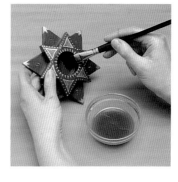

2 Cut out the two star shapes and sand any rough edges. Stick together with wood glue to form a twelve-pointed star. Paint with white undercoat and sand lightly when dry. Cover with a base coat of dark green acrylic paint, then paint on the design. Seal with a coat of matt varnish.

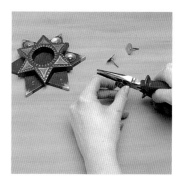

3 Using a spike, make six holes for the copper disc rivets. Trim the stems of the rivets with wire-cutters and push into the holes.

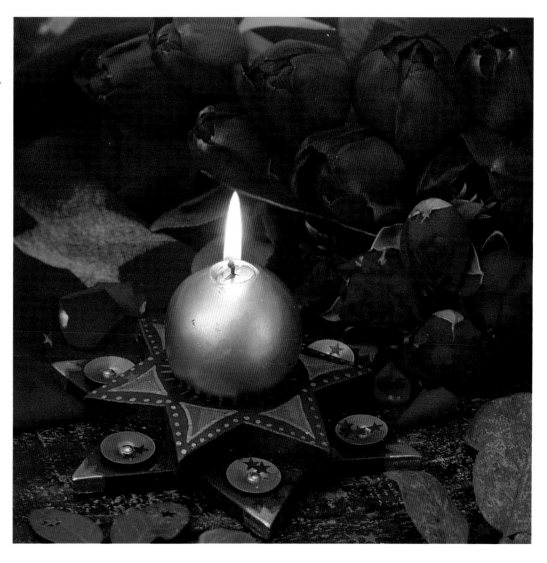

• Wood, Wire and Tinwork •

Painted Tin

This project does not require you to learn the somewhat specialized brushstrokes used in traditional tin-painting, although the colours and antiquing will ensure that it blends in well with any other painted pieces.

You Will Need

Materials
metal primer
large metal tin with a lid
emulsion (latex) paints:
black, brick-red
and maize-yellow
tracing paper
masking tape
shellac
clear varnish
raw umber artist's acrylic paint
clear satin varnish

Equipment
paintbrushes
hard and soft pencils

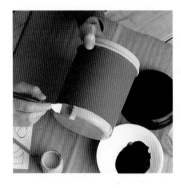

1 Prime the tin, then paint the lid black, and the tin brick-red with yellow stripes.

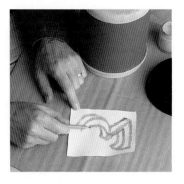

2 Trace the template on this page, enlarging if necessary. Cross-hatch over the back of it with a soft pencil.

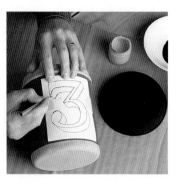

3 Tape the pattern in position on the tin and draw over it with a hard pencil to transfer the design.

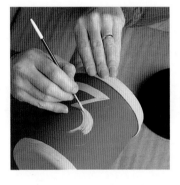

4 Fill in the main body of the "3" in yellow.

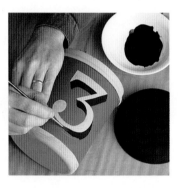

5 Fill in the shadow of the "3" in black.

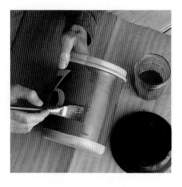

6 Varnish the tin with shellac to give it a warm glow.

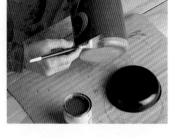

7 Tint the varnish with some raw umber paint and apply it to the tin. Then apply a coat of clear satin varnish to seal the surface.

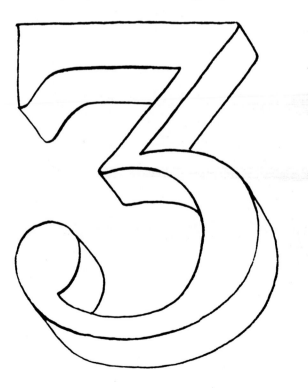

208

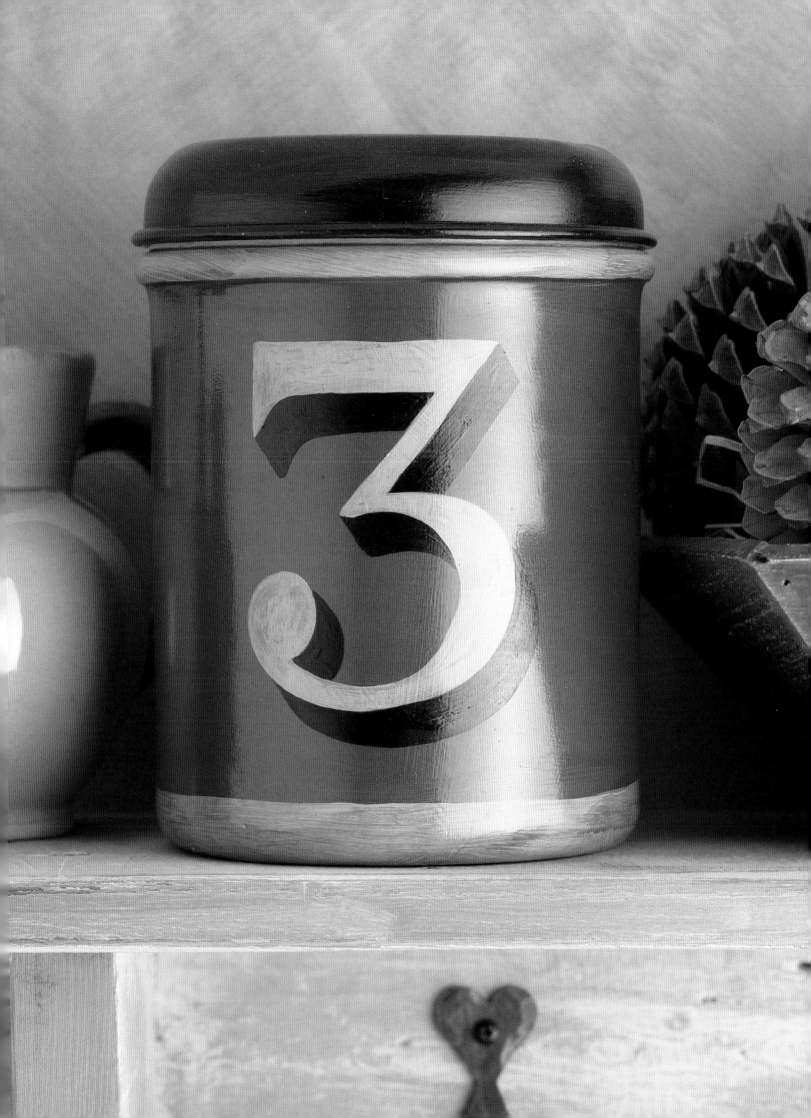

• Wood, Wire and Tinwork •

Lantern

This tin can lantern is reminiscent of Moroccan lanterns that have similar curlicues and punched holes. A cold chisel and heavy hammer are used to cut ventilation holes out of the metal on the lantern roof.

You Will Need

Materials
large tin can
thin aluminium sheet
sheet of chipboard
scrap of thin tin
flux
fine wire

Equipment
tin opener
magic marker
protective gloves
tin shears
pliers
file
pair of compasses
pencil
protective goggles
cold chisel
hammer
nail or centre punch
soldering mat
soldering iron and solder
protective mask
wire-cutters

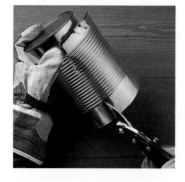

1 Using a tin opener, remove one end of the tin can. Make an aperture for the door by marking a rectangle on to the front of the tin. Wearing gloves, cut out the rectangle.

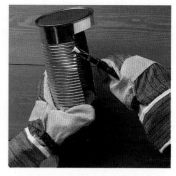

2 Turn over the door edges with pliers to make the aperture safe. File away any remaining rough edges.

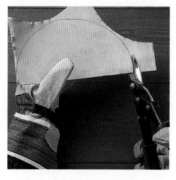

3 To make the lid, draw a semi-circle on a scrap of aluminium sheet. The radius should be equal to the diameter of the tin. Cut out and file the edges smooth.

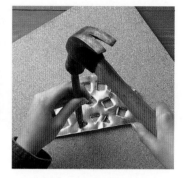

4 Lay the lid on some chipboard. Wearing goggles, cut ventilation holes in the lid using a cold chisel and hammer. File any rough edges.

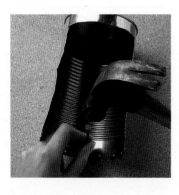

5 Using a hammer and nail or centre punch, punch holes around the top edge of the lantern and around the bottom of the curved edge of the lid. File away any rough edges around the holes.

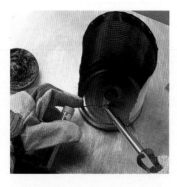

6 To make the candleholder, cut a strip of tin. File the edges and curve the tin around to make a circle. Place the lantern on a soldering mat. Apply flux to the join. Wearing a mask and goggles, solder the holder inside the lantern.

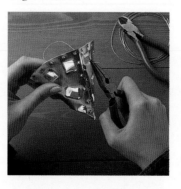

7 Curve the lid around to make a cone. Using a pair of pliers, thread fine wire through the holes in the lid to join the sides together.

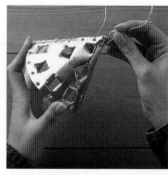

8 For the handle, cut a length of fine wire, then cut two shorter pieces. Make a loop in either end of the shorter pieces, then centre them on either side of the longer wire and solder in place. Curve them, then thread the ends through the holes in the top of the lid and twist them into tight spirals inside.

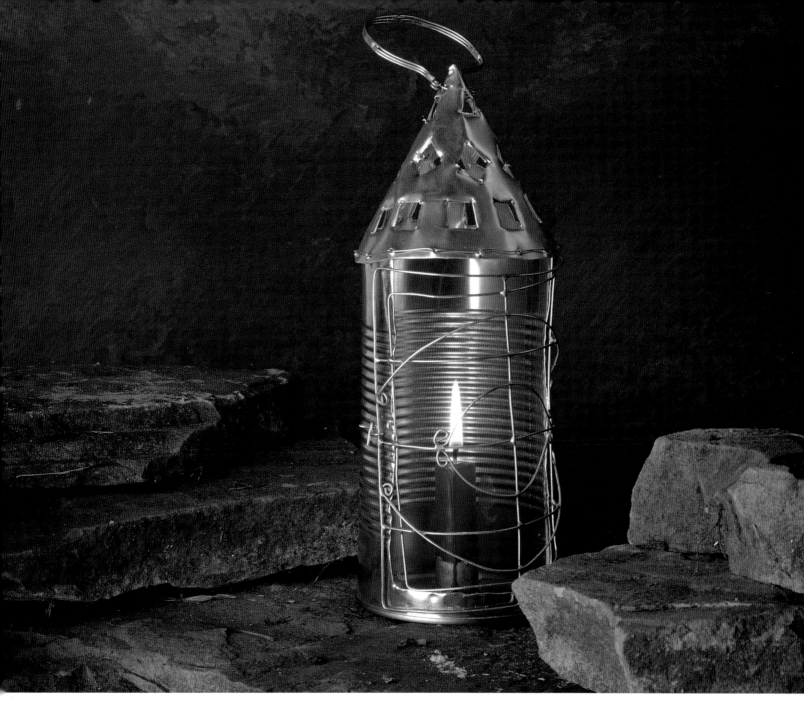

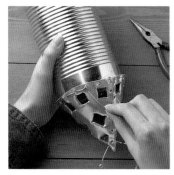

9 Attach the lid to the lantern using fine wire. Pull the wire tight using pliers.

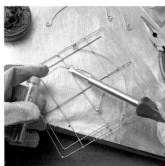

10 For the door, make a decorative rectangular frame from lengths of wire. The frame should be slightly taller and wider than the aperture. Lay the frame on a soldering mat and solder all the sections together. When the door is complete, curve it to the shape of the lantern.

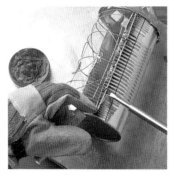

11 To make hinges, bend two short lengths of wire into "U" shapes. Bend each end of the "U" into right angles. Solder one end of each hinge to the lantern. Place the door inside the hinges so that it rests on them and doesn't drop down. Solder the other end of the hinges to the lanterns.

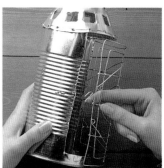

12 For the latch, make a hook and a "U"-shaped catch from short lengths of wire. Solder the catch to the side of the lantern and attach the hook to the door frame.

Wooden Dish

This wooden dish would be good for serving candies or nuts. It's very easy to make, if you take the time to measure, draw, and cut accurately.

You Will Need

Materials
5 mm/¼ in birch-faced plywood sheet
2.5 cm/1 in pine slat
double-sided tape
tracing paper
wood filler (optional)
sandpaper
wood glue
white undercoat paint
acrylic paints: red, green, yellow, white and brown
matt varnish

Equipment
pencil
fretsaw or coping saw
ruler
drill, with medium bit
paintbrushes
paint-mixing containers

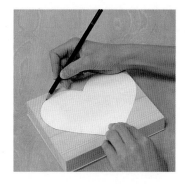

1 Attach the plywood to the back of the pine with the double-sided tape. Trace the template on this page, enlarging if necessary. Place the template on the pine and draw around it. Cut out the heart shape from the plywood and pine with the fretsaw or coping saw.

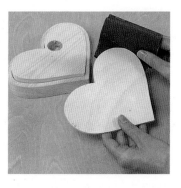

2 Detach the plywood heart. On the pine heart, mark a line 5 mm/¼ in from the edge (make a smaller template and draw around it). Drill a hole for the saw blade. If you can't do this easily, saw through from the side and repair the cut with a little filler. Cut around the inner outline and detach the smaller heart. Sand the two pieces smooth.

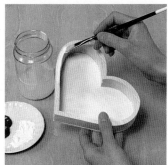

3 Line up the plywood heart exactly with the pine one, as a base. Glue it in place and allow to dry. Sand around the edges again. Paint with white undercoat and allow to dry. Lightly sand again, with fine-grade sandpaper, and decorate with acrylic paints. When dry, finish with a coat of varnish.

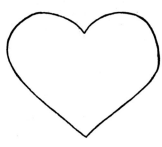

• Wood, Wire and Tinwork •

Painted Garden Sticks

These cheerful sun and moon faces are very simple to make and will really brighten up the garden. Use them to enhance the festive atmosphere when you are having a barbecue or garden party. You could also put them into a border or bed, or use them to give height and structure to plants in a container.

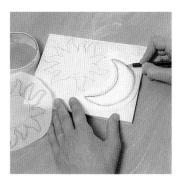

1 Draw the sun and moon shapes freehand on tracing paper and transfer the outlines to the plywood. Cut out the shapes with the saw and sand the edges smooth. Drill a hole in the edge of each shape for the sticks.

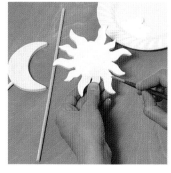

2 Paint the sticks and shapes all over with undercoat. Allow to dry. Sand lightly with fine-grade sandpaper. Glue the sticks in place.

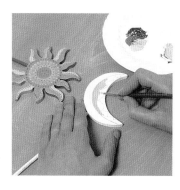

3 Decorate the sticks with acrylic paints and allow to dry thoroughly. Finish with a coat of varnish.

You Will Need

Materials
tracing paper
5 mm/¼ in birch-faced plywood sheet
medium- and fine-grade sandpaper
garden sticks or canes
white undercoat paint
PVA (white) glue
acrylic paints: red, yellow, brown, blue and white
gloss varnish

Equipment
pencil
coping saw or fretsaw
drill
medium and fine paintbrushes
paint-mixing container

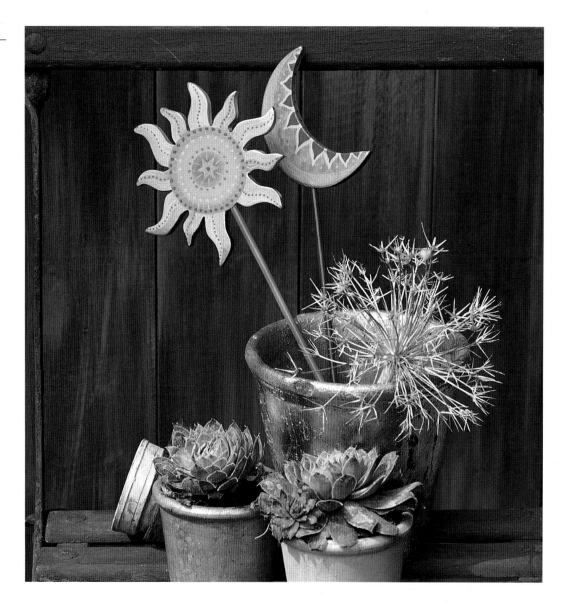

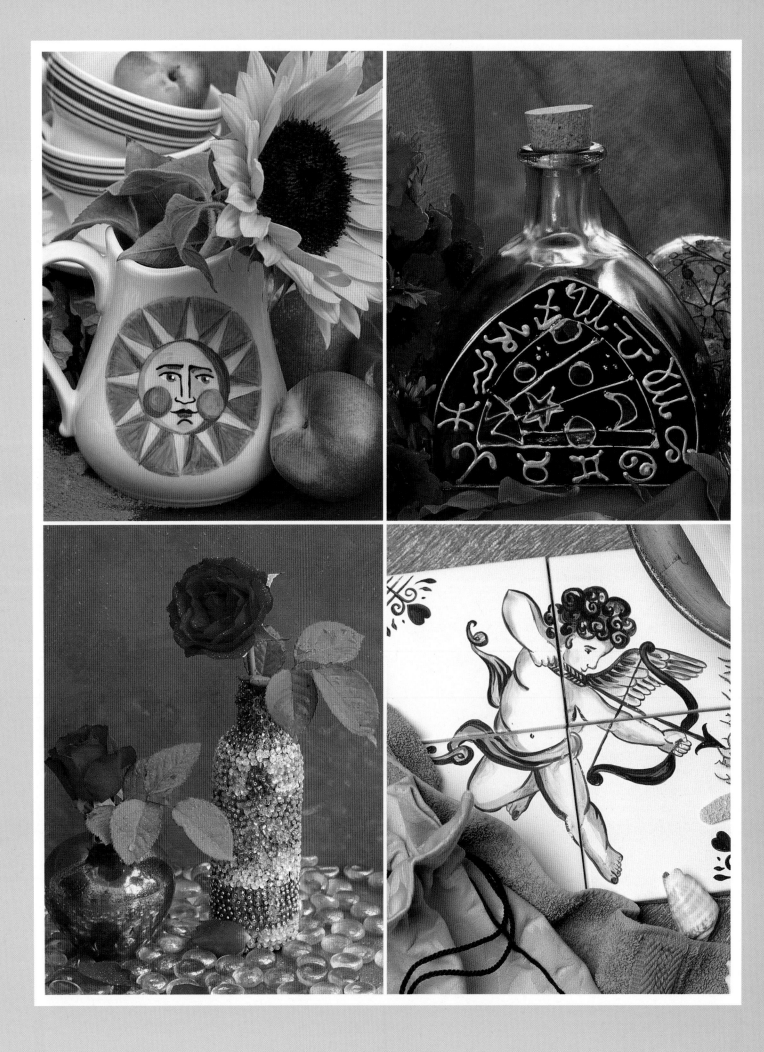

Decorating Glass and Ceramics

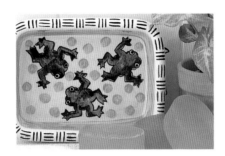

Painting glass and ceramics is a straightforward craft that can be as simple or complex as you like. Using a wide range of special paints in different colours and finishes, you can produce a truly varied and dynamic set of glassware, crockery and decorations for around your home, or to give as gifts. Start by experimenting with a single plain tile, then progress as your confidence grows to decorate a whole tea service.

The important thing to remember about this craft, is that the surface to be treated must be totally clean and free from grease. Once that has been seen to, you can set to the task of transforming the object to an individual style of your choice. Don't be constrained by the templates and motifs offered here – just follow the steps carefully for the technique, then develop your own personalized style.

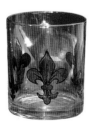

• Decorating Glass and Ceramics •

Materials and Equipment

You probably already have most of the materials and equipment you need for painting glass and ceramics among your household supplies. However, materials such as paints do have to be specially purchased.

As well as considering the aesthetic qualities of a particular type of paint, you should also consider the practicalities; whether, for instance, it can withstand the level of wear and tear it will receive. You should also consider any safety implications, and always read the manufacturer's instructions before applying paint to a surface. This is of the utmost importance if the end product is to be used for food or drink.

A variety of paints can be used on glazed and fired surfaces and specially formulated paint ranges are available from specialist suppliers for application on glassware and ceramics. These include the following.

Solvent-based cold ceramic and glass paints are specially designed for use on ceramics and glass. They are called "cold" because they are not fired. The solvent evaporates, once applied, to leave the colour in place as painted. When painted on to a non-porous surface, such as glazed white tiles, they can be wiped off with a solvent. They take about 24 hours to dry.

Water-based ceramic paints are special paints that are brighter than their solvent-based counterparts, come in a wide range of colours and can be mixed to achieve yet more colours. They have a thermal resin acrylic which, when heated, renders the paint indelible. Though water-based, the paints should not be diluted more than 20 per cent with water. Once the painted object is dry, the object can be baked in the oven to fix the paints. Always follow the manufacturer's instructions.

Acrylic paints A wide range of these can be used on ceramics and glass, though they are not specifically designed for such use. They include rich, opaque colours available in glossy, matt or a pearly finish. Acrylic paints adhere well, but are for decorative use only and are best coated with at least one coat of polyurethane varnish.

Enamel paints work well on glass and ceramics, and they give a hard, smooth covering. However, some of them do contain lead and so are unsuitable for any piece of tableware. They are very durable, with a great range of colours.

Polyurethane varnish and glazes come in matt or gloss finish. Always read the manufacturer's instructions before use and use in a well-ventilated room. Apply the finish evenly, using a large, flat brush and stroking in one direction. The more coats you apply, the more durable and washable the surface, but keep each coat thin, allowing a minimum of four hours' drying time between coats. Polyurethane varnish is unsuitable for surfaces that may come into contact with food or the mouth.

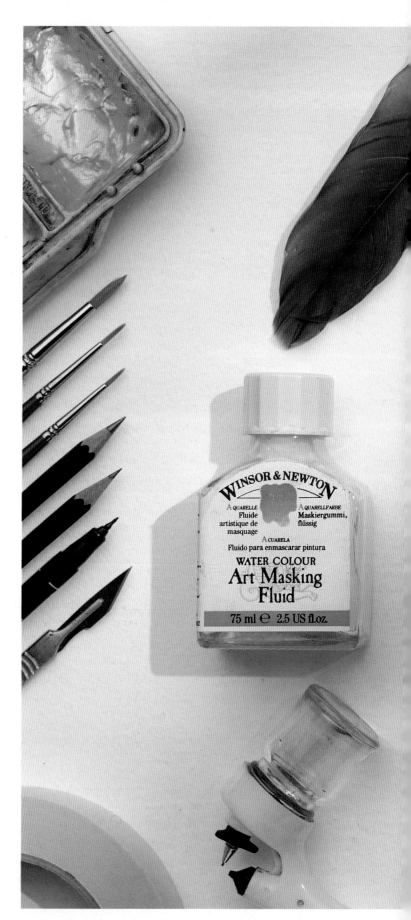

RIGHT *A selection of tools and materials you'll need to create your own decorative glass and ceramic projects.*

• Decorating Glass and Ceramics •

Materials and Equipment

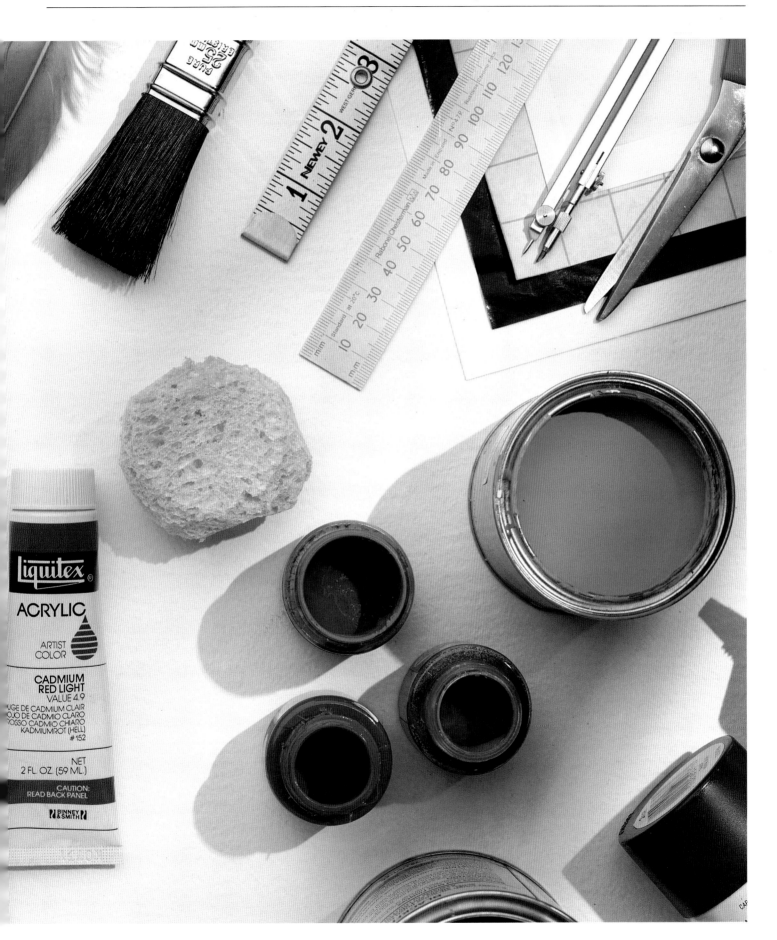

Lemon Tiles

You could paint this fresh, graphic design on individual tiles to make focal points on the wall or create a repeating design by setting decorated tiles in groups or rows. Reserve some tiles to paint with a simple "filler" design like the checks used here. Use solvent-based ceramic paints that do not need to be fired.

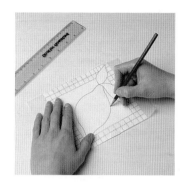

1 Trace the template on this page, enlarging it to fit your tiles exactly. Copy it on to paper and decorate the border with squares, if liked.

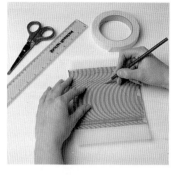

2 Place a sheet of carbon paper on the tile, then the paper template, and secure with masking tape. Draw over the outlines with a sharp pencil to transfer the design.

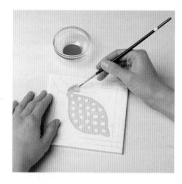

3 Mix up enough ceramic paint in each colour to complete all the tiles you need, adding ceramic paint medium to give transparency. Paint the tiles, allowing each colour to dry before applying the next.

You Will Need

Materials
tracing paper
plain white ceramic tiles
paper
carbon paper
masking tape
ceramic paints
transparent ceramic paint medium

Equipment
pencil
ruler (optional)
scissors
paintbrush

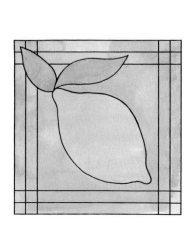

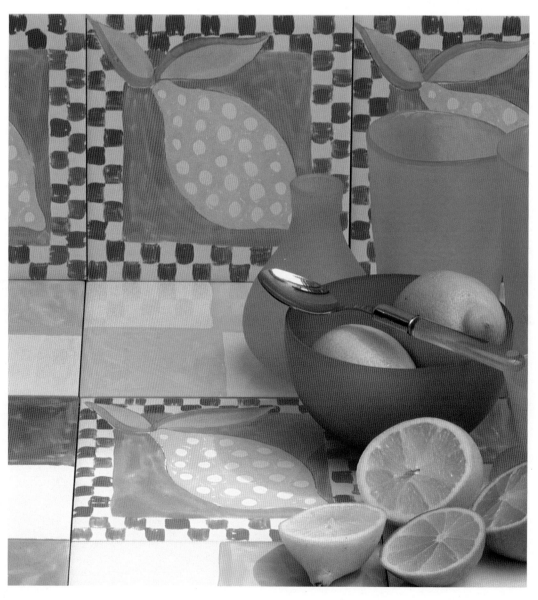

• DECORATING GLASS AND CERAMICS •

Japanese Glass Vase

Transform a plain vase with some highly effective and attractive stamping in a calligraphic style.

You Will Need

Materials
*high-density foam,
25 x 10 x 5 cm/10 x 4 x 2 in
black acrylic enamel paint
washed plain glass vase*

Equipment
*set square
felt-tipped pen
craft knife
plate*

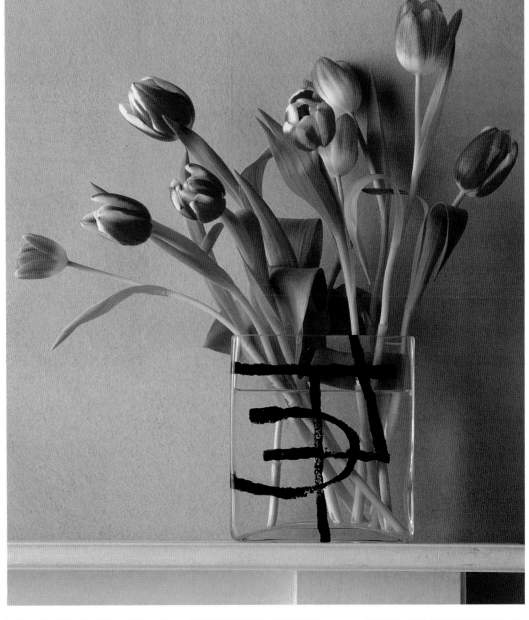

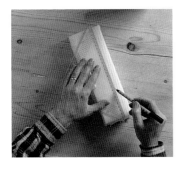

1 Using a set square and pen, draw lines 1 cm/½ in apart on the foam. Cut along the lines with a craft knife, then part the foam and cut through.

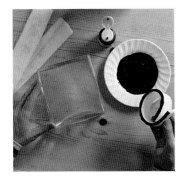

2 Spread an even coating of paint on to a plate. Curl up a strip of foam and dip it into the paint.

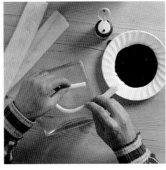

3 Curl the foam strip into an open-ended shape. When the curve looks right, press it on to the vase. Lift it off straight away to avoid smudges.

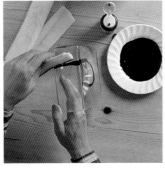

4 Press a straight strip of foam into the paint, then use it to continue the line around the side of the vase.

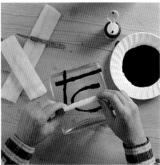

5 Complete the calligraphic pattern with a series of these straight lines. Applying the pressure unevenly will give a more authentic effect.

Soap Dish

Inspired by the colours of bright glycerine soap, this dish, with its green, yellow, black and white aquatic theme, adds a fresh and humorous note to a bathroom.

You Will Need

Materials
glazed dish with sides
ceramic paints: yellow,
black and bright green
tracing paper
carbon paper
masking tape

Equipment
paintbrushes
hard and soft pencils

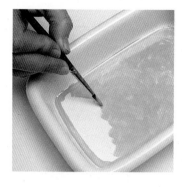

1 Paint the base of the dish yellow. Using a fine paintbrush, paint around the inside edge of the base, then use a larger brush to fill the middle. Spread the paint thinly. Fix the paint following the manufacturer's instructions.

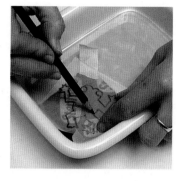

2 Trace the template on this page, enlarging if necessary. Place some carbon paper on the underside of the tracing, position on the dish and tape down. Trace around the frog three times to create a triangle of frogs.

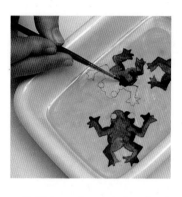

3 Using a fine paintbrush, paint the frogs black from the outline in, spreading the paint thinly to achieve a watery effect. Fix the paints as before.

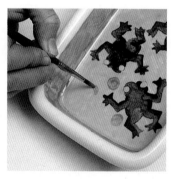

4 Paint the inner sides of the dish green. Start from the yellow edge, working the strokes along and up and stopping where the sides curve above the rim. Allow to dry. Paint green dots randomly over the yellow base.

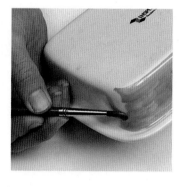

5 Paint the outer sides of the dish green. Paint along the edge under the top rim, working the strokes along and down, and tackling a small area at a time. Allow to dry. Fix the paints as before.

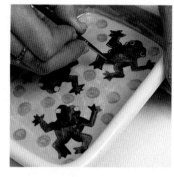

6 Using a fine paintbrush, paint a black outline around the frogs, leaving small gaps of yellow here and there. If you like, paint circles with central black dots for a frog spawn effect.

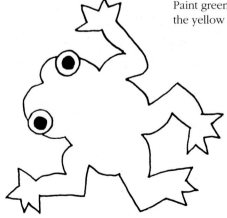

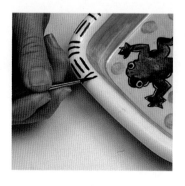

7 Using a soft pencil, mark a stripe motif at the four corners on the rim, then complete the rim pattern one section at a time, following the photograph. Paint the stripe motif in black. Allow to dry, then fix the paints as before.

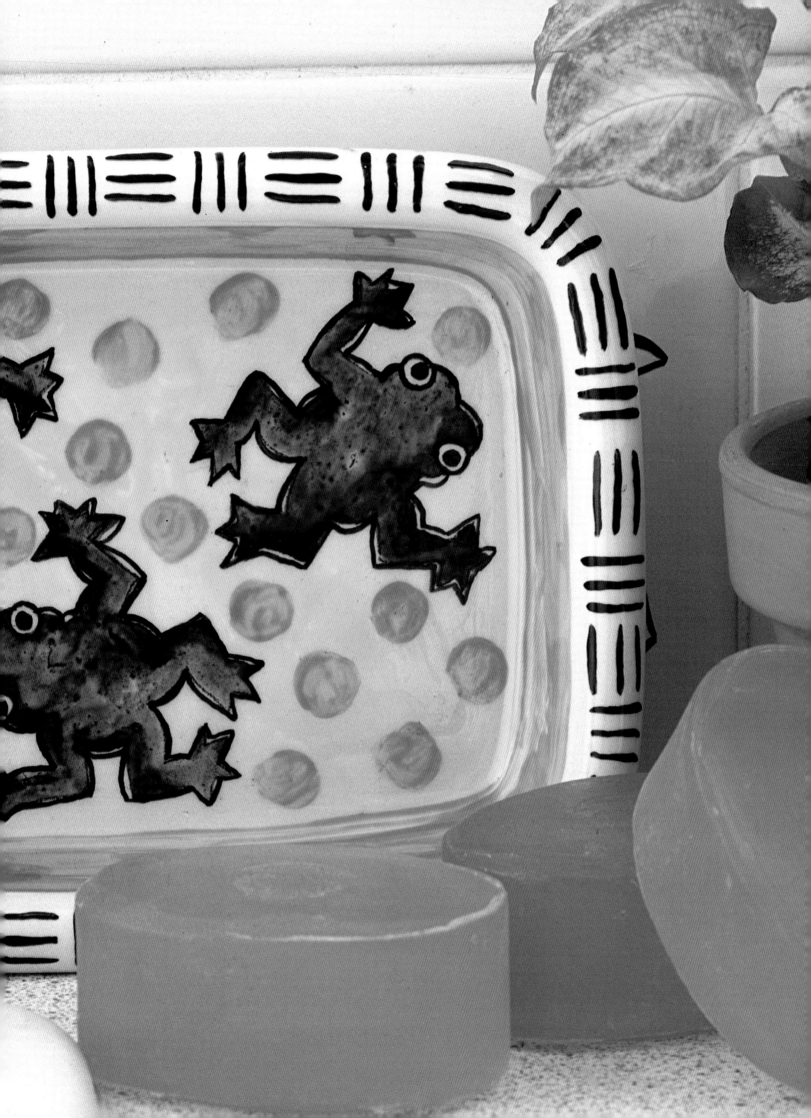

• Decorating Glass and Ceramics •

Gilded Fruits

The colours of the fruit really glow in transparent glass paints. Relief gold outliner defines the design like the leading in a stained-glass window.

You Will Need

MATERIALS
*glass bowl
gold glass-painting outliner
solvent-based glass paints:
red, green and yellow*

EQUIPMENT
*methylated spirit
paper towels
packing material or
bean-bag
paintbrushes*

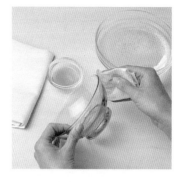

1 Wash the bowl in hot, soapy water and dry thoroughly. Wipe over the surface with methylated spirit to remove any remaining traces of grease.

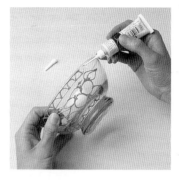

2 After a few practice runs, draw the design carefully with the gold outliner. It is easiest to do this in sections, leaving each section to dry for at least 12 hours before moving on to the next.

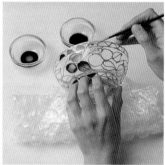

3 Prop the bowl on its side, supported by packing material to keep the section that you are painting horizontal so that the paint does not run. Apply the glass paint thickly to avoid streaky brushstrokes.

4 Leave each section to dry overnight before beginning the next. If you are a beginner, stick to single blocks of colour. More experienced glass painters could try blending two or more colours into each other to achieve an attractive effect.

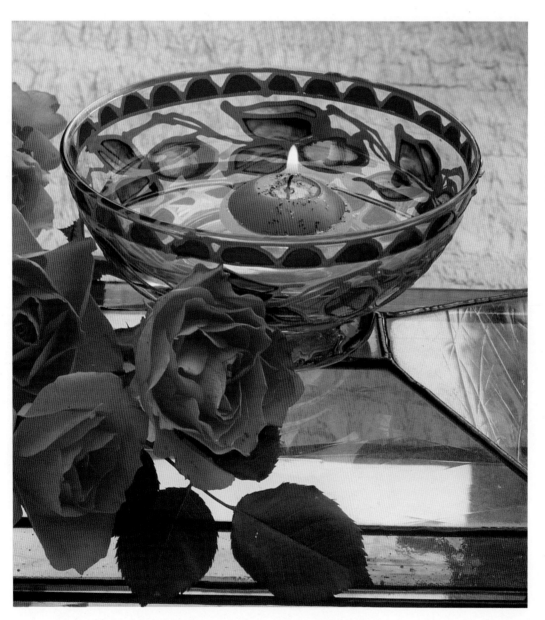

Candle Jar

A straight-sided jar is a good shape to choose if you haven't tried painting glass before, as the flow of the paint is easiest to control on a flat, level surface. As the candle burns down inside the jar, the jewelled colours of the design will really start to glow.

You Will Need

Materials
glass jar, with a candle
gold glass-painting outliner
solvent-based glass paints:
red, green and purple

Equipment
methylated spirit
paper towels
paintbrushes
white spirit

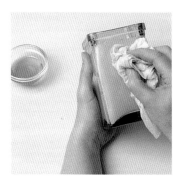

1 Wash the jar in hot, soapy water and dry thoroughly. Wipe over the surface with methylated spirit to remove any remaining traces of grease.

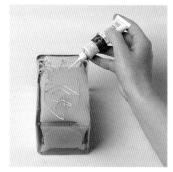

2 Lay the jar down on its side. After a few practice runs on an old jam jar, draw the design carefully with the gold outliner. Allow this to harden for at least 12 hours before starting to colour your design.

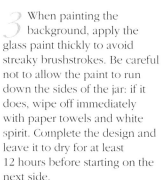

3 When painting the background, apply the glass paint thickly to avoid streaky brushstrokes. Be careful not to allow the paint to run down the sides of the jar: if it does, wipe off immediately with paper towels and white spirit. Complete the design and leave it to dry for at least 12 hours before starting on the next side.

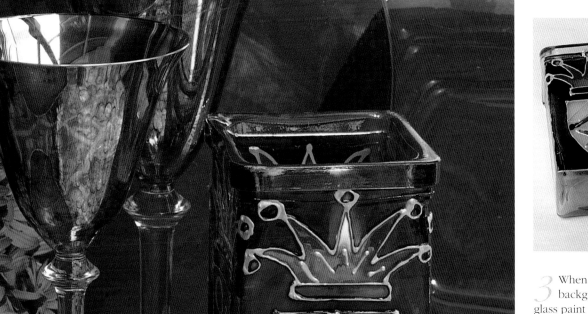

• DECORATING GLASS AND CERAMICS •

LOW-RELIEF JUG

Ceramics with low-relief decorative motifs are ideal for beginners to paint. Like children's colouring books, the shapes are all set out for you to colour in, and as there are no clearly defined outlines, minor mistakes are not noticeable. Reproduction Victorian white relief pattern and contemporary Portuguese pottery make the ideal base for this work.

YOU WILL NEED

MATERIALS
white glazed low-relief jug
ceramic paints: acid-yellow, golden-yellow and light, medium and dark green
polyurethane varnish

EQUIPMENT
paintbrushes

1 Paint some lemons on the jug in acid-yellow. Vary them to give one group two acid-yellow lemons, the next group one, and so on. Leave a narrow white line around each lemon and leave the seed cases and small circles at the base of the fruit white. Allow to dry.

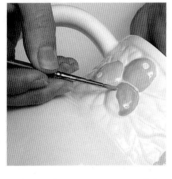

2 Work your way around the relief pattern, painting the remaining fruit a rich golden-yellow. Leave a narrow white line around each fruit. Allow to dry thoroughly.

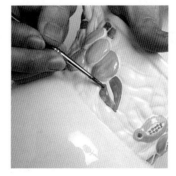

3 Use the three shades of green for the leaves. Start with the palest green, painting roughly a third of the leaves, evenly spaced apart. Leave the central mid-rib of each leaf white and a narrow white line around each leaf. Allow to dry.

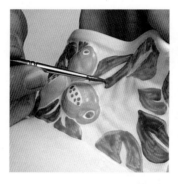

4 Paint a third of the leaves medium green, again spacing them evenly around the jug. Paint the narrow base of the jug green, and allow to dry once more.

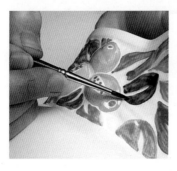

5 Paint the remaining leaves dark green and allow to dry. Fix the paints according to the manufacturer's instructions.

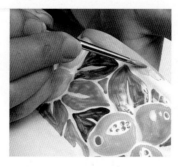

6 Paint the rim or the handle in acid-yellow, leaving a narrow white line at the lower line. Once dry, varnish the jug.

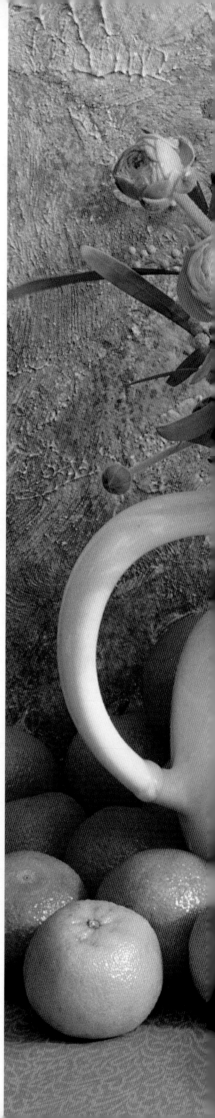

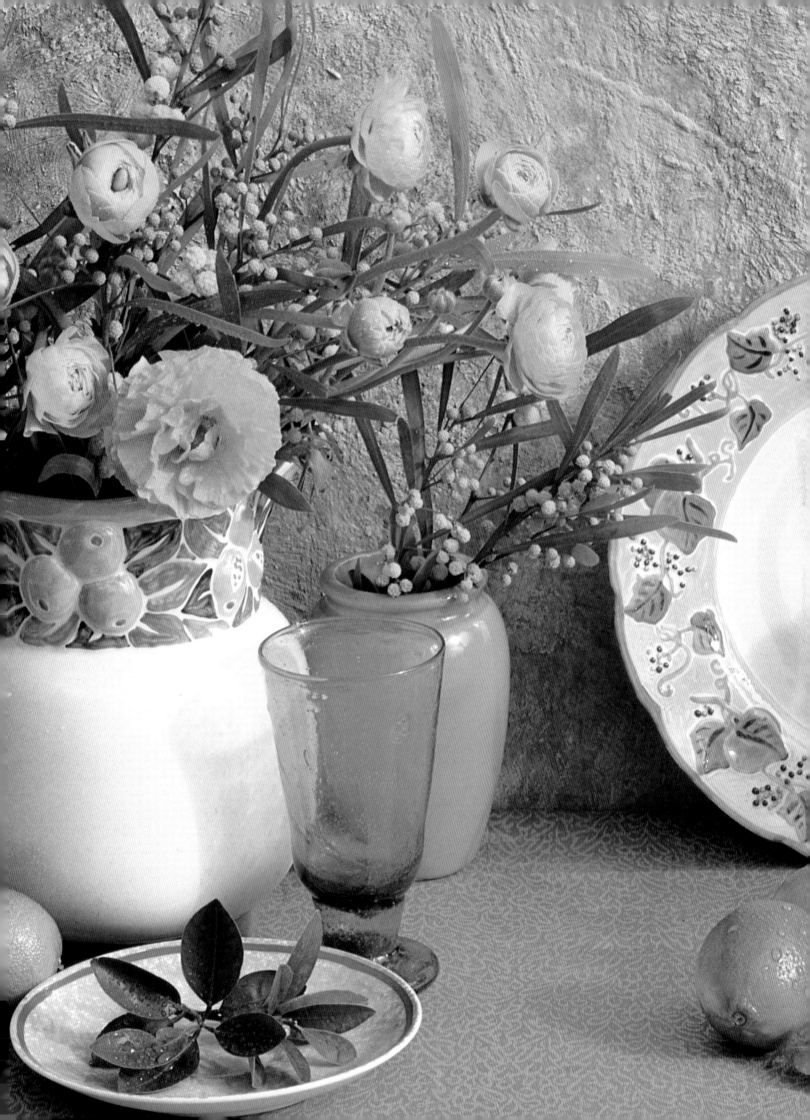

• DECORATING GLASS AND CERAMICS •

GILDED BOTTLE

A corner of a star forms the motif on this lovely, glowing bottle.

YOU WILL NEED

MATERIALS
*flat-sided glass bottle or jar
gold glass-painting outliner
solvent-based glass paints:
red, blue, green and yellow*

EQUIPMENT
*methylated spirit
paper towels
paper
paintbrushes*

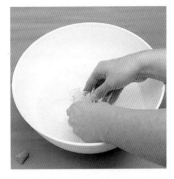

1 Wash the bottle or jar in hot, soapy water and dry thoroughly. Wipe over the surface with methylated spirit to remove any remaining traces of grease.

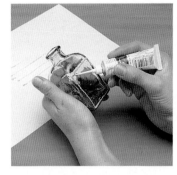

2 Lay the bottle or jar on its side. Practise with the gold outliner on a piece of paper first, then draw on the design from the back of the book. Allow to dry for 12 hours.

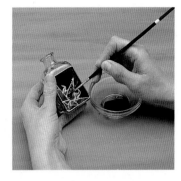

3 Apply the glass paint between the outlines, brushing it on thickly to avoid streaky brushstrokes. Leave the bottle or jar, lying on its side, to dry for at least 36 hours before starting the next side.

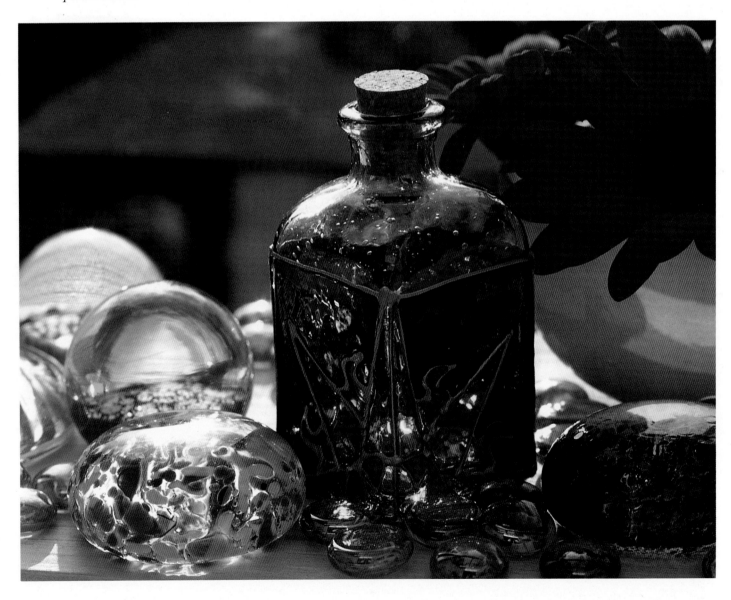

• DECORATING GLASS AND CERAMICS •

MARITIME TILES

Four plain ceramic tiles combine to make a striking mural design, reminiscent of Japanese crafts in its graphic simplicity and clear, calm blue and white colour scheme. There are many different brands of ceramic paint available. Some are fixed by baking in the oven, while others can just be left to dry.

YOU WILL NEED

MATERIALS
tracing paper
masking tape
4 white glazed tiles,
15 x 15 cm/6 x 6 in
ceramic paints: mid-blue,
dark blue and black

EQUIPMENT
soft and hard pencils
china marker
small and fine paintbrushes
paint-mixing container

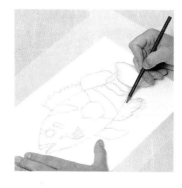

1 Trace the template from the back of the book, enlarging if necessary. Tape the tracing to the tiles, positioning it centrally. Transfer the outline to the tiles with a hard pencil.

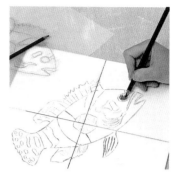

2 Trace over the outline again with the china marker. Draw the border freehand, and add any extra details to the fish. Follow the finished picture as a guide.

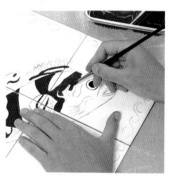

3 Using the ceramic paints, fill in the fish shape. First, paint the main part of the fish in mid-blue.

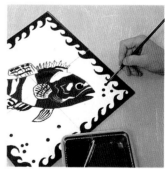

4 Paint the detail and the border with dark blue. Highlight the scales with black. Fix the paint following the manufacturer's instructions. The tiles should withstand gentle cleaning.

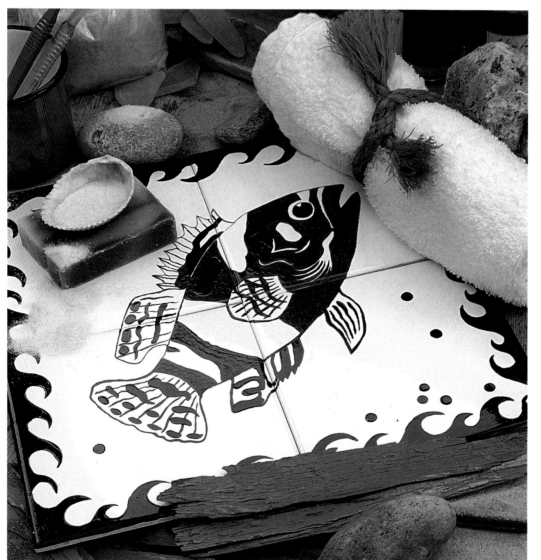

• DECORATING GLASS AND CERAMICS •

ITALIANATE TILES

These Florentine-style tiles are based on ceramic decoration of the Renaissance. They are painted with easy-to-use enamel paints that are fixed in the oven. A single tile could be a focal point in a bathroom, but when several are arranged together, interesting repeat patterns are formed. Adapt the colours to fit in with your own decor.

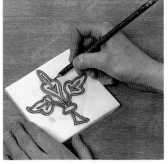

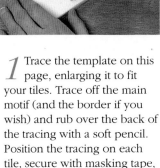

YOU WILL NEED

MATERIALS
tracing paper
washed white square tiles
masking tape
enamel paints: mid-green,
dark blue-green, rust-red
and dark blue

EQUIPMENT
soft and hard pencils
paintbrushes
paint-mixing container

1 Trace the template on this page, enlarging it to fit your tiles. Trace off the main motif (and the border if you wish) and rub over the back of the tracing with a soft pencil. Position the tracing on each tile, secure with masking tape, and draw over the outline with a hard pencil.

2 Paint the leaf in mid-green enamel paint and allow to dry. You may need to mix colours to achieve the shades you wish. Using a dark blue-green, paint over the outline and mark in the veins. Paint a dot in each corner of the tile in the same colour.

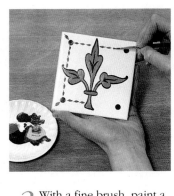

3 With a fine brush, paint a border of rust-coloured leaves and a slightly larger leaf in each corner. Paint a curved scroll to either side of the large leaf in dark blue. Repeat with the remaining tiles. When the paint is dry, fix it following the manufacturer's instructions.

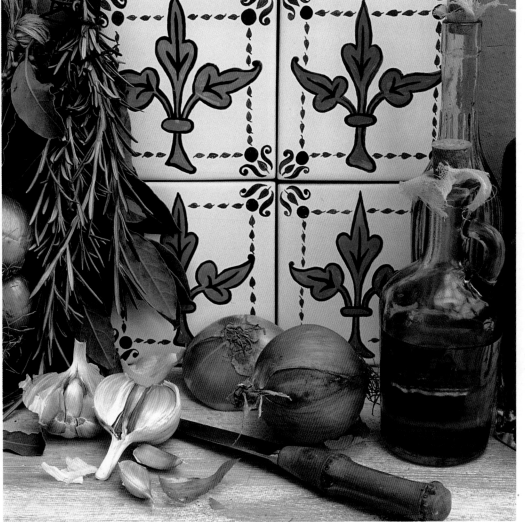

• DECORATING GLASS AND CERAMICS •

Whisky Glass

The fleur-de-lys was the heraldic emblem of the kings of France from the twelfth century. Use the template to make two sizes of fleur-de-lys. Paint each motif in a different combination of colours, matching them with small motifs on the opposite side.

You Will Need

MATERIALS
*whisky glass
black cerne relief outliner
tracing paper
masking tape
solvent-based glass paints:
red, blue and yellow*

EQUIPMENT
*methylated spirit
paper towels
pencil
fine black pen
paintbrushes
craft knife*

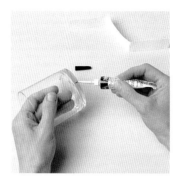

1 Wash the glass in hot, soapy water and dry thoroughly. Wipe over the surface with methylated spirit to remove any remaining traces of grease. Divide the base of the glass into three equal sections and mark them with cerne relief.

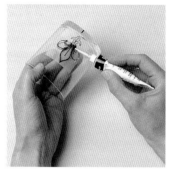

2 Trace the template from the back of the book, enlarging if necessary, and tape it inside the glass. Draw the design with the black pen in each of the three sections. Leave each section to dry for at least 12 hours before moving on to the next. Outline small motifs opposite in this way.

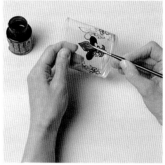

3 Colour the first large motif, using different colours for each section, and allow to dry overnight before turning the glass for the next motif. Paint each small fleur-de-lys in colours matching the motif on the opposite side of the glass. When you have finished, scrape off the reference marks on the base and allow the paint to dry before washing.

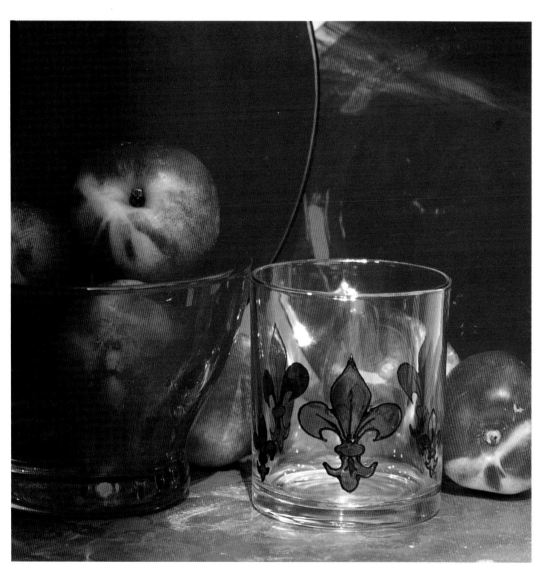

· Decorating Glass and Ceramics ·

Decorated Tea Service

If you are bored with your plain tea cups and saucers, why not cheer yourself up with some pretty stamped patterns in vibrant colours?

You Will Need

Materials	Equipment
tracing paper	pencil
paper or thin card	eraser
spray adhesive	craft knife
white china tea service	cutting mat
ceramic paints: orange, blue and black	piece of glass

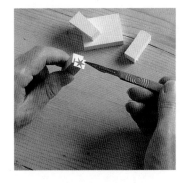

1 Trace the template from this page, enlarging it if desired, and transfer to paper or thin card. Spray the template with adhesive and stick it on the end of an eraser.

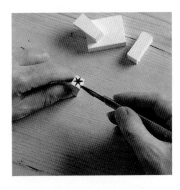

2 Cut around the outline of the star, making sure that the points are sharp.

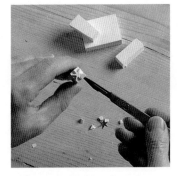

3 Cut horizontally into the eraser, to meet the outline cuts, and remove the excess. The star shape must have points of even lengths, so make a test print and adjust any obvious flaws with a craft knife before you work on the china.

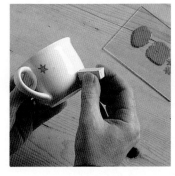

4 Spread an even coating of orange paint on to the glass and press the star stamp into it. Make a test print to ensure that the stamp is not overloaded, then begin stamping widely spaced stars. The inked stamp will tend to slide on the glazed surface, so compensate for this by dotting it on and removing it directly.

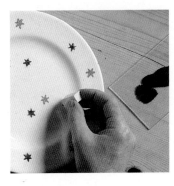

5 Stamp blue stars in the same way, leaving space for the final colour.

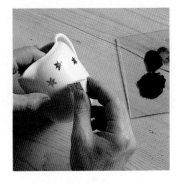

6 Stamp black stars in the spaces so that the three colours form an all-over pattern. Allow to dry, then fix the paints according to the manufacturer's instructions.

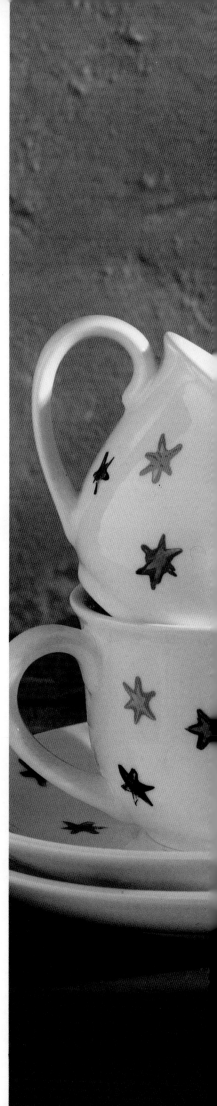

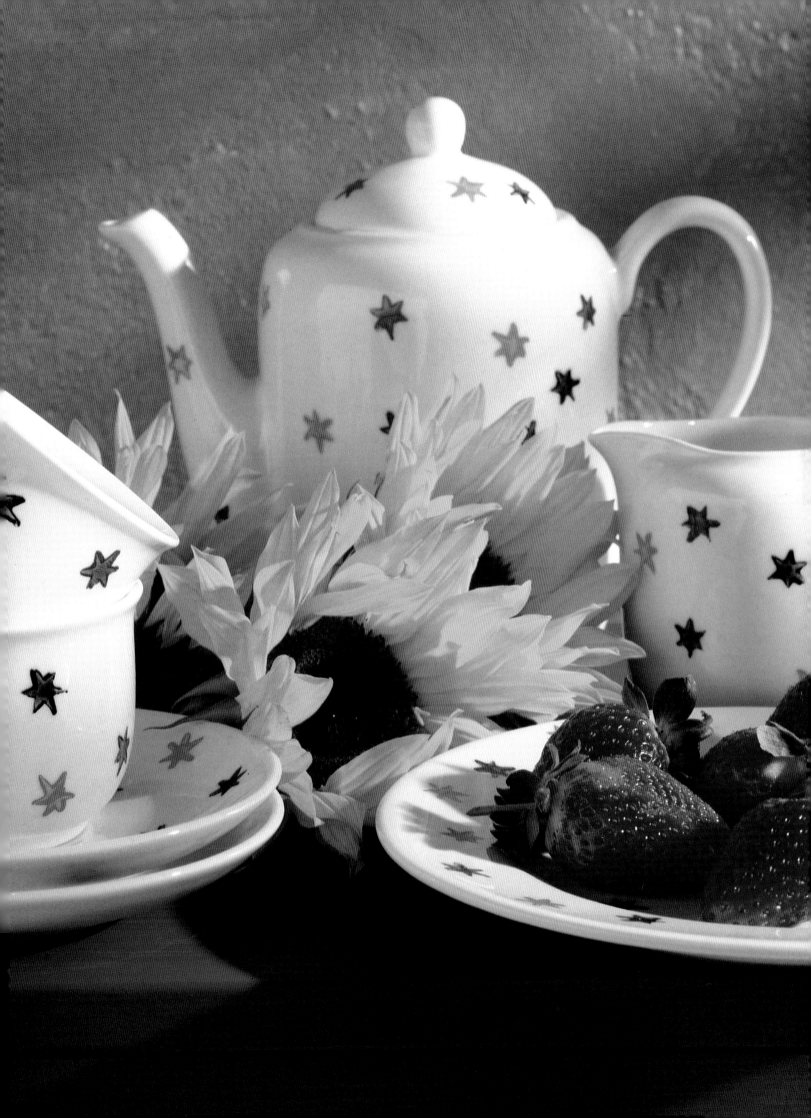

• DECORATING GLASS AND CERAMICS •

SUN JUG

A good way to brighten up a plain jug is to use china paints to apply a vivid and bold motif. This cheerful sun face would be particularly welcome on the breakfast table. The colours could be adapted to suit your other china.

YOU WILL NEED

MATERIALS
tracing paper
washed white ceramic jug
masking tape
ceramic paints: black, bright yellow, ochre, blue, red and white

EQUIPMENT
soft and hard pencils
scissors
fine paintbrushes
hairdryer (optional)

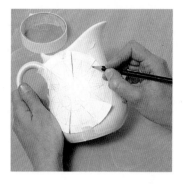

1 Trace the template from the back of the book, enlarging if necessary. Cut it out roughly and rub over the back with a soft pencil. Make several cuts around the edge of the circle, so that the template will lie flat against the jug, and tape it in place. Draw over the outlines with a hard pencil to transfer the design.

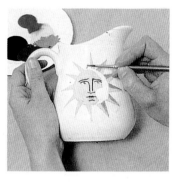

2 Using and mixing the paints according to the manufacturer's instructions, paint the sun. Go over the outline for the features in black first of all and allow the paint to dry completely; a hairdryer can speed up the drying process. Paint the main face and the inner rays in bright yellow and then paint the cheeks and the other parts of the rays in ochre.

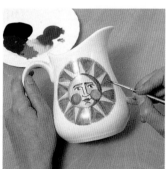

3 Paint the background in blue and then add fine details to the sun face, to give it a sense of depth. Finish off by painting a white dot as a highlight in each eye. Fix the paints according to the manufacturer's instructions.

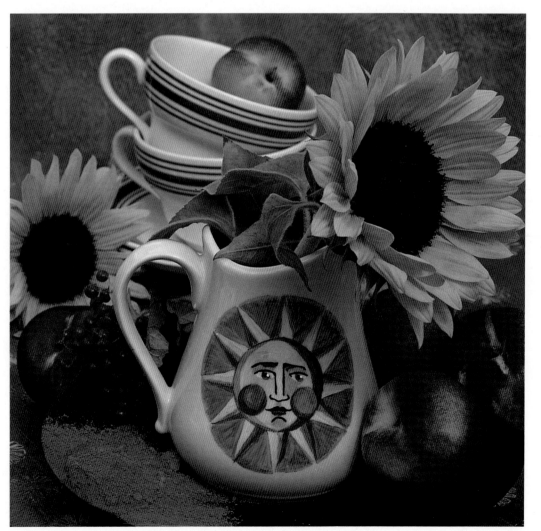

• DECORATING GLASS AND CERAMICS •

HANDPAINTED FLORAL TILES

This is a great idea for decorating plain ceramic tiles, which could then be framed and hung on the wall.

YOU WILL NEED

MATERIALS

*tracing paper
masking tape
washed white glazed tiles
ceramic paints: green, yellow, red and blue*

EQUIPMENT

*soft and hard pencils
scissors
paintbrushes
paint-mixing container*

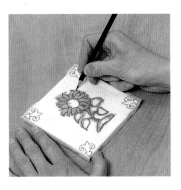

1 Trace the template from the back of the book, enlarging if necessary. Turn the paper over and rub over the outline with a soft pencil. Tape the transfer to the tile. Draw over the main flower outline with a hard pencil, to transfer the motif to the tile.

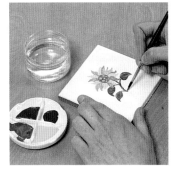

2 Using a medium brush and thin layers of paint, colour in the leaves and petals. Fix the paints according to the manufacturer's instructions.

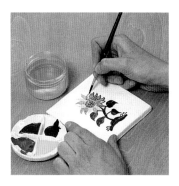

3 With a fine brush and blue paint, draw in the outline and detail of the petals, leaves and stalk. Paint tiny dots in the centre of the flower. Transfer the four corner motifs in the same way and with a fine brush, paint them blue. Fix the paint as before.

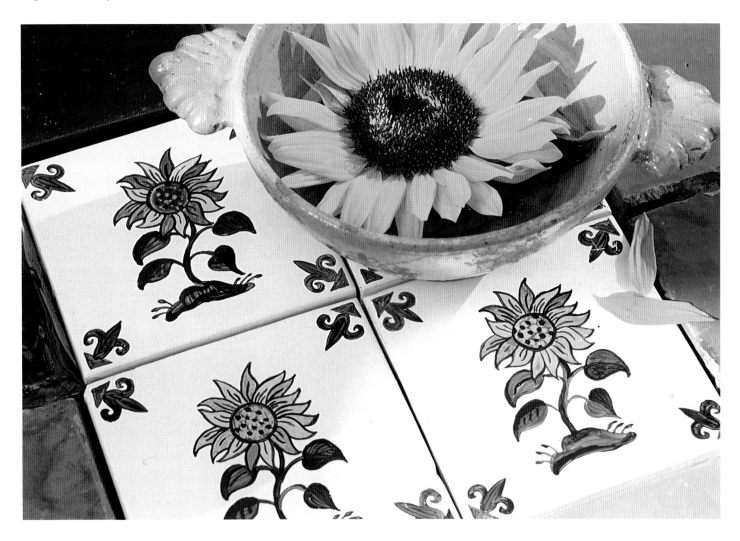

233

• DECORATING GLASS AND CERAMICS •

STAR-SIGN BOTTLE

Create a container fit for a magic potion using glowing glass paints to enhance a gilded design. This beautiful bottle would look stunning catching the light on a bathroom windowsill, but make sure the contents don't obscure the jewel-like colours.

YOU WILL NEED

MATERIALS
*flat-sided glass bottle
gold glass-paint outliner
scrap paper
solvent-based glass paints:
red, blue, green and yellow*

EQUIPMENT
*methylated spirit
paper towels
paintbrush*

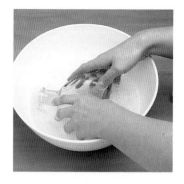

1 Wash the bottle in hot, soapy water and dry thoroughly. Wipe over the surface with methylated spirit to remove any remaining traces of grease.

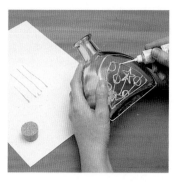

2 Practise using the gold outliner on paper before drawing the outline design (as seen in the picture) on one side of the bottle. Allow to dry for at least 24 hours.

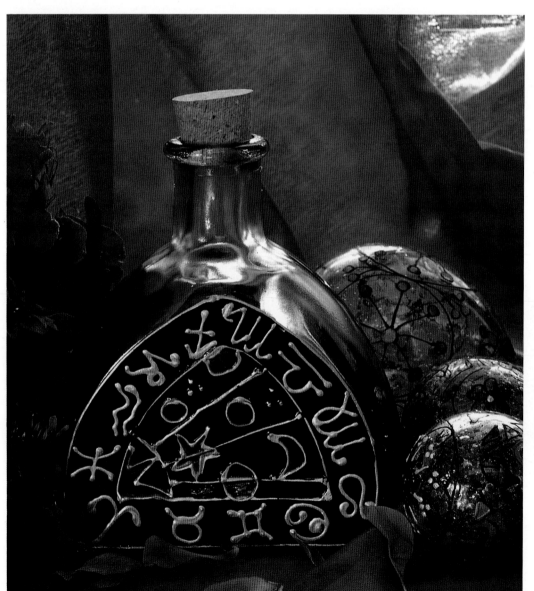

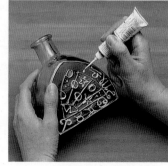

3 Apply the glass paint between the outlines, brushing it on thickly to achieve an even coating. Leave the bottle on its side to dry for at least 24 hours.

4 Using the gold outliner, draw the astrological symbols (see template section) around the design. Allow to dry completely before repeating the design on the other side of the bottle.

• Decorating Glass and Ceramics •

Majolica-style Tiles

Majolica is glazed or enamelled earthenware, noted for its bright colours. These tiles imitate the style very effectively, making use of ceramic paints on crisp, white ceramic tiles.

You Will Need

Materials
tracing paper
4 white square ceramic tiles
ceramic paints: dark blue, yellow and red

Equipment
pencil
fine paintbrushes
paint-mixing container

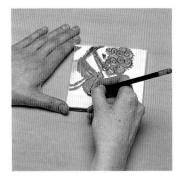

1 Trace the template from the back of the book, enlarging it to fit your tiles. Transfer a quarter of the design on to each tile.

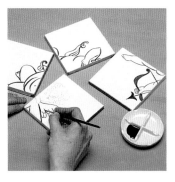

2 With a fine brush and dark blue paint, paint over the main outline on each tile. Fix the paint according to the manufacturer's instructions.

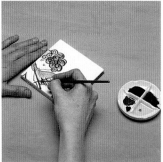

3 Fill in the wings, hair and drapery with yellow. Allow the colour to dry. Mix the colours to add darker tones, using the finished picture as a guide. Fix the paints again, to prevent the colours smudging.

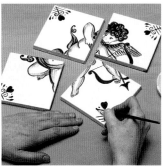

4 With diluted blue paint, mark in the shadows on the cupid's face and body. Go over any areas that need to be defined with more blue paint. Paint the corner motifs freehand and then fix for the final time.

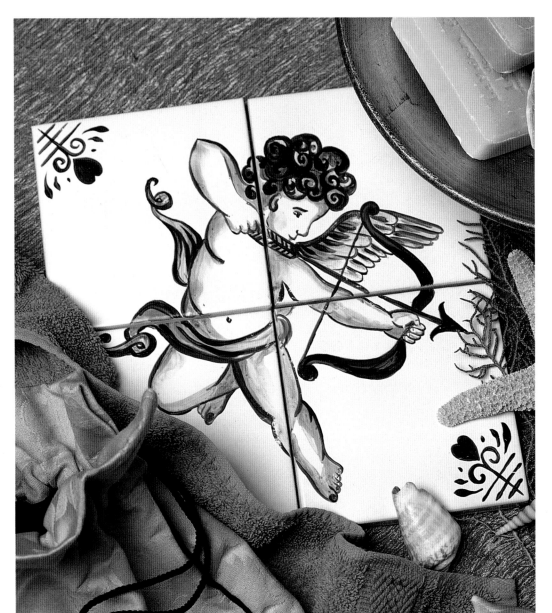

• DECORATING GLASS AND CERAMICS •

FROSTED JUG

If you love the effect of frosted glass but don't like the rather banal designs often found in shops, this technique is for you. You can use the same technique to make a set of glasses to go with the jug.

YOU WILL NEED

MATERIALS	EQUIPMENT
paper	pencil
sticky-backed plastic	scissors
washed glass jug	soft paintbrush
etching fluid cream	rubber gloves

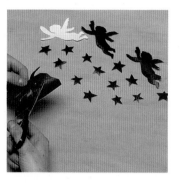

1 Draw a cupid and star freehand on to paper and cut out. Trace around the shapes on to sticky-backed plastic and cut out.

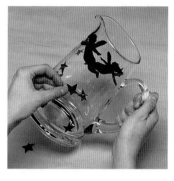

2 Peel the backing off the plastic and stick the shapes around the jug.

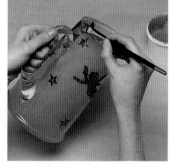

3 Follow the manufacturer's instructions to paint the etching fluid cream on to the outside of the jug, avoiding the handle. Leave to stand for about ten minutes.

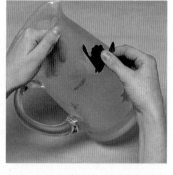

4 Wearing rubber gloves, wash the cream off the jug in warm water and leave it to dry. If there are any unfrosted patches on the glass where the cream hasn't taken, simply repeat step 3. When you are satisfied with the frosted finish, peel off the shapes.

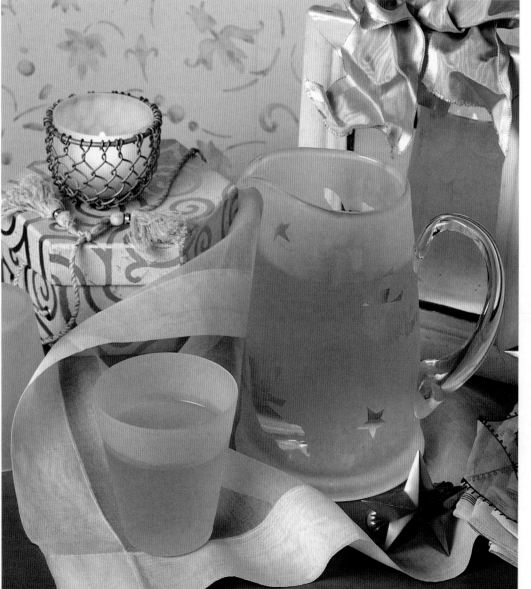

• Decorating Glass and Ceramics •

Rosebud Jug

If you are a beginner at painting on glass, you might find it easier to trace the template (see back of book) on to paper and fit the paper inside the jug. Then trace the design with the outliner.

You Will Need

Materials	Equipment
tracing paper	methylated spirit
glass jug	paper towels
old jam jar	pencil
gold glass-painting outliner	packing material or
solvent-based glass paints:	bean bag
red and green	paintbrush
	white spirit

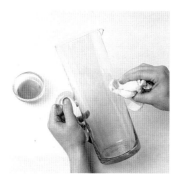

1 Wash the jug in hot, soapy water and dry thoroughly. Wipe over the surface with methylated spirit to remove any remaining traces of grease.

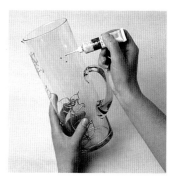

2 Controlling the flow of the outliner can be tricky, so have a few practice runs on an old jam jar. Draw your design on to the jug. This is easiest to do in sections and each section should be left to harden for at least 12 hours before you begin the next.

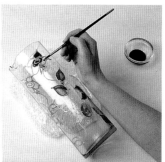

3 To fill in the design, prop the jug up on its side on the packing material or bean bag. Try to keep the area that you are painting horizontal, to stop the paint from running. Carefully paint in a section, applying the glass paint thickly, to prevent streaky brushstrokes. Remove any excess paint with the brush. Leave each section to dry overnight before turning the jug to do the next section. Clean the brush with white spirit each time.

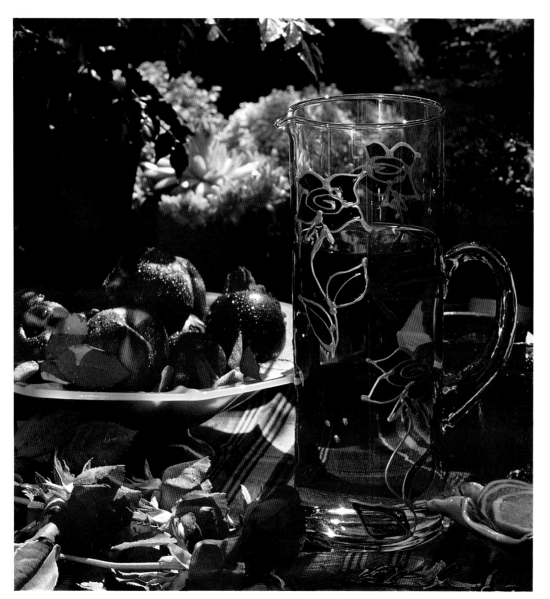

• Decorating Glass and Ceramics •

Mosaic Dragonfly Plaque

Very effective mosaics can be made using broken china, then fixing the pieces with ceramic adhesive and grouting just as you would when laying tiles. The old, chipped plates you were going to throw out may be just the colours you need.

You Will Need

Materials
*tracing paper
plywood, 51 x 51 cm/
20 x 20 in
PVA (white) glue
acrylic primer
dark green acrylic paint
electric cable
selection of china
tile adhesive
coloured tile grout*

Equipment
*pencil
fretsaw or coping saw
bradawl
paintbrush
sandpaper
cable strippers
tile nippers
rubber gloves
nail brush
cloth*

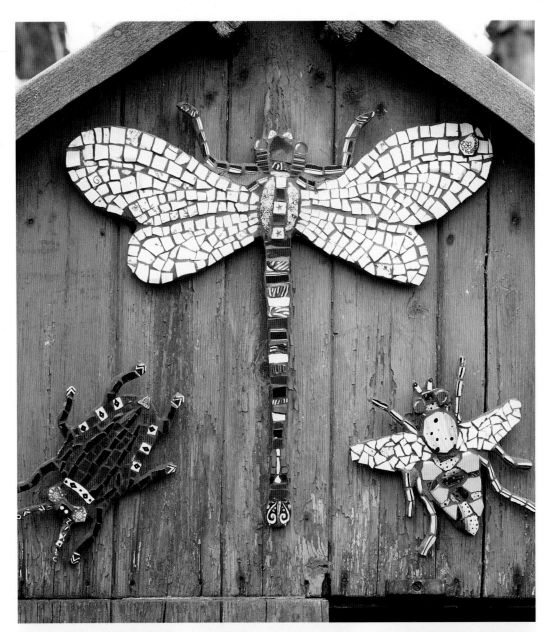

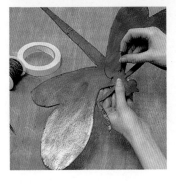 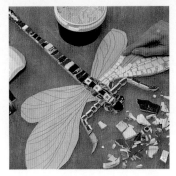 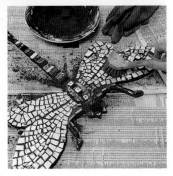

1 Trace the template from the back of the book, enlarging if necessary. Transfer it to the plywood. Cut out the dragonfly and make two holes at the top of the body with a bradawl. Seal the front surface with diluted PVA (white) glue and the back with acrylic primer. Allow to dry. Sand the back surface and paint green.

2 Strip some electric cable and cut a short length of wire. Push this through the holes on the dragonfly and twist together securely.

3 Cut the china into regular shapes using tile nippers. Dip each piece into the tile adhesive, scooping up a thick layer, and press down securely. Allow to dry overnight.

4 Press the grout into the gaps between the china. Allow to dry for five minutes, then brush off the excess. Leave for another five minutes, then polish with a cloth.

• DECORATING GLASS AND CERAMICS •

MOSAIC SHIELD PLAQUE

This plaque uses simple square tiles to build up the design. By carefully mixing light and dark shades, you can give the impression of the curved edge of a shield without having to cut the glass pieces.

YOU WILL NEED

MATERIALS
*5 mm/¼ in medium-density fibreboard, 23 x 30 cm/ 9 x 12 in
tracing paper
PVA (white) glue
glass mosaic squares, 2.5 x 2.5 cm/1 x 1 in
white grouting
2 screw eyes
picture wire, 20 cm/8 in*

EQUIPMENT
*pencil
ruler
paintbrush
damp cloth
soft, dry cloth*

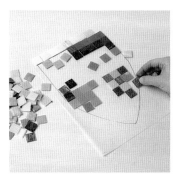

1 Draw a line 2.5 cm/1 in in from each edge of the board. Rule a line down the centre of the board. Draw a horizontal line 11.5 cm/4½ in from the top, then mark in a gentle curve in each lower quarter. Trace a shield shape on to tracing paper as a base for working out the design. Take time to find a satisfying arrangement of colours.

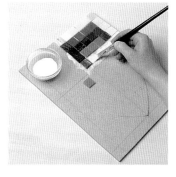

2 Paint a thick layer of glue in a top quarter of the shield and stick on your chosen tiles. Surround these with a single row of white around the outside edge, and a darker colour along the centre lines. Repeat with the remaining quarters of the shield.

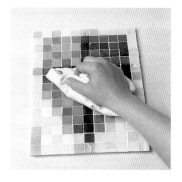

3 Leave overnight for the glue to harden, then fill in the spaces between the tiles with white grouting. Wipe off the surplus with a damp cloth and, when dry, polish with a soft cloth. Fix the screw eyes into the back and attach the wire for hanging.

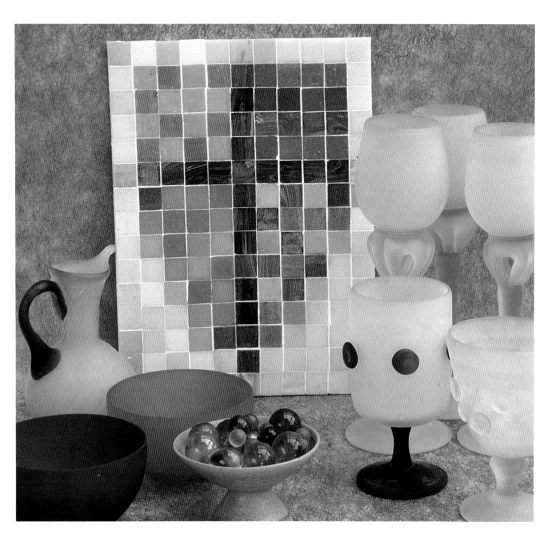

• Decorating Glass and Ceramics •

Sequinned Rose Bottle

This ingenious technique could be used to decorate any kind of container, but it is particularly suited to a tall, narrow bottle, which might otherwise be hard to work on. The rose motif shown here would make a very suitable decoration for a special gift bottle of fragrant rosewater!

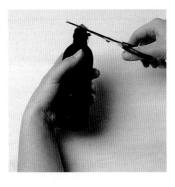

1. Place the bottle in the toe of one leg of the tights. Thread a needle, wrap it around the neck of the bottle, secure it and trim away the excess fabric.

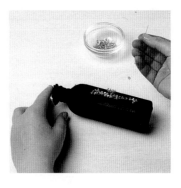

2. Thread the beading needle with invisible thread and work the rose motif: firstly, thread a sequin and then a bugle bead, bring the needle down and then up next to the first stitch and continue working like this.

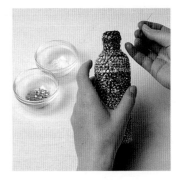

3. Draw the stripes with the marker and fill them with sequins and glass beads, in the same way.

You Will Need

Materials
glass bottle
tights
matching thread
invisible thread
sequins
bugle beads
glass beads

Equipment
needle
dressmaker's scissors
beading needle
fabric marker

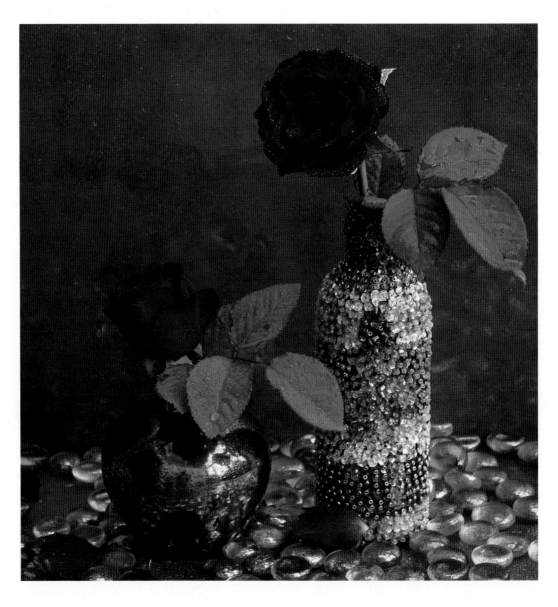

240

PAINTED VASE

Painted glassware was a popular folk art from Europe, with bright figures used to adorn bottles of spirit and drinking tumblers from France to Hungary. Try to find old glasses in junk or antique shops for this project as imperfections won't show.

YOU WILL NEED

MATERIALS
tracing paper
glass
masking tape
enamel paints: red, green,
yellow, blue and black
enamel paint thinner

EQUIPMENT
pencil
scissors
cloth
paintbrushes
paint-mixing containers
elastic band

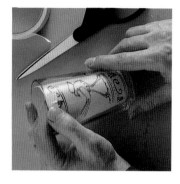

1 Trace the template from the back of the book, enlarging it to fit inside your glass. Cut out and secure it with masking tape.

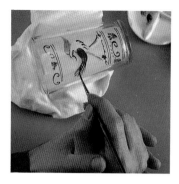

2 Rest the glass on a cloth and support your painting hand with your other hand as you paint. Make sure the paints are thinned enough to make them flow nicely as you paint the pattern on.

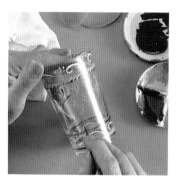

3 Add the dots and motifs to suit your glass. Allow to dry, then place an elastic band around the glass to guide you as you paint stripes of colour.

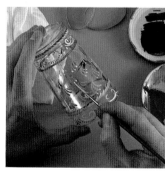

4 Introduce some individuality by adding embellishments of your own, perhaps just a few squiggles, some dots or even your initials.

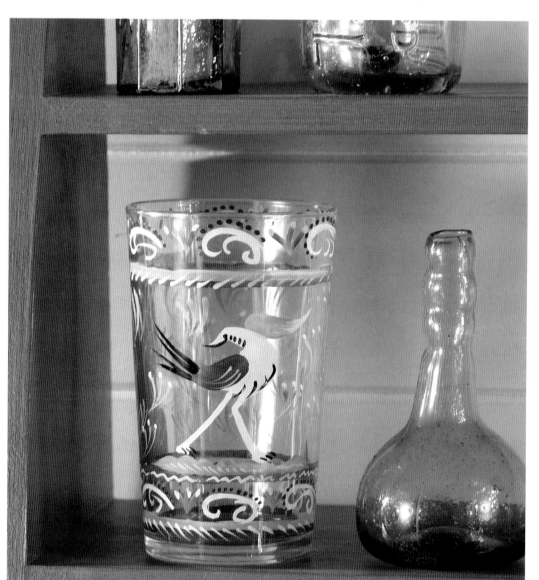

• DECORATING GLASS AND CERAMICS •

FRUIT BOWL

*T*his is a freehand project, and the loosely drawn oranges, leaves and flowers do not demand sophisticated artistic skill. You can substitute apples, pears, pineapples or lemons for the oranges.

YOU WILL NEED

MATERIALS
*white-glazed bowl
ceramic paints: orange,
lilac, lime-green, dark
green, burgundy and black
polyurethane varnish*

EQUIPMENT
*black magic marker
paintbrushes*

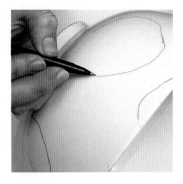

1 Draw four or five whole oranges on to the bowl, leaving space for the leaves and flowers. Draw four or five cut-off oranges along the top rim and base.

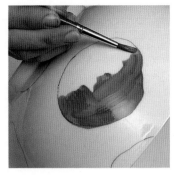

2 Paint the oranges, spreading the paint thinly. Allow to dry.

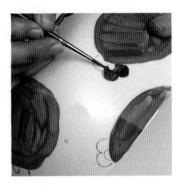

3 Draw flowers peeping out from behind the oranges, as shown, and paint them lilac, leaving the centres white.

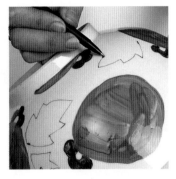

4 Draw leaves, one small and one large, for each orange. Space them so there are no big gaps in the background. Draw half leaves going off the bowl.

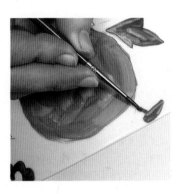

5 Paint the small leaves in lime-green and the large leaves in dark green.

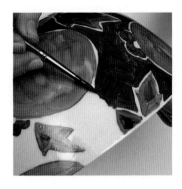

6 Paint the background burgundy, leaving a thin white outline around the motifs. Spread the paint thinly so the brushstrokes remain visible for textural variety.

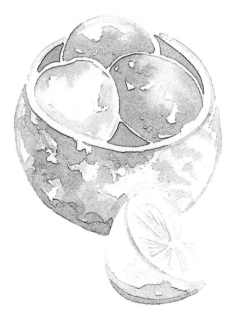

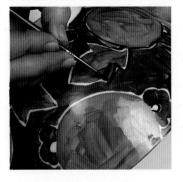

7 Paint loosely around the motifs in black. Vary the pressure on the brush so the line is sometimes thick and sometimes thin. Paint the midribs in the leaves and the circular centres in the flowers.

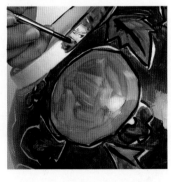

8 Paint the rim at the bottom in dark green, spreading the paint thinly to emphasize the hand-painted quality of the design. Allow to dry, then varnish the bowl.

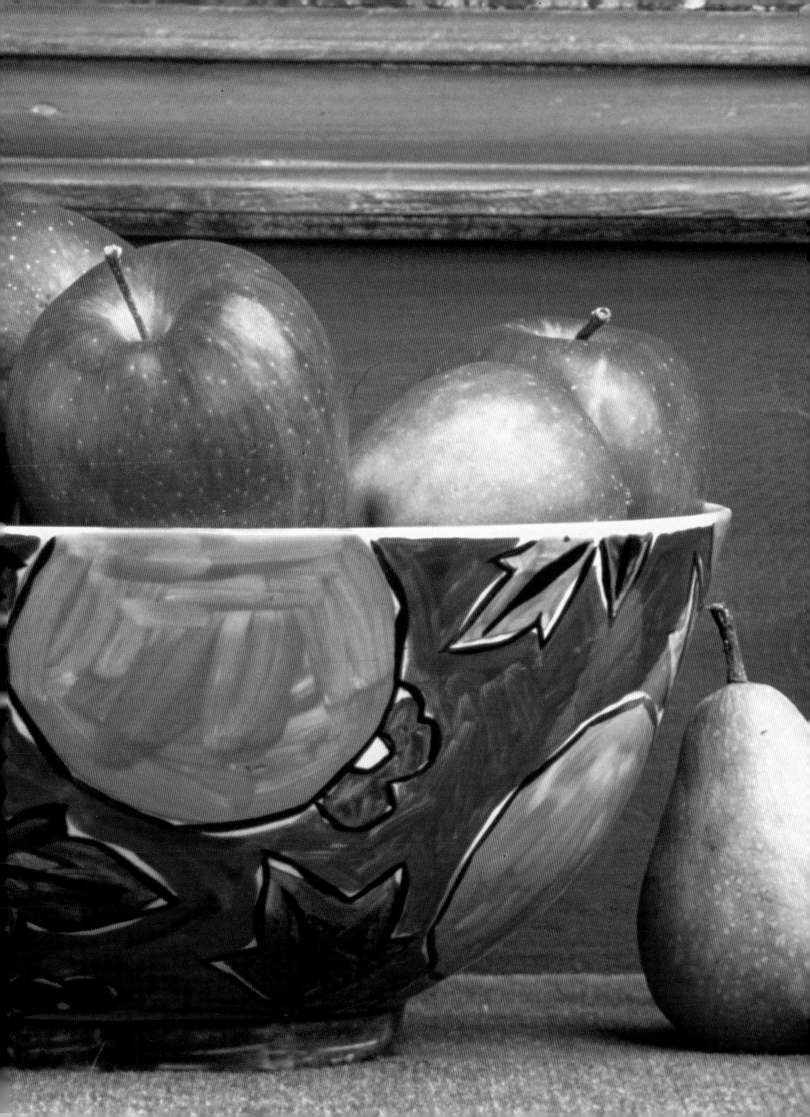

· DECORATING GLASS AND CERAMICS ·

HOLLY PLATTER

Display this festive painted plate heaped high with Christmas tree balls, repeating the chosen colour scheme, or a mixture of tree balls and pine cones, spray-painted in metallic colours or left natural. For a children's party, heap the platter with sweets and wrapped chocolate coins.

YOU WILL NEED

MATERIALS
white-glazed plate
masking tape
paper or thin card
ceramic paints: green, red, maroon and gold
gold spray
polyurethane varnish

EQUIPMENT
pencil
craft knife
cutting mat
paintbrushes

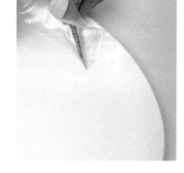

1 Mask off the centre of the plate with masking tape, leaving the outer rim clear.

2 Draw two or three holly leaves on to paper or thin card. Cut out the leaves and their centres.

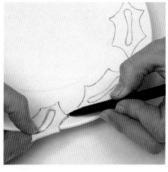

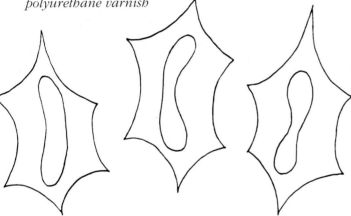

3 Lay the leaf stencils to fit around the rim of the plate, leaving space for a border, if liked. Mark on where the first stencil starts, then trace the leaves on to the plate.

4 Add some straight and curved stems to the leaves. Some can be single, and others should join to form sprigs. Fill the gaps with berries.

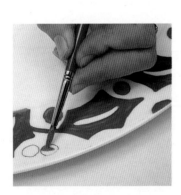 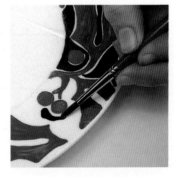 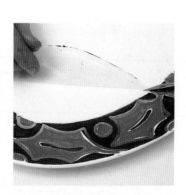 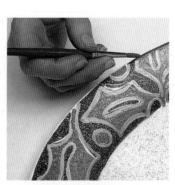

5 Paint the leaves and stems green, leaving the central mid-rib white. Allow to dry, then add touches of green to highlight. Allow to dry, then paint the berries red.

6 Paint the background maroon, using a fine brush to go around the motifs first.

7 Paint a gold outline around the leaves and berries and along one side of the stems. Try to leave as much white outline as possible. Use the edge of a craft knife to remove the masking tape from the plate.

8 Lightly spray the plate gold, then paint a narrow red band around the rim, if liked. Allow to dry, then coat with a layer of varnish.

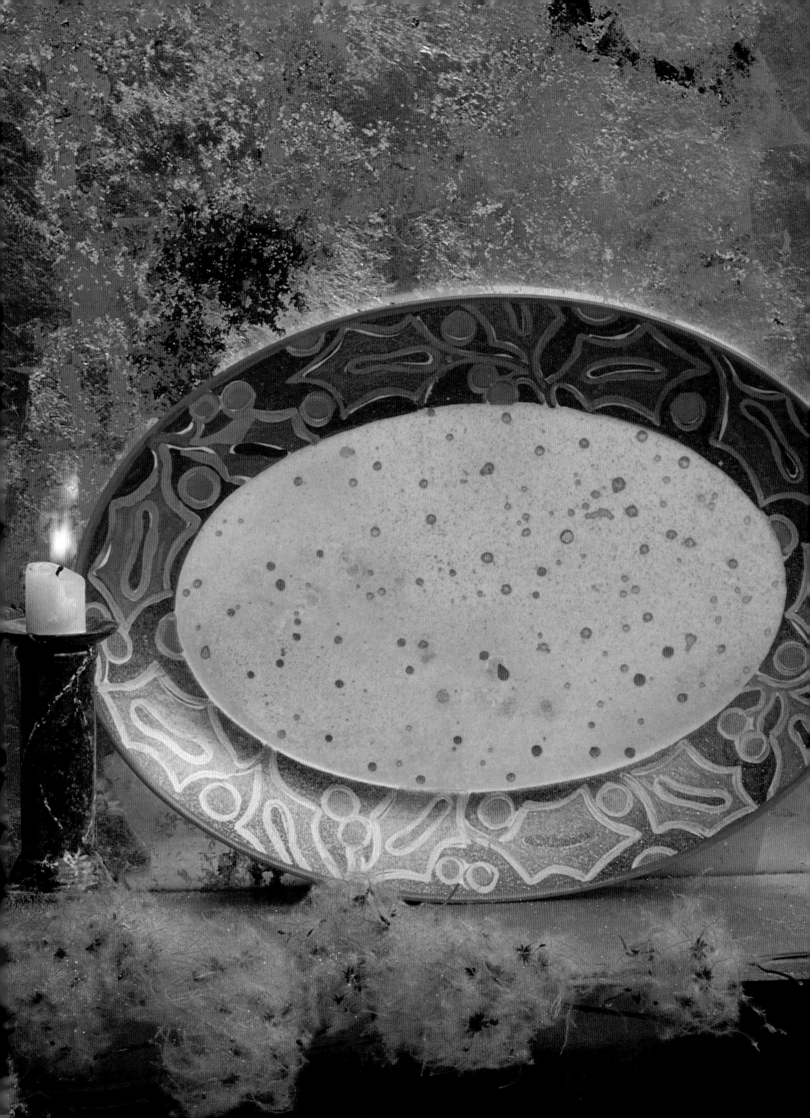

Templates

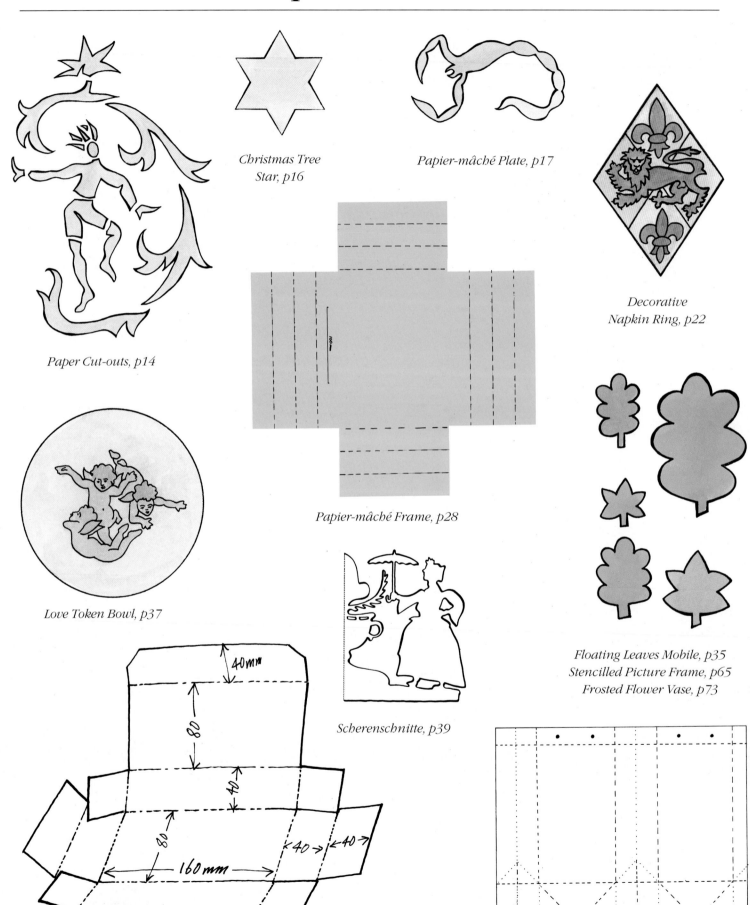

Paper Cut-outs, p14

Christmas Tree Star, p16

Papier-mâché Plate, p17

Decorative Napkin Ring, p22

Papier-mâché Frame, p28

Love Token Bowl, p37

Floating Leaves Mobile, p35
Stencilled Picture Frame, p65
Frosted Flower Vase, p73

Scherenschnitte, p39

Cardboard Gift Boxes, p40

Carrier Bags, p42

· Templates ·

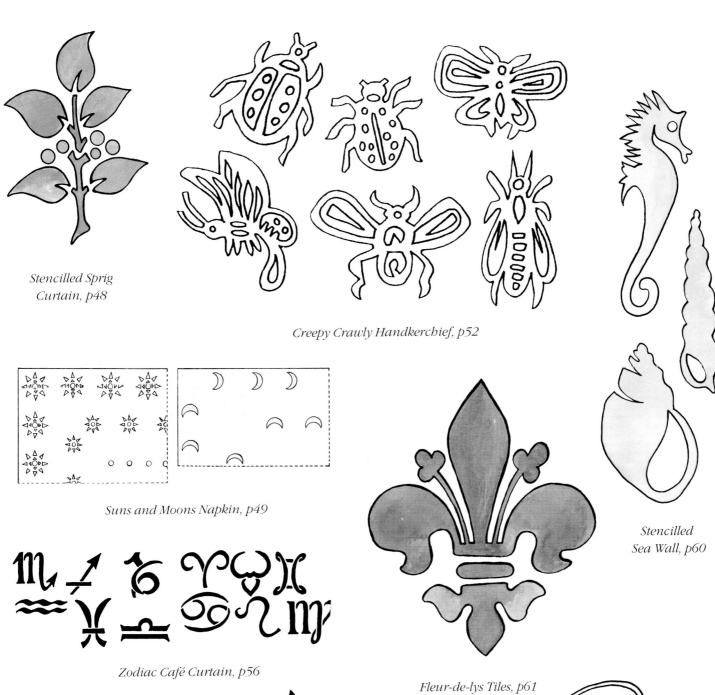

Stencilled Sprig Curtain, p48

Creepy Crawly Handkerchief, p52

Suns and Moons Napkin, p49

Stencilled Sea Wall, p60

Zodiac Café Curtain, p56

Fleur-de-lys Tiles, p61

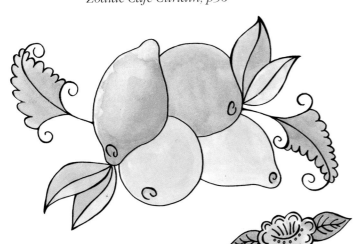

Mexican Citrus Tray, p66

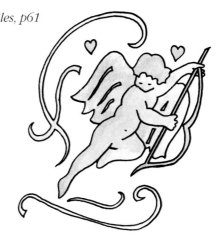

Cupid Linocut, p67

· Templates ·

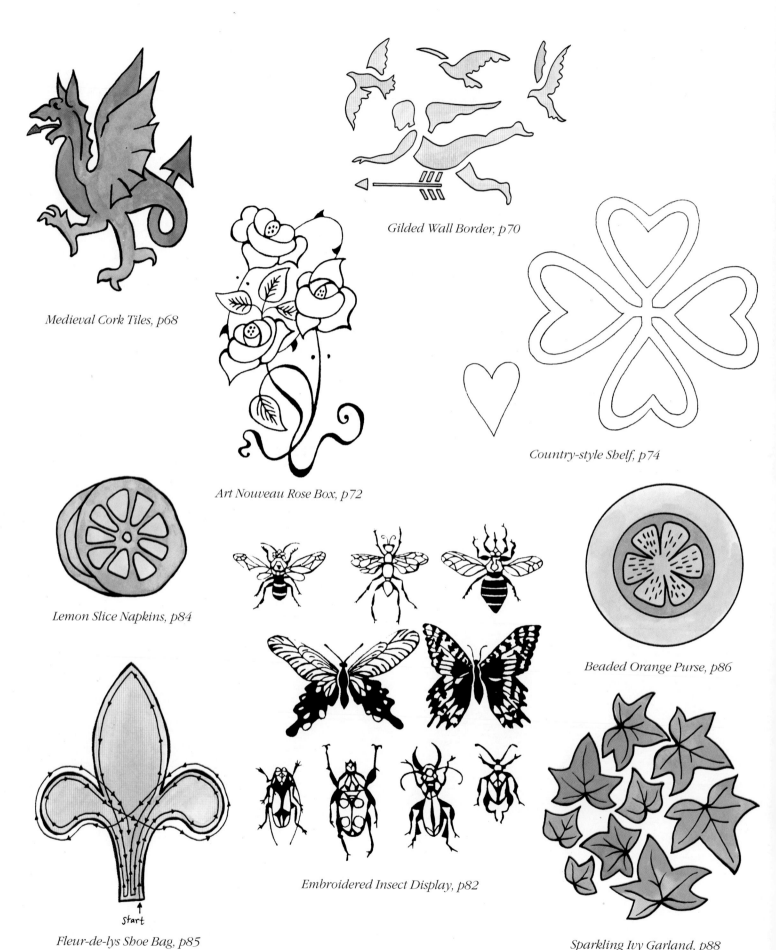

Medieval Cork Tiles, p68

Gilded Wall Border, p70

Art Nouveau Rose Box, p72

Country-style Shelf, p74

Lemon Slice Napkins, p84

Beaded Orange Purse, p86

Fleur-de-lys Shoe Bag, p85

Embroidered Insect Display, p82

Sparkling Ivy Garland, p88

· Templates ·

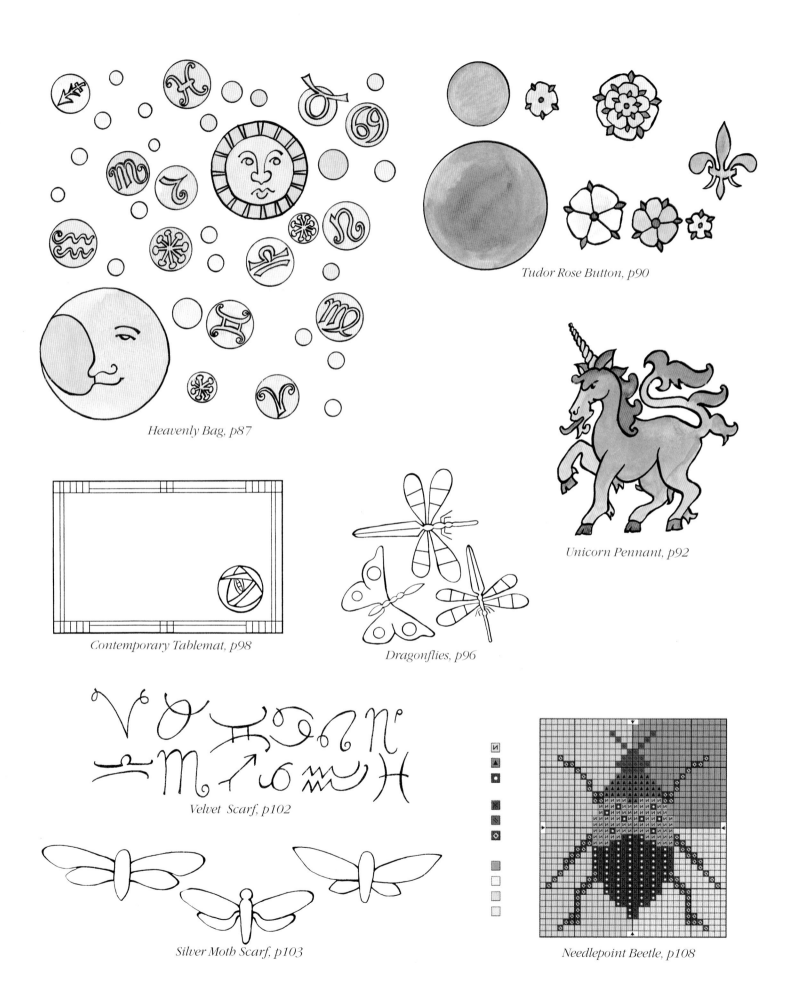

Heavenly Bag, p87

Tudor Rose Button, p90

Unicorn Pennant, p92

Contemporary Tablemat, p98

Dragonflies, p96

Velvet Scarf, p102

Silver Moth Scarf, p103

Needlepoint Beetle, p108

· Templates ·

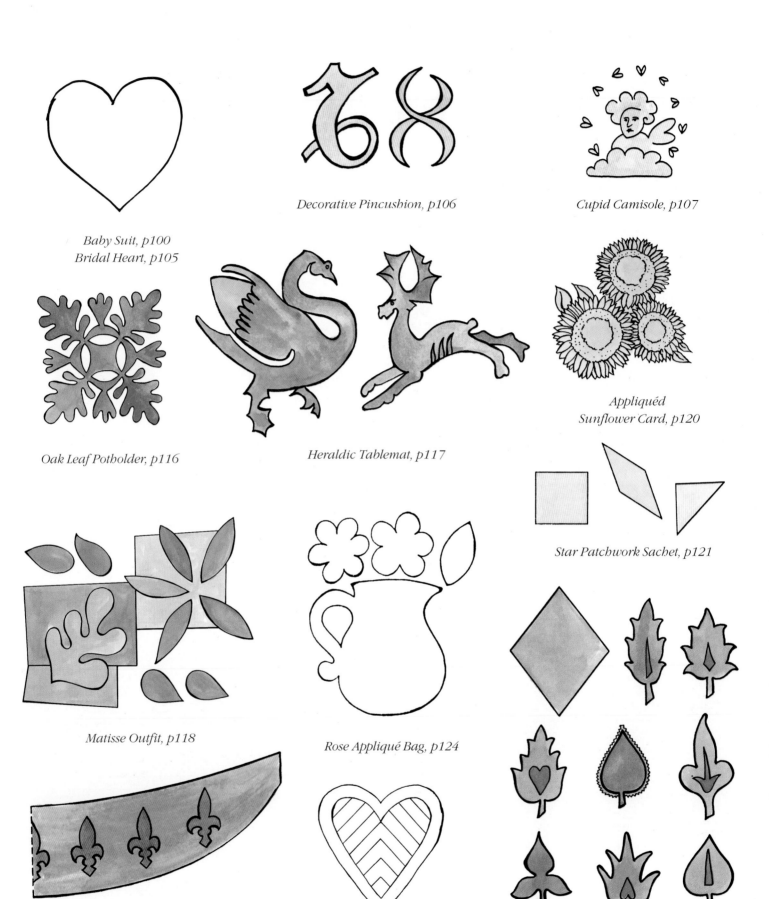

· TEMPLATES ·

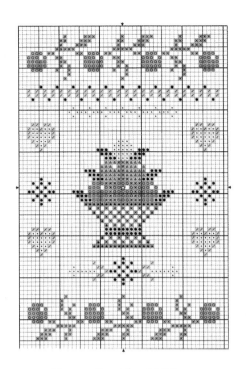

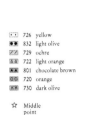

Star-spangled Banner, p132

Star-spangled Scarf, p131

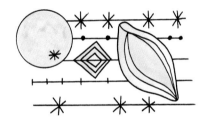

Oranges Tea Towel, p136

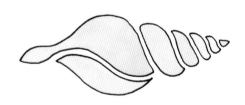

Seashell Beach Bag, p130

Orange Sampler, p127

Appliqué Star Card, p139

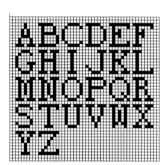

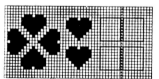

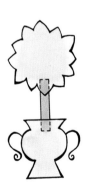

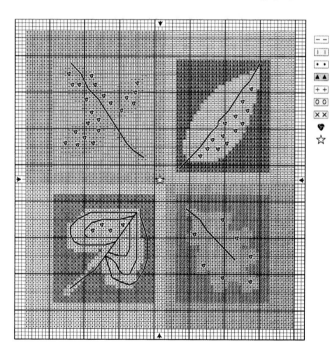

Shaker Towel, p137

Appliqué Notebook, p140

Needlepoint Mat, p138

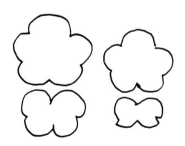

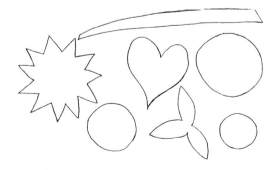

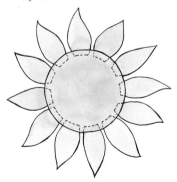

Hand Towel and Washcloth, p141

Appliquéd Sheet and Pillowcase, p142

Child's T-shirt, p143

251

· Templates ·

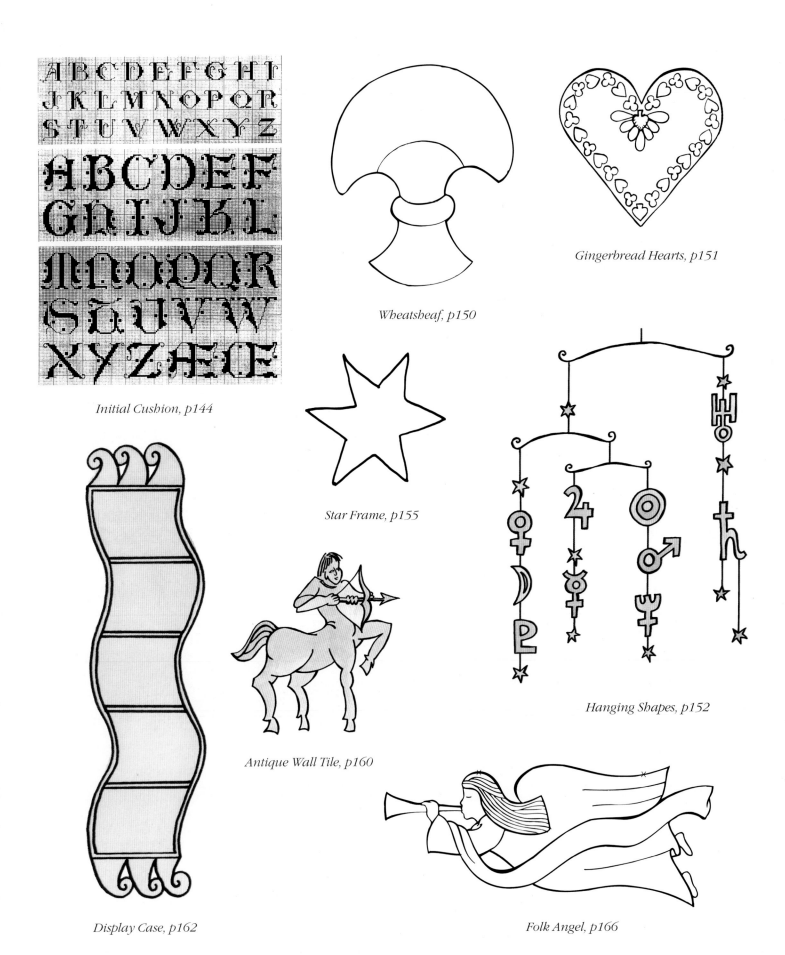

Initial Cushion, p144

Wheatsheaf, p150

Gingerbread Hearts, p151

Star Frame, p155

Hanging Shapes, p152

Antique Wall Tile, p160

Display Case, p162

Folk Angel, p166

· TEMPLATES ·

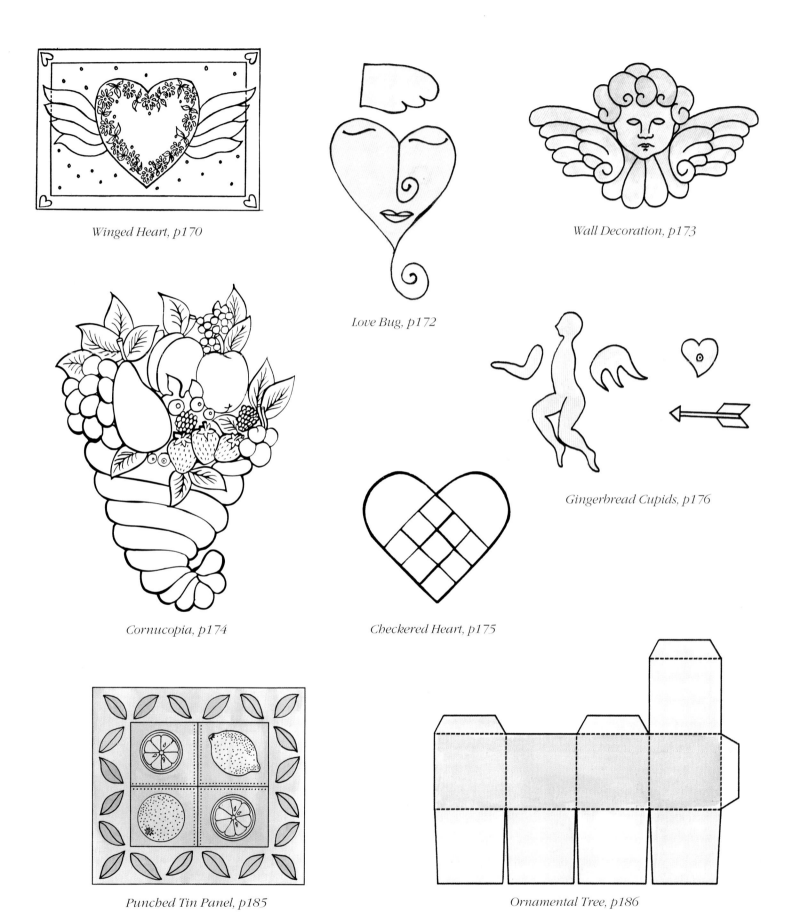

Winged Heart, p170

Love Bug, p172

Wall Decoration, p173

Cornucopia, p174

Checkered Heart, p175

Gingerbread Cupids, p176

Punched Tin Panel, p185

Ornamental Tree, p186

· Templates ·

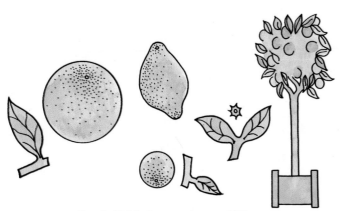
Exotic Table Decorations, p188

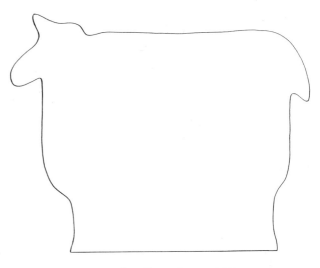
Wooden Sheep Sign, p187

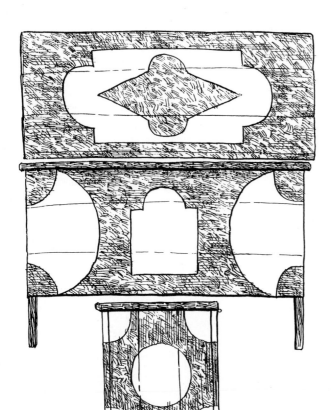
Painted Chest, p196

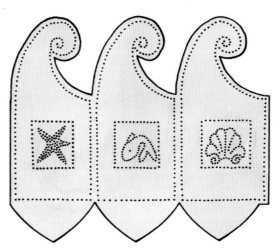
Tin Candleholder, p192

Woodburning, p190

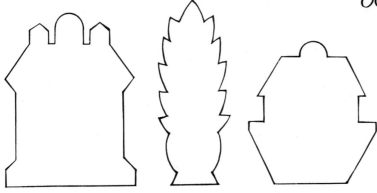
Christmas Decorations, p202

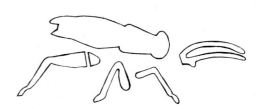
Grasshopper on a Stick, p206

· TEMPLATES ·

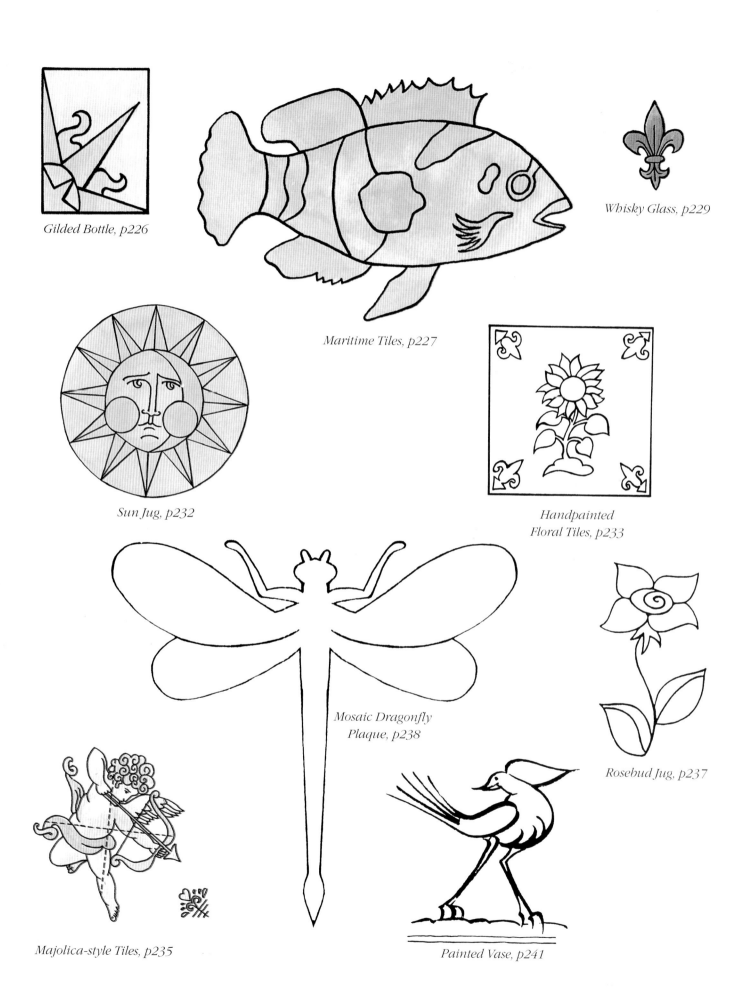

Index

Appliqué 115
  Appliqué Notebook 140
  Appliquéd Sheet and
    Pillowcase 142
  Appliqué Star Card 139
  Appliquéd Sunflower
    Card 120
  Appliqué Throw 122
Art Nouveau Rose
  Box 72

Bags
  Carrier Bags 42
  Crepe Paper Bags 42
  Fleur-de-lys Shoe
    Bag 85
  Heavenly Bag 87
  Rose Appliqué Bag 124
  Seashell Beach Bag 130
Beaded Orange Purse 86
Bowls
  Fruit Bowl 242
  Gold-rimmed
    Bowl 33
  Love Token Bowl 37
  Metal Embedded Bowl
    178
  Orange Bowl 23
  Sunburst Bowl 24
Boxes
  Amish Sewing Box 184
  Art Nouveau Rose Box
    72
  Cardboard Gift Boxes 40
  Decorated Box 36
  Mirrored Keepsake Box
    34
Bridal Heart 105

Candles
  Candle Collars 195
  Candle Jar 223
  Tin Candleholder 192
Cards
  Appliqué Star Card 139
  Appliquéd Sunflower
    Card 120
Checkerboard Potato
  Print 54
Checkered Heart 175
Christmas Decorations
  202
Christmas Tree Star 16

Clothes
  Baby Suit 100
  Child's T-shirt 143
  Colourful Hat 95
  Cupid Camisole 107
  Matisse Outfit 118
Cornucopia 174
Country-style
  Shelf 74
Crackle-glazed
  Print 30
Cross stitches 114
Cupid Linocut 67
Curtains
  Stencilled Sprig
    Curtain 48
  Zodiac Cafe
    Curtain 56

Decorated Tea Service
  230
Decorative Pincushion
  106
Decoupage Rose Eggs
  15
Dishes
  Love and Kisses Soap
    Dish 189
  Soap Dish 220
  Wooden Dish 212
Display Case 162
Dragonflies 96

Embroidered Hem 99
Embroidered Insect
  Display 82
Exotic Table Decorations
  188

Fishy Ornaments 104
Fleur-de-lys Tieback 126
Floating Leaves Mobile 35
Foam-block Printing 76
Folk Angel 166
Frames
  Copper Frame 200
  Engraved Mirror Frame
    156
  Papier-mâché Frame 28
  Star Frame 155
  Stencilled picture frame
    65
  Twisted Paper Frame 26

Galvanized Trivet 191
Gilding
  Gilded Bookmark 18
  Gilded Bottle 226
  Gilded Candleholder
    207
  Gilded Candlestick 204
  Gilded Fruits 222
  Gilded Glass 234
  Gilded Wall Border 70
Gingerbread Cupids
  176
Gingerbread Hearts 151
Grasshopper on a Stick
  206

Hanging Shapes 152
Holly Platter 244

Initial Cushion 144

Jugs
  Frosted Jug 236
  Low-relief Jug 224
  Papier-mâché
    Jug 27
  Rosebud Jug 237
  Sun Jug 232

Lantern 210
Leafy Espresso
  Cups 62
Leafy Pencil Pot 57
Linen
  Appliquéd Sheet and
    Pillowcase 142
  Country-style Pillowcase
    145
  Cradle Quilt 128
  Creepy Crawly
    Handkerchief 52
  Stamped Bedlinen 58
Love Bug 172

Materials and equipment
  12, 80, 182, 216
Mats
  Contemporary Tablemat
    98
  Heraldic Tablemat 117
  Needlepoint Mat 138
Midnight Sky Picture
  101

Modelled Mirror 158
Napkins
  Decorative Napkin Ring
    22
  Lemon Slice Napkins 84
  Suns and Moons Napkin
    49
Needlepoint Beetle 108

Oak Leaf Potholder 116
Orange Sampler 127
Ornamental Tree 186

Painted Chest 196
Painted Garden
  Sticks 213
Painted Tin 208
Paper Cut-outs 14
Paper pulp 13
Papier-mâché Plate 17
Pierced Tin Shelf 194
Plaques
  Beaming Sun Wall
    Plaque 20
  Mosaic Dragonfly
    Plaque 238
  Mosaic Shield Plaque
    239
  Wall Plaque 38
Punched Tin Panel 185

Salt and Pepper Pots 168
Salt Dough Basket 164
Salt Dough recipe 149
Scarfs
  Embroidered Organza
    Scarf 83
  Silver Moth Scarf 103
  Star Spangled Scarf 131
  Velvet Scarf 102
  Wild Rose Chiffon Scarf
    94
Scherenschnitte 39
Seashore Spongeware Set
  53
Sequinned Rose Bottle
  240
Sgraffito Eggs 64
Shaker Hand 167
Sparkling Ivy Garland 88
Spice Scented Pot Stand
  134

Spider Buttons 154
Stamping techniques 47
Star Patchwork Sachet 121
Star-sign Bottle 234
Star-spangled Banner 132
Stencilled Sea Wall 60
Stitches 81
Storage Canister 198
Stylish Lampshade 50
Sunflower Magnet 203
Sweet Hearts 110

Templates 246
Tiles
  Antique Wall Tile 160
  Fleur-de-lys Tiles 61
  Handpainted Floral
    Tiles 233
  Italianate Tiles 228
  Lemon Tiles 218
  Majolica-style
    Tiles 235
  Maritime Tiles 227
  Medieval Cork Tiles 68
Tin Can Insects 193
Towels
  Hand Towel and
    Washcloth 141
  Oranges Tea Towel 136
  Shaker Towel 137
Tudor Rose Button 90
Trays
  Garland Tray Cut-outs
    19
  Mexican Citrus Tray 66

Underwater Picture 91
Unicorn Pennant 92

Vases
  Frosted Flower Vase 73
  Japanese Glass Vase 219
  Painted Vase 241

Wall Decoration 173
Wall Sconce 199
Water Bearer's Shrine 32
Wheatsheaf 150
Whisky Glass 229
Winged Heart 170
Woodburning 190
Wooden Sheep
  Sign 187

256